The most neglected story in modern health care, the Story of the Chemical Elements and their need in correctional nutrition for the prevention, reversal, and healing of disease.

The Chemistry
of
Man

2nd Edition

Bernard Jensen, PhD, ND

Second Edition

First Printing: 2007
Second Printing: 2012
Third Printing: 2014

Copyright © 2007 Whitman Publications
ALL RIGHTS RESERVED

WHITMAN
PUBLICATIONS

Whitman Publications
220 Parker Street
Warsaw, IN 46580

Library of Congress Control Number: 2006940836
ISBN: 1-885653-24-7

Printed in the United States of America.

Dedication

To those men in every science and art who are investigating the properties of the chemical elements, their structure and their application for the betterment of the physical temple of man's well-being. I dedicate this book. To know the dust of the earth in the form of vitamins, enzymes, protein, starches, fats, prostaglandins and mineral supplements in foods is to understand the source in Nature from which health and well-being spring. I dedicate this book to my friend and teacher, V. G. Rocine, whose research into food Ichemistry and the chemistry of man gave me the incentive to investigate and apply this work in my sanitarium practice.

—Bernard Jensen, Ph.D.
October 1983

This compilation of the works of Dr. Bernard Jensen in the field of nutrition as applied to his sanitarium practice reveals the research studies of Dr. V. G. Rocine, whom he considers one of his greatest teachers.

Dr. Jensen verified the teachings of V. G. Rocine by demonstrating, through over 50 years of sanitarium work, the effectiveness of nutrition in restoring patients to normal health.

Biography

Born on March 25, 1908, to Eugen and Anna Jensen, Jorgen Bernard Jensen was raised in Stockton, California, then a small rural town in one of the richest agricultural valleys of the state. The unexpected death of his mother at age 30, from tuberculosis and consumption, left three children to be raised by the father, a chiropractor.

At the age of 18, he entered the West Coast Chiropractic College, supporting himself working at a dairy. Long hours of work and study, along with poor food habits, took a heavy toll on his health, which collapsed shortly after his graduation from college. Doctors diagnosed his condition as bronchiectasis, an often fatal lung condition, with no known cure at the time. "There is nothing we can do for you," they told him.

The young man refused to give up, searching out a Seventh Day Adventist doctor who taught him basic nutritional principles, told him to leave junk food alone and put him on a healthy diet. He began taking breathing exercises with Thomas Gaines, once an instructor for the New York City Police Department. His health slowly, but surely, responded.

Dr. Jensen opened his first office practice in Oakland, California, in 1929. He later moved to Los Angeles and expanded his practice to include branch offices at Long Beach and Santa Monica, with several chiropractors working under him. Such success had not come about overnight.

Beginning from the Standpoint of chiropractic, Dr. Jensen added nutrition and then began exploring related drugless healing arts and specialties, studying with some of the best teachers in the United States and Europe. He learned iridology from Drs. F. W. Collins and R. M. McLain, and traveled to the Battle Creek Sanitarium in Michigan to study bowel care with Dr. John Harvey Kellogg. He studied the water cure at Father Kneipp's famous baths at Worischofen, Germany, while from Drs. John Tilden and George Weger, both MD's, Dr. Jensen learned how to use fasting to purify the body and speed up the healing process. He studied reflex therapy with Dr. Major De Jarnette, polarity work with Dr. Randolph Stone, glandular balancing with Dr. Melvin Page, nutritional balancing with Dr. Weston Price, sanitarium work with Dr. Ralph Benner of the Bircher-Benner Sanitarium in Zurich, Switzerland, homeopathy with Dr. Charles Gesser in Florida and many other subjects including herbology, diets, personology, acupuncture, craniopathy and other aspects of the wholistic approach to health. Dr. Jensen has taken over 6,000 hours of graduate course work during his career.

In the 1930s, Dr. Jensen attended a lecture that profoundly changed the direction of his work. Dr. V. G. Rocine, a Norwegian homeopath, claimed that excess or deficiency in any of the primary chemical elements needed in human nutrition could account for most diseases and psychopathic mental symptoms known to man. Thus, Rocine believed that food (along with essentials such as fresh air, sunshine, rest, etc.) was man's best medicine. Dr. Jensen studied and worked with Dr. Rocine off and on for ten years in Oakland, California, Portland, Oregon and Chicago, Illinois. Rocine regarded him as his best student.

Dr. Jensen used Rocine's work as the basis for the programs used in his sanitariums—first a 25-bed sanitarium in San Leandro, California, then others in Ben Lomond and Altadena, and finally an 85-bed sanitarium at Hidden Valley Health Ranch in Escondido, California. The sanitariums, quite successful, demonstrated the effectiveness of Rocine's ideas and their practicality in working with patients.

Proper nutrition, together with sunshine, rest, exercise, fresh air and positive attitudes helped thousands of patients at Dr. Jensen's sanitariums leave behind the symptoms of chronic diseases that they had developed. After working with over 350,000 patients, he concluded that nutrition is the single most important therapy to be used in the healing arts.

Patients came from all over the world, some to stay at his sanitariums, others for outpatient consultations and still others to attend his classes in Rejuvenation and Food Studies. Thousands of New Zealanders formed clubs to follow his dietetic advice, filling out the 350,000, which accumulated over the years. He acquired a multitude of experiences from these people individually and in group studies, acquiring information and summing it up for use.

Over the years, Dr. Jensen has traveled to over 52 countries, lecturing, teaching and searching for health and longevity secrets to bring back to his sanitarium work. He has visited many of the oldest men and women of the world, one of whom was 153 years old, to find out how they stayed healthy, active and clear-minded so much longer than the average person.

He visited the Hunza Valley, where disease, doctors, dentists and hospitals were practically nonexistent and where there were no jails, prisons or police, because there was no crime. He visited the Caucasus Mountains in the USSR to meet a 153-year-old man who had stopped riding horseback a few years earlier only because of his doctor's orders. He traveled to Vilacamba, Ecuador, where heart patients were able to recuperate so marvelously. Everywhere he went, he brought back some new remedy or approach to integrate into the system he taught his patients.

Author of over 25 books on health and nutrition, Dr. Jensen published *The Science and Practice of Iridology* in 1952, and it quickly became a classic in its field, establishing him as one of the top world authorities on the subject. His most recent book, *Iridology: Science and Practice in the Healing Arts, Volume II,* has received international acclaim, not only for its subject matter, but the beauty of its photographs and illustrations.

In 1977, Dr. Jensen sold the 100-acre portion of his Hidden Valley Health Ranch prior to retiring from active practice. Several times each year, seminars are held for limited numbers of students at the 25-acre portion of the Ranch on which his home, offices and classrooms are located. At the same time, the doctor is developing a computerized system for analyzing the iris, using space-age technology to standardize analysis techniques and interpretation.

Retiring from active practice in 1978, Dr. Jensen has devoted himself to teaching, writing and lecturing on the subjects of nutrition, rejuvenation and iridology. He has recently completed work on a soon to be released two-hour feature film, tentatively titled *World Search for Health, Happiness and Long Life,* narrated by Dennis Weaver.

Dr. Jensen received his Ph.D. degree at age 75 from the University of Humanistic Studies, San Diego, CA.

Awards and Honors

Dr. Jensen has received many honorary degrees and awards, not only from his own country, but nations such as France, Portugal, Italy, Ecuador, Belgium and others. Several awards were presented to him for the basic work he was doing with the chemistry of man.

Not all honors have been of the traditional sort. Twenty years ago, a New Zealander, Mr. Wally Archer, came to the Hidden Valley Health Ranch with little life left in his body. After a dramatic recovery of health, he brought Dr. Jensen to New Zealand to lecture. He later launched the "Dr. Jensen 729 Health Clubs," the 729 refers to the fact that there is only one doctor for every 729 people in the area. These health clubs taught their members proper nutrition, exercise and other components of health by presenting Dr. Jensen's books and tapes, so they could avoid ailments and diseases. There are now 11 such clubs in New Zealand and Australia.

New Zealand 729 Club members revised their district school lunch program to follow Dr. Jensen's ideas, and the results were spectacular. Teachers reported less absence and tardiness, better study concentration. Parents said their children had fewer colds, no more constipation and considerably improved well-being.

On another more recent occasion, Dr. Jensen was deeply touched when, after a lecture at the University of Canton in the People's Republic of China, a professor invited him to his office. As they entered, Dr. Jensen said, "Those students seemed to know quite a bit about my work." The Chinese doctor smiled and pointed to a bookshelf. "This is why they are familiar with your work." There were all of Dr. Jensen's books—with Chinese translations beside them. "I could not believe my work was being used even in China," he said.

In 1954, Dr. Jensen was honored with the Doctor of the Year award in Portland, Oregon.

An Academy of Science in Paris awarded Dr. Jensen a medal in 1971 for exceptional services rendered to humanity, and in the same year, he received an honorary doctorate from the Center for the Study of Human Sciences in Lisbon, Portugal.

At a ceremony in San Remo, Italy in 1973, he was presented the Ignatz Von Peczely International Iridology Gold Medal by the World Congress of Scientific Medicine, an organization embracing many medical and health disciplines.

A congress of health professionals at Aix-en-Province, France, in 1974, recognized Dr. Jensen with an award for his "valuable contribution in the field of iridology." The following year, the International Naturopathic Association honored him for his service to mankind through his work in the fields of health, iridology and nutrition.

Knighted into the Order of St. John of Malta in 1978 for his humanitarian work, he was awarded the cross of St. John at a special ceremony in New York City.

In 1981, at the Fifth Annual Herb Symposium, the Agnes Arber Distinguished Service award was presented to him for his contributions to the current "herb renaissance."

In 1982, the National Health Federation honored Dr. Jensen with its Pioneer Doctor of the Year award at its annual convention in Long Beach, California.

Most recently, Dr. and Mrs. Jensen traveled to Brussels, Belgium to accept the 1982 Dag Hammarskjold award of the Pax Mundi Academy, an international organization which presents annual awards to those in the arts and sciences who have made outstanding contributions in their fields. The award, in the category of scientific merit, was for "the exceptional services rendered to collective humanity...toward international cooperation and solidarity...." The doctor was personally congratulated on his award by U.S. Ambassador, Charles Price.

A moment with you

In coming to *The Chemistry of Man*, we take an advanced look at nutrition, nutritional deficiencies and types of people. For the student or the nurse, for the doctor who wants the proper information to teach his patients, for the person who is ready for a new path, this is a book that will provide a broad-based rationale for changing our old habits of life. It will show that nutrition is probably the greatest of all the health arts, and it is necessary for us to know this art in order to keep well.

While we say nutrition is most important, it is not everything. But, we must realize that when we apply the mental, physical, mechanical and chemical therapies in the healing art, it will be to no avail unless the nutritional foundation has been properly laid. No therapy can ultimately be successful unless we have the nutritional art working with it.

We have brought out in this volume that our bodies are made of the dust of the earth, so we must live close to the earth, the vegetables, fruits, nuts, berries, flowers and herbs that transform the chemicals of the earth into living biochemicals, fit for our use. We cannot go amiss in seeking out the values in this direction. We can pray, and we will pray amiss, unless we realize that we must follow the natural path of living to experience the level of health and vitality we are made for.

Much research has gone into *The Chemistry of Man*. Diet after diet has been explored and many of them have brough forth. Some have turned out to be unhealthy and have been discarded. However, as we go through the chemistry of man, we want you to realize that man lives as much on what he expresses as what he eats. It is his expression that gives him a philosophy and awakens his consciousness to seek the greater things in life. So, as we touch on the various symptoms that come from chemical

shortages in the body—let us realize that this is one department that needs to be explored to a greater extent than we have previously gotten into.

While many diets can balance our body and while many diets can make up for chemical shortages, a great number are useless. There are about as many diets as there are doctors. The most important question is what is the makeup of a particular diet? We must inquire whether there is adequate nutrient variety and density to replace and rebuild the chemical structure of the human body. The human temple which is made up of the dust of the earth must be understood.

When we recognize that we have to have the dust of the earth, that includes everything between the earth and the heavens, too. And, it is to this end that we must go deeper into the body and find out what we are made of—where we have come from and what is possible to become in the future.

Food science has brought out in many directions today that we cannot understand nutrition without knowing the chemical structure of foods and the chemical needs of the body. And, we must know that our bodies are as different as every gem found in the earth. We start by realizing that only the chemical elements found in the topsoil can be utilized by plants. Depleted soil means depleted foods. It is very necessary that we know what is in our carrots; what makes a plum; why the oxalic acid in rhubarb can be of harm. Then we need to look at symptoms in terms of body chemistry. When we see how every symptom in our body can be from a chemical shortage and how symptoms can be eliminated from the body by taking foods to restore what we have burned out in our body, we begin to understand how carrots and plums can be our "medicine." It is then that we realize how a deeper study has to come along to explore what will help to make this human body all that it is possible to be.

This volume is for the advanced student or health professional. It points directly to that which will change the body, replacing old tissue with new. By now, most people should recognize that foods have effects on the body, and there is more to diet than just putting together a conglomeration of edible substances. Poor foods can have undesirable side effects just like drugs. Good foods, balanced and in the right proportion, assist the body in healing itself and in moving us onward and upward to high-level well-being. To truly enjoy life, we must have all of the elements which are so necessary in order to have a full-grown, beautiful, lovely body.

I owe so much of this work to V. G. Rocine, who has been the one teacher whom I believe has given me more to think about, more to work with in my sanitarium practice than any other. I was able to see those people who were ailing leave their problems behind; I was able to see those who had poor mental attitudes change for the better; I was able to see the alcoholic kick the habit; and those who had a tendency toward violence became more relaxed and mellow again through the proper changes in nutrition and activity. Above all things, we hope that the chemical dynamics of the body are sufficiently shown here to point to what we need to understand and do in order to bring the body to a full and whole expression of health—physically, mentally and spiritually.

While we have spent many years in many dieting procedures, we recognize that there is the spiritual, mental, ethical, moral side to the eating programs, but we cannot be well with a prayer in one hand and a cola drink and a frankfurter in the other. This book is slanted toward the most important thing we can think of and that is the chemical story. This is the most neglected part in most diets and it is from this viewpoint that we have built a healthy way of living that takes in the jobs, marriages, finances, environment, types of people, the kind of foods we eat, the values in those foods so that we may become a whole person, and having high-level function in every organ, every system and every tissue in the body. This book is taking up what we are neglecting in the chemistry of man. The neglect is as much a sin toward the human body as the neglect of the spiritual philosophy.

Dr. Jensen's thoughts:

The true responsibility for the handling of disease should be put directly in the hands of those who are dedicated to preventing diseases.

We spend a great deal of time and money patching and fixing up a broken-down physical vehicle that was designed to be self-repairing, self-rebuilding, self-rejuvenating. If we would only take care of it properly in the beginning, it wouldn't develop so many problems.

Every disease takes time to develop. To eliminate a disease properly it is necessary that we spot it and take care of it in the beginning.

Our American cancer society says that it takes at least 20 years to develop many types of cancer. Where is the doctor who can diagnose and take care of these diseases in the beginning? People need prevention and early treatment, not such a late diagnosis that there is little that can be done.

A body that is chemically well-balanced will normalize itself. Every disease, every symptom, discharge, pain, indicates chemical imbalance in the body.

Eighty percent of all diseases treated in the U.S. are chronic. I am sure that half of these problems could be corrected by developing the proper nutritional balance in our eating program.

Author's preface

In the course of my life, I have had the privilege of working with some of the great pioneers of health and nutrition—men like Dr. John Harvey Kellogg of the Battle Creek Sanitarium, Dr. John H. Tilden of Denver, Colorado, Dr. Henry Lindlahr of Chicago, Dr. Ralph Benner of the Bircher-Benner Sanitarium in Switzerland and Dr. V. G. Rocine. These were men who mastered their particular specialties through years of sanitarium experience. From such men, I harvested the best of the nature cure knowledge in foods and dieting, fasting, homeopathy, water cure, herbal remedies, colonics, bowel care, iridology and other specialties. Then I put these ideas to work in my own sanitariums.

Sanitarium practice is much different from the office practice most doctors prefer today. The average doctor with an office practice sees most patients only a few times a year and has no idea whether they are following his directions, whether they are experiencing adverse side effects from his prescriptions or whether they are living in such a way as to ruin the health he is trying to restore. In a sanitarium, on the other hand, the patients follow a certain regimen, eat what is served at meal times, exercise as directed and see the doctor frequently. When you live with your patients, you must face your successes and failures every day. If a certain program isn't working, you change it until it is working.

I can think of no better way to learn the many facets of healing work and to correct the poor living habits of many patients than through sanitarium work. This is verified in my own experience. My patients have been my textbooks; and I have learned much from them. Thousands of men and women have been able to return to their homes and jobs rejuvenated and revitalized, not so much because of what I have done for them, but because of what nature has done for them. Nature cures, but sometimes she needs a helping hand—especially with those who have departed so far from her ways.

We find that 9 out of 10 patients seek out practitioners of the drugless healing arts for three basic reasons. Often they have tried the methods of Western medicine and have not been helped. Some of them don't believe in drugs and surgery, and others are afraid of them. These are not the "average" patients found in the waiting rooms of medical doctors. The fact that so many of them have found the help they were seeking at my sanitariums is a testimony to the effectiveness of the methods I have followed.

V. G. Rocine was my greatest teacher, a Norwegian homeopath who taught me much of what I know about foods and nutrition. I can truthfully say that nutrition has been the single most powerful technique in my work with patients. Every branch of the healing art tree has its proper use, but we find that the tissue of the human body cannot be restored or rejuvenated without the proper foods. Food, wisely used, is the key to health and well-being.

*The purpose of **The Chemistry of Man** is to open the door to all who wish to enter to survey the array of findings that has made my work what it is. It is primarily about nutrition and its role in the human body. In quite another sense, it covers issues that we need to understand in order to use foods wisely and well.*

We have strayed so far from a natural, pure and wholesome way of living that we are confronted with the need to turn around and see what has thrown us off the path.

The environment that Nature provided for us has undergone dramatic changes at the hands of man. Modern agriculture, determined to seek maximum harvests and maximum profits by any means available, has changed the nature of what is being presented to us as food. The food processing industry has carried this a step farther by presenting us with a vast array of attractive, appealing, tasty substances that are so devitalized, so deficient in vitamins, enzymes, fiber, certain biochemical elements and nutrients that we can scarcely call them foods any more. Our bodies were not designed to ingest and assimilate these foodless foods or the additives that give them eternal shelf life in the supermarket.

Lacking proper foods, deficient in the chemical elements needed by the cells, the human body molds to this state of affairs by responding the only way it can—by sickness and disease.

God intended us to work with Nature, not against her, for our own good. We need to return to a simpler way of life. We need to get closer to Nature and to live a more natural life. This may mean changing jobs, moving to a different climate, solving the marriage problem, spending more time in the sunshine and eating proper foods. Health is not achieved by taking remedial action as our bodies malfunction over and over again. Health is a way of life in which we experience high-level well-being—physically, mentally and spiritually.

To assist in telling this story, I am reintroducing some of the basic wisdom, in terms of the 16 primary minerals, as it is revealed in the works of Victor G. Rocine, who was my teacher, doctor and confidante—my best friend. Many of my successes and revelations are in debt to Rocine's work with the natural chemicals, and inspired by what he called "Bionomy"—the science of life.

I include this information from Rocine as a kind of flag waving from a mountain top. It is for all students and indicates that there is more to know about the correlations of body, mind and the subtle energy bodies than any of us currently are practicing. Clearly, Rocine was far in advance of his age and even this age; yet for the sake of future science based on wholistic thought, I share with you what we still have. Unfortunately, much of the Rocine work is lost forever; but we are trying to bring some of his work back so that others may benefit from his wisdom. Such is the case with many other important works of healers of the past who were far in advance of accepted 20th century understandings.

During the past few years, I have shifted from concentrating heavily on treating patients to teaching and writing activities, and this has been a period during which I have published several books aimed at how to heal oneself. With **The Chemistry of Man** I now turn to the doctor and the healing profession itself, to the academic, humanistic world, and to the world at large in need of healing. This book is meant to be a companion volume to my second volume on iridology titled **Iridology: The Science and Practice in the Healing Arts, Volume II**. These works, I hope, will aid the science of Iridology as it comes of age, and help a new profession come forward—iridology, nutrition and the wholistic healing arts.

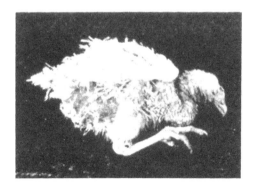

BEFORE

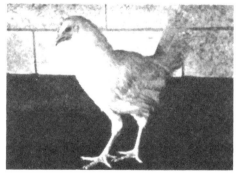

AFTER

The pictures of the chickens indicate what can be done with nutrition. When fed on diets improperly balanced chemically, the animals are small, scrawny and weak; while those fed on a diet properly balanced with the chemical elements necessary for proper growth are strong well-developed and free from disease.

FOREWORD

The title of this book, *The Chemistry of Man*, is taken from a talk I have given thousands of times. I call this story the greatest story ever told on earth. As a practitioner of the natural healing arts for more than 50 years, I have tried to apply natural and spiritual laws to teach the patient how to restore balance within him/herself and become firmly set on the path toward good health. It is the perplexing **im**balances that reveal themselves as "dis-ease" manifestations or as **diseases** as we more conventionally refer to them. My treatment combines nutritional counseling with the art and science of iridology, which analyzes the human ailments through the iris. It is an analytical diagnostic tool which focuses on health and ill health of the whole person.

At the current stage of development in Western medicine, the majority of practitioners are most successful in the area of acute **conditions, rather than in prevention, and levels of imbalance. But in my long history of daily** practice, I have often been able to treat patients who have come to me as "a last resort," purely by improving diet and lifestyle. Thus, I have practiced without the use of 20th century technological medical inventiveness such as chemical drug intervention or the dominant modes of surgical procedures lying outside my practice. I must quickly add, however, that I am not opposed to advances in 20th century medicine. I would like to see these advances balanced with the natural healing laws and methods which have existed since the beginning of recorded and prerecorded history.

Made up of body, mind and spirit, we humans must realize that all of these dimensions are important for healthy and harmonious living. Through the study of iridology, we come to understand not only the workings of the body but the workings of the inner self, and it is from

this study that we can begin the tremendously important work of rebuilding people's lives and even society itself.

The eye is the window to subtle orders of energy by which we can observe inherent weaknesses in body systems and proceed to match them with individual mineral requirements. Specific minerals represent specific functions in the organs where they are dominantly stored. Moreover, there are mental and spiritual characteristics which correlate with these minerals, for, on the deepest levels, each mineral is a conductor or transmitter of specific kinds of brain/mind activity, or what we might call vibration.

As we apply the missing chemical elements through improved nutrition and interrelated lifestyle, we can clearly see changes in the weak organs as reflected in the iris. Shifts in coloration from dark to light indicate that there is a reverse activity in the body as it moves from chronic to more acute states. Indeed, to the degree a person lives in accord with natural and spiritual laws, the eye itself "comes clean." It becomes clearer and clearer—murkiness disappears. Dark and light areas specifically relate to tiny lesions or holes, which fill in with lines or fibers as the rebuilding process develops and the healing lines intermesh. It is through this intermeshing that the lesions fill in and lighten up; this can be very clearly seen when the eye is examined.

Improper mental attitudes and unhealthy foods can burn out the body reserves faster than minerals can be built up in the body, and it is this lack of reserves which shows up in the lesions. Each lesion relates specifically to an organ and to a body system of energy, reflected as a magnetic-electrical quality of expression. The dark lesion areas represent aspects of us where the life force, which can only be carried by a dynamic electrical movement, has not entered fully. Where there is light there is life, movement and activity.

If we add a well-ordered, pure and natural diet to a person with dis-ease, we can see within a three-month period the physical manifestation of movement both in the irides and in the physical body of the patient. The shifts from dark to light clearly relate to constructive changes and improved mental outlook. In fact, to the degree that the person adapts to a whole, pure and natural diet, personality itself will change, for whole foods inspire wholeness and wellness in a person.

The Chemistry of Man is by no means a completed story, yet it introduces the vital bridges that must be built to understand the nature-cure wisdom of the past and the medicine of tomorrow. There are many paths in the wholistic healing art—nutrition, acupuncture, reflexology, herbs, water treatments, color therapy, music, sound, spiritual wisdom and others, and *The Chemistry of Man* is just one of them. To present the story of the 16 chemical elements, I am acting as coauthor with my late teacher, mentor and friend, Victor G. Rocine, whose inspiration was responsible for a great deal of my success. Many of my own subsequent discoveries and revelations are linked, to some extent, to what I learned from Dr. Rocine, particularly through what he called "Bionomy," the science of life.

I include this information from Rocine as a kind of flag waving from a mountain top. Dr. Rocine was a prolific writer/educator for lay people. He taught and believed that a new day had dawned in the healing art, through food chemistry capable of bringing in both physical and mental healing. He was a very well educated man. Personally, I like to measure a man by his studies, his work and the books he reads. Rocine knew ten languages, and the books on his library shelves showed familiarity with a broad array of subjects from nature-cure work and food chemistry to theosophy. He was balanced in his knowledge of body, mind and spirit.

Clearly, Rocine was far in advance of his age and even this age; yet for the sake of future science based on wholistic thought, I share with you what we still have. Much of Rocine's work is lost forever, but I am bringing some of his work back so that others can benefit from it.

Rocine presented his material in books and from the lecture platform. I brought it down to the practical level in my sanitariums with patients. It works beautifully, as thousands of my patients can attest, in many cases where all other treatments had failed.

During the past few years, I have shifted from concentrating heavily on treating patients to teaching and writing activities, and this has been a period during which I have published several books aimed at how to heal oneself. With *The Chemistry of Man* I now turn to the doctor and the healing profession itself, to the academic, humanistic world, and to the world at large in need of healing. This book is meant to be a companion volume to my second volume on iridology titled *Iridology: The Science and Practice in the Healing Arts, Volume II.* These works, I hope, will aid the science of Iridology as it comes of age, and help a new profession come forward—iridology, nutrition and the wholistic healing arts.

I should make very clear, however, that while I have tried to include only constructive ideas in this book, I recognize that some people will misconstrue my intentions. Much of the material will be new. In many clinics, it will be automatically opposed because it may appear too simple; it may take study; it may require extra effort in counseling and teaching.

Once again, what is written here is not the entire story, covering every situation. But it certainly belongs in the consciousness of the person who wants to live correctly and have a new path to follow. I cannot see why any doctor would object to anyone wishing to learn ways and means of taking care of himself or herself.

But there are people who may have difficulty understanding this book and should remain under a doctor's supervision. Similarly, there are those with special needs, such as mechanical manipulation, constructive surgery, acupuncture, and so forth. In such cases, it is better that a patient procure the proper advice and guidance of a qualified practitioner and have the supervision of that person in whatever cures are undertaken.

I am giving out the knowledge contained here because it has meant so much to the patients of my last 53 years of office and sanitarium practice, and it has also been the means of their getting well. I aim to speak of the highest good and the finest materials possible in all my studies. My main objective is to help people get well, and so I direct this work to the new doctor and the people who would like to put health problems for themselves and their families in their own hands. This group, of course, includes mothers and cooks, because it is in the kitchen that so much disease begins. The new healing profession will have its starting point right in the home.

I hope that this book will find its way to every college and university. It should be on the shelf in every doctor's office. It may help alleviate the problem which has many people clamoring for the knowledge it contains.

The day will come when people will provide for their own wellness by living correctly. Until then, we need doctors who will help patients to get involved with their own healing. An agreement is needed between doctor and patient, in which the doctor shifts responsibility back to those who are not living and eating properly, in order to keep their bodies well. As it is, the patient, who considers his health problems no further than cost and the nuisance of prescriptions, depends entirely on the doctor to do the healing. The truth is—as it has been said in the past—the doctor dresses the wounds and nature heals.

The tendency is to ask, "What is this treatment going to do for me?" It is better to ask, "What can I do for myself?" We must recognize that good health comes from within and that we have a responsibility to ourselves that begins at home. Until the day comes that we are effectively able to care for ourselves, we need a doctor committed to the principles to be found in this book. It is through doctor and patient talking together, feeling together, and working together that we can acquire the very best of health. Getting well may be a matter of educating rather than medicating.

Definitions from Webster's New World Dictionary:

FOOD. Any substance taken into and assimilated by a plant or animal to keep up its life and growth; nourishment. Solid substances of this sort: distinguished from drink. A specified kind of food. Anything that nourishes or stimulates (food for thought).

NUTRITION: A nourishing or being nourished; esp., the series of processes by which an organism takes in food and uses it in living and growing and in repairing tissues. Nourishment; food. The science or study of proper diet.

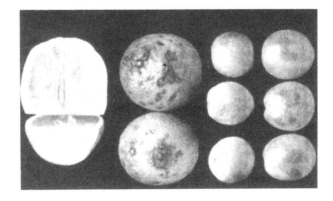

When the soil has been depleted and the soil structure is unbalanced, then we grow plant life which is diseased and undeveloped such as we find in the picture of these oranges. By making a more fertile and well-balanced soil, we are able to change these diseased conditions.

Contents

III A vital course on foods

What the chemicals do in the body; vital lessons in the chemical story.

IV The proof is in the healing

Special color section with case histories

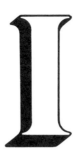

We are the dust of the earth

It is said we are made of the dust of the earth, the same basic chemical elements of which the earth is made. Yet, spectrophotometric analysis has shown the same elements are present in the stars, so it can also be said we are made of stardust. In any case, we are matter evolved to its highest vibratory state on this planet—living, thinking, breathing matter—a structure so magnificent and complex that it would take a computer the size of the Woolworth building to simulate its brain functions.

The chemical elements of which we are made are a fascinating study in themselves. Scientists can tell what elements are in the stars because each one emits a certain characteristic frequency or vibration of light.

The colors and physical properties of gems are due to the crystalline structures of their chemical elements in certain combinations. Diamond is crystallized carbon. An emerald is beryllium aluminum silicate, a green form of beryl. (The color of beryl may be green, yellow, pink or white, depending on slight changes in the crystal structure.) Rubies and sapphires are aluminum oxide, while turquoise is copper aluminum phosphate. Particular chemical elements, in combination with others in a certain crystalline structure, determine the type, color, clarity and hardness of any gem. Remove a certain element from a gem, and its properties and beauty disappear.

Just as gems are made of the chemical elements, so are we—only man is much more complex. Our bones and teeth are primarily calcium and phosphorus structures. The skin and hair are primarily silicon organs, and iron is the centrally important element in the blood. Each organ and specialized tissue type in the body needs certain chemical elements to do its job, to play its part in the overall functioning of the human body. When we are lacking in certain needed biochemicals, the corresponding body organs and functions are damaged and impaired. Since every organ, tissue and microscopic cell contributes to the well-being of the whole body, chemical deficiencies lower our state of wellness. On the other hand, when we take in chemical elements which do not belong in the body—such as lead or strychnine—cell destruction takes place.

Man cannot take in nutrients directly from the earth but needs the higher-evolved biochemicals. Plants, with the help of sunlight, take the basic chemical elements from the earth, air and water and raise the vibratory levels of those elements so they can be assimilated by higher life forms such as man. The sequence of living things that provide food for one another—plants, insects, birds, fish, animals and man—is called the food chain. As chemical elements are passed along up the food chain, they may become higher evolved, a finer food for man because of the raised vibratory level.

The human body is a complex structure of billions of specialized parts and electrochemical processes, constantly moving, flowing, changing, in the state of dynamic equilibrium we call life. The average lifetime of a red blood cell is 120 days, and when it dies, it is replaced by new ones. As long as we provide the body with the biochemical nutrients it needs, the various organs and tissues can rejuvenate themselves indefinitely—provided we also get enough exercise, fresh air, sunshine, rest and recreation.

On the other hand, if the body is not given the biochemical nutrients it needs, cells break down and die before their appointed time. If it is given substances it can't digest, use or completely excrete, they remain in the body as toxic settlements in the tissue, reducing the ability of some organ or tissue structure to do its job. We must have the right foods to build and sustain high-level wellness.

To understand how to get rid of or prevent disease and achieve high-level wellness, we must have a basic understanding of what foods are composed of and what they do in the body.

I have spent over 50 years searching for the keys to good health and long life, traveling throughout the world looking for vital health secrets. I have spent many years in sanitarium work, observing first hand what foods and therapies did for patients with varying health problems. This is a subject I know well from direct experience.

Without a balanced diet of wholesome, nutritious foods, wellness cannot be achieved and sustained, no matter what else we do.

We draw our foods from different parts of the food chain. Meat animals are at the top of the food chain, and they draw their nutrients from grasses, grains and other members of the vegetable kingdom. We also eat grains, seeds, nuts, vegetables, fruits and other foods which are below animal protein on the food chain. On the bottom of this food chain, we find single-celled organisms such as algae, which produce as much as 80% of the world's oxygen—and provide food for many species of germ life, insects and other small life forms which, in turn, provide food for large creatures until we come to the species which serve as food for man. All plant life derives its nutrients from earth, air and water. All other life forms, including man, derive theirs from plants or other living things that eat plants.

Soils vary in composition and quality. So do the plants and trees that grow in them. That means we must know something about foods and soils to get all the right nutrients to have healthy bodies. We will get into that more in Chapter 1, but for now, it is necessary only to realize how important it is to have integrity in the food chain which provides us with life.

When soils or any other part of the food chain suffer loss of integrity through pollution or lack of certain chemical elements, everything above it on the food chain is affected—including man. For most modern cultures, a peculiar and artificial component has been introduced into the food chain—the food processing plant. Simply put, a food processing plant adds something to, takes something away or alters the chemical structure of some food as made by nature. We find there are many other ways in which man has introduced toxins or created chemical deficiencies in parts of the food chain.

All disease conditions originally begin with a chemical deficiency or a toxic substance taken into the human body. Keep in mind, however, that deficiencies can be induced by stress, and toxins can be accumulated from the body's own internal processes due to chronic overwork (fatigue) or psychosomatic factors such as bitterness, hatred, unforgiveness or worry.

Simple examples of deficiency, toxic addition and psychosomatic effects are: goiter, caused by iodine deficiency; anemia, caused by iron deficiency; hardening of the arteries, primarily due to too much salt and greasy or fatty foods; and ulcers due to excess acidity caused by worry.

Health, then, is restored by getting rid of toxins, by eating food with the right chemical elements, and by changing to positive attitudes and emotional patterns.

This book is about the basic chemical elements needed by the body, the foods that provide them and the role of foods in taking care of tissue conditions leading to or accompanying various diseases. This work is based upon the principles and teachings of my former instructor, the late V. G. Rocine.

We must obtain and continue using the elements required for health in order to care for this bodily instrument properly.

2

one

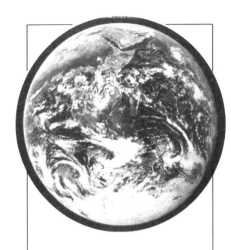

Man, his environment and the elements

What follows in this book is the history of man's past and an invitation to a better, healthier future. We cannot continue to do as we have been doing or the next generation will fall. All of our responses, from our minds to our bones to our digestive systems will become weaker, unless we change our ways. Health of body and mind and spirit derives from proper food, correct living and high thoughts, which is a very simple concept but one frequently overlooked.

My studies and findings on this subject follow throughout the remainder of this book. I wish to say at the outset that what I have learned has been proven through my extensive sanitarium experience. My experience not only benefitted my many thousands of patients, but became my own university. My patients were my books and my teachers. What they taught me is that drugless healing has a place in the healing arts. Indeed, the priceless education of my sanitarium experience forms the foundation for what I wish to convey in this book.

I was confronted with mechanical, chemical and psychological problems, which meant that my staff and I had to find a way to heal, through observation and consultation, so as to help our patients. Observation was essential. Then, we pigeon-holed various experiences, recorded them, took them out for study and comparison.

Was a particular problem primarily mechanical or psychological? Was it the fear that came before the glandular problem? We had to learn how to "clear" the patient and, afterwards, teach him or her to drop old and develop new habits. We had to learn that there were many ways of taking care of problems besides the merely orthodox healing methods.

There were some people with the vitality to overcome their troubles very quickly simply by taking the sunshine. Some were in need of association with others, having been lonely, love-lost, depressed or confused. They were looking for a way out of their low vitality because they were sick of being sick. It was a matter of showing them a new life, of giving them a window to see through.

Sometimes, a person without the ability to digest or breathe or eliminate or metabolize found himself next to a person moving along into a new day. Each patient was different. Each one's digestion was different.

Some patients were mean and others beautiful in their soul expression. Some were lost because they didn't realize that, through soul expression, they could make changes in their physical bodies.

My sanitarium experience led me to certain findings which are explained in greater detail later in this book. For example, I found that potassium eliminates water and balances sodium.

I wanted to impress on some people that the chemical structures of the body could be balanced if they would make certain changes. I saw how calcium could ground a mentally distressed person who was nearly ready to "fly the coop" and I saw how calcium gave him the power and energy to repair his nervous system. I saw how iron attracts oxygen. I found that unless a patient had the proper amount of iron in his body, no amount of proper breathing would attract sufficient oxygen from the air.

I saw that silicon carries magnetism from the brain through the tissues of the body and that the nerve force was lowered when there wasn't enough silicon in reserve. Additionally, the skin, which is a silicon organ, is always in a state of distress. Mental expressions changed with sufficient silicon so that the sick look left a person.

Each of us is an electrical dynamo, a factory of a million strings to be fed and rejuvenated so that we can operate at the highest efficiency. In my studies of chemical elements, each with its own vibratory rate, I learned that sulphur has somewhat the same vibratory rate as the skin. When sulphur was used in packs and salves, there was always a positive reaction in the skin. I became convinced that sulphur has a vibratory effect on the body and has a vibratory and vital effect on every disease of the body. From here, I proceeded to studies in the electrolytic and colloidal activities taking place in my patients. I saw that, through this finite, almost gaslike activity, new life is made. The construction of a new body for a patient led to the most intense and minute considerations of human processes.

I began to do color experiments to find what effect color had on plantlife. I created a red "greenhouse" and saw how plants in their early

stages grew twice as fast as they did in the regular greenhouse. Then I put plants in a blue "greenhouse," which caused them to be stunted. I felt that there was a story coming out in the use of colors. I wondered why someone hadn't been using colors in a therapeutic way.

I thought about the expressions we use that include color—and this is true in every language. We are blue with cold and someone has a red hot temper. Red signifies sexual life and the lower chakra, which concerns the emotional body and sex life, and the red light district. Further, the Red Revolution. Also, experiments have been done to show that people work twice as hard in a room that is painted red—but in three hours they are fighting!

I was one of the first in the United States to use music in order to study changes that could come about in the body. The glands responded and the heart would either calm down or speed up, depending on the type of music. Could it be possible that vibrations could be thought about in an abstract way and we could not see or feel or measure what the music therapy achieved?

There seemed to be some applications of these findings to my sulphur studies. For example, I wondered why I saw areas of sulphur color many times in the iris of the eye?

The answer lies in the electro-chemical activity of the body. The sulphur mystery is solved if we understand that vibrational activity working colloidally with vibrations through the nervous system is responsible for a certain result.

We may think it is difficult to observe the vibratory factor of a crude sulphur when it is carried throughout the body, but it is not. Drugs are carried in a very definite way by vibrations to the various organs and built back into a chemical state definitely related to the original chemical used.

We cannot understand what is going on in the body unless we study color, vibrations and nature. We must realize that crises come and are natural. In my sanitarium work, there were times when patients experienced toxic eliminations so strongly that I wondered whether I was bringing another disease to a person. But then I began to see how diseases differ from healing crises. A healing crisis is an elimination process in which a vital principle is at work. The body wants to get rid of catarrh and we should not stop that elimination.

My work clearly illustrated Hering's law of cure, which states, "Healing occurs from the head down, from inside out, and in reverse order as the symptoms have first been acquired." I discovered the value of biochemicals in breaking down chronic and acute conditions. I began to use tonics, soups and broths high in certain chemicals in order to neutralize acids in the body. In other words, bodies were rearranged chemically by means of foods containing important chemical elements. I found present symptoms—called diseases—would leave of their own accord without any medical treatments. I advised exercises, nutritional assessment and change and mental readjustment.

It is this vibratory story—the food story—which needs to be considered when caring for a patient. The sanitarium years clearly demonstrated that nature works for us if we work with it. There are some very positive moves that we can make. It is not so much what we give up that counts, but what we take up.

Food as a Medicine

When we had gone over so many experiences with patients in which symptoms were taken care of by homeopathic cell salts, I began to wonder if there was a better way to supply chemicals needed by the body. These cell salts in tablet form were put up in a milk sugar base. They worked well enough, it is true. But I wondered if there was a more natural way to accomplish the same or better results.

I sought out Dr. V. G. Rocine, who taught me that foods were our best medicine. He showed me how to use honey and how to make soups and broths, how to make special food preparations for certain organs in the body and for certain symptoms that were expressed in the body. I built up my repertoire of food routines to such a point that when a person spoke about dizziness, I knew that he needed sodium and chloride. If there was a dry mouth, I knew sodium chloride was needed. If we had a dry skin, I knew we needed sodium and a chloride.

So, it got to the point whenever any one of the symptoms came up I could tell that there were certain elements that were lacking. We could tell when a patient was anemic. If a patient lost her pink cheeks and suffered menstrual disorders, she needed iron. We found that if calcium was lacking, there would be hemorrhages, nasal hemorrhages. When we found ears were itching and flaky substance would come from them when scratched, we knew that phosphorus was lacking.

With Dr. Rocine's examples and teachings and by getting acquainted with foods, I was able to tell what foods would help which symptoms in the body. This was the channel in which I was particularly interested. In this book, I am giving you many food remedies that have been used as healing agents. As concentrated food substances, with a specific attraction and affinity, they are earmarked for certain organs in the body. We begin to see that there is a direct relation between the need for these chemical elements (when we are short of them) and the particular place in which a person resides.

There are parts of this country that are very high in certain chemicals and low in others. In parts of Colorado, you can see the fluoride ring in a person's teeth because they have excess fluorine. When there is no hardness in the teeth at all, fluorine is lacking.

So it is a matter of knowing the symptoms. In knowing the body, we were able to tell what chemical elements a person lacked.

Next, in the study of iridology, we got into the study of inflammation of the body as revealed by signs in the iris. From our knowledge of what foods aided certain organs and symptoms, we could tell what particular elements were necessary to remove those inflammations from particular parts of the body. When we found the inflammations in certain organs, we could recommend the biochemicals needed to take care of various stages of inflammation settled there.

This is a work so important that I would like to see it carried on. The most simple and effective way of taking care of our health is via the kitchen. We can still return to nature and by way of solarized and potentized juices, tonics, soups and broths, we can get concentrated elements that rebuild the body and eliminate the symptoms usually treated by pills, potions, etc.

Tissue cell salts have been used with good results for many years. While there are many salts that can be used to good effect, we have found that there are foods that provide these salts in concentrated form. Certain vegetables, fruits, berries and nuts have concentrated salts and they can be used as medicine. Some are high in certain chemical elements that can be used for chemical shortages in certain organs of the body. For example, one of our high copper foods is apricots. One of the high sodium foods is celery. High calcium and phosphorus content are found in turnip greens.

Magnesium is in yellow cornmeal. Manganese is in Missouri black walnuts, potassium in watercress, iron in asparagus, spinach, parsley.

We can go still further and find that there is a definite activity in certain foods that will promote a greater activity to certain organs, such as black cherry juice for liver disturbances, asparagus for kidney disorders, whey for stomach disorders caused by lack of sodium. There is an affinity between some of these foods and certain organs. The nutrients they provide are earmarked to go to certain cell structures of the body. Yet, there is more to it than that. Our body chemistry is so designed that the bloodstream will pick up the elements we need from the digestive system and will distribute them to the proper place as they are needed by the various organs of the body. This is what naturally happens when these chemicals are washed over tissues lacking any of the chemical elements. These elements are needed to help all organs to repair, rebuild and to regenerate. This is why we say that we dress the wound; we feed the tissues; but nature does the curing.

All nature needs is an opportunity and the body will repair and regenerate itself without any help from human hands. What we have to do is to supply the deficiencies in our bodies, not to treat the disease symptoms. The deficiency is overcome by the application of foods, not by the use of drugs. Drugs cannot build new tissue. Only food can do that. This method of treating the body cannot, in any way, be construed as the practice of medicine. It is strictly nutrition. Yet, all doctors, including medical doctors, should understand how to use food as medicine, how to use food to overcome ailments.

In this book, we offer ways to take care of the stomach, to take care of the heart and to take care of the various orther organs in the body. We are going to discuss herbs that provide some of the elements that may be necessary. We are going to present charts that show you what foods and what elements are necessary to overcome shortages and to build a balance in the body.

We find that nature, in foodstuffs, always has the chemical salts in minute quantities. We find that small quantities of the salts are much more easily assimilated and, consequently, act much faster than the large quantities of crude chemical elements found in our drugs.

It was Professor Liebig who said, "It happens that a tissue in chronic disease reaches such a degree of density, becomes so clogged, that the salt solution of the blood cannot enter to feed and nourish; but, if for therapeutic purposes, a solution of salt be so triturated and given, so diluted, that all its molecules are set free, it is presumable that no definite hindrance will be in the way of these molecules to enter the abnormally condensed part of the tissue.

We find this true when we use food salts, vegetable and fruit salts, and use them in the form of tonics, soups, broths and so forth. In using them, the clogged arteries are helped. Hardening in the arteries is gradually reduced. Arthritis calcium deposits and spurs are dissolved. Ulcers of the stomach are relieved. Certainly, that should be proof enough that cell salts found in foods reach their destination in the appropriate tissue and do their work.

When an adequate supply of food salts is lacking over a long period of time, we find that the blood cannot compensate for this or prevent deterioration of the tissues. If this deficiency affects the intestinal tract, so important to digestion, mal-assimilation may occur, and the intake of nutritious foods will not bring improvement. Before foods can be useful to the body, they must be digested.

We find in using the cell salts in a triturated form by drinking juices that they are of such character that they are assimilable directly into the bloodstream. They are very easily digested and the process starts right in the mucous membranes of the mouth.

Those people suffering from arthritis, diabetes, Bright's disease, paralysis and other slow-recovery diseases, should absolutely abstain from drinking tea, coffee and cocoa.

It is only ignorance that hinders the healing of any disease or condition, and the cure for

6

ignorance is knowledge. I wonder if we really have all the knowledge we need to help our patients with their problems, large and small, as we are meant to in the healing art? How many people will listen to this story and try what is recommended here? I know how right it is because my experience has shown it to be so. It has been proven by effective results in a large number of cases with my sanitarium patients. This work presents a right way of going, a clean way of going, that will lead to high-level wellness for many, if not most. It may not cure every disease, but the percentages of people getting well that I have personally observed indicates it must be seriously considered. Don't stop reading and don't stop thinking. Don't stop!

IN A GARDEN
The kiss of the sun
    for pardon,
The song of the birds
    for mirth, —
One is nearer God's heart
    in a garden
Than anywhere else
    on earth.
DOROTHY F. B. GURNEY

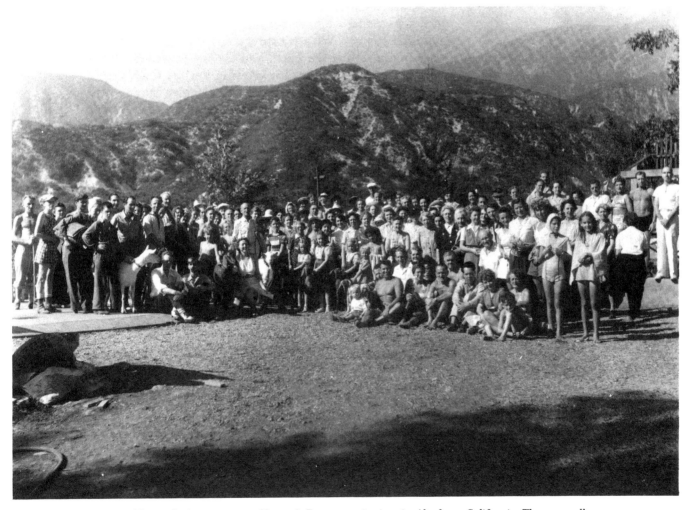

This gathering was at my Nature's Retreat sanitarium in Altadena, California. They were all studying to find out more of what Mother Nature was able to provide in the way of health.

two

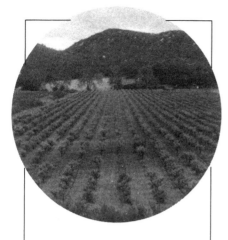

Soils, minerals and seeds

The laws pertaining to building healthy soil are the same as those for building a healthy body. Good health in either case is made up of all the required chemical elements the soil and body need. Of course, soils and bodies are different. There are different kinds of healthy soils which build different kinds of plants. There are different chemical types of people who build different kinds of bodies, each based on a different chemical balance. Good health comes from having a balance of the elements we need in soil and body.

Healthy Bodies, Healthy Soils

Unfortunately, civilization has been proceeding at such a pace that we have become inconsiderate of our natural resources. We are approaching the bankruptcy stage in plundering the Earth and leaving ourselves with improper conditions for growing healthy food. Our number one problem is topsoil erosion, which may trigger a food shortage in the 1980s. This condition is on us **at this moment**. Erosion is caused not only by rainfall but also by a lack of plantlife which, through root systems, holds the soil together. Additionally, improper soil replenishment contributes to the disappearance of soils vital to the production of food.

Food does not enrich itself automatically without proper soil care. To create one inch of topsoil, nature labors anywhere from 100 to 1000 years, as decaying material from leaves, animals and droppings is processed to become organically rich humus. This material is not only rich in minerals, but able to retain water and, through porosity, admit air to the roots of plants. This kind of naturally healthy soil is a living soil, filled with friendly bacteria and having resistance and power. These qualities are passed on to the humans and animals eating the plantlife derived from this vital soil.

In the past, the dust bowls of the Middle West have been caused by wind-blown topsoil being carried away by the Mississippi and various rivers to the ocean. Our bread and butter, so to speak, lies on the ocean floor. We **must** take care of this problem.

Some 80 years ago, topsoil totaled 80 inches. Now, on an average, in the United States, that 80 inches has been reduced to 8 inches. Additionally, the tendency of our farmers today is to avoid traditional soil-renewal methods. No longer is it common practice to allow land to lie fallow or to be refurbished through a cover crop to restore nitrogen and other key ingredients. The drive to produce more and more farm produce is responsible for this change, combined with the increased use of artificial fertilizers—an average of 200 pounds per acre per year.

This failure to replenish topsoil gradually uses up the resources of our croplands. The forecast is for an 8% reduction in American farm yields over the next 50 years. Recent news reports support these findings. A study conducted by Lester Brown, head of the World Watch Institute, concludes that possible food shortages in the 1980s could outdo the oil shortages of the 1970s. World food output has doubled since 1950, but only at the expense of serious injury to our soils, specifically the loss of topsoil mentioned above. The consequence of this loss is a severe decline in productivity. American cropland, for example, is down 34%. The United States Department of Agriculture has estimated soil losses of 14.1 tons an acre in Tennessee; 11.4 tons an acre in Missouri; and 10.9 tons in Mississippi. Increasingly, countries of the world are dependent on the United States and Canada for grain shipments, a demand which has created problems because farmers have responded with boosts in production at the expense of their soil.

Failure to Replenish the Soil

Such production demands have led to the increased use of chemical fertilizer, which has risen in production from 14 million tons in 1950 to 113 million tons in 1980. But what is the nature of this fertilizer? If the proper chemicals are not replaced in the soil, the Wheel of Life and Health is not taken care of. The Wheel of Life is the natural cycle of things in which decaying matter is absorbed by the earth, and then returns to the plant finally becoming food. The Hunzas in Pakistan recognize that whatever life has passed away eventually returns to the soil. But in the United States, most of our cattle and pigs are shipped to Chicago and Kansas City, either for export or preparation for consumption. The bones and other materials of the animals do not return to the soil, another reason that there is no longer the chemical balance we have had in the past.

Because more and more artificial fertilizers are being used to grow our plantlife, the result is unhealthy plants, lacking the proper chemical elements. In this way, it is possible to starve with a full stomach, because foods are being grown from depleted soils. Deprived of necessary, organically derived chemicals, such plantlife makes a wonderful food for pestilence, the Mediterranean fruit fly and other pests. The plantlife may look healthy to the average person, but it does not compare to the best crops coming from well-balanced soils. It is through the chemicals found in plantlife that our body structure is built. What we eat today will walk and talk tomorrow.

Without the proper elements coming out of plants and into human tissue, each organ will not be balanced as it should be and will not function properly. Each will be subject to an invasion of germlife. Most people think that we "catch" germs; however, all diseases come about from a lack of proper chemical balance. For example, when there isn't enough boron in the soil, avocado leaves turn brown, citrus fruits become pithy and their peelings look as though they have psoriasis. California soils have 25% less calcium than soils of other states. On the other hand, celery coming out of Utah has 25% more sodium than celery grown elsewhere in the country. If the soil doesn't have the proper balance, the plants cannot have it and neither can man. Eventually plants and humans end up with shortages which invite diseases due to improperly balanced chemical structure.

Dr. Albrecht's Experiments

I have spent some time studying with Dr. William Albrecht, one of the most important agricultural scientists this country has had. He made valuable contributions to my understanding of the chemical story while he was a professor at the University of Missouri and his work has stood up against considerable opposition. He has shown that plants grown on properly chemicalized soil can be strong, may develop into much larger sizes and also will have a greater amount of power and resistance. When not adequately chemicalized, on the other hand, they can have a greater water content and possibly be dry and pithy.

In one of his experiments, Dr. Albrecht used two pots of soil. In one pot, he removed the manganese, boron and other vital chemical elements inherent in the soil. Beside that pot he set another one, fully chemicalized, and planted two sister plants, one in each pot. They grew together, one entwined about the other on a trellis. The plant in the pot missing the chemical elements was a very light green color that was almost transparent. But the other plant was dark green. The one which was light in color was filled with bugs and parasites, whereas the dark green plant had no bugs whatsoever on it. He explained the reason the bugs had not invaded the dark green plant: "Disease preys on an undernourished plant." I have never forgotten that lesson.

On my own, I have been able to see plants respond according to the way the soil is tended. Placing different chemical elements in the soil has determined what kind of plant grows. Lacking certain elements, a plant will grow with very little green in the leaves and its buds will drop off with the least amount of wind playing against it. And, as with Dr. Albrecht's experiment, when healthy plantlife is grown entwined with unhealthy, diseased plants covered with bacteria and parasites, even direct contact fails to transfer the disease from one plant to the other!

Pollution Adds to the Problem

Pollution of our atmosphere is obviously adding to the problem of growing healthy plantlife and human beings. Pollution not only creates unhealthy air but also cuts out the ultraviolet rays from the sun which are vitally necessary to the healthy growth of all living things on the surface of the planet. Pollution has spread to 90% of our water, and contamination creates acid rain even in remote and once beautifully pure lakes. Additionally, along with artificially doctoring the soil, we have developed powerful pesticides to doctor our plants.

But it is very poor thinking to do this doctoring by developing stronger chemical compounds. Instead, to be free of pests, we must live in harmony with the laws of nature. That we

can kill one form of life, an insect which is part of nature, and not have harmful accumulated effects on our health through association with herbicides and pesticides is also poor thinking. Chemicals have aggravated as many pest problems as they have alleviated. Dr. David Pimentel, Professor of Entomology and Agricultural Science, has reported that 65% of the pesticides used in the United States are applied by aircraft and 50 to 75% of this amount ends up in the environment generally, with only 25% attacking the intended target.

Famine in the Seeds

Additionally important to consider is the way we are handling today's seeds. We have developed so many hybrids that it is very difficult to get original nonhybrid seed. This hybridization is the making of foods to fit the pocketbook. Squash, for example, is being made ten times bigger than it should be. Most of our vegetables have derived from herbs, but they no longer have the essence and pungent odors of those herbs. They are increasingly losing their power and effect in the human body.

If squash is made larger, we are eating more pulp instead of chemical elements. The same chemical elements found in a small squash are diffused into a squash ten or twenty times bigger. To get a chemical balance, we have to eat the whole of this larger squash. The same is true for the large versus the small banana. We should be getting our chemical elements in concentrated form, as it was before our nuts, seeds, fruits and berries were hybridized. Hybrid plants are sterile, meaning that seeds must be purchased for every planting. This may be good for the seed companies but not for the seeds. The nonhybrid seeds produce crops with immunities to pests and blights, through the struggles of nature. Those seeds survive.

In modern times, thousands of varieties of seeds have been replaced with hundreds, and these hybrids are vulnerable. The problem with this is that most of the crops grown in the United States are derived from hybridized seeds of very few varieties. As the National Research Council of the National Academy of Sciences has indicated, many of our crops are so genetically uniform that they could easily be hit by disastrous disease epidemics.

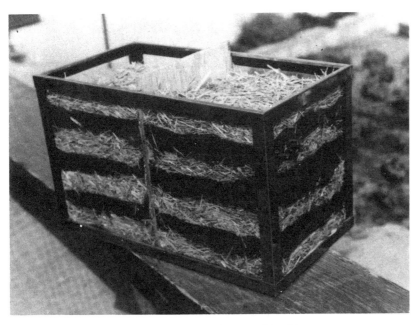

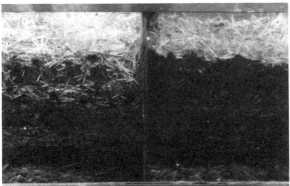

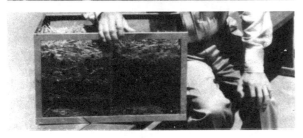

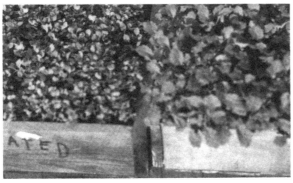

Compost in picture A represents start of experiment in which worms were added to the right side of the box. B. shows the work of lthe worms in breaking down compost. Worms are the rancher's and farmer's best friends, C. In D, unfertilized soil at left grew inferior plants.

11

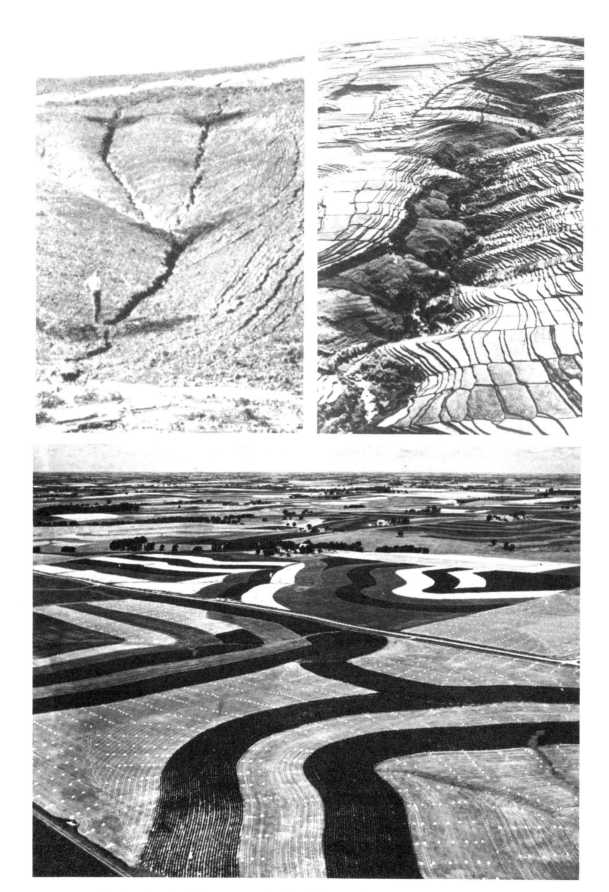

Erosion is reduced by contour plowing, following the natural curves of the land, and by terracing in mountain regions, such as the Hunza Valley. Erosion washes topsoil into the sea, and plant life grown on the depleted soil left cannot make healthy tissue in the human body.

Prior to 1950, the world could rely upon vast seed reserves from underdeveloped countries, but this is no longer true. Hybridized seeds were adopted in large quantities while the native seeds disappeared. The Los Angeles Times reported in 1974 in Sri Lanka, 90% of the rice crop derives from only three or four new varieties of seeds, replacing thousands of indigenous forms.

But we do now have a seed bank in the United States located at Fort Collins, Colorado. The government stockpiles billions of seeds representing all known varieties of food crops in the world. However, as indicated by the New York Times in 1981, this facility is operated inefficiently, with inadequate packaging and insufficient regard to the age of the seeds, which lose viability after five years. It is obvious from all this information that the world is highly vulnerable to famine and blight due to the monopolistic, greed-oriented system of controlling the world seed supply.

Additionally, we have entirely forgotten the importance of consuming seeds. The navel orange, for instance, was originally a little berry no larger than a cherry, with a hundred seeds in it. Yet today, we have produced a large orange that is seedless. We have taken away the glands from this food, which gave it great power to reproduce and continue. We should be eating watermelon seeds instead of spitting them out, because they aid greatly such conditions as hypertension, nephritis and kidney disturbances. Eating whole foods means eating the seeds also in most cases. But now, many of these seeds are available only at special herb stores.

It has been found that seeds carry a male and female hormone. The date seed is very high in the male hormone. Grapefruit and orange seeds are very high in the female hormones. Humans need both, but often today, are suffering from an imbalance because our glands are not being fed properly as we grow and develop. Similarly, we have been getting away from whole foods by failing to live on a whole cereal and getting the needed vitamin E. We haven't been living on whole rice, rye or wheat, which give us lecithin, the brain and nerve fat, as well as glandular food. We have, in short, only

been taking half a loaf of bread and expecting to be whole. We must pay attention to those matters if we are to produce the next generation successfully. We must stop destroying the foundations of our lives.

Plants and People

It is extremely important that we see to it not only that the table is full of food but that the food is full of nourishment. We mold ourselves to the food we put in our bodies. We are what we eat. We grow, build and repair. We need strength and power to overcome disease and the complexities of everyday living. We need resistance as does the plant. In our repair work, the old is thrown away and the new takes its place. What we eat finally finds its way to every cell and organ in the body. Made from earth's chemicals, our blood bathes every organ. A healthy bloodstream builds a healthy body, while a poor bloodstream builds disease.

When we have the balance of elements our bodies require, just as with the plants, we are living in accordance with the laws of nature given to us. Both plants and people must balance the building up and breaking down processes that the organisms require in order to be clean inside.

Obviously, all organic structure depends on the soil for its very life. We can develop a dried-up orange due to the lack of certain chemical elements in our soil and we can produce skin diseases on the exterior of the fruit. The same holds true for humans. Our systems can be dried up and we can produce blotches on the skin through the lack of needed chemical elements. We are also able to produce these conditions in animals. Truly, we are all dust of the earth, and that is why we need soil doctors! It is possible that in the future we will set up a system of doctors with different doctoring functions, and Doctor No. One for our health will be the "Doctor of the Soil." He will know that without calcium, iron and sodium in the soil, we might as well be trying to use the alphabet without A, I and U. If the soil structure is depleted and unbalanced, we grow diseased and underdeveloped plantlife. Through doctoring the soil, we *can* change these conditions.

three

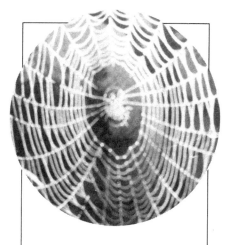

Nature to the rescue

The 1960s gave birth to a social phenomenon some have called "environmental awareness." Scientists presented strong warnings about the destructive streams flowing from the toxic industrial wellsprings of our nation, warnings about the consequences for the future due to our increasingly polluted air, earth and water. Biologists began to toss around terms like "ecology" and "symbiotic relationships," and great numbers of people insisted that our government do something about pollution.

"Clean air" laws were passed. Automakers were required to install emission control devices on new cars, and the oil companies were told to come up with an unleaded gasoline. Logging practices were regulated to prevent undue damage to the land. Cigarettes had to have warning labels on the packages. Land use became more strictly regulated to preserve natural resources and prevent abuses, and entire communities turned out to pick up litter in their areas, dispose of unslightly trash and develop "green belts" and parks.

The "Back to the Land" Movement

One consequence of this environmental awareness phenomenon was called the "back to the land movement," people returning to farms and rural areas to grow foods the natural way and to build up the soil organically. They believed that to live healthy lives and have healthy children, it was necessary to eat wholesome, natural food obtained from healthy soils. This move-ment had its precedent in an earlier tradition of organic gardening and farming representing a much smaller, although deeply devoted, following. Perhaps the best known spokesman for this tradition was the late Robert Rodale, whose son continues to run the publishing company his father started. Organic gardening and farming in this country, of course, had its roots in an older tradition in Europe and England.

Organic methods are not new or experimental, excepting in the sense that new discoveries continue to emerge. One enthusiastic married couple bought a dilapidated farm on the East Coast with soil so depleted that the previous owner had given up farming. For three years, this couple planted soybeans on the devitalized land, plowing the crop into the ground repeatedly, a process called "green manuring." They were determined not to use chemical fertilizers or pesticides on their farm. Their purpose in restoring life to the soil was to raise organic beef cattle. The second year, an infestation of caterpillers invaded their soybean crop and were consuming it at a rapid rate. Following a tip by a friend, the couple gathered several buckets of caterpillers, ground them up and let them sit in the sun until they were certain that bacteria had multiplied in the concoction. Then, diluting the ground-up pests with water, they sprayed the strange mixture on their soybean crop. The caterpiller infestation was soon destroyed, and the crop was saved. Eventually they achieved their goal of raising fine beef cattle, feeding them on their own organic soybeans, supplemented with a little seaweed trucked in from the coast. The seaweed provided the salt, iodine and trace minerals the cattle needed. No antibiotics, steroids or commercial feeds were used. The meat from these animals was considered so exceptionally good and high in quality that it brought excellent prices.

There are many other success stories that could be used to prove the viability of organic farming. It is possible to restore healthy topsoil to much of this nation's farmlands, despite the contentions of the big agribusiness corporations that it would be too costly. What are our costs now, in terms of lowered vitality and epidemic levels of heart disease, cancer and other conditions due to inferior depleted foods? What will our costs be when our nation's topsoil is even more depleted, and our stores of chemical fertilizers run out or skyrocket in price?

The Wheel of Life

Organic farming is patterned after nature's way of building up and maintaining soil, called the Wheel of Life. A wonderful work was done by Dr. McCarrison and Sir Albert Howard, who demonstrated that the quality of the soil was dependent on the principle of return. The death of plant life basically undergirds the life of the soil. Leaves, twigs, grasses, dead trees and other matter form a layer on top of the soil and begin to decay. To this is added animal waste, bird droppings and wind-blown debris. Not only are the biochemical elements restored to the soil, but the layer of decaying organic matter serves

as a mulch, protecting the root systems of young plants and holding in-ground moisture. Each new generation of plants and animals lived, died and returned to the soil to become life for the next generation. This is what the Wheel of Life represents.

Man's imitation of nature's way of building soil is called composting. Sir Albert Howard's recipe for compost is two parts barnyard manure to six parts vegetable waste. He experimented with different methods, arrangements and quantities of organic material to find the fastest and best way of producing compost. He worked out his method at Indore in Asia, building compost heaps in different ways to see what worked.

Through glass observation windows embedded in the soil, earthworms were observed. They found that 300 pounds of worms could work their way through 30-40,000 pounds of soil in a single year, tremendously enriching the soil in the process as well as aerating it. Earthworms utilize the decaying material at the bottom of the compost heap, adding their own rich castings to the nutrients from rotted vegetation. Through the Indore method, compost is ripe and ready to use in 12 weeks, whereas the process of natural decay of vegetation can take up to two years. I have heard that even faster methods of composting have been developed more recently.

One simple method of composting is to dig a trench 2 feet wide, 2 feet deep and as long as desired. Mix 1/3 manure; 1/3 leaves, kitchen garbage, straw or any chopped or shredded organic matter; and 1/3 soil. The remaining soil can be added in as the compost decays and shrinks, together with more leaves, manure and so forth. Keep it wet and continue adding to the top of the pile. Worms can be put on top and covered with a thin layer of soil.

Natural soil fertility in America, whose healthy, virgin prairies and valleys have been exploited and depleted through ignorance or greed, is almost a thing of the past. A true natural topsoil is alive, not only containing the proper chemical elements and decayed vegetation, but bacteria and worms which play an active role in increasing the soil fertility. When the bacteria and worms are gone, the soil is simply dead, inert matter. It has been estimated that worms, in a healthy area of ground, may contribute up to 120 tons of nutrient-rich castings per acre each year. Composting is one of the few methods for bringing a depleted, dead soil back to life and fertility. Generally, nature can do nothing—at least in a few short generations—to restore land stripped of its natural vegetation, depleted of its natural nitrogen, potassium and phosphorus by intensive single crop farming, and left barren and dead.

Soil deprived of nutrients and repeatedly doused with chemicals is often acidic, and composting is often not sufficient to change the acidity. Most fruits, vegetables, grains and other food crops grow best in an almost neutral soil. So, alkaline salts must be added to sweeten it. I have seen experienced farmers pick up a pinch of earth and taste it, able to tell if the soil needs sweetening in that way. Lime or potassium carbonate is often used to neutralize or sweeten an acid soil.

Animal urine, high in urea which contains a good deal of nitrogen, is collected in the feeding stalls by Swiss farmers and is sprinkled either on their compost piles or directly on the soil. Farmers in other countries who live near the sea add seaweed or sprinkle sea water on their compost piles to make sure the trace elements and iodine are there. Goiter, due to a lack of iodine is relatively common in countries far from the ocean.

Besides the type of composting we have described, there is green composting or manuring, as discussed in the story of the couple who plowed under their soybeans to enrich the soil. Besides soybeans, you can use any type of legume or plant which stores the nitrogen it fixes from the air in nodules on its roots.

Worms—Nature's Soil Conditioners

It may be necessary to bring worms to soil which has lost its vitality. This is usually best done after composting the land has been started.

There are different kinds of earthworms. The ordinary gray worm is found in most gardens. However, cross-breeding has resulted in new species which are particularly good for speeding up the breakdown of compost. Those who have their own "worm farms" often use red worms. They may travel as much as 100 feet in a single night. Eggs are laid every 9 to 21 days,

each egg producing about 20 little worms. Unless there is enough "food" for them, the baby worms will migrate elsewhere in search of it.

Ground-up straw mixed with a little molasses has been used to feed worms, which grow to maturity in 90 days. Rabbit manure is excellent, because it doesn't draw flies. Some species of worms, if fed properly, are said to live as long as 15 years, burrowing as far down as 12 to 15 feet.

Worms can bore into red clay or adobe soil, eventually breaking it up and aerating it as they improve the nutrient composition. Each worm produces its own weight in castings about every 24 hours.

The Miracle of Life

Plants require soil, water, carbon dioxide and sunshine to turn inorganic chemicals into living matter. Through the action of sunlight on the chlorophyll in green leaves, food is manufactured by the plant. The action of sunlight on chemicals potentizes them to the higher biochemical form in plants, raising the vibratory level to the point where they can be utililzed and absorbed by insect and animal life. The nutrients manufactured by plants include protein, carbohydrates and lipids in varying amounts. Animals acquire these substances only by eating plants or other animals.

The roots hold the life of the plant in their grasp. Water and minerals are drawn from the earth by the root system and carried to the leaves where they are combined with other elements in the process of photosynthesis. Tiny root hairs, almost invisible, extend outward from every part of the visible root system. Researchers carefully measured and added the lengths of roots and root hairs on a single oat plant and came to a total of 3,000 miles. Agricultural experts have found that alfalfa roots can penetrate as deep as 250 feet in the ground, bringing nutrients from far underground to be transformed in the leaves. Alfalfa can reach through several feet of depleted soil to obtain the nutrients it needs from richer soil below.

Foods manufactured by plants may be stored in the root, leaves, fruit, nut or seed; and it is these foods which contain the chemical elements transformed into more evolved substances—biochemicals with higher vibratory levels than inorganic chemicals.

Animals feeding on vegetation raise the vibratory level of biochemicals another step higher. Unlike plants, animals cannot build up complex nutrient molecules from inorganic chemicals. So they must eat plantlife or other animals. I have a great deal of respect for vegetarianism, and I don't like to say this, but nearly all of the oldest people I have encountered in my travels around the world were meat eaters. In animal flesh, we find the proteins concentrated and in a higher-evolved state; the carbohydrates and lipids are more easily assimilated. Meat, taken in moderation, can benefit the body. What we are considering here is the way nature—and only nature—can lift the chemical elements to the higher-evolved states where they provide the most benefits in our diet. The phosphorus used by the bones, for example, does not have to be as highly evolved as the phosphorus needed by the brain.

Let's have a look at the basic nutrient groups needed by man. Protein, essential for growth, tissue building and repair of tissue, is found in the protoplasm of every cell in our bodies. Protein is made up of amino acids in which nitrogen is the key ingredient, in combination with carbon, hydrogen, oxygen, phosphorus, sulfur and iron.

Carbohydrates and lipids are carbon-based nutrients, and each is made of carbon, hydrogen and oxygen. Carbohydrates are the sugars, glycogen (animal starch), vegetable starches, dextrins and celluloses. Fats or lipids are our most concentrated energy food, and fatty acids are needed for growth. Lipids form part of the cell membrane and carry fat-soluble vitamins throughout the body. Where do the other chemical elements come in? The structure of vitamin B-12 reveals a cyanide group, an amino group and a cobalt atom, and other vitamins bring in other elements. Milk products provide calcium and phosphorus needed by the bones, nerves and brain. So we recognize that although protein, carbohydrates and lipids are primary sources of biochemicals, we need other biochemicals to survive and thrive as well. It is interesting that vitamin C is made of the same chemical elements as fats and carbohydrates. The difference lies in the number of atoms of carbon, hydrogen and oxygen in the molecular structure and in their arrangement.

Following Nature's Way

Nature can do wonderful things in terms of selecting the chemicals right for each plant, the right plants for each animal to eat and so on. Nature is a wonderful soil builder through the buildup and decay of organic matter and the activities of worm life and soil bacteria. Nature purifies air by means of rain, and water by means of movement. Water is purified as it runs over natural gravel and rock beds at certain rates of speed in rivers and streams. Clean air and water and pure wholesome foods are necessary for the reversal of disease and the restoration of high-level wellness in man. As we learn to cooperate with nature and nature's laws, we can have healthy bodies, healthy societies and a healthy world.

Since the dawn of science, technology and industry in the last few centuries, we have prodded, poked, polluted and provoked Mother Nature. Our soils have been depleted from ignorance and greed. We have created convenience foods, fast foods and preserved foods—trying to save time, energy and money through bypassing nature's ways. The result? More and different diseases, more chronic diseases than ever before in the history of man.

The greatest casualty of "progress" has been man himself.

When we stop and think about it, violating or ignoring the principles of nature has brought about nearly every ill wind that blows in modern society. Disease, crime, violence, perversion, mental illness, war and all other forms of imbalance are unnatural.

Only nature can come to our rescue. Only cooperation with nature and nature's laws can restore mankind and the conditions on this planet necessary for mankind to survive. Nature, not our science laboratories, holds the secret of life in her hand.

In my view, the path to wholeness and high-level wellness starts with nutrition and nutrition starts with the chemical elements—and the way nature puts them together for our use.

17

four

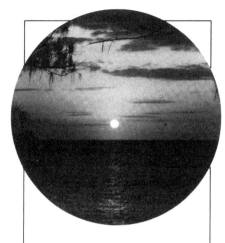

Living in the light ages

The next step out of darkness, the step into light, will occur when we recognize the significance of color, and vibration and light itself. We are just beginning to discover color, a development no doubt leading us toward a more highly-evolved expression of our humanness.

Eventually, we will know more of the colors beyond the visible range, the colors about which we know nothing, as yet. We will study the mind and soul by highly-refined photography, which will read our vibratory levels in relation to color and show how to attract colors to us. All this activity will assist us in establishing clearly that man is not just biochemical elements. He is not to be engineered in the laboratory. There is something beyond man that puts all the elements together to make the living being.

As we saw in the previous chapter, light from the sun (comprised of colors, each with its own vibratory rate) will pick up a "vehicle," or physical form, as the vehicle becomes ready for this energizing force. A sodium mineral vehicle, for example, has been "potentized" by the color of the light and the resulting vibration due to its union with light. Through a food such as celery, sodium is taken into the body as a powerful biochemical to become part of our ability to neutralize acids, and part of the tendons, joints and stomach wall.

What remains of that food comes out of the body in a form of sodium chloride that is no longer potent. You can taste it in the sweat of the body. The potentized material has been used up and the rest must go back to the dust of the earth, where it will again be empowered by the sun and evolve into organic material usable by man.

Man, The Alchemizer

Man, then, is not merely his biochemical elements but the potency that comes from the sun. The body is a miraculous alchemist that changes the coarse structures derived from the earth into living tissue. Foods go through the intestinal tract by way of the mouth. The foods must be prepared and absorbed. They have to be warmed and transmuted to reach us as essences. They have to be broken down into the most minute forms we can imagine, and these are what is made into the human body.

Man, the alchemizer, transfers color and vibration from his food to himself—and that is his aliveness, his vitality. A corpse has all the chemical elements, but you can't bring him back to life. The essential life of man is in the vibration that is man, and this life force is carried with the mineral elements in their response to the light of the sun.

The Path of the Soul

First of all, before he evolves to physical form, man is a soul, which exists both before and after his physical presence. The pattern of the soul—each soul is one of a kind—exists in the smallest possible particle, just as the essence of calcium exists waiting to evolve. Again physical form is created through light, which, as the ultimate creative force, is guided by God's intelligence. Utilizing light, God creates everything from an ant to a human being and provides a path of wisdom to follow.

Light guides the soul in its evolution through man and woman toward its physical destiny which starts when a person is born and begins the struggle to express his or her uniqueness. Again the human alchemizing system is at work, forming new life out of the elements which come from the dust of the earth. By using the body as a vehicle for physical expression, the soul demonstrates a second way in which man is more than his chemical elements. In fact, by virtue of his soul, man is a living akashic record with the memory of the complete past—our starvation periods, our biorhythms and various cycles of activity. All these form the expression of each one of us, a pattern set in the brain but first set in the pattern of the soul. Each of us works out this unique life pattern.

Eventually, we shed the body and the physical elements go back to the earth, but we still remain as something. The soul continues. It takes on other qualities and we see ourselves naked, so to speak. We won't have ears; we will hear through vibrations or light. Nothing will hinder us in travel, understanding or development. We will, however, be hindered if we have not been following the path toward higher understanding, which only comes through study and growth.

Vibratory Rates and Foods

Light is a spiritual quality in the deepest sense, both forming and symbolizing the spirit of man. A sick person is without spirit or light and is likely to be without color. To get rid of these troubles, a person must eat foods carrying the correct light and material to make a new body. Upon doing so, light and life return. We have too many people on crutches; too many who cannot walk, run or think clearly. Taking a job is too much for them, and marriage kills them. Acquiring good health and vitalilty however, means not getting only the physical elements from somewhere, but also receiving the light and vibrational energy that goes with these elements. These qualities come only from plant life or from other higher forms of evolved, transmuted elements.

Vibratory rates and color make foods what they are. A broad leaf will get more sunshine, whereas a thin leaf will take less, and this factor will affect each one's color and energy. Some foods develop from chemical elements existing only in certain parts of the earth where the sunlight is of a particular intensity. Forms and colors of foods exist in abundance, from the skins of potatoes, peaches and string beans to the bark of many trees. We can take sap from one tree for a particular effect, then sap from another for an entirely different effect. Chemically breaking down these foods may leave us mystified as to why they have specific functions, but further study will bring us answers and a share of God's wisdom.

It might be difficult to see distinctions between a blade of grass and a geranium, yet there is a world of difference due to subtle dimensions beyond measure. The green color of the geranium contrasts to the green of the blade of grass, indicating the presence of more nitrogen, oxygen and calcium. The blade of grass contains more silicon, because it is likely to grow where the wind will blow on it, and the silicon will contribute to its resilient quality. Such subtleties in plants are transferred to us when we consume them.

Color guides us to the properties of plants. Magnesium, for example, is found in its highest concentration in yellow corn. Yellow has its own vibratory rate which is attracted to the corn because of its chemical makeup. Yellow

19

indicates magnesium, which in organic form, becomes a laxative. All laxatives in nature are yellow. Thus, by noting the presence of the color, we know something about the different qualities and properties in the physical object.

I can look at a food and recognize it as a high sodium food which will make a stomach more alkaline. Then I can use that food instead of bicarbonate of soda or a drug. I see that particular food as medicine ready to be transferred to and alchemized in the laboratory of the human body. Foods can be earmarked and directed towards specific parts of the body. For every symptom you can mention, there is something in nature to transform the body, either adding to it or subtracting from it in order to balance it. Then the symptom will disappear.

A person needs potassium in the muscle structure, so plants with potassium are valuable. But to live on such foods entirely and go brainless, is to deprive the system of balance when there is another plant fueled with the chemical structure earmarked for the brain and with the vibratory force and all the color energies the brain requires.

We find that sulphur, effervescent as it is, tends to explode, but it accomplishes things. It is found mostly in the brain. The brain also needs phosphorus, the "light bearer." Phosphorus in the brain expresses a vibration entirely different from the way phosphorus expresses itself in the bones. These two kinds of phosphorus may appear exactly the same to the chemist; yet they have evolved differently through plantlife to suit different purposes.

The differing effects from the chemical elements must be kept in proper balance or else we have problems. Imbalances will lead one person to have dizziness; another may have insufficient sex drive traceable to a lack of zinc or to eating foods without all the inherent color they are intended to have in their natural state. A person can have liver problems from a lack of iron or spleen problems from a lack of sodium. A person may not "explode" enough—that is, be unemotional or unresponsive due to insufficient sulphur. Such a person needs to become aware of the sulphur-bearing plants such as cabbage, broccoli, garlic and onions.

Relearning the Foods

To become wiser, we must know plants and what they can do for us. We need to know every

food source that grows on the face of the earth, but today we are woefully ignorant of these foods. Man doesn't even know what's in a tomato. He doesn't know there is an enzyme in pineapple which is a valuable digestant. He doesn't know the proper time to pick apricots because he buys them from the market picked 8 days too early. He eats grapefruit picked 2 months early. He doesn't know that his bones need calcium that has been taken from rock, gone through a transformation in the vegetable kingdom, alchemized in the body, and made into a material earmarked for the building and repair of bone. Very few people recognize these differing alchemical processes—they don't see the whole story.

You can take groups of rats and feed them on natural foods, and then take rats fed on foods that have been fried, preserved, processed and confused in their chemical makeup (where the light values are gone and the vibratory rates have been distorted) and we find that these rats live only half as long. What is the reason for this?

Today, we are doing a tremendous amount of scientific investigation in a variety of areas, but we have never looked, thoroughly into nature. Nature, of course, has already done the experimentation to answer why natural foods are superior, in terms of proper combinations of vibration, color and light.

Man doesn't know his potentials because he doesn't know how to eat. My best advice, therefore, is to relearn the natural foods and what they are intended to do to build healthy bodies. We have foods specifically for the stomach, the brain and various mental centers. We need to be cautious of the vibratory rate of meat, which is very stimulating to the ego centers of the brain, and which can be very destructive. There are cooling foods and heating foods, which should be taken properly in terms of the seasons. We have foods for many purposes to help us to be healthy and to reach forward to our potentials.

Reaching Toward Potentials

Man is always praying to God to take his troubles away but is seldom able to look to his experiences as a stepping stone to enlightenment. We have many people who actually are crippled through negative attitudes.

They tend to spend too much time and energy on unhappy moments, without realizing their latent potentials to be healthy and dynamic. Once understanding this problem, a person has to start down a new soul path. Spirit, attitudes and body must all work together.

We have a potential faculty to have dominion over ourselves, but we cannot have dominion over anything unless we have the ability to invent, to construct and to be practical. Without joy, we destroy our progress, because we lack incentive. All these faculties are developed as we eat properly. Merely eating certain combinations of foods can either detract from or add to brotherhood. With a lack of iodine, one can become mean. Indeed, because we are not eating in a way that supports a nurturing, peaceful society, we have crime, turbulence and eagerness for war.

Despite all these problems, we live in a world of abundance. We think we're limited by the amount of gasoline we have, but we are only limited by our minds. We have never really touched our potentials. These include our intuitive and psychic possibilities, which are only going to come to us when we are ready for them and can handle them.

A man in Florida, for example, has used large rocks to construct buildings. He handles them entirely by himself, without a crane. It seems that no one could lift such huge and heavy rocks without the use of a crane. One day, a man drove up and backed his truck in. He wanted to take away a rock weighing two or three tons. The man who lifted rocks told the trucker to walk around the corner. When he returned, the rock was on the truck. This man who lifted the rock onto the truck keeps his secret to himself, but he would seem to have the power to control gravity.

In contrast to such a marvel, the average man today is likely to be heavy and distressed— out of harmony with his foods and his environment. He is preoccupied with acquiring more money and possessions. He tends to compromise himself and live in fear. If he is starving, he says, "I can't live like this," and he is ready to steal or rob, commiting violence, if necessary. Others feel that someone or something is out to harm them, and the only way they can attain a comfortable, secure old age is by making a fortune. Then they leave the fortune

to their children and never enjoy it anyway. All this time they are in conflict with what is good for them.

The Coming Light Ages

At the moment, we are still in the Dark Age, in comparison to what is possible. You can see this Dark Age reflected in our television advertising. We are told to take a particular drug to stop a cough for five or six hours. Another drug can suppress the symptoms of a cold for four or five hours. No correction is considered nor is it offered. Sugary, lifeless foods, presented to us with misleading images and messages about their nutritional value, are followed by advertising for drugs to relieve us from the pains induced by the foods we have just been encouraged to consume!

In contrast, developments are taking place which show us the way toward a better age. Commercial production of a new protein-rich food developed by modern methods of biotechnology has tremendous importance for world hunger problems. This product is a protein foodstuff made from carbohydrate raw materials using a fermentation process. The concept here is to convert what is plentiful into what is not in order to assist the less developed countries which are short of protein and faced with escalating costs in food production.

Indeed, the world shortage of food doesn't disturb me, because man, as the highest of all creations, will do whatever he can to alleviate the problem. Billboards in India and the Orient, stressing fewer but healthier and better educated children, are doing part of the job. Japan, with more people per acre than any other country in the world, is stepping forward to develop new food supplies. One of these is an alga that man can live on almost entirely with no supplement. It is easy to grow and a powerfully nutritious food.

These enlightened ways will help us. I have seen many advances in my many years of practice, and have faith that many more are yet to come. I have seen an alcoholic of 18 years' abuse take on new life by changing his food. I have seen a person with 13 leg ulcers that were running green-yellow pus for 3 years become healed in 15 days just by changing the diet. I've seen people with ulcers of the stomach who have cured themselves by changing their attitudes about life, work and marriage. They've also changed their harshness and criticalness, and the need to be a dominating person. In some cases, they have changed from being timid and fearful. I've seen one stutterer cure himself through spiritual inspiration, and another helped by treatment with minerals alone.

The enlightened surgeon of tomorrow will not consider operating on a patient unless he knows that person will be physically able to recuperate. He will know the wounds heal beautifully only if the necessary biochemical elements are there to be used. Instead of using suppressive drugs, he will use foods as medicine, knowing that pain can be eliminated in this way.

Instead of patching up the body all the time, the enlightened doctor will make new tissues and a new body in place of the old one by prescribing foods.

Another step to bring on the New Age will come when we go into our prisons and realize that men there are starved for certain nutrients, and that much of their disturbed behavior is due to their imbalanced bodies. We're going to find that divorces are, to a great extent, influenced by the foods we eat. Lifeless foods produce lifeless marriages, where magnetic current fails to flow between the partners. And we're going to find that the enlightened person is not only healthier and good for society but much happier within him or herself.

Released from a concentration camp after World War II, this 27-year-old man appears more in his 60s or 70s due to malnutrition. Malnutriton hastens the aging process.

Health and nutrition are international priorities, and I have found eager audiences wherever I have lectured around the world. The new age doctor will do more educating than medicating.

five

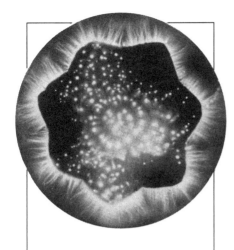

The finer forces

Research has shown that 80 percent of what we learn comes through vision, but what we don't see is as important, in many cases, as what we do. The force of gravity, the air we breathe, the electromagnetic waves all around us are examples. The finer forces play a fundamental role in life and health.

When I was a young man, I met George Starr White, MD and Dr. Arrums, a San Francisco radionic technician. These men told me each disease had a specific electromagnetic expression, a specific vibrational frequency. I was fascinated. But, how can such things exist? What do they mean?

A physics professor once told me that every object on earth has a certain vibrational frequency that can destroy it completely, cause it to fly apart. Opera singers can break wineglasses by hitting high notes. Marching soldiers break step when crossing a bridge to avoid damaging it structurally. A plucked string on one guitar can cause the string on another guitar a few feet away to start vibrating. Is it so strange to think that a disease would have a certain vibration?

Kirlian Photography

According to Dr. David Sheinkin, Kirlian photography, which captures on film the auras around many objects, may provide a tool for the early detection of disease. Unlike conventional photography, Kirlian photography requires no camera or lens but involves placing an object such as a leaf or human hand directly on top of the film. The exposure is produced by a high voltage, high AC frequency electric power supply attached to a nonferrous plate. Dr. Sheinkin believes changes in the extent and density of the flared corona around a finger on a Kirlian photograph may be used to signal the subclinical conditions preceding a particular disease.

It is evident that dis-ease vibrations would cause a change in the body's energy field, and we would expect this change to show up in a Kirlian photograph. With normal people, a Kirlian photograph of a finger or hand shows a full corona surrounding it. Disease changes it. It is known that alcohol consumption causes corona flare. A pneumonia patient had no corona at all around the fingertip. In many illnesses, the border between the image (of finger or hand) and its aura becomes hazy. There is much left to be researched in this area, but a beginning has been made. Perhaps one day the Kirlian technique may help identify specific diseases.

Acupuncture and the Body's Energy Field

Acupuncture points on the meridians of the body have long been known to have a different electrical resistance than other areas of the skin. This may imply that the electromagnetic field lines of the body go through the points. Dr. Irving Oyle, author of *The New American Medicine Show*, has used high-frequency sound on the appropriate acupuncture points of patients, with good results. We might speculate that the high-frequency sound on the acupuncture points restored the electromagnetic vibration natural to this area. The absence of the electromagnetic field there may have been what was blocking the corona in Dr. Sheinkin's Kirlian work with illnesses. To an extent, we are seeing pieces of a puzzle from two different studies that fit together well.

Electromagnetic Vibrations in Foods and Chemicals

If we persist in looking for the effect of finer forces in healing and disease, we may find that an organ or tissue area which is lacking in a needed chemical element, or one which is irritated and inflamed by toxic accumulations, has an altered electromagnetic field, a changed vibration.

We can say that certain foods, because of their vibrational qualities, respond in a rejuvenating, restoring, healing manner to tissues with certain chemical shortages or toxic burdens. The vibrations of the food raise the vibrations of the tissue, so to speak. There would be other substances—additives, sprays and drugs—which could lower the vibrational level of tissues.

Now, we can take this a step further.

We know that each chemical element has its own unique frequency or vibration, and where these elements serve in molecular compounds or complex chains, the entire molecule will have a certain characteristic frequency or vibration. In

the human body, so long as these molecular chains are complete, they would generate one type of electromagnetic vibration—but when incomplete they would generate another type. Could this be what attracts the biochemicals needed by a particular tissue site from the supply of nutrients in the blood and lymph? Is it possible that the targeting of certain biochemical nutrients to starving tissue areas is done via the "linking" of the two vibrations— one indicating a need, the other indicating the potential fulfillment of the need?

Doubtless there are other factors involved. Osmotic pressures at cell membranes, RNA patterns, electrochemical processes and neurogenetic brain reflex activities affect what we digest, what we assimilate and whether an organ or tissue can take in the biochemicals its cells need.

Brain Activities

When we consider brain activities and functions, we enter another domain in which the finer forces operate. Thoughts, emotions, attitudes and beliefs can raise the level of health and vitality or drag it down. I have often said, we cannot think sour thoughts and expect to have sweet digestion and assimilatin. Rather, sour thoughts are likely to stimulate acid conditions in the stomach or duodenum which eventually result in ulcers. Anger, bitterness, hate, jealousy, unforgiveness and other negative feelings, attitudes and expressions give forth vibrations that influence the body chemistry and glandular functions. It has been well established that negative expressions can lead to and sustain conditions which we called psychosomatic diseases. Ulcers, asthma, cancer and heart disease, to name a few, have been found to have psychosomatic components in many cases.

There are brain centers that rule over each part of the body, from sensory-motor functions to autonomic functions. The brain needs to have the right nutrients to exercise proper control over the tissues, organs and glands of the body. I believe the brain is sensitive to what happens in the external environment, the internal environment and in its own consciousness. We can be driving down a smoggy freeway, thinking of a beautiful mountain meadow and aware of a pain in the left foot, all at the same time. These

24

mental activities have an effect on every cell in the body, to some degree, by their effect on other brain and nervous system activities and by the shift in body chemistry due to related endocrine gland secretions.

We find there are also brain centers that rule over certain conscious activities, such as a center for business. Dr. V. G. Rocine was the master teacher on the subject of these brain centers, and we cover them elsewhere in this book. Many other aspects of brain function are presented in my book *Iridology, Science and Practice in the Healing Arts, Volume II.*

Spiritual Values

In the realm of the finer forces, the spiritual level is the finest level of all. It has been said that man is a spirit being who has a soul and lives in a body. In my experience, integration, balance and harmony are essential in all three—spirit, soul and body—to get on the path to high-level wellness.

When I was young, I came home and shared with my mother how I'd learned God's commandment to love our neighbors as ourselves—and even to love our enemies. "Listen, son," my mother said. "It isn't so much for their sakes God wants us to love them, but for our own sakes." If we are filled with loving thoughts toward others, we won't have room for hate, bitterness and that sort of thing, with the dis-ease producing vibrations that go along with them. Love is for our own good.

The important breakthrough that has come through wholistic health is the recognition that we must take care of the spirit, mind and body to be in good health. We can't have a sick mind and a healthy body or healthy spirit. Sickness in one infects the others. That is why I say, "Health is a way of life." You can't get it from a drug, an operation or a week-long crash diet. We earn health by the way we treat others, by what we think, by the way we eat, work, sleep, exercise, relax and enjoy the fresh air and sunshine. We must bring in the highest and finest forces to experience high-level wellness.

Over the years, I have learned that our spiritual values have a great deal to do with disease and wellness. My book *Arise and Shine* tells about my spiritual studies and the fascinating experiences many of my patients have had as they learned to deal with obstacles on the path of life.

Beauty, Art and Music

For many years now, doctors have recognized that beauty, art and music have healing power of some kind, an ability to elevate the mind, soul and spirit to a place where there is peace and harmony.

Flowers, waterfalls, the serenity of a lake at dawn, the rosy hues of a magnificient sunset, a vista of distant mountains, the music of the wind in the pine trees—these expressions of natural beauty carry healing and restoration by touching something deep inside us. Beauty is one of the finer forces with great healing power and uplifting vibrations. Just as there is proper food for the body, there is proper food for the mind, soul and spirit.

Ugliness, confusion, conflict and disarray carry the opposite vibration—there is dis-ease in the wings of these things, although they say, "Beauty is in the eye of the beholder." I find little peace and comfort in litter-strewn streets, crumbling buildings, turned-over garbage cans and junkyards. Those who do must be especially and unusually blessed.

Similarly, there are types of music and art that I do not care to be around, although some people claim to be crazy about them. I believe frantic music creates frantic people, confused art breeds confused people and sad, lonely art and music create sad and lonely people.

Music and art communicate to us, via sympathetic vibrations, a certain mood and emotional response. Soothing, melodic music or inspiring works of art lift us up. Viennese waltzes have a wonderful healing power. Paintings by the Old Masters of Europe or early American artists—especially their pastoral or natural scenes—are uplifting and healing. Anything that jangles the nerves or brings on sadness, anger or depression should be avoided like the plague.

Every artist and composer puts something of his soul and spirit into his work. If he is a mean-spirited person, the work will express that quality in its vibrations, and it will drag others down to that level. If he is a more spiritually developed person, his art or music will tend to lift others. We need to be aware of such things.

In more recent years, experiments have shown that pure colors and pure musical tones stimulate and speed healing in hospital patients.

The Peace Gland

The pineal gland, for many decades, has been a mystery gland to Western medicine. Some have speculated that it is a vestigial organ, active in some past stage of man's evolution but now inactive. Mystics have referred to it as the "third eye," the organ of spiritual vision or intuition. More recent research, however, shows that the pineal gland plays an active role in health and wellness at the mental and physical levels.

The pineal gland, scientists theorize, is a light-sensitive organ which requires stimulation from electromagnetic impulses from the optic nerves. Sunlight enters the eye and triggers retinal nerve impulses which travel to the pineal gland. From there, the resulting nerve impulses from the pineal gland are fed to the hypothalamus and pituitary, which control, mediate or affect many of the vital functions of the body. Additionally, only the pineal gland makes melatonin from serotonin, a process which operates strictly according to day-night cycles. Melatonin formation is stopped by light and proceeds in darkness. So, we find the pineal gland, because of its sensitivity to light, has a profound effect on the biorhythms of the body. It is a kind of biological clock that affects the timing of certain physiological functions.

Melatonin works together with tryptophan in the brain to regulate the sleep/wake cycle. Experiments have shown that melatonin induces sleep with vivid dreams and increases alpha wave activity in the brain, as measured by EEG. We find that alpha is the healing state of the conscious, awakened mind, while sleep interspersed with vivid dreams is known to be a wonderful restorative. The pineal gland, in other words, may be called the "peace gland" because of its biochemical role in rest, relaxation and healing.

All the patients who come to me with serious conditions are tired, fatigued, low in energy. They need rest and relaxation, and we know the pineal gland plays a vital role in that process.

Because of the role of light in the functioning of the pineal gland and, indirectly, many vital activities of the body, we find the pineal to be one of the mediating organs by which the finer forces act on the body and mind. Dr. Mark Altschule of Belmont, Mass. has found that extracts of animal pineal substance given to schizophrenics or depressed patients have had a beneficial result on most. The activity of the pineal gland has psychological as well as physiological consequences, and there is more.

Because the pineal gland strongly influences the brain-wave pattern and sleep-wake cycle, we can be sure it is involved in coming to the state of consciousness in which spiritual processes take place, and this, too, profoundly affects health. Dr. Rocine often spoke of "exalting the Great Within." The life of the spirit is a fundamental harmonizing factor, a guiding factor in leading us to that path in life that is uniquely ours. It is in the "quiet place" within that we meet with God to seek the wisdom we need for right living and right understanding. Here is the fountainhead of truth, and when we "exalt the Great Within," this truth comes down through the soul and body to manifest in our lives. When we seek that place of peace and quiet within, stilling the noise of the mind, truth works in us.

The Finer Forces and Man

We find that different individuals are differently attuned to the finer forces, although all are influenced by them. In my experience with the various personality types, I have noticed that people range from coarse to fine on many levels.

There are people so attuned to the coarse physical level of matter that you almost have to hit them with a brick to get their attention. There are others so finely attuned to the spiritual or mental level that they can hardly keep their feet on the ground. A critical remark throws some persons into torrents of tears, while others may respond with anger or indifference. Many people have difficulty handling praise and keeping their mental balance at the same time.

Among the greatest marriage problems I have encountered is the pairing of a coarse person with a fine person. Perhaps the man might be a big, muscular fellow who tramps across the living room rug without wiping his boots outside, who loves loud music and who is not much interested in conversation. The wife may be a quiet woman who loves soft music, who keeps house beautifully (despite the bearish behavior of her husband) and who has very sensitive feelings. This is often a sad combination because of the difficulty these two types will have in understanding one another. The differences are apparent, not simply at the personality level, but also in terms of vibration.

We will discuss Rocine's types in a later chapter, but what I want to make clear here is that all people have a certain vibratory quality at the level of the finer forces, and some types do not mix—at least not easily. Conflict can lead to health problems.

I believe that the vibratory level and quality of people can make them susceptible to certain chronic diseases, particularly if in their work or family life they are forced to be around people with whom they cannot harmonize, people who hate, scorn, dislike or disapprove of them. We need to be around people who love us. We need to have jobs which make good use of our natural gifts and talents. We need to find that unique path in life in which harmony can be expressed at all levels.

The finer forces have a tremendous import on our lives and on our state of health and well-being. To come to the place of high-level wellness, we must pay attention to and learn to harmonize with the finer forces.

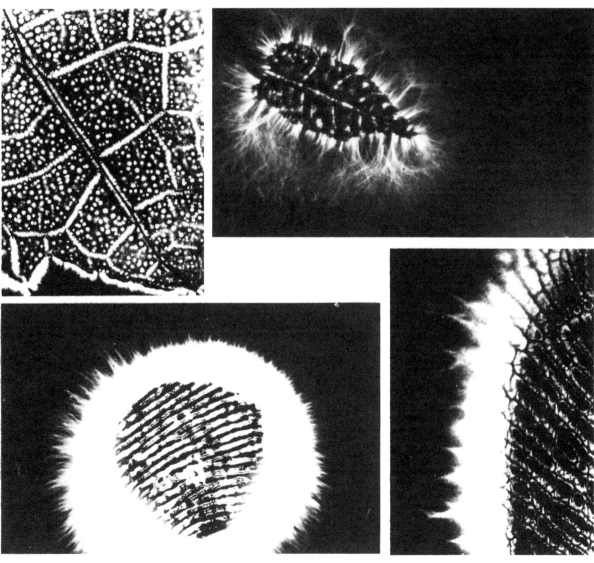

These Kirlian photos of leaves and fingertips show that living things have electromagnetic fields which are related to the life force in them. Notice how the energy flares discharge from the fingerprint pattern on the bottom right photo.

six

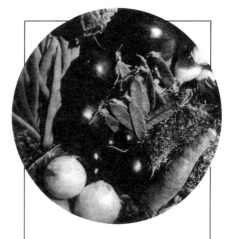

Food is more than meets the eye

As the new day comes in the healing arts, nutrition is beginning to gain recognition as particularly important for wholistic health care. Nutrition today, however, is quite incomplete, recognizing calories, vitamins, proteins, carbohydrates, acids, alkalines, raw or cooked foods and so forth, without considering that evolved biochemical elements—what we might call "the dust of the earth"— make up our frame and muscle structure and every part of our body. We must dig deeper into the true nature of food and what we are doing to ourselves with our injurious habits in food growing and preparing.

Each tissue structure, function and regenerative activity is driven toward fulfillment of perfection as encoded in the DNA and RNA of the cells and in the functions of the brain. This can occur only when the appropriate elements of the earth are present within us to work on our behalf. As already indicated, these chemical elements are found in the earth in the form of inorganic materials. They eventually become biochemical or life-giving as they evolve through plantlife via seeds, fruits, berries, greens, salads, juices, tonics and whatever else we set before ourselves on the kitchen table.

At the deepest levels, food is vibration, just as all matter is vibration. What appears solid to the eyes is the movement of energy at lower or higher frequencies or rates of vibration. Some of these rates of vibration are healthy for us, but others are not. In foods not grown according to the laws of nature, the vibration is not healthy. In short, health and dis-ease are to be understood in terms of vibrational states within the body, with improper vibrational conditions leading to disharmony or dis-ease. The iris clearly reflects nerve rings which indicate the impact of unharmonious vibrations upon us. Indeed, all vibrations— from food, music, color and so forth—are related and affect our bodies, thoughts and emotions. To harmonize this concert of energies is to bring body, mind and spirit into perfect balance.

Thus, we need to be aware that food is more than protein, carbohydrates, fats, pulp and fiber. It is a level of deep thought. If we want to raise our bodies to a higher level of health, we must go to the food vibrations our bodies should have and which are found in the whole, pure and natural foods. Does our diet feed us the biochemical elements we need in order to create new tissue in our bodies? **New tissue perfectly functioning in every organ in the body is the ideal we are all working to attain.**

What Our Foods Are Made Of

Foods are made of the chemical elements like everything else on this planet, but special combinations of them have distinct functions in the body. These are proteins, carbohydrates, fats, enzymes, vitamins and minerals (chemical elements assimilated individually into the body). We will discuss the chemical elements in some detail later, so only the others will be presented here.

Proteins found in the human body are made up of various combinations of twenty amino acids. These are compounds made of carbon, hydrogen, oxygen and nitrogen primarily, while certain amino acids also contain sulphur, iron, phosphorus, zinc and copper. Proteins are used in tissue building and repair and make up about half of the dry weight of the body. They help form enzymes, antibodies and hormones and can be broken up and joined to other chemicals to make neurotransmitters and neuroinhibitors which are vital to brain and nervous system function. Proteins make up antibodies like gamma globulin and blood proteins such as albumin, fibrinogen, globulin and hemoglobin. About half of the amino acids can be broken down for producing heat and energy. There are eight amino acids that can only be obtained through foods. The rest can be manufactured in the body.

Essential	Nonessential
Threonine	Glycine
Leucine	Alanine
Isoleucine	Aspartic acid
Valine	Glutamic acid
Lysine	Proline
Methionine	Hydroxyproline
Phenylalanine	Cystine
Tryptophan	Tyrosine
	Serine
	Arginine*
	Histidine*

*Essential in growing children.

Carbohydrates are formed by green plants and are a basic source of energy. Commonly, we refer to them as sugars or starches, and they are made of carbon, hydrogen and oxygen. They are converted in the body to glucose, which is immediately usable, or to glycogen, the storage form. Ribose, one of the most important sugars, is used in the nucleic acids DNA and RNA. Processed carbohydrates such as white flour, white sugar and products made of them are not useful to the body and are most often harmful. We should obtain our sugars and starches from fruits, vegetables, seeds, nuts and whole cereal grains, often referred to as complex carbohydrates.

Fats, perhaps surprisingly, are among the most useful of foods but are also among the most abused foods. They provide an efficient source of energy, carry the fat-soluble vitamins to the cells, are necessary for hormone production and make up the myelin sheath that covers and protects many of the nerve cells in the body and brain. The average American diet is made up of about 50% fats, mostly saturated fats (the kind that harden at room temperature, in general—mostly animal fats), and these are blamed for the high incidence of heart disease, along with several other factors. We hear a great deal about cholesterol and the triglycerides as contributing to heart disease, yet both are essential to the body in certain quantities. There are three essential polyunsaturated fatty acids necessary in human nutrition which come from grains or seeds, and these are linoleic, linolenic and arachidonic acids, forms of which make up triglycerides. The triglycerides provide most of the fat-derived energy for the body. Cholesterol comes from eggs, meat and milk products but is also manufactured in the body in much greater quantities than from our food intake. Cholesterol is important in hormone production, myelin sheath makeup and in every cell of the body (along with lecithin). It seems that when lecithin is taken in sufficient quantities, it balances the cholesterol, keeps it dissolved in the blood and prevents it from coating artery walls. We destroy lecithin at cooking temperatures and seldom eat enough uncooked lecithin-containing foods to get the amount we need.

Lecithin, a waxy substance found in egg yolk, soybeans and other foods, is the main source of choline which is needed to form the neurotransmitter acetylcholine. Fats, like carbohydrates, are made of carbon, hydrogen and oxygen but with less oxygen. We can keep our body's fat intake in balance by avoiding all fried foods or foods cooked in fat, minimizing our intake of animal fats, taking lecithin supplements and getting enough exercise.

Enzymes are complex proteins that assist in chemical changes in the body without being changed themselves. Technically, they should not be called foods since their only function is to help change one substance to another in the body's metabolism. They are especially important in digestion. There are enzymes that help break down proteins, carbohydrates and fats and others that help the breakdown products from chemical bonds with other substances.

Vitamins, as most people realize, are essential to health because they serve as regulators of metabolic processes and sometimes as coenzymes in the biochemical reactions of the body.

Minerals are the chemical elements that our bodies need singly, not necessarily in compounds or complex groups as found in proteins, carbohydrates, fats, enzymes and vitamins.

The Refining of Wheat

The processing and refining of many of our foods today effectively destroys biochemical elements when they are altered from their natural state. Man has changed his food through milling, polishing, processing, bleaching, preserving, canning, seasoning, flavoring and coloring. In the refining and preserving of wheat, for example, the vital life elements are destroyed. The starchy part of the wheat remains, void of the mineral and vitamin balance needed for proper heart action, bowel regularity and other body functions. Vitamin E is known as a definite help in many cases of heart trouble, assisting the heart function to become normal. It is found in the germ of the wheat which is part of the seed's outside covering. But much of the flour we eat today is devitalized because the refining process removes this

outside hull and the valuable wheat germ. We are eating a "heartless" flour and have been doing so for years! We have been building up heart conditions through the habit of using devitalized flour, and when we finally get our heart trouble we rush to the store to buy vitamin E made from wheat germ. Why didn't we eat the whole thing in the first place?

Many of our chronic diseases today, like heart trouble, have developed through eating devitalized foods. Heart trouble is, of course, recognized as being at the top of the list of diseases causing death. The problem comes not only from deficiency of vitamin E but also a lack of calcium, potassium and other vital elements needed to maintain tone in our muscles. The heart is an organ made up principally of muscle tissue. When the heart action is hindered, all vital organs must be affected, because every organ depends upon the blood pumped from the heart. All the organs must have a proper balance of vital biochemical elements instead of being subjected to dietary starvation.

White Sugar

Natural foods such as vegetables, fruits, honey and grains are easily metabolized by the body. Refined foods such as white flour and white sugar are not adequate to meet the body's needs for nutrients. They provide mainly taste and calories. White sugar, processed from sugar cane or sugar beets, is not merely neutral in its effect on the body—it is actually harmful.

Among the detrimental effects of white sugar are the following:

It promotes tooth decay.

It leaches calcium from the body so that the delicate balance between calcium and phosphorus (normally 2.5:1) is destroyed.

It causes a deficiency of B vitamins.

Vitamin B must be present in the alimentary canal for sugar to be digested, but because the B vitamins normally present in sugar have been removed in the refining process, the digestive organs must draw the needed B vitamins from other areas of the body. The result is a deficiency which may lead to nervous problems, nervous breakdown and mental illness. Such a deficiency may also lead to heart problems, constipation, mouth and skin disorders and in the extreme, beriberi and pellagra.

White sugar also contributes to low blood sugar, a condition brought about primarily by a diet of refined carbohydrates. Eating refined sugar causes the release of insulin from the pancreas, which signals the liver to convert blood sugar to glycogen for storage. The glucose from the refined sugar is rapidly used up and the liver simply cannot break down glycogen fast enough to bring back a normal blood sugar level when it is needed. A low blood sugar condition causes people to be nervous, tired, restless, dizzy and hungry. They may ultimately develop migraine headaches, asthma, alcoholism or epileptic seizures.

Indirectly, consumption of white sugar contributes to all diseases caused by deficiency of protein, minerals or vitamins, because the more sugar one consumes the less interest he has in eating good foods, and hunger is reduced in general. Artificial sweeteners are not the answer for those who seek to eliminate white sugar from their diet. In fact, artificial sweeteners contribute nothing at all to the body nutritionally. They are manufactured from coal tar and unquestionably have been proven harmful to the body.

Bodies Do Not Thrive on "Junk Foods"

We should further note that sugars are often highly concentrated in foods, particularly candies, to such a degree that our taste buds are unable to warn us to stop eating (which they would if we were consuming too much sugar from oranges, for example). Continuing to eat sugar-filled food reduces hunger for proper food. We have people today living on a very heavy carbohydrate diet and breaking down the kidney structure. A high carbohydrate, fatty and protein diet can sometimes consume the tooth-building material and weaken the will. Excessive diets of sweets and starches make us obese and plethoric. A heavy protein diet fills us with autotoxins, whereas a fatty diet leads to fatty degeneration.

We must recognize that some of the foods we eat today, such as sugar-coated dry breakfast cereals, will not build a genius. We cannot feed a brain on potato chips, and we cannot rebuild and repair tissues properly on junk foods. The intelligence we try to get from coffee, the kidney building we try to get from buns, bagles and noodles, the strength we try to get from gouty sausages and embalmed meats—are purely illusory. We are not going to find our way to health with these foods. We are not going to improve our memories or build the highest efficiency for ourselves through the ice cream and the saccharin that people are hoping will not be taken away from them.

Although we have developed our awareness of polluted water and air and have tried to control these problems, we have done very little about polluted foods. Many people will point out that pasteurized milk is clean, pure and free of bacteria, but is its biochemical balance what it should be?

Here, then, is the problem. Refined and processed foods, along with junk foods, not only do not have the biochemical elements with which they started, but may introduce toxic chemical additives into the body. White sugar contains some 40% less calcium than raw sugar. There is 25% less calcium in white flour than in whole wheat flour and most white bread has preservatives added. When the biochemical balance is thrown off in this way by lack of nutrients or addition of toxins, the body is no longer functioning harmoniously. It begins to experience disharmony or dis-ease. A disease is an indication of toxic accumulations or of a shortage—perhaps a **starvation**—of one or more of the biochemical elements. In this way, disease is seen to be a form of starvation.

In an experiment conducted by Dr. Diana Fishbein, professor of criminology at the University of Baltimore, a group of inmates at a Florida prison had all refined carbohydrates—junk food—removed from their diet. As a result, disciplinary problems and violence in this group dropped dramatically, as compared to a control group on the normal prison diet. When the group returned to the usual prison fare, they noticed changes in their own behavior, outlook, anxiety levels, sleep patterns and aggression. Many asked to be allowed to continue the experimental diet. A similar experiment was conducted at a juvenile facility. Sugar was removed from the diet. Soft drink machines were taken out and replaced with machines that dispensed unsweetened fruit juice. Sugary snacks and deserts were replaced with popcorn, fresh fruit, nuts and peanut butter. The number of trouble-prone juveniles dropped 90%. These experiments simply confirm what I have known for years, that what we eat determines, by and large, how we behave.

Chemical Additives

It used to be possible to:

Drink a glass of milk knowing it was pure, raw milk straight from the cow.

Buy fruit grown without pesticides and chemical fertilizers.

Eat a breast of chicken without wondering what had been added to its feed or injected into it.

There were no unknown quantities or questionable ingredients in breads, cereals or even candies. Today, however, we have to be food chemists to determine the composition of much of what is marketed under the general but misleading term of "food."

Since 1930, food additives have become increasingly common in American products. Chemicals are added to preserve, soften, harden, color, stabilize, inhibit mold, thicken, flavor, alkalize, acidify, bleach and, of course, enrich various food products. There may be as many as ten or more such additives in a single package of instant casserole or breakfast cereal. The average consumer has neither the time nor the training to mean that you have all the chemical elements you need with the vegetarian way. So we're going to build a healthy way of living, a variety of foods sufficiently flexible for the average person to adapt to and enjoy. If you want to go further, it is perfectly alright. However, you need to understand that nearly all the vegetables and fruits are alkaline. Nearly all the starches and all proteins are acid. There are a few exceptions, but not many.

I want you to see that if you have six vegetables and two fruits then you are having eight of the alkaline foods. And if you are having one starch and one protein, then you are having two of the acid foods. I told you that it should be 80% alkaline and 20% acid. This diet is very nearly 80% alkaline and 20% acid. Have you got that idea? That's the way it should be.

We have to have 60% raw foods every day. You can have raw fruits or even dried fruits. You can have raw almonds and other raw nuts. They cannot be toasted or roasted. They have to be raw. It is the raw foods that have the enzymes, the digestive elements, and 60% raw foods is not hard to put into practice. Some people say, well, if 60% is so good, then why not go 100%? There are people who are 100% on raw foods. But we find that it is most difficult to go with 100% raw foods. I'm not teaching that because the average person can't or won't go that way. I'm offering you something you can start with, and if you want to go farther, one of these days, you can.

There are a few precautions to observe. I don't want you to eat lima beans raw. I don't want you to have artichokes raw. Don't eat potatoes raw. Do you understand? There is a right way of doing things and my job is to take you one step at a time. Some people can go farther in the more extreme diets, but it depends upon what kind of body they have, what type they are. If we go 60% raw, that's a healthy way. That's a way of variety, and variety is very necessary. Baked potatoes are nice—but not two meals a day of them.

If we have a variety of vegetables, we will get them from different soils and from different parts of the country. If you get fruit and vegetables from California, they may be short in calcium. Vegetables, fruits and nuts from other places may be short of other things. Variety is one of our main principles.

Some people immediately think that variety is going to be difficult, but it isn't. If you have a salad, you have quite a variety of vegetables right there, don't you? What kind of salads should we eat? Rainbow salads. Think of rainbow colors in the foods that you eat because every color represents a different chemical element or combination, and the variety that you see in all of these colors will help you get the chemical elements you need. You won't have to remember them all. When you have a colorful plate of food, many of the body's functions will be taken care of. With yellow vegetables, you're going to have a natural laxative; with the greens, you're going to have the blood builders for anemia; with the reds, you're going to have an arterial stimulant. Each one of these vegetables does different things for you; each of the fruits does different things for you. These are little things, but they are useful and important. I've studied foods and their effects on people for years in my sanitarium work—this has been my life.

At times, I had to sit down and take care of a person who had come in very sick, feeding him a teaspoon of broth every hour in order to bring him back. And, I do know what brings people back. Because foods give such wonderful results, we all need to know these things.

Let's Avoid Overeating

After variety, the next thing we must look at is eating. The average person overeats. I do too. Sometimes I can't help it. A charming hostess says, "Oh, I made this especially for you, Doctor." If I don't eat it, I'm in trouble. People try to bribe us with foods. Did you know that? "I made a special dessert for you," they say. "I can't eat another thing," I reply. "You can't mean it, Doctor," they say. "I hear that only at the cemetery." I really don't know where I'll put it in these cases.

I've heard parents tell their children, "If you finish your meal, you can have dessert"; or "I'll give you a quarter"; or "I'll take you to the circus if you'll finish your spinach." Bribery works, but what is often the result? Overeating. Once I went to one of those all-you-can-eat smorgasbords with my friend, Sam. Sam kept going back through the line, and the fourth time, I said, "Sam, you're going to kill yourself with all that food!" He said, "I'm paying for it." All right, so he'd paid for it. That didn't mean he needed to abuse his body to get his money's worth. He was really paying twice—once in money and a second time in consequences to his health.

Many years ago, I had the privilege of dining with the late great George Bernard Shaw and a number of his acquaintances. When one of the men couldn't finish his dinner, he offered it to the famous British philosopher and wit. "Don't give it to me," Shaw retorted. "I don't intend to make a garbage can of my stomach."

None of us should eat excessively just to prevent food waste. Most things can be refrigerated and saved at least a day or so.

I believe overeating can really kill us. One of the secrets of life is right there. If you eat too much, it is hard on the digestive system because it doesn't have sufficient digestive juices to take care of the load. As a consequence, the body must use extra energy to handle the surplus, which depletes energy resources. It is far healthier to end a meal a little bit hungry than stuffed up to the ears. During my world travels in search of the secrets of longevity, I found that many men and women over 120 years of age lived on diets that most us would consider too small. Yet, they were obviously healthy and vigorous.

For those who are overweight and would like to reduce—all you have to do is cut off a little bit of each meal. Now, I don't mean that as an excuse to eliminate the things you don't like. I mean to eat a little less of everything in your meals—just a little bit off the six vegetables, a little bit off the two fruits, a little bit off the starch and the same with the protein.

Of course, this diet would apply mainly to moderate climates. When you get down into the tropics with hot weather throughout the year, you can have more fruits and less vegetables.

Replacing Lost Biochemicals

In the tropic heat or when we get vigorous exercise, we perspire a good deal, losing sodium chloride in the perspiration. Salt tablets are often taken to replace the salt we lose under those circumstances. But, that isn't the kind of salt we should put back into our body. Inorganic salt is not a replacement for biochemical salt.

One of my patients was a prominent professional basketball player. He had gone through four operations because the cartilege in his ankle was breaking down and not repairing and rebuilding itself the way it should. So when this big 6 ft 11 in. basketball player came to me, I said, "You know, you haven't fed that ankle the way you should." And he said, "What do you mean, I haven't fed that ankle?" I said, "That joint material hasn't been fed. It needs sodium. Has anyone told you about the sodium foods, getting the sodium back into your diet?" He said, "No." I asked him, "How much weight do you lose in a game?" He said, "As much as 15 pounds." What is the 15 pounds he loses? Water and salt—sodium chloride. It comes out through perspiration in playing these professional games. Now he is getting some of this weight back. Depletion is a very serious thing. His doctors were trying to take care of a bad joint, but it wouldn't hold; it wouldn't stay. It was due to a lack of sodium—a lack of salt. But what kind of salt? Too many people disregard the distinction between inorganic salt and the biochemical elements we get from a food standpoint. But, experience reveals the difference.

Another common way of losing important biochemicals is during menstruation. By now nearly everyone knows that iron is lost at this time. But we also find a good deal of calcium is lost, and calcium is equally as important as iron. Both must be replaced. How many women do we find with lower back problems? The percentage is very high. The spine is one of the bony structures of the body from which calcium is drawn when this biochemical has become depleted in the body. When calcium is lost during the menstrual cycle and not replaced, it is drawn from the spine. At some point the spine becomes too weak to hold its alignment, and it goes out. The resulting misalignment is painful and limiting. Often, we find that chiropractic adjustments do not hold in these cases. The back keeps going out. What do we do? We must feed calcium to the spine and we do that by going to the calcium foods and calcium supplements, if necessary. When we take calcium supplements, it should always be with phosphorus in the ratio two-and-a-half parts calcium to one of phosphorus. Calcium can't be used in the bony structure of the body without phosphorus.

Combining Foods

I believe that we pay too much attention to combinations. Some people say, "You can't combine this and that." I suppose they are saying Nature hasn't shown much wisdom at making combinations. Let's look at beans for example—20% to 30% protein and the rest is starch. Even wheat is 12% to 14% protein, even though it is generally listed as a starch. Very few foods are completely starch or completely protein. Some are heavier in starch; some are heavier in protein. Too often we go too heavily with one thing.

We need to consider how to handle the heavy proteins and the heavy starches, and this is what I do. We're going to have three vegetables at noon and three vegetables at

night—a starch at noon and protein at night. This is the ideal way. But, for practical reasons, my combinations may not be perfect for breakfast, so I'm going to say that we can have a little starch and a little protein with fruit and a health drink. This will work out all right if you have a chance to work it off during the day. Vigorous physical exercise builds a healthy appetite, good digestion and good assimilation, even with foods that may be better to eat separately. If you can do the right thing 2 out of 3 meals a day, and only one meal is off, I believe it is alright.

We need to understand that melons do not mix well with most starches, with the grain cereals, but they will mix fairly well with fruits— with most fruits. Personally, I don't believe the wet fruits and the dry fruits mix well. But it is the heavy starches and heavy proteins that really bring in the problems. Meat and potatoes make a poor combination, and most of these heavy combinations should be avoided, especially by sensitive people who can't take these foods together.

Many people are concerned about combinations, but I have not found them of great significance in my work. Other things are more important. I think combinations should be put on the bottom of the list. We have paid too much attention to this. The most important law is to have natural, pure, whole foods in correct proportions; 20% acid and 80% alkaline; 60% raw; a variety of foods; and avoid overeating. I would rather know you are eating natural, pure and whole foods not mixed properly rather than trying to take canned foods with fried foods, or some other combination. I'm exaggerating, but only to show you that I think combinations should be at the bottom of the list.

Foods in the "Average" Diet

I used to make my patients write down their diets for one week and bring them to me. I've gone over many of these diets and found that what we might call the "average" diet has certain foods in common. Many people select foods they think are healthy but which, in fact, are not. Let's have a look at some of these foods and investigate their value.

The "average" diet generally includes: orange juice, iceberg or head lettuce, wheat bread (usually white), milk and milk products, beef and pork, coffee and tea, salt, pepper and sugar.

Orange Juice. Most people had orange juice with breakfast every day, often the frozen concentrated juice, sometimes fresh squeezed. Neither has the food value we've been led to believe it has. Oranges are picked green for commercial juicing purposes and for sale to markets. Those sent to the market are generally processed with a special gas to turn the outer peel a bright, attractive orange color, to give the impression they are "tree ripened." But, they are not. So, we have unripe oranges picked too early for proper development of the vitamin C.

When oranges are juiced, most of the pulp which contains the calcium is lost, and it is calcium which neutralizes the acids in the fruit. The pulp also helps provide the bulk needed for the bowel. We lose the pulp and most of the calcium when we only drink the juice of the orange and pectin.

To get some good from the orange, we should have tree-ripened, organically grown fruit, untouched by chemical sprays. They should be peeled and eaten in sections.

How often should we have oranges? Every day is too much. We need to take the principle of variety seriously. Nature offers us cherry juice, papaya, pineapple, grape, berry, prune, apple and many other wonderful juices. It is enough if we have an orange once a week for breakfast.

Iceberg or Head Lettuce. This is the most commonly used salad ingredient in the average diet, and it is almost worthless, nutritionally. This type of lettuce is often gas forming and tends to slow down the digestion. Once the outer green leaves are discarded (which most people do), the chlorophyll-containing part is gone and only the crisp, pale interior leaves remain—mostly water.

There is a hundred times more iron and much more potassium in leaf lettuce than head lettuce. Once people change over to the various leaf lettuces—romaine, red leaf, butter lettuce and so forth—they tend to prefer the taste.

Wheat Bread. The average family has bread with every meal. It is not unusual for many people to have a dozen slices a day. When we add pastries, pies, cakes, crackers, cereal and other wheat products, we find that wheat makes up a large portion of the American diet—29% according to U.S. government figures.

White bread and white flour products are the worst offenders among wheat products. Nearly all baked or toasted wheat products are constipating, but white flour products are the most constipating. I worked with Dr. Sidney Shellburg, the New York colonic specialist, and I always knew which people were the heavy bread eaters. They were the ones with the sluggish bowels, the ones with serious constipation problems. The making of white flour involves throwing away the bran or outer husk (which would have provided healthy bulk for the bowel) and the wheat berry at the center (which contains enzymes). Bleaching kills other vitamins. White flour products, then, may be regarded as dangerous to the health, not simply worthless, nutritionally speaking.

Whole wheat products are better. But, in all baked products, we must realize that natural oils and lecithin are destroyed by the heat. Lecithin is not only used by the nerves, brain and glands, but together with natural oils it serves as a lubricant in the bowel. Baked products are somewhat constipating for this reason.

According to the U.S. Government, one-fourth of the American diet is wheat. Again, we find the principle of variety being violated. We have millet, brown rice, rye, yellow cornmeal, barley and oats—all nourishing grains—and we need to make use of them. Each individual's body chemistry and nutritional needs are different, and only when we take in a variety of juices, fruits, vegetables, grains and so forth can we be sure of getting the essential nutrients our bodies need. We can't rely too much on one food or we risk failing to provide our body with the right balance of nutrients.

I don't advise telling people to cut out bread entirely when they have been eating a dozen slices a day for years. Cut it down to two or three slices. People can live with that. Later, if they want to eliminate it completely, they can.

Milk. Milk and milk products—cheese, butter, cottage cheese, yogurt, ice cream and many others—rank high in the average diet. The government tells us that 25% of the American diet is milk and milk products. Together with wheat, that makes a total of 54% of the average daily food regimen! Again, we run into problems when we ignore the principle of variety. With all the wonderful foods in God's garden, surely we can choose a more healthy range and variety of foods.

Among the highest paid and busiest men in the medical arts are the allergy specialists—those who deal with hay fever, asthma, bronchitis, catarrhal troubles and other allergy related conditions. What are two of the most frequently found allergens? Milk and wheat. These men make their living on wheat-logged, milk-logged people.

We don't need to rely so much on milk products. There are many other good sources of protein, calcium and phosphorus around. If we must use milk, it is well to look toward goat's milk rather than cow's milk. And, it should be raw milk.

Pasteurization may have been justified during the period in history when sanitation was such a threat to health, when tuberculosis and other diseases were passed along by way of diseased milk cows and unsanitary conditions in milking, handling, storing and distributing milk. But, pasteurization kills important enzymes and reduces the nutritional value. We also find scientific research indicating that homogenized milk may be one of the contributing causes to atherosclerosis.

We will be going more thoroughly into goat's milk later, but in my experience, it is more easily digested and assimilated than cow's milk, without generating the heavy catarrh so often produced by cow's milk. We also have seed and nut milk drinks that produce no catarrh whatsoever. Use these as substitutes for milk when heavily laden with catarrh.

Beef and Pork. Red meat fried in grease is a common part of the average American diet. Two of our country's favorite fast foods are hot dogs and hamburgers; and ham, bacon or sausage is considered by many to be an essential part of breakfast. Heavy, fatty meats are also likely to be contributing factors in heart disease, cancer and other chronic diseases, according to researchers.

Because pigs are basically omnivorous—willing to eat garbage, carrion—I consider pork a high-risk meat. Trichinosis is transmitted through improperly cooked pork. The pig is not a clean animal, and I recommend eliminating pork from the diet.

Frying meat (or anything else) in hot fat causes unnatural chemical changes which our bodies are not designed to deal with. Roasting, baking and broiling are preferable to any kind of frying. We should consider throwing out the frying pans.

We find that red meat is often not completely digested, especially by people who lack adequate hydrochloric acid in their stomachs. The incompletely digested protein is treated as toxic waste by the body, eliminated through the bowel or deaminated by the liver and excreted through the kidneys as nitrogenous waste.

I do not advocate complete elimination of meat from the diet, although I have great respect for the vegetarian way and believe the vegetarian way may be the best way to go. However, in my worldwide travels in search of the secrets of longevity, I found that the great majority of those who lived past 100 years of age had some meat in their diet—usually fish, fowl or lamb and bone soups. There were very few vegetarians among them.

Any fish with fins, scales and white meat is a good source of protein. Chicken, turkey, quail and other fowl can be eaten. I found that lamb was one of the meats favored in Turkey, the Caucasus Mountains of Russia and other areas where old men and women were still strong and vigorous. These meats are among our best sources of protein.

Again, we can't always persuade the person who has eaten beef and pork all his life to eliminate them entirely from the diet right now. This goes especially for men, who tend to be more stubborn about retaining a good deal of meat in the diet. So, we recommend cutting down. Twice a week for a while. Then once a week. At some point, it will be possible to drop beef and pork from the diet completely. One can live well without meat if he desires and knows how.

So, our goal, in summary, is to eliminate orange juice, head lettuce, white bread (and most wheat products), cow's milk (and most of its products), beef and pork. We are going to substitute other foods for these, and one of our aims is greater variety.

Keep in mind that what we are discussing here is based upon my sanitarium experiences, where people were my textbooks. I lived with my

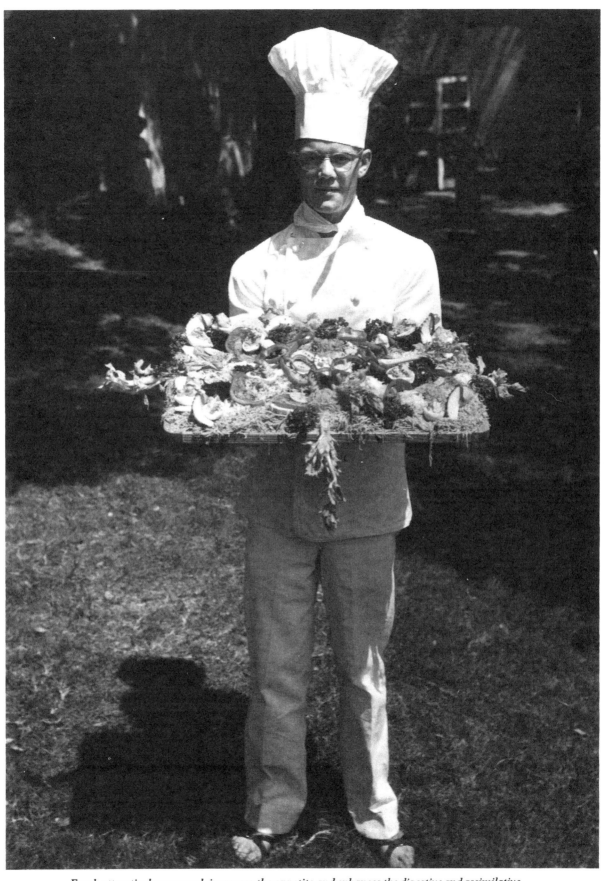

Food, attractively prepared, increases the appetite and enhances the digestive and assimilative functions. I have always insisted that Ranch meals be as attractive as possible.

patients, day in and day out, and I could see what was helping them and what was holding them back. Doctors don't find these things out with an office practice because they can't follow the effects of food and diet changes on both a day-to-day and long-term basis. At the sanitarium, we knew what people were eating to bring about positive results and progress. What we are presenting here is not theory but actual results.

Coffee and Tea. The number of coffee and tea drinkers in the United States must be phenomenal, not to mention consumers of the many caffeinated "soft drinks" available. Because many coffee and tea drinkers add white sugar to their beverage (the "soft drinks" come already loaded with sugar), we find several unnatural chemical jolts delivered to the body. The caffeine acts as a stimulant, signaling the liver to convert glycogen to glucose, increasing the heart rate and constricting blood vessels. Sugar goes directly into the bloodstream, triggering the release of insulin from the pancreas, which signals the liver to reverse the caffeine stimulus (convert blood sugar back to glycogen). When the sugar is gone, the blood glucose drops dramatically, causing the adrenal glands to pump adrenaline into the system to raise the energy level. Acid from the coffee, tea or soft drink irritates the lining of the stomach and bowel.

Any artificial stimulant places an unhealthy burden on the body, but when this happens three to five times every day it becomes a dangerous habit. The stress put on a particular organ or set of organs over a period of time renders it vulnerable to disease-producing conditions.

Healthy people don't need stimulants. Herbal teas are refreshing without irritation to the body. So are fruit juices. I advise shifting to herbal teas and fruit juices from coffee, tea and other caffeine-laced beverages.

Salt, Pepper and Sugar. These three things are always on the dining room or kitchen table of the average family, and all three are harmful in direct proportion to the quantity used.

We have already discussed what is wrong with white sugar, and I will simply add that the relatively high percentage of those with diabetes and hypoglycemia in this country indicates that excessive intake of sugar is raising havoc with the pancreas.

Salt, basically, is not a food but an inorganic chemical compound—sodium chloride. The body responds differently to table salt than it does to the sodium naturally found in green vegetables, whey and other foods. Excess salt (it doesn't take much) contributes to hardening of the arteries and imbalance of calcium and potassium in the body.

Dr. Martin Filmer of South Africa observed that healthy natives who moved from rural villages to the cities soon got into the habit of eating meat and vegetables boiled in pots with large quantities of salt. The cooking water, which picked up vitamins, minerals and other nutrients from the overcooked contents, was usually thrown away. He observed a remarkable rise in heart disease and high blood pressure among urban South African blacks from the villages and attributed it to the shift in their food habits, including excessive salt use.

I have found that salt and other spices and condiments are not needed when we have fresh, whole nourishing foods. There are herbal and vegetable seasonings which add wonderful flavor to soups, meats, vegetables and grains without stressing or irritating the digestive tract, the heart and other vital organs. If you must use salt, try a little sea salt. But, aim at eliminating salt altogether from your diet.

Black pepper is a liver irritant, and it is easy to replace with cayenne pepper. Cayenne, or red pepper, is just as spicy but without the harmful effects of black pepper. Cayenne pepper drives the blood and functions as a gentle, natural stimulant. Again, be conservative in its use. Large amounts of anything can irritate the body, especially spices.

Perhaps the point to be emphasized most here is that fresh foods, properly prepared, taste wonderful without salt, pepper, sugar or anything added. If we are accustomed to salt and spices, food will taste bland for a while before we get used to the new taste. If we persist, the reward is worth the effort in terms of both health and enjoyment of our food.

A Word About Diet

When we look at the foods that turn up regularly on the average American table, we find significant basic pattern which is related to the rise in the chronic diseases found in our time. Adding up their effects, we can begin to understand what a burden the body must carry when these things are a regular part of the diet.

Orange juice, coffee, tea, cola drinks, bread, pastries, cakes, pies, sugar, salt, pepper, head lettuce, milk, butter, cheese, cottage cheese, yogurt, cream, beef and pork—these are the main items we need to eliminate or reduce in our diets. If we reduce milk and wheat products to 6% or so of our total diet, we will be all right. I don't advocate going to the extreme, but I realize this is already extreme for many Americans accustomed to eating so many of these things regularly.

What we are searching for, what we are moving toward, is not a new diet but a right way of living. I don't like the word "diet." It implies, too often, special restrictions or special purposes; on the other hand, it is so nonspecific it can mean anything we eat. We can have coffee and donut diets, cake and hamburger diets, reducing diets, elimination diets, weight-gaining diets—anything.

Our perspective here involves looking at our overall food pattern as a structure, a building program whose purpose is to contribute to high-level well-being. Specific foods are the building blocks that make it up, and our goal is to take out those blocks which weaken the structure or fail to contribute energy and substance and replace them with blocks that serve us well. The better building blocks are made up of the dust of the earth, raised or evolved to higher vibratory levels to match the nutrient needs of our bodies. We want to match our food intake with metabolic needs, vibration by vibration, block by block, until we are functioning at our highest and best level.

Only foods can build new cells, new tissue structures, but not all foods—or at least what we call foods—can do that. So, we must sort out the worthless from the worthwhile. When doctors learn to do more educating, they will be able to do less medicating.

It isn't what we eat once in a while that counts, it is our overall food pattern, what we eat regularly. A cup of coffee and a donut won't kill us, and a good salad won't heal us. But, if we have these things every day over a period of years, consequences develop, and we are "married" to these consequences, so to speak, for a considerable time. Let's learn to make right food choices, because we know we'll enjoy the results.

Good Foods—The Building Blocks of Wellness

We are going to look at an array of what I consider the best foods and examine the reasons why. Keep in mind, these are not the only good foods. There are others, and we will mention some of them as we go along. You may know of others, but I have noticed the best results from these in my sanitarium work.

The Best Starches. I feel the best starches are: millet, brown rice, rye, yellow cornmeal.

We can use buckwheat, oats, barley, soybeans and a baked potato once in a while as well, but I consider the first four the best.

Millet is one of the basic foods used by the Hunza people, who have been among the healthiest people on this earth. I visited the Hunza Valley some years ago and was amazed at the vigor and energy of the people. Men in their 80s, 90s and 100s were still working in the fields.

Brown rice is a high-quality starch, because we have the whole grain, as we do with all four of the top starches. The Chinese and Japanese eat a great deal of rice, and you seldom see a fat person in those countries. You do see glossy hair, smooth skin, quickness of thought and movement.

Rye is our third cereal grain. Just as wheat builds fat, rye builds muscle. The Scandanavian countries use a lot of rye, and we can gain an idea of its results from their athletes. The Scandanavians are excellent skiers, gymnasts and runners—especially the Finns. The Finns have sent out some of the finest Olympic runners. The Russians use a great deal of rye too, and their athletes do well in the Olympics. A Russian has won the gold medal in Olympic weight lifting for several games consecutively.

Yellow cornmeal is our fourth cereal, and we find it is high in magnesium. The American Indians used corn, as did the Aztecs of Mexico, who developed one of the most advanced cultures on the American continent.

Buckwheat and oats are acceptable, but we find some catarrh formation from them. Soybean flour, many times, can be used as a substitute for wheat flour. It combines easily with other flours for making muffins or bread. Barley is an excellent grain for winter cereal and soups because it heats the blood nicely. Another good starch is a baked potato, but we must eat it with the skin.

Just as a farmer rotates his crops to make the best use of his land, we need to rotate the starches in our diet. Keep in mind that many of the organs and specialized tissue structures of the body have individual nutrient needs. By using a variety of starches, we can be sure our bloodstream carries the right nutrients to meet these individual needs.

Cooking. There are many ways of cooking grains, but, in principle, we aim at selecting methods that will keep them as close to the natural state as possible. We can cook many grains whole, rolled or coarse ground, the latter taking less time. For whole grains such as rye, millet, barley, oats, buckwheat and rice, there are two basic methods we use.

First, the vapor method requires a double boiler. In the upper section, use three parts water to one part grain, keeping in mind that the cooked grain will expand to 3 or 4 times its uncooked measure. One-third measuring cup of grain is usually adequate for a single portion, but we may wish to cook more and store the leftover amount in the refrigerator for later reheating. Bring the water in the lower part of the double boiler to a rapid boil, then turn it to low and allow the grain to heat slowly for six to eight hours or until sufficiently soft to chew. Different grains require different cooking times, and rice may require more water in the upper boiler than the usual 3 to 1 ratio. We do not cook whole, hard-kernel corn because of the excessive time required to soften it sufficiently. Buckwheat cooks more quickly than most others.

The overnight method requires a broad-mouth thermos. Soak the grain in water for 12 hours, pour off the water and place wet grain in thermos. Cover grain with boiling water, seal the thermos and allow to stand for 12 hours. Be sure to leave enough room for the expansion of the cooked grain—up to 2 or 3 times the space of the water-soaked grain.

Brown rice and millet (dry) can be cooked directly in a stainless steel pan with a tight lid. Bring two cups of water to a boil, add one cup

brown rice or millet and turn heat down to low for approximately 45 minutes.

Cornmeal can be purchased in many natural food stores coarse ground for cereal purposes, as can some of the other grains. We find oats either whole, rolled or steel-cut, and the steel-cut takes the least cooking time. The advantage of using coarse ground grains is to reduce cooking time, but keep in mind that some nutrients are lost in grinding and storing any cereal grain.

Coarse ground grain also takes a ratio of 3 parts water to 1 part grain, except rice which takes 4 to 1 and cornmeal which takes 5 to 1. The milled grain can be cooked by the vapor method, overnight or directly over low heat. For the direct cooking method, bring water to a boil in a stainless steel pan, add cereal grain, turn heat very low (or off if room is warm) and let cook 20 minutes. The cooking in the double boiler is also greatly reduced over the time required for whole grains.

Whole unpearled barley is wonderful in soups. The Danish make a soup of green kale and barley which is an excellent winter soup.

Any of the grains used as morning cereals can be sweetened by adding raisins, chopped dates or figs.

Barley is high in sodium and is excellent for feeding the nerves, muscles and joints. It is also fattening and must be used in moderation. Barley and cornmeal are easily digested, and corn contains an oil which helps lubricate the bowel for good elimination. Yellow corn is about 4% phosphate which helps keep calcium in solution and in the body. Oats are high in silicon, an element necessary for good tone in the muscles and nerves and for healthy skin and hair.

The starches are of great value when there are problems on the left side of the body. In all heart conditions, more carbohydrates are needed. Be aware that when left-side disturbances are found, starches may generate gas in the bowel. We find that starches are not as hard on the kidneys as proteins.

Energy comes primarily from carbohydrates, and I consider the starches more as winter foods because they heat the body and tend to be fattening. If we overuse grains in the winter and gain weight, it is advisable to go on an elimination diet in the spring. This is especially true for those who live in cold climates. Grains stored for long times lose some of their natural oils through oxygenation, so it is best to buy fresh grains when possible. It is also best to have them ground at the time of purchase, if that service is available. You may wish to consider buying a small hand operated or electric mill for grinding your own grains.

The Scotch people who eat a great deal of natural oatmeal and oat cakes have fine, strong bodies. Scottish shepherds are away from home for long periods, walking miles and miles, and much of their diet is from oats.

We can make gruels from many of our grains and I believe combining grains for this purpose is all right on occasion.

The Best Proteins. Just as starches are our primary energy foods, not only for work and play but also for driving the thousands of metabolic processes going on in the body, proteins are our primary building materials for replacement and rejuvenation of tissue. Proteins are made up of amino acids which form the substance of much of our bodies, and they are vital. We must realize that very few foods are 100% protein; most starches have some protein, and most proteins have some starch.

When we look to the protein foods, we must take several factors into consideration. We must consider purity, for much of what passes as protein in the supermarket is adulterated or processed to an extent which makes it unfit for tissue building. We must consider completeness in terms of the essential amino acids, of which 10 have been identified to date. Digestibility is of primary importance, since we can only use what we can digest. Our three criteria for foods—pure, whole and natural—apply to proteins but can be more difficult to determine in the supermarket. We must be careful and discriminating in our shopping.

Meat is the food highest in usable protein. Without intending any offense to vegetarians, I simply must point out that the biochemicals in meat are higher evolved than those in plant life. As we go up the food chain, we find the biochemicals in the foods at each step being raised to a higher vibratory level. The phosphorus we get from vegetables is not the same quality as the phosphorus we find in meat, eggs, cheese and so on, and the latter is more

suited for use by the brain, which requires the highest evolved phosphorus we can find. The same principle holds for the other elements.

I am not saying we must eat meat and I am not telling vegetarians they must include animal proteins in their diet. If vegetarianism is working well for you, stay with it. But, I believe the vegetarian way is not for everyone, and here, as I have mentioned before, we are taking the middle way, a way most people can live with and can adjust to family-wise and to the society they are used to living in.

For reasons I have mentioned before, I do not recommend beef or pork, and we must consider the possibility of impurity in any of the supermarket meats. We must be particularly concerned about steroids such as stilbestrol, often used commercially to speed weight gain. Stilbestrol is a sex stimulant which has been linked to cancer formation. We also need to consider possible chemical spray residues, antibiotics and other chemical substances in the commercial feed given to animals. Keep in mind also that excess consumption of proteins can lead to urea buildup in the body, with associated toxic effects. Too much protein is hard on the liver and kidneys.

On the positive side, my study of the factors contributing to longevity among the oldest people in the world revealed that most all were meat eaters to some extent. I would like to say there were vegetarians among them, but there were not. Many of them ate lamb, which is perhaps the least stimulating of the meats. Others had a little poultry or fish in their diets. None ate large portions of meat at a single meal, and moderation is one of the key factors.

Poultry, lamb and fish with fins, scales and white meat are the best of the meat proteins. All meat eaten should be lean, easily digestible, clean and as nonstimulating as possible. Meat should always be baked, broiled, roasted or boiled (if for soups and stews), never fried in grease or cooked in hot oil. Choose longer cooking times at lower heat whenever possible and do not overcook. Do not make white flour-based gravies with the fat and juice in the broiling pan.

Men accustomed to having meat three times a day can have difficulty adjusting to a low meat diet of say, once or twice a month. I advise the ladies to be patient with their husbands, cutting back gradually and making a special effort to prepare attractive, delicious meals without meat a few times a week to generate interest by the husband. Use meat substitutes—good protein sources.

Eggs, milk and cheese are the foods next highest in protein. I consider eggs the perfect protein because they have the finest balance of essential amino acids, matched closely to the needs of the bloodstream.

In an experiment some years ago, Alexis Carrell, a medical doctor, kept a chicken's heart alive for 29 years with egg yolk. I have heard of no comparable experiment with any other protein source, supporting living tissue so long in that way. That's another reason why I believe eggs are the highest quality protein source.

The egg is a whole food. It builds the whole chicken—brain, bones, flesh, sinews, nerves, skin—and it is natural and pure. The only way an egg, particularly the yolk, can be impaired in nutrient quality is if the chicken is not getting the right foods. If we put cayenne pepper in chicken feed, the egg yolk comes out red. If the yolks are light yellow, we can give the chickens greens and get a nice, dark orange egg yolk. Give a hen a basically decent diet and it will produce excellent eggs. The best eggs come from chickens that have the freedom to walk around and peck and scratch for bugs in the dirt, according to their nature.

Doctors tell us to skip eggs because of the cholesterol. But the egg also has lecithin, which balances out the cholesterol in the body. We find that the brain and nerves need both cholesterol and lecithin, so again the egg comes out on top. One word of caution: high heat destroys lecithin, so the egg must be soft-boiled, poached or raw.

One of the finest nerve drinks is an egg yolk in black cherry juice. This makes a high iron drink with balanced amino acid nutrients in it. The liver, an iron organ, takes the combination very well. It's good for the liver, good for rheumatism, good for the nerves.

Next after eggs, the best protein source is milk, preferably clabbered raw milk. I may have a glass of milk a day, half a glass at a time mixed with carrot juice. The problem with cow's milk is that most often we find it pasteurized, which not only kills harmful bacteria but many of the enzymes nature put there as well. Another thing, cow's milk is a heavy catarrh producer for many people. If we digest milk easily, without forming excess catarrh, we should have it raw and "as close to the cow" as possible. Often, those who can't tolerate cow's milk will do well with goat's milk, which is high in fluorine, the resistance element. We also have fine milk substitutes—the nut milks, seed milks and soy milk—which we'll talk about later. These produce no catarrh whatsoever.

When I'm busy working at the Ranch, I often say, "Just give me my drink," because I may not have time to sit through a meal. My drink consists of raw goat's milk or soy milk (1-1-1/2 tbsp soy milk powder to a glass of water), a tablespoon of sesame seed butter or almond nut butter, a teaspoon of honey and a sliver of avocado or half a banana. This makes a whole nutritious drink. At times, I ask for an egg yolk in with it.

Just behind milk, the next best protein is cheese—raw cheese. Get goat milk cheese if possible, and if you can't, the Tillamook Company of Oregon makes a nice raw cheese from cow's milk. We can often find the raw goat milk cheese in natural food stores, usually from the Briar Hills Dairy in Chehalis, Washington or the Altadena Dairy in California, at least in the western states.

Why do we recommend goat's milk and goat's milk products? Basically, this wisdom is founded on experience that goes back thousands of years. If you take a drive in the country and see a farm with goats, you'll receive an interesting surprise if you stop and ask the people why they have goats. They'll say, "Because my child had tonsil troubles," or "My wife had a digestive disturbance," or "My husband had ulcers and nothing else would help." They always have the goats for health purposes. I believe about 60% of the world today is living on goat's milk products and one or more cereal grains. And, if you want to know what sort of milk God meant in the Bible where the "land of milk and honey" is mentioned, it is goat milk.

The best cheese is aged cheese, cheese that crumbles easily.

Seeds and nuts are wonderful proteins, and I recommend seeds as the best of the vegetarian's protein foods.

Sesame seed is the king of the seeds, widely used in Turkey where we find the strongest people in the world. I saw a 75-year-old Turk carry a piano on his back for nine blocks. While I was visiting that country, I found out the champion wrestler was also 75 years old. The Turks are high in energy, including sexual energy. Their families mean a lot to them. One of their foods is made with concentrated grape juice and ground sesame seeds, and that is wonderful for the sex life, they say.

We can take the seeds best in the milk drinks or the butters, and I'll give the recipes at the end of this section. We always use the hard-shelled nuts which keep the oils fresh.

I am often asked about tahini and halvah, two of the popular sesame seed products in the natural food stores. First, we find that many times halvah has corn syrup and cane sugar in it. Secondly, I would say it is best to make the seed and nut products fresh to get the most good out of them. Nature puts hulls and shells on them to protect the nutrients inside, and once these have been broken down, the enzymes begin to deteriorate. Tahini from stores often goes rancid very rapidly.

Other seeds I recommend are sunflower and alfalfa. We are seeing the apricot seeds used more now in this country. In the Hunza Valley they eat apricot seeds, but only if they are sweet. Here, they are often sold without regard to whether they are bitter or sweet, which is something to think about. In the Hunza Valley, they chop down a tree which produces bitter seeds. They consider it poisonous.

We hear a lot about the laetrile in apricot kernels as a cancer-preventing or cancer-fighting substance, but we need to realize that cancer is caused by so many substances and processes that it is doubtful whether a single seed or nut ingredient could do much for it. This is a cancer age. We live in the midst of carcinogen-producing chemicals, products and activities. I don't doubt that apricot kernels do some good, but let's not give them more credit than they deserve.

Now we go on to the nuts. The almond is the king of all nuts, the only alkaline nut we have. But we can use many of the other nuts— Brazil nuts, pecans, Missouri black walnuts (highest in manganese, the memory element), macadamia nuts and others. The nuts must have hard shells to protect the kernel inside, and we must make them into butters or milk drinks to

digest and assimilate the nutrients. Nuts with thin shells lose their oils and moisture by evaporation. They do us little good. Lecithin, a valuable brain and nerve fat, is found in these oils.

Why do I say we must have the butters and milk drinks rather than eating the nuts? Because we don't chew them long enough or well enough for proper digestion and assimilation. I have given so many colonics that I know from experience how incompletely masticated nuts pass right through the bowel.

Seed and Nut Butters and Milks

We make the seed and nut butters simply by putting them through a Champion Juicer, available at many health and natural food stores.

Sesame Seed Milk. 1/4 cup sesame seeds to 2 cups of water, raw milk or goat milk. Place in blender and blend 1-1/2 minutes. Strain through fine wire strainer or 2-4 layers of cheesecloth. This is to remove the hulls. Add 1 tablespoon carob powder and 6-8 dates. For flavor and added nutritional value, any one of the following may be added to this drink: banana, stewed raisins, apple or cherry concentrate, date powder or grape sugar. Your own imagination or taste may dictate other combinations of fruits or juices. Whenever adding anything, run in blender again to mix. This milk may also be used as the basis for salad dressings.

I believe that sesame seed milk is one of our best drinks. It is a wonderful drink for gaining weight, for lubricating the intestinal tract, and its nutritional value is beyond compare, as it is high in protein and minerals. This is the seed used in the making of Tahini, a sesame seed oil dressing. This also is the seed that is used so much in Arabia and as a basic food in East India.

Other uses for sesame seeds: Salad dressing, added to vegetable broth, added to fruits, mixed with nut butter of any kind, for after-school snacks; use on cereals for breakfast, add to whey drinks to adjust intestinal sluggishness, twice daily with banana to gain weight; add supplements such as flaxseed meal or rice polishings.

Almond Nut Milk. Use blanched or unblanched almonds. Other nuts may be used also. Soak nuts overnight in apple or pineapple juice or honey water. This softens the nut meats. Then put 3 ounces of soaked nuts in 5 ounces of water and blend for 2 to 2-1/2 minutes in the liquefier. Flavor with honey, any kind of fruit, concentrates of apple or cherry juices, strawberry juice, carob powder, dates or bananas. This can also be used with any of the vegetable juices.

Almond nut milk can be used with soups and vegetarian roasts as a flavoring. Use over cereals, too. Almond milk makes a very alkalilne drink, high in protein, easy to assimilate.

Pumpkin Seed or Sunflower Seed Milk. The same principle as is used for making nut milks can be employed to make sunflower seed milk; i.e., soaking overnight, liquefying and flavoring with fruits and juices. Use in the diet the same way as the almond nut milk. It is best to use whole sunflower seeds and blend them yourself. However, if you do not have a liquefier, the sunflower seed meal can be used. Add seeds or nuts. NO peanuts!

Soy Milk. Soy milk powder is found universally in health food stores.

Add 4 tablespoons soy milk powder to one pint of water. Sweeten with raw sugar, honey or molasses, and add a pinch of vegetable salt. For flavor, you can add any kind of fruit, apple or cherry concentrate, carob powder, dates and bananas. You can add any other natural sweetener.

Keep in refrigerator. Use this milk in any recipe as you would regular cow's milk. It closely resembles the taste and composition of cow's milk and will sour just as quickly. Therefore, it should not be made in too large quantities or too far ahead of time.

Beans and Legumes have the least protein and are at the bottom of our list. There is more starch than protein in them, and it is not hard to gain weight on beans and legumes.

The champion of the legumes is lentils. It has the finest fiber and the hull is not such an irritant to the bowel. It has been discovered that the gas produced in the bowel by beans and legumes comes from the hulls, not the contents. We find there are many kinds of lentils, many colors, but my criterion is primarily size. The smallest are the best. The same is true of beans,

nuts and seeds. The smallest ones are always the best because the concentration of the vital essence is higher.

Fats and lipids are also necessary in the diet. The wonderful thing about a diet of fresh, whole foods is that we get our essential fats and lipids the natural way. We get the vegetable oils from the whole grains, nuts and seeds. We get cholesterol and lecithin from egg yolk and we get the animal oils from fowl, lamb and fish.

BALANCED DAILY EATING REGIMEN

Make a habit of applying the following General Diet Regimen to your everyday living. This is a healthy way to live because, when followed, you do not have to think of vitamins, mineral elements or calories. The best diet, over a period of a day, is two different fruits, at least four to six vegetables, one protein and one starch with fruit or vegetable juices between meals. Eat at least two green leafy vegetables a day. Fifty to sixty percent of the food you eat daily should be raw. Consider this regimen a dietetic law.

Rules of Eating

1. Do not eat fried foods or foods cooked in heated oils.
2. If not entirely comfortable in mind and body, do not eat.
3. Do not eat unless you have a keen desire for the plainest food.
4. Do not eat beyond your needs.
5. Be sure to thoroughly masticate your food.
6. Miss meals if in pain, emotionally upset, not hungry, chilled, overheated and during illness.
7. Have citrus fruit in sections only, never in juice form.
8. Have a limited amount of bread (with bowel trouble, no bread).

Food Healing Laws

1. Natural Food: 50-60% of the food eaten should be raw.
2. Your diet should be 80% alkaline and 20% acid.
3. Proportion: 6 vegetables daily, 2 fruits daily, 1 starch daily and 1 protein daily.
4. Variety: vary proteins, starches, vegetables and fruits from meal to meal and day to day.

5. Overeating: you can kill yourself with the amount of food you eat.
6. Combinations: separate starches and proteins. One at lunch and the other at dinner. Have fruits for breakfast and at 3 pm.
7. Cook without water: cook at low heat. Cook without air touching hot food.
8. Bake, broil or roast: if you eat meat, have it this way. Have lean meat, no fat, no pork. Use unsprayed vegetables, if possible, and eat them as soon after being picked as possible.
9. Use stainless steel, low-heat cooking utensils: it is the modern health engineered way of preparing your foods.

Before Breakfast

Upon rising and 1/2 hour before breakfast, take any natural, unsweetened fruit juice, such as grape, pineapple, prune, fig, apple or black cherry. Liquid chlorophyll can also be used, 1 teaspoon in a glass of water.

You can have a broth and lecithin drink if you desire. Take 1 teaspoon of vegetable broth powder and 1 tablespoon of lecithin granules and dissolve in a glass of warm water.

Between fruit juice and breakfast, do the following: skin brushing, exercise, hiking, deep breathing or playing. Shower. Start with warm water and cool off until your breath quickens. Never shower immediately on rising.

Breakfast

Stewed fruit, one starch and health drink or two fruits, one protein and health drink. (Starches and health drinks are listed with the lunch suggestions.) Soaked fruits, such as unsulphured apricots, prunes, figs. Fruit of any kind—melon, grapes, peaches, pears, berries or baked apple, which may be sprinkled with some ground nuts or nut butter. When possible, use fruit in season.

Suggested Breakfast Menus

MONDAY
Reconstituted dried apricots
Steel-cut oatmeal - Supplements
Oat straw tea
Add eggs, if desired, or
Sliced peaches and cottage cheese
Supplements - Herb tea

TUESDAY
Fresh figs
Cornmeal cereal - Supplements
Shave grass tea
Add eggs or nut butter, if desired, or
Raw applesauce and blackberries
Coddled egg - Supplements - Herb tea

WEDNESDAY
Reconstituted dried peaches
Millet cereal - Supplements
Alfamint tea
Add eggs, cheese or nut butter, if desired
or
Sliced nectarines and apple
Yogurt - Supplements - Herb tea

THURSDAY
Prunes or any reconstituted dried fruit
Whole wheat cereal - Supplements
Oat straw tea
or
Grapefruit and kumquats
Poached egg - Supplements - Herb tea

FRIDAY
Fresh pineapple slices w/shredded coconut
Buckwheat cereal - Supplements
Peppermint tea
or
Baked apple, persimmons,
chopped raw almonds with
Acidophilus milk - Supplements - Herb tea

SATURDAY
Muesli w/bananas and dates
Cream - Supplements
Dandelion coffee or Herb tea

SUNDAY
Cooked applesauce w/raisins
Rye grits - Supplements
Shave grass tea
or
Cantaloupe and strawberries
Cottage cheese - Supplements - Herb tea

Preparation Helps

Reconstituted dried fruit. Cover with cold water, bring to boil and leave to stand overnight. Raisins may just have boiling water poured over them. This kills any insects and eggs.

Whole grain cereal. To cook properly with as little heat as possible, use a double boiler or thermos to cook your cereal.

Supplements. (Add to cereal or fruit.) Sunflower seed meal, rice polishings, wheat germ, flaxseed meal (about a teaspoon of each). Even a little dulse may be sprinkled over with some broth powder.

10:30 a.m. Vegetable broth, vegetable juice or fruit juice.

Lunch

Raw salad or as directed, one or two starches, as listed and a health drink. Get salad suggestions from **Vital Foods for Total Health**.

Raw vegetable salad: Tomatoes (citrus); lettuce (green, leafy type only such as romaine); celery, cucumber, beansprouts, green peppers, avocado, parsley, watercress, endive, onion (s), cabbage (s). (s) indicates sulphur foods.

Starches

Yellow cornmeal, baked potato, baked banana (or at least dead ripe), barley (a winter food), steamed brown rice or wild rice, millet (have as a cereal), banana squash or hubbard squash.

Steel-cut oatmeal, whole-wheat cereal, Dr. Jackson's meal, whole grain, Roman meal, shredded wheat bread (whole wheat, rye, soybean, cornbread, bran muffins, rye krisp, preferred).

Drinks

Vegetable broth, soup, coffee substitute, buttermilk, raw milk, oat straw tea, alfamint tea, huckleberry tea, papaya tea or any health drink.

Note: If following a strict regimen, use only one of the first seven starches daily. Vary the starch from day to day.

Suggested Lunch Menus

MONDAY
Vegetable salad
Baby lima beans - Baked potato
Spearmint tea

TUESDAY
Vegetable salad (with Health Mayonnaise)
Steamed asparagus
Very ripe bananas or steamed unpolished rice
Vegetable broth or herb tea

WEDNESDAY
Raw salad plate w/Sour cream dressing
Cooked green beans
Cornbread or Baked hubbard squash
Sassafras tea

THURSDAY
Salad w/French dressing
Baked zucchini and okra
Corn-on-the-cob - Rye krisp
Buttermilk or herb tea

FRIDAY
Salad
Baked green pepper stuffed w/eggplant/tomato
Baked potato and/or bran muffin
Carrot soup or herb tea

SATURDAY
Salad
Steamed turnips and turnip greens
Baked yams
Catnip tea

SUNDAY
SALAD w/lemon-olive oil dressing
Steamed whole barley
Cream of celery soup
Steamed chard
Herb tea

Salad Vegetables

Use plenty of greens. Choose four or five vegetables from the following: Leaf lettuce, watercress, spinach, beet leaves, parsley, alfalfa sprouts, cabbage, young chard, herbs any green leaves, cucumbers, beansprouts, onions, green peppers, pimentos, carrots, turnips, zucchini, asparagus, celery, okra, radishes, etc.

Vital Foods for Total Health, Nature's own cookbook by Dr. Bernard Jensen, is a complete food guide. Tables for vitamin and mineral guidance, acid and alkaline tables—with complete instructions for perfect combinations to assure you a correct daily balance—designed to get and keep you well.

This book shows how to cook, prepare and serve foods healthfully, the natural food way. It is illustrated with charts and recipes.

3:00 P.M.

Health cocktail, juice or fruit.

Dinner

Raw salad, two cooked vegetables, one protein and a broth or health drink, if desired.

Cooked Vegetables. Peas, artichokes, carrots, beets, turnips, spinach, beet tops, string beans, Swiss chard, eggplant, zucchini, summer squash, broccoli (s), cauliflower (s), cabbage (s), sprouts (s), onion (s) or any vegetable other than potatoes. (s) denotes sulphur foods.

Drinks. Vegetable broth, soup or health beverage.

Proteins

Once a Week. Fish—use white fish, such as sole, halibut, trout or sea trout.

Three Times a Week. Meat—use only lean meat. Never pork, fats or cured meats. Vegetarians: Use meat substitutes or vegetarian proteins.

Twice a Week. Cottage cheese or any cheese that breaks.

Once a Week. Egg omelet.

If you have a protein at this meal, health dessert (allowed but not recommended), *never* eat protein and starch together. (Note how they are separated.)

You may exchange your noon meal for the evening meal, but follow the same regimen. It takes exercise to handle raw food and we generally get more after our noon meal. That is why a raw salad is advised at noon. If one eats sandwiches, have vegetables at the same time.

Vegetarians: Use soybeans, lima beans, cottage cheese, sunflower seeds and other seeds, also seed butters, nut butters, nut milk drinks and eggs.

Suggested Dinner Menus

MONDAY
Salad
Diced celery and carrots
Steamed spinach, waterless cooked
Puffy omelet - Vegetable broth
Herb tea

TUESDAY
Salad
Cooked beet tops
Broiled steak or ground beef patties
Tomato sauce
Cauliflower
Comfrey tea

WEDNESDAY
Cottage cheese - Cheese stix
Apples, peaches, grapes, nuts
Apple concentrate cocktail

THURSDAY
Salad
Steamed chard - Baked eggplant
Grilled liver and onions
Persimmon whip (optional)
Alfamint tea

FRIDAY
Salad
Yogurt and lemon dressing
Steamed mixed greens - Beets
Steamed fish w/slices of lemon
Leek soup - Herb tea

SATURDAY
Salad
Cooked string beans - Baked summer squash
Carrot and cheese loaf
Cream of lentil soup or lemongrass tea
Fresh peach gelatin w/almond-nut cream

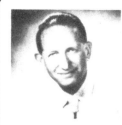

A RETURN TO A MORE NATURAL WAY OF LIFE

As life becomes more complex, man, in his scurry for convenience of living, forgets that, especially in food, there are basic rules of nature by which we all are governed. At HIDDEN VALLEY HEALTH RANCH, we practice and teach a more natural way of living. We invite you to return with us to a more serene and sensible way of life!

Dr. Bernard Jensen, NUTRITIONIST

ACCOMMODATIONS

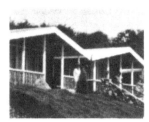 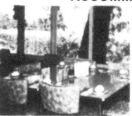 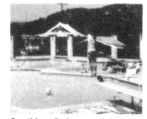 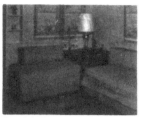

Comfortable Cottages are nestled in the shaded surroundings for the ultimate in relaxed living. A rustic and restful tenting and camping area is also available year 'round, by day, week, month or year.

Magnificent Meals are provided for guests in the light and airy dining room overlooking the Ranch's garden area. HEALTHFUL, NATURAL FOODS, tastefully prepared in a stainless steel kitchen, are the keynote of every meal.

Soothing Swims under a temperate sun are relaxing and therapeutic. The pool and game area is centrally located and constantly maintained.

Restful Rooms provide comfortable area where guests may refresh and rejuvenate both mind and body. Accommodations are available for an individual or a family.

This is one of our earlier brochures when the Ranch was going full swing. It was a different way of life for most who came there.

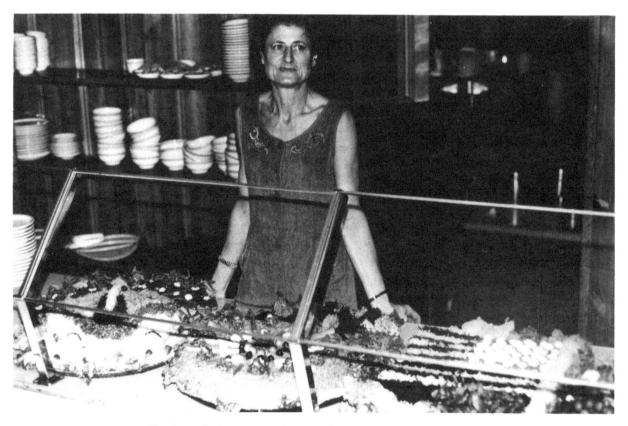

We always had many compliments about the food at our sanitarium.

48

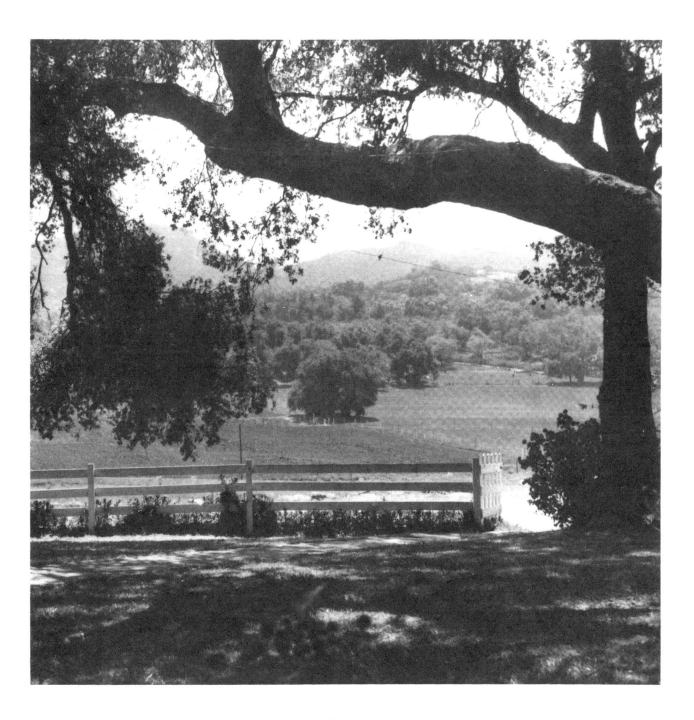

Hidden Valley Health Ranch was the fulfillment of a dream—a dream of a peaceful valley where the air was pure and clear, where the soil was fertile, where birds were singing in the trees— where people could come to leave the disease way of life behind and learn how to live.

SUNDAY
Salad
Steamed diced carrots and peas
Tomato aspic
Roast leg of lamb w/mint sauce
Herb tea

Vegetarians: Use vegetarian dishes in place of meat dishes.

Survival Foods

Chlorophyll. The greatest blood cleanser and blood builder is chlorophyll, found in all green plants. The process of photosynthesis, in which the energy of sunlight interacts with chlorophyll in the manufacture of plant food in green leaves, is the basis for life on this planet as we know it. Chlorophyll is a purifier in the blood, eliminating heavy metals, drug residues and other toxins. Iron, found in all green plants, works with chlorophyll to build the blood. A young lady from Canada came to the Ranch with pernicious anemia, her red blood cell count dangerously low. She was a vegetarian and couldn't take liver or other animal sources of iron, so we gave her liquid chlorophyll—a great deal of it. With a disciplined use of chlorophyll, she raised her red blood count to 4,800,000 (normal) in three months. This is evidence of its incredible effectiveness.

They say the U.S. Army has tested chlorophyll and found that it helps cleanse the body of radioactive contamination. Other researchers have claimed that it clears toxic heavy metals out of the body including arsenic. It may be possible one of these days to introduce chlorophyll into the bloodstream directly to increase the blood count.

Two of our top chlorophyll foods worthy of being ranked among the top survival foods, are spirulina and chlorella—single-celled microalgae with 50 to 60% protein and good quality carbohydrates and lipids. They are high in vitamin A, several of the B vitamins, calcium, phosphorus and iron, and are increasingly appearing in natural and health food stores. The whole plant, in this case a single cell, is eaten. A man in Japan is said to have lived for fifteen years on chlorella alone so we must take this alga seriously as an excellent survival food.

Seeds. I rank seeds highly as a survival food because we eat them whole; they are high in quality protein, pure and uncontaminated, good for the reproductive system and contain vitamin E. The best, as I have said, are sesame seeds, but we should not underestimate others.

Watermelon seeds are wonderful for kidney problems, high blood pressure and stress relief. We can take the seeds from pomegranates and make a wonderful seed milk drink for the genito-urinary tract and kidneys.

When we understand that something like 80% of the men over 60 years of age in this country have had prostate operations, and a high percentage of the women have had hysterectomies or serious female problems of other kinds, we realize we must learn to feed the glands, to keep the life force going. And this is done with the life force values in seeds. Seeds have all the life-giving vibrations in them to give birth to a whole plant.

We find that we are as young as our glands. I don't mean just our sexual vitality, although that is an important factor; I mean the skin, the muscle tone, the countenance, the energy and vital force for work, for play, for life in all its variety.

Sprouts. Experiments in vitamin research, conducted in different parts of the world have shown that sprouts of grains and legumes develop liberal quantities of vitamins—especially vitamins A, B and C. Certain legume sprouts, in fact, develop so much ascorbic acid, which is part of the vitamin C complex, that a single serving of the sprout as a salad may supply half of the daily requirement of ascorbic acid for an adult. So, it has been pointed out, no one in any part of the world, land or sea, need suffer from the lack of this essential vitamin if there are seeds available for sprouting. The great survival value of sprouts is that they are pure, whole and have the activated enzymes from the "mother" seed. Whole foods are valuable sources of balanced nutrient groups. With sprouts, we don't have to worry about chemical sprays or depleted soils. They are a pure, clean food with high nutritional value.

I believe many people do not realize what a simple process seed-sprouting is. It can be easily done in your own kitchens. Including sprouts in your diet seems to me so important that I feel it is wise to pass along more detailed information on this subject.

I recently was sent a pottery device for sprouting seeds. This porous vessel keeps the seeds in the right state of moisture by capillary action, producing vitamin-rich sprouts in three to five days.

Seeds for sprouting should be clean and free from broken seeds, as the latter will fail to sprout and only swell and ferment, interfering with the germination of other seeds by the production of alcohol and the growth of molds.

Place the appropriate amount (as indicated in the following table) of cleaned seed in a cup of warm water and allow it to soak for the length of time indicated. Then pour off all water and place the seeds in the porous bowl or in a shallow vessel, such as a glass pie plate or a cake tin. Pour one-half inch of warm water, and then set the porous sprouting chamber in the water, putting on this vessel a cover that will exclude light, but not air.

Ordinary room temperature is usually ideal for sprouting, but in cold climates, it may be necessary to place your container on a warm part of the stove to maintain a suitable germination temperature. The next day, when you look at the seeds, you will find they are swollen and have probably begun to produce fine roots. Pick out any broken seeds which may show up after swelling, and if you have left too much water on the seeds the first day and much is still present in the sprouting vessel, carefully pour it off. Experience will soon teach you the proper amount to leave.

By the third day, you will find the sprouts and the rootlets are larger. It is usually a good plan to wash bean sprouts with cool water, by filling the vessel and then very carefully, without disturbing the sprouts, pouring the water off. The water in the bottom of the vessel should be changed on the third day.

Care should be taken not to leave the sprouting container uncovered for any great length of time, as the production of ascorbic acid (vitamin C) is reduced by exposure to light.

By the fourth day, most of the sprouts will be ready for use, though the Mung beans (Chinese bean sprouts) may require an additional day. Remember, seed sprouts are the freshest vegetables you can eat. They continue to grow even after they are on the salad plate, so one is sure of getting the utmost of vitamin value. They may be stored in the refrigerator, but in that process some vitamin C is lost.

Wheat and alfalfa seeds are wonderful sources of protein of high biologic value, and whole wheat contains large quantities of blood-building iron as well. These two are perhaps the best to start with in your seed-sprouting adventure. Sunflower seeds are also a fine source of protein.

Another procedure for growing sprouts is to soak the whole seed in water for twenty-four hours, then place this moistened seed between folds of soft flannel, folded loosely to allow for the swelling of the seed to several times its original size. Keep these flannel encased seeds in a warm place and sprinkle each day with lukewarm water, but allow for drainage.

If you wish to obtain a green color in the sprouts, expose the seeds to the sun for a short period every day during the sprouting time. These sprouts will grow to two inches or three inches in a period of from four to six days. After the sprouts are developed, they should be kept in a cool place, like any other fresh vegetable. They are delicious in raw green salads, Chinese dishes or added to scrambled eggs.

If used in hot dishes, sprouts should not be added until just a few minutes before serving, as they lose their crispness. A delicious breakfast cereal is made by grinding or blending together one cupful of sprouted wheat and ten dates or any fruit desired.

	Correct Amount for One seeding	Soaking Time	Ready to Use
Radish	2 teaspoons	4 hours	3-5 days
Alfalfa	1 teaspoon	8 hours	3-5 days
Red clover	1 teaspoon	8 hours	3-5 days
Grains	2 tablespoons	8 hours	3-4 days
Mung beans	1/4 cup	8 hours	3-6 days
Lentils	1/4 cup	8 hours	3-6 days

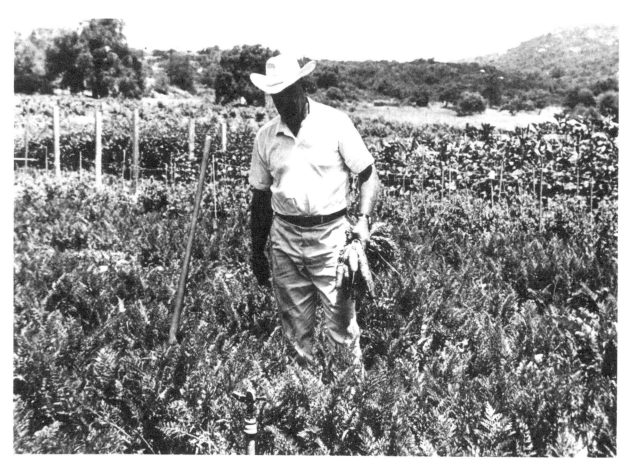

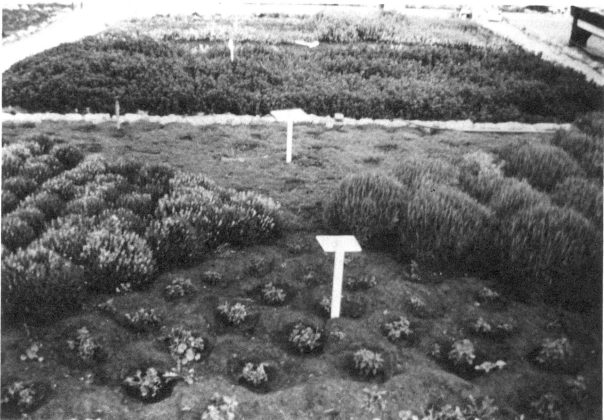

Nutrition is the proper basis for all sanitarium work. Foods should be whole, pure and natural.

52

I highly recommend the use of sprouts in the diet as we receive full mineral and chemical content of the seed before it has had a chance to deteriorate. By sprouting these seeds as you need them, you always have a fresh supply.

At the Ranch, we have an old ice box that has a temperature regulator in it such as used in a chicken incubator, and we keep the temperature regulated at 85 degrees. We use a shallow dish of pottery or some other porous material with a lid that does not fit too tightly. We place in this a teaspoonful of alfalfa seed, cover it with water and let it sit for 12 hours at room temperature. Carefully pour off water. Place dish with seeds into larger dish which has small amount of water in it. Cover top dish and place in refrigerator which is set at 85 degrees. Keep at this temperature. Keep water in lower dish. Seeds will sprout in 2 to 3 days. For soybean sprouts, let stand in water for about 20 hours before draining.

A diet of vegetable juices and bean and seed sprouts has been found to be tremendously helpful in cases of multiple sclerosis.

Browne Landone was one who also believed in the value of sprouts. He realized that as they were grown in darkness, the power that was used and developed in these seeds to come into light is the power and electrical energy we need for our bodies. This is the great life force that is found in the proverbial grain of mustard.

Berries. I chose to include berries on my survival list because they are among the least tamth of our food sources. Many of the commercial agricultural food sources—fruit, nuts, grains, vegetables and so forth have been hybridized and tampered with genetically to increase size, improve color and taste, allow for mechanized harvesting and add shelf life. We can hardly be sure what the remaining nutritional values are. Man's tampering with mother nature seldom—if ever—works out well.

Berries are still relatively wild, as natural as we can find in the fruit realm. The ratio of pulp to liquid in berries is not far from the ratio of "pulp" to "liquid" in man. The percentage of iron in the blackest berries is very close to the percentage in the human liver. Whereas most iron tonics are constipating, berries are not (with the exception of blackberries).

We find that berries are loaded with seeds, which are high in oils and enzymes that feed the glands and help us retain youthful looks and vigor.

Different parts of the country and world have different berries, but we can almost always find blackberries, logan berries, black and red raspberries, strawberries, gooseberries and ollalie berries in most parts of this country.

Making Food Patterns Work Right

In my work, I have been a little different than other nutrition teachers. Some of them are so exacting and demanding that they almost succeed in making a dis-ease out of trying to be well. The anxiety level shoots up like a rocket. They generate discomfort, stress and dis-ease by laying down the law about foods, requiring so much discipline and such difficult standards that you begin going through life uptight. I think that seeking good health should be a relaxed and enjoyable way of living. So if you tend to be a food extremist, one who "goes to the edges" as they say in London, I try to keep away from that. I have been called a compromiser—and, yes, I do compromise. When I say that I compromise, it is because I have found out that you can't focus seriously on health 24 hours a day without losing the point of the whole thing, which is to move into a right way of living. When we become obsessed with nutrition and health matters, we become addicts—healthaholics— and I wonder if Nature doesn't give in just a little bit.

There has to be some compromise, some bending in life. If you're going to do everything with military precision, you're going to have to become a hermit; you're going to have to go off by yourself. Eventually, you'll find that the world is not built this way. Now I believe a long life lived is not good enough, but a good life lived is long enough. The main point is to educate yourself and establish health patterns that allow you to be active mentally, high spiritually and vitally alive physically. That's what I call high level well-being.

Balance in life is most important. It is a high priority. I've had so many patients come to the Ranch, especially women, and you know they go home with some nice ideas that I give them. What happens then? They drive their husbands and children crazy by demanding instant food enlightenment from them. "You can't do this, you must do that, you've got to change." Who is going to live by that kind of stuff? The poor husband says, "Do I have to eat this?" The kids ask, "Do I have to eat that?" The first thing you know, all the nice things I've shared with them have been turned into homemade disaster.

Now it would be best to do it in degrees. It would be well to take your time in changing your way of life. Don't jump into it. I was a strict vegetarian 25 years, but I've backed up a little bit. Before, I didn't believe in milk; I didn't believe in cheese. There were so many things I didn't believe in that I found myself stuck in a place where I couldn't go out to eat with anyone. To this day, if my wife and I go out to eat, I am very selective about where I go. It must be a nice place to eat, a place where the chef knows about foods. I'm not so choosy about what sort of theater I go to. You can take me anywhere. But you can't take me to just any restaurant.

The same standard holds in our home. The food has to be good. I tell my wife to spend all the money she needs on foods, because if we don't spend it on good food, it will be spent on doctors. Doctors make their living on the mistakes we make in the kitchen; the mistakes we put on our dinner plates; the mistakes we eat. However, we don't need to be so perfect that we become perfectly rigid. We need to bend with the wind once in a while. At my son's birthday party, my wife brought out a dozen cookies and asked him to pass them around. David started passing them out to the 12 children, and when he came to the last child, there was only one cookie left on the plate. I remember him looking at that cookie and saying, "You know, I think I'd better take this cookie. I can eat it because I've been living on health foods." If we're healthy, we can take a break once in a while without seriously compromising our way of life. Let's face it, if you try to keep your kids away from cookies and away from everybody who might give them cookies or candy, including grandma and grandpa, I'll tell you, you're going to have a difficult job.

If you want to be a strict vegetarian you can go that way. If you want to live on lettuce leaves, you can go ahead. I'm not going to try to persuade you to do anything against your will. I believe you should eat in such a way that your meals are attractive and pleasant, that the foods you eat assist in promoting good bowel movements, in getting rid of skin problems and in bringing you to a level of vitality you enjoy. How you do that, how far you go, is your business. Mine is the middle road.

I don't exactly like health foods. I eat them because I've learned they keep me well and I learned the hard way. I was born into a Danish family. I was raised on rich Danish foods, coming out of a lifestyle where Danish pastry and 20 cups of coffee a day was the custom. When people talk about coffee today and coffee substitutes, I'll tell you there is no substitute for coffee. It is the real thing as far as I am concerned. On the other hand, I don't drink it. I know it's not good for me. But I had to find it out for myself. I *did* find it out, and I also found out many other things along the way. I discovered we need phosphorus and calcium for our bones. We need silicon for the skin and hair. We have to have sodium for the stomach wall. Each organ and each tissue structure has its own needs.

In the process of evolution, we find that grasses come first, then herbs. From herbs, vegetables emerged. Originally, all vegetables were herbs. And, each vegetable, fruit, herb and grass brought out a certain combination of biochemicals from soil, water and air. The human body, also made of biochemicals, needs the right elements to replace the cells that grow old and die. All disease conditions are characterized by lack of one or more of the chemical elements.

The Four Most Needed Chemical Elements

Looking back on over fifty years of working with patients, the four most important chemical elements I find lacking in nearly everyone who has come to my office are:

Calcium
Iodine
Sodium
Silicon.

Calcium. The nickname for calcium is "the knitter." If you break a bone, you must have calcium or you can't knit. If you have a leg ulcer that won't heal, you must get calcium into the body before it will begin to improve. When a person comes to me feeling sick, calcium is the first element I think of. Without calcium, you can't heal anything in the body.

Calcium provides energy, tone and power. On the physical side, we associate it with strength; on the mental side with courage. Those who don't have sufficient calcium, tend to be fearful, cautious, timid. They have great difficulty meeting problems and facing difficulty. A deficiency in calcium can hinder or prevent a person from having the drive and determination to become a success in life. To be a success, a person can't remain a "milktoast." We need the calcium to move out and take charge.

The new lady president of the Parent Teacher's Association in town had just finished her inaugural speech. When the applause ended, she pointed to the front row and said, "Now, I'd like to introduce my husband. Squeak up, dear."

To get past the "squeak up" syndrome, we must have calcium. There are people who can't make decisions due to the effects of calcium deficiency. Paranoia, unfounded anxiety and stuttering can result from a lack of calcium in the body.

We must get our calcium from foods. Nuts, seeds, grains and milk products are high in calcium. The metabolic control of calcium in the body is balanced by green leafy vegetables and by getting enough iodine. Because calcium works with phosphorus, we must make sure we have a balance. We need two-and-a-half times as much calcium as phosphorus in the bloodstream.

Some years ago a patient came in with 13 leg ulcers running green and yellow pus. The ulcers had appeared 3 years before, and this lady had spent a great deal of time and money at well-known medical clinics trying to get rid of them. The main problem had been diagnosed as pellagra, calcium deficiency. There was no knitting going on, despite the fact that one clinic spent three months trying to get calcium in her. She couldn't assimilate the chalk-like form of calcium they gave her.

At another clinic, she was given iodine in an attempt to stimulate or develop control over calcium. They had the right idea, but they were giving her inorganic calcium instead of the biochemical form, and the iodine didn't work.

She wanted to try a diet approach, so I began trying to figure out what to do. I'd been reading about the Hunza people who had no disease and many of whom lived to the ripe old age of 120 or so with every tooth still in their heads. "What a great calcium diet they must have had," I thought to myself. Long lives, no pigeon chests, pronated ankles or other calcium related problems. And, about two-thirds of their diet was greens, vegetables that grow in the sunshine. I thought about the time I had to take care of a child with pronated ankles. I used a sun lamp, a mercury-arc lamp and the results were wonderful. I thought, if direct sunshine can help develop calcium control, why wouldn't indirect sunshine work just as well through the green vegetables? I'm telling you, the idea really came through to me.

I put this lady on greens. This was in the day before liquefiers and juicers, so I had her cut the green leafy vegetables very fine with a knife, then put them in water to soak for an hour or two. Straining the mixture through cheesecloth and squeezing the pulp, she drank the juice. I kept her busy doing this every day. As the weeks passed, the pus stopped draining and new pink skin began to form. We didn't stop the juice program at this sign of progress, because even then I felt that healing an imbalanced body chemistry was a long-term program. Yet, can I say I was delighted? Can I say that seeing those multiple leg ulcers heal completely made a believer out of me? When you begin to understand the healing power of foods by seeing it happen before your eyes, it really awakens you.

Iodine. Possibly the most dramatic symptom of iodine deficiency is goiter, enlargement of the thyroid gland. The thyroid gland is an iodine organ. Its two secretions, thyroxin and triiodothyronine, are powerful hormones containing iodine, and when the thyroid gland is deprived of iodine, it enlarges to filter more of the bloodstream to pick up as much iodine as possible. This enlargement is called goiter.

Nations far inland from the sea, like Switzerland, are those most prone to goiter. Iodine is a sea element, found in abundance in seaweed, fish and all seafood. The Japanese, who depend on the sea for much of their food, have no problem with goiter.

Why is iodine so important? The thyroid is an extremely sensitive gland, exerting a great deal of control over the metabolism of the body and taking part in at least 20 biochemical processes. The thyroid, called the "emotional gland," is under the control of the pituitary, the "master gland" of the endocrine system. But, no matter how well the pituitary functions, the thyroid can't do a thing without iodine. The speed of all basic cell functions—food assimilation, tissue building, waste elimination and others—depends on the thyroid. The thyroid and parathyroid glands together regulate calcium, the "knitter." Through its effect on the metabolism and the regulation of calcium, iodine plays a key part in healing and in high level well-being.

We find two common conditions of imbalance in the thyroid. In hyperthyroidism, the thyroid is speeded up beyond normal and uses up iodine rapidly. In hypothyroidism, the thyroid is functioning below normal, often because of lack of iodine. To take care of either condition, iodine is needed in the diet.

The hyperthyroid person is nervous and easily excitable, while the hypothyroid person is sluggish, both mentally and physically. Hypothyroid women may have menstrual problems, and hypothyroidism generally results in dry skin and puffiness of hands and face.

Healing, we can see, is powerfully affected by the thyroid gland. Because it is so sensitive to the emotions, I always emphasize positive attitudes to my patients. Positive attitudes, together with adequate iodine intake, work wonders in healing many conditions.

I was once called to a home in Bremerton, Washington, where a three-year-old baby girl had a sore about the size of a half dollar at the end of her spine. The parents said she was born that way. Checking the irides of the mother and father, I could see where a weakness in the thyroid area of each indicated problems with holding enough iodine. The baby had inherited the condition, so I knew she needed iodine.

The little girl began taking 30 dulse tablets, rich in iodine, every day. Within a month and a half, the sore had healed. To see the iodine increase the healing rate and control the calcium was a wonderful thing.

Sodium. When I talk about sodium in front of my classes, someone always asks about table salt, which is common inorganic sodium chloride. Table salt presents us with a classic difference between inorganic and organic sodium compounds. We find that excessive use of salt can bring calcium out of solution, leading to arthritis and calcium deposits in the joints. Inorganic table salt has been linked with heart disease, hardening of the arteries and other conditions, and yet many of these same people show a lack of sodium in the gastrointestinal tract. They need organic sodium—the "youth" element—the kind we find in whey, goat's milk, celery and other foods. Table salt can't supply that need because its vibratory rate is too low. We need the elements as evolved in foods, not as mined from rock salt and processed at high temperatures in factories. No one needs inorganic table salt, but we all need plenty of sodium in our foods.

In my sanitarium work, I noticed one of the most common problems with all of my patients was an underactive bowel. The science of iridology, the analysis of tissue conditions in the body as revealed in the iris, always shows the stomach and bowel to be the most underactive organs in the body. These are sodium organs. When sodium is depleted in the gastrointestinal system, we know it is depleted elsewhere in the body. The deficiency is affecting all organs and tissues that need it in greater or lesser degree.

Sodium performs many vital functions in the body. It buffers acids in the stomach and intestine and assists in the transport of nutrients through the walls of the small intestine. If there wasn't a lot of sodium in the stomach wall, the hydrochloric acid would eat a hole right through it. We have to have an alkaline stomach wall. A high concentration of sodium is found in the fluid surrounding the cells of the body, while potassium is the main element inside the cells. The electromagnetic interaction of these two biochemicals controls the distribution and movement of water in the tissues, and a related interaction of the same two elements is vital in nerve impulse passage through synapses, the gaps connecting nerve cells. The amount of sodium in the body is regulated by the gastrointestinal tract, kidneys, adrenal glands and skin.

What do people do when they have stomach problems, digestive problems? They take bicarbonate of soda, an inorganic sodium compound. Antacids are the wrong way to go in getting sodium into the body. It must be brought in by foods to have the proper activity, the proper vibrational quality for assimilation and use by the tissues.

Both physical labor and mental stress can deplete sodium from the body. When we work or exercise hard, we perspire, and perspiration carries sodium chloride with it. When we work at Ulcers, Inc. or worry over a bad marriage, we lose sodium as a consequence of overworked adrenal glands. I've seen some people get married and go downhill from the first day, becoming anemic, chemically deficient and imbalanced in their metabolism. Others get married, and their health blossoms. Personality clash triggers biochemical imbalance, while harmony and love promote high level well-being.

Sodium is the element we need most to keep young and active, pliable and limber in the joints. After the gastrointestinal system, the next highest sodium structures in the body are the joints. When a patient comes in who can't move his fingers, who has stiff and painful joints with calcium deposits around them, what does he lack? Sodium. That's what rheumatic pains and troubles are all about—extreme deficiency of biochemical sodium.

Where do we get sodium? In whey. Cheesemakers take milk and make cheese by separating the whey from it. They throw away the whey and sell us the binding part—cheese. Whey is the laxative part of milk, and we don't get enough of it.

Rheumatism and arthritis indicate chemical shortages, chemical imbalance. The people who have these conditions either haven't been getting enough sodium in their diets, or they have been burning it out through hate, bitterness, unforgiveness, resentment, resistance and a life out of harmony.

There is a myth going around that arthritis is a disease of old age. An elderly lady, so the story goes, went to see her doctor about arthritis pains in her left knee. "How old are you?" the doctor asked. "I'm 65," she said. "I'm 65 and I have arthritis, too," the doctor told her. "There's no cure for it. Just go home and chalk it up to old age." And this little old lady looked at the doctor and said, "I want to tell you something. My right

knee is the same age as my left knee, and it doesn't have arthritis!"

Arthritis is not a matter of age, it is a matter of body chemistry.

A ten-year-old girl from Salt Lake City was carried into my office by her mother just as a 92-year-old patient was leaving. The youngster could scarcely move due to arthritis, while the older man was as spry and limber as a colt. The young girl couldn't walk or clothe herself. I have heard of cases of infants with arthritis. It is not a condition confined to the elderly.

Arthritis Can Be Overcome at Any Age

Ethel Lesher, 98, has been on the Johnny Carson television show and has her own dance band in Cottonwood, California. She played the piano on one of our recent shipboard cruises and is a living inspiration to anyone who has had arthritis.

At the age of 76, Ethel came to see me at the Ranch with a bad case of arthritis. "I've been healthy most of my life," she said, "but I became run-down from doing too much. I was working hard on the ranch and was actively involved in five organizations. I took a trip in 1961 and when I came back, I felt weak and my knees were swollen. My doctor told me I had arthritis. He said we all get it as we grow older and that I'd just have to live with it. That kind of stirred me up. I didn't want to live with it. I tried different ways, looking for something that would help, but it just got worse."

Remembering a lecture of mine given in Redding, California, years before, Ethel decided to come to my Ranch in Escondido to find out what she could do. I put Ethel on a program that included vitamin B-12, jacuzzi baths, the cold water Kneippe baths, barefoot grass walks and a food regimen with some of the high sodium foods such as whey, celery and okra to bring the calcium into solution in her body. It took her two years to get rid of the arthritis.

"I thought I would never play the piano again," Ethel said. "But gradually I was able to get back to it."

She began playing with a band—drummer, tenor sax and banjo player—for senior citizen groups. The local Veteran's Hall asked the band to play at a dance, and their music was so well liked that they played there Saturday nights for

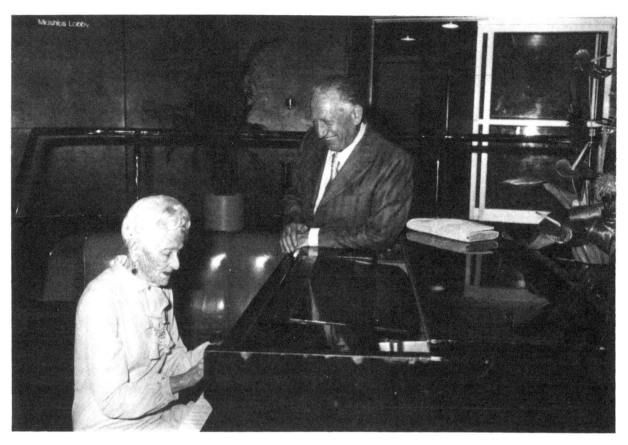

Dr. Bernard Jensen with Ethel Lesher, 98, at the piano. To grow old and yet retain youth, we must keep active and interested in life.

SECRETS OF OVERCOMING HEALTH PROBLEMS

The Ethel Lesher story is among the most satisfying of my career, but there are many others I could mention. I have seen patients come off their death beds and continue to improve until they were able to resume full, normal lives. There are a few secrets to this kind of success, and not all the credit goes to the doctor.

The best doctor can do little for an uncooperative patient. So much depends upon the patient's determination to get well, upon his or her willingness to make major lasting life changes, that a great deal hangs on the patient's attitude. It is only now, in recent times that people have begun to learn that they are primarily responsible for taking care of lthemselves, for eating right, getting enough rest, exercising and so forth. Once a person has grasped this principle, a giant step forward has been taken.

On the doctor's side, I believe there is much more to take care of than the patient's body. Especially among those with chronic conditions, every resource at the patient's disposal, body, mind and spirit, must be considered and brought to lbear on the healing process if the patient is to get well. A positive attitude is a must. Willingness to work with the doctor is a must. And perseverence through what is often a long, routine program of cleansing and rebuilding is a must. Everybody is looking for a good doctor, but I look for good patients. A good patient is one who will do whatever is necessary to leave the disease or ailment behind.

Perhaps the most useful art a doctor can have is to touch that part of the patient, something deep inside, that engages the will to live and get well at all levels of the person. This, I believe, is one of the greatest keys to the wholistic healing art.

58

three years. The crowd that came to dance tripled in that time. Johnny Carson heard about the Ethel Lesher Band and asked her to appear on the Tonight Show, a crowning touch for a woman in her 90s once almost crippled by arthritis. Ethel is able to dance—she danced with the ship's social director on our cruise—and to keep up with all the usual household tasks.

Ethel Lesher watches her foods carefully and closely follows what she learned at my Ranch, eating a variety of fresh vegetables and fruits with eggs, poultry and fish as her main proteins. She keeps her bowels regular, is physically active and has many friends. "I think the mind needs activity as much as the body," she says. Many of those she grew up with have passed away or live in convalescent homes. The remarkable thing about Ethel Lesher is that she has shown how a person can remain healthy, happy, vigorous and active—even youthful—by following the path of right living.

With the proper diet, exercise and other factors taken care of, 25% of my arthritis patients become free of all symptoms. Another considerable percentage are helped.

I don't claim to have a special touch. The answer is nutrition. Nature does the curing. All we can do is give nature a helping hand.

Goat's milk is a high sodium food. Have you ever watched goats? They are among the nimblest animals on earth, jumping and playing on rocks as if it were effortless. Their joints are superbly limber. Cows, on the other hand, are calcium animals. Their hides are thick, their bones are heavy and they are plodders. There is no quickness, grace or limberness in them. I have seen goats climb on the roof of a low barn. You'd have to use a crane to get a cow up there.

We find sodium in fruits, especially citrus. In my younger years as a hygienist, I used to recommend citrus highly. But when I moved to the citrus belt of California and found they pick citrus two months early, I backed off. Green fruit is not good for us. Now I tell patients to avoid it unless they can find tree-ripened citrus.

Okra and celery are high in sodium, as is the veal joint broth Rocine recommends which is made as follows: Get a clean, fresh, uncut veal joint and wash in cold water. Put into large cooking pot, cover half with water and add the following, cut finely:

1-1/2 C. apple peelings
2 C potato peelilngs
Small celery stalk
1/2 C. okra, canned or fresh
1 large parsnip
1 onion
2 beets, grated
1/2 C chopped parsley

Simmer all ingredients 4-5 hours; strain off liquid and discard solids. Drink warm or hot. Store leftover broth in refrigerator.

Silicon. We call silicon the "magnetic" element, because the silicon type is a charming, "magnetic" personality, graceful in movement, a good dancer. Glossy hair and healthy skin and fingernails result from adequate silicon in the diet. On the other hand, those with hair and skin troubles, catarrhal problems, people who seem to have two left feet when dancing—these things show a need for silicon.

Once when I was sick as a young man, a homeopath prescribed Avena sativa, a homeopathic cell salt, for my condition. I paid $15 for a small vial. After I became acquainted with Dr. V. G. Rocine, a homeopath, I asked him what Avena sativa was. "It's an extract from oat straw, high in silicon," he said.

"Oat straw!" I exclaimed. "Is there any way of getting this stuff any cheaper?" I was a student then, and money wasn't growing on trees.

"There certainly is," Dr. Rocine said. "You just get oat straw and boil it for ten minutes. Drink 2 or 3 cups a day, and in six months, you'll have your results."

Dr. Rocine taught me that the biochemicals in foods are naturally triturated and potentized, just like the cell salts and other remedies of the homeopaths. He taught me foods are our best medicines, and I have lived by that philosophy.

Just as calcium is stored in the bones, and sodium is stored in the digestive system, silicon is stored in the skin and hair. The ladies want "the skin you love to touch." That comes from silicon. The nervous system and glands also require silicon.

For acne, skin breaking out and boils, silicon is needed. For itching rectum, itching skin, psoriasis—any skin problem—it is most likely a lack of silicon. For falling hair, cracking nails and running ears—silicon. People come to me, and almost before they begin to describe their symptoms, I'm thinking, "Silicon, silicon, silicon...." The effects of silicon deficiency are very clear cut.

One of my patients had seen about 24 doctors before he was 27 years old, trying to find someone who could help him take care of a severe case of psoriasis.. No one seemed to be able to do a thing for him. A special diet high in silicon foods and a tissue cleansing program finally helped him. Improvement was evident in a few months. Now, he's doing very well, although he still has more work to do.

Can you understand how important the chemical elements are to the body? Who can tell us what happens when they are lacking? Who can tell us what to do? The average doctor doesn't know this. The average parents don't know this. I'm sorry to say, my family didn't know a thing about it. Every sick person has a lack of one or more chemical elements.

Silicon is in flaxseed, used a good deal by the Irish in their diet. The Irish often have beautiful hair.

When I buy a horse or a goat, I always feel the hair. I don't want a drab-coated horse or a dull-haired goat. I'm looking for sleek, glossy coats, animals with spirit and magnetism. The milk from the goat is affected by every organ in its body, and if it doesn't have silicon in it, it isn't going to feed me properly. You can't draw an element from a goat that doesn't have it.

The same principle applies to human child bearing. A mother gives life to her child, drawing from all the nutrients in her body. In a sense, the child draws its calcium from her bones, its sodium from her stomach and joints, its iodine from her thyroid, its silicon from her hair and skin. What the mother doesn't have, the child can't get, and any deficiencies will affect the child's health.

When we marry, we don't want to marry an "old goat" with falling hair and no magnetism. Of course, hair loss can come from a glandular disturbance, an imbalance of male over female hormones. Overwork, poor circulation, clogged blood capillaries and adhesions under scalp can cause baldness. We need our hair, because our hair is our antenna. But, we must also have silicon to have a good skin, good nerves and good glands. Without enough silicon, you can't wink and mean it.

The food highest in silicon is rice polishings, followed by sprouts, seeds and beans. Oat straw tea and potato peeling broth are high in silicon, and yet we so often throw the potato peelings away. It is found in bran, in the outer coatings of all grains. That is one of the reasons I tell people to eat the whole thing, the whole food.

Foods for Specific Conditions

Working with V. G. Rocine taught me a lesson that has been a wonderful principle in all my work over the years: food is our best medicine. Food is the only thing that can build new tissue, build a new body.

Before any disease settles into a body, catarrh is encountered. The mucus, phlegm and catarrh being expelled from the body are signs that toxic elimination is taking place. We should never stop a catarrhal flow nor suppress it with drugs, but eat foods and take drinks that assist in catarrhal elimination. Likewise, there are antitoxic foods, foods which contain various specific biochemicals and essences, foods with solvent properties and foods which are antipsoric and antiscorbutic to take care of the skin and to prevent or eliminate scurvy. The following sections list foods which have been found to be helpful in these conditions. The last section in the group provides health tips for many specific conditions.

Foods and Conditions which are Beneficial for Catarrh

Alfalfa tonic
Antibacterial foods for infections
Blackberry juice
Bone broth
Boneset tea (for flu, catarrh)
Calcium food
Chlorine food (for phlegm, mucus, catarrh and pus catarrh)
Clam broth
Cucumber broth
Dry climate and heat
Eggshell broth (for ovarian catarrh)
Egg white, beaten
Fish roe

Fluorine (for lung trouble)
Formic acid food (for starch catarrh)
Grindelia blossom tea
High altitude
Iodine food (for watery catarrh)
Iron food
Low protein food
Magnesium (for eye catarrh)
Mangoes
Milk and eucalyptol tonic
No meat or milk diet
Nonstarch diet
Nonsugar food
Oat straw broth
Oatmeal dishes
Onion poultice (for throat)
Onion syrup (for sunset catarrh)
Onion tonic
Redweed tea
Russian raspberry tea (for exophthalmia)
Salad greens
Silicon food (for pleural catarrh)
Sodium food (for pus, catarrh)
Strong sunlight (for germ catarrh)
Tannic acid food
Tartaric acid food
Vegetable juices
Wheat straw tea

Foods Which Are Antitoxic

Foods often contain toxic matter from vegetable, meat or fish sources. Manufactured foods contain many harmful toxins. In addition, toxins are generated by the body itself, from body impurities in bones, tissues or brain or from decaying leukocytes in the blood. The liver is the organ which breaks down such toxins. When the liver is not functioning properly, toxins may be conveyed to the brain and may ultimately cause brain disease or insanity. Toxins may also damage the blood, the kidneys and glands, affecting secretions.

Almost all vegetables, grains, nuts and drinks such as tea, coffee, chocolate and colas contain toxins. A few contain no toxins—eggs and milk, for example. Certain other foods help to neutralize and fight toxins in the body. These toxin fighters are able to help purify the blood

and usher toxic gases and bile products out of the body. Such antitoxic foods include:

Alfalfa tonic
Bitter greens
Blackberry juice and products
Black raspberry juice
Cherries
Cherry juice
Dewberries
Dewberry juice
Dwarf nettle broth
Grindelia tea
Highly laxative and harmless foods
Hop tea
Leak greens
Magnesium foods
Mangoes
Pichi leaf tea
Pomegranates
Raspberry juice
Sage tea
Sage tea with clam broth
Spearmint
Tamarinds
Tamarind whey
Tannic acid food
Tartaric acid foods (some)
Wild cherry juice

Foods Which Are Antiseptic

Some foods are known to be antiseptic, while others are antitoxic and still others are both. Foods which are always antiseptic and healing are lime foods and silicon foods or broths. The latter are particularly beneficial in soothing mucous areas which have become ulcerated. The most highly antiseptic foods are:

Bramble berries
Boneset tea
Burdock leaf tea
Cashew nuts
Chervil
Cucumber
Currants
Eggshell broth
Eucalyptol
Grapefruit
Grapes: Concord, green, white
Iodine food
Lemons
Lime food

Mangoes
Mulberries
Nettle broth
Oat straw broth
Pineapple juice
Plums, all 300 varieties
Prickly pears
Salty, hot drinks
Silicon food
Sodium foods
Sorrel
Sulphur food
Spearmint tea
Tamarinds
Tartaric fruit acid
Tomatoes
Tomato poultices
Veal joint jelly
Wheat straw broth
Wintergreen

Foods Which Contain Various Chemical Elements and Essences

Essences contained in foods may be either harmful or helpful to our bodies. Food should not be poisonous or drugging in its effect; it should be beneficial, medicinal.

Each of the following food chemicals affects the body in a particular way. We need to know how, what and when to eat, as well as how to combine our foods to obtain maximum benefit from our diet and enhance our health and beauty.

Alcohol: beer, wines, liquors
Alkaloids: kola nuts, peppers, colas, cocoa, chocolate, tea, coffee, tobacco
Alliol: chives
Allyl: leeks
Amygdaline: bitter almonds, sometimes edible almonds
Anethol: dill
Anthriscin: chervil
Apiol: celery, parsley
Arachin: peanuts
Aroma: quince
Arsenic: egg yolk, grapes, raisins
Artocarpin: bread fruit
Asparagin: asparagus, beans, peas, romaine
Avenin: barley, oats

Berberin: barberries, blackberries, bilberries
Betaine: beets, mussels
Bitters: endive, hops, sage, birch bark and leaves, senna
Brassin: all cabbage
Caffein: coffee
Capsicum: red peppers, paprika
Caracin: papaya
Cardol: cashew nuts
Carotene: carrots
Celtin: hackberries
Caratonin: carob
Chamol: clams
Cholin: meat muscle
Cinnamic aldehyde: cassia, cinnamon
Cinnamon: cassia
Citrin: limes
Citrol: citron
Cucumin: cucumbers
Ergot: grains, often rye
Essence: bananas, sassafras, tangerines
Ether: cardamon, peaches
Eucalyptol: eucalyptus honey
Eugenol: cloves, allspice, pimentos
Euonymin: strawberries
Ingluvin: gizzard
Iodine: green turtle, oysters, crabs, herring
Juniperol: juniper berries
Lactucarium: wild lettuce
Lactucerin: lettuce
Laurin: coconut oil
Leontodin: dandelion
Lupulin: hops
Menthol: spearmint
Myristin: coconuts, nutmeg
Nut toxin: nearly all nuts
Opuntin: prickley pears
Origanin: marjoram

Essences:
Pagurin: sea crab
Panacin: millet
Pectenol: shellfish
Pelletierin: pomegranates and their roots
Piperin: black and white pepper
Prunin: prunes
Quercin: acorns
Ranin: frog legs
Resin: mace
Ribin: currants, gooseberries
Ricin: caster oil
Sabalol: serenoa

Salicin: wintergreen
Salviol: sage
Sambucin: elderberries
Scolymin: artichokes, cardoons
Secalin: rye
Sequiterpene: pimentos
Sinalbrin: white mustard
Sinigrin: black mustard
Solanin: potatoes
Sovariol: butternuts
Tannin: chicory, nettles, greens, tea, pimentos
Thein: tea
Theobromin: chocolate, cocoa
Thiol: nasturtium, onions
Thiosinamin: horseradish
Toxid fumes: bleached flour or foods
Triticin: couch grass, green wheat

Foods Which Affect the Skin

The primary food elements which heal and nourish the skin are sulphur, potassium, silicon, calcium, fluorine and iodine foods. An excess of food sulphur is irritating to the skin and may cause eruptions. Food sulphur deficiency results in itching, psoriasis and exanthemata, particularly in babies whose mothers were sulphur-starved before the birth.

Some fatty material also enters the skin. Fats (meat, butter and oils) in excess may cause prolific boils on the skin. Sunlight, heat, cold and air affect the skin as well. Psoriasis is benefitted by a warm sunny climate, a high lime diet and concurrent flaxseed poultices and certain other foods.

Food elements necessary for the health and integrity of the skin are supplied by bone broth, oat straw broth, eggshell broth, goat cottage cheese, lemons and veal joint jelly. An antiseptic, anesthetic oil (thymol) which is helpful to the skin is contained in thyme or its broth. The skin is protected against bacteria and parasites by sulphur, calcium, silicon, fluorine and potassium foods.

It is, of course, necessary to ascertain first what skin elements are lacking or in overabundance, and then eat foods which supply or counteract the abundance. The appearance of the skin, pain, eruptions and other symptoms give us clues as to which

elements are out of balance. For instance, sulphur is related to pellagra and beriberi. Silicon protects and insulates the skin.

Foods Which Are Antipsoric and Antiscorbutic

Antipsoric foods counteract skin ailments and itching while the antiscorbutic foods are high in vitamin C and counteract scurvy. There are, of course, differing causes of psora, psoriasis and other skin and itch ailments in different people. Scurvy is nearly always caused by lack of fresh fruits and vegetables. Here we mention only the foods which are known to have a particular effect on the skin.

Apple peeling broth
Apricots
Artichokes
Baker's yeast
Barberries
Bergamot
Bilberries
Birch bark tea
Bitter teas
Blackberries
Blueberries
Bone broth
Burdock leaf tea
Cloud berries
Cold baths
Cranberries
Currant juice
Dandelion
Dewberries
Eggshell broth
Endive
Elderberries
Flaxseed poultices
Gelatin dishes
Goat cottage cheese
Gooseberries
Grapes
Guavas
Hackberries
Huckleberries
Juice from greens
Juniper berries
Kale broth
Leek greens
Lettuce (head)
Lemons
Lemon-milk curd

Limes
Loquats
Mandarines
Mangoes
Mangosteen
Nectarines
Mulberries
Oat straw broth
Okra
Opuntia (prickly pear)
Oranges
Oregon grapevine tea
Oysters
Pineapple
Plums
Pear peeling broth
Pine needle tea
Raspberries
Roebuck berries
Rutabaga
Saffron tea
Sassafras tea
Sorrel
Sunlight
Spearmint tea
Spinach
Swiss chard
Tamarinds
Tangerines
Tomatoes
Thyme
Turnip leaves
Veal joint jelly
Watercress
Wheat straw broth
Whortleberries

Foods Which Have Solvent Properties

Certain foods are known as solvent foods. For example, food lime dissolves oxalic acid. Sodium is solvent to lime. Salicylic acid and heat keep uric acid in solution. Food magnesium acts to maintain an open bowel. Formic acid food lowers inflammation in diseased tissues, forestalls congestion and acts on starch ferments, tumors and pus. Food sulphur is able to promote the flow of bile, maintain the balance of phosphorus in the body, aid elimination and stimulate the cells. Food silicon is able to build and repair membranes, walls, linings and canals and protect them from parasites, bacteria and infection. Chlorine is a germicide which, with sodium, slows blood clotting, cleanses the body, and aids in keeping blood, albumin, fibrin and casein in solution.

Foods which contain the above elements in generous quantities are solvent and cleansers. They help eliminate hardenings, crystallizations, cysts, fibroids, gout rheumatism, calculi, tumors, ossification and they counteract degenerating eyesight and hearing caused by hardening.

If we only knew how to eat, from birth to death, we would, no doubt, be in perfect health. But we do not even pretend to know all the details of food chemistry, diet and nutrition, nor the chemistry of men and diseases. The areas to be studied and researched are many and different. Foods affect people in different ways, and there are many kinds and causes of tissue hardening and stone formation.

We do know that the most solvent foods, broths and teas seem to be these:

Alonyl
Apollac
Arbutus (Calif. variety)
Asparagus shoots
Ash leaf tea
Avocado
Beets (red, white, yellow)
Bile-producing food
Bone broth
Black willow bark tea
Beet skin and root broth
Bilberries
Blueberries
Celery cabbage
Celery juice
Citron
Cloudberries
Condensed goat's whey
Cowberries
Cranberries
Currants
Custard apples
Dandelion broth
Dewberries
Dwarf nettle broth
Duckweed broth
Eggshell broth
Eucalyptus honey
Formic food acid
Goat milk whey

Gooseberries
Grapefruit
Hot milk applications
Kumquats
Kale broth
Lactic food acid
Lemons
Limes
Mandarin oranges
Mangoes
Nectarines
Oranges
Oyster broth
Papaya
Pineapple
Plums
Pomegranates
Prune juice
Pine needle broth
Red clover tea;
Romaine juice
Raspberries
Seronoa
Strawberries
Sugar beet leaves
Tomato broth
Tomatoes
Tomato poultices
Veal joint vegetable jelly
Wheat straw broth
White clover tea
Willow leaf tea
Wintergreen tea

Health Tips and Home Remedies

Acid stomach: alkaline foods and small meals.
Albuminuria: protein-free diet and mild broths.
Anemia: iron, sodium and chlorine foods, high altitude.
Beriberi: citric juices, lime and bran foods.
Boils: fat-free diet, low sulphur food, onion poultices.
Brain (fatigue): fish roe and fish broths.
Breasts (caked): butter applications and tight bandages.

Chillblains: birch bark decoction as a wash.
Chills: hot, strong mixture of clam broth and sage tea.
Colds: hot, strong mixture of clam broth and sage tea.
Congestion: hot drinks of condensed goat whey.
Convulsions: hot drinks of condensed goat whey.
Feet (sore): olive oil rubbed on; tomato poultice.
Flu: hot juice of baked lemons, to be drunk hourly until system is saturated; then boneset tea to be drunk until fever breaks.
Gallstones: white beet broth, beet (sodium) diet, pumpkin seed broth. Magnesium foods, water through osmosis purifier.
Gas: hot drinks of condensed goat whey, hot salty drinks.
Gout (calcic): calcium-free diet with high sodium diet.
Hay fever: high calcium diet, fish roe in quantity, higher altitude.
Hemorrhages: eggshell broth, gelatine dishes, veal joint jelly, bone broths.
Insect bites: lemon slice tied to area.
Ivy poisoning: Grindelia tea, drunk often.
Kidneys: lukewarm water in rubber bag to be lain on; milk-whey to be drunk often.
Piles: Virgin olive oil as daily wash.
Stomach ulcer: Bed rest for 30 days, no food other than broths with 2-3 tablespoons raw milk added to be drunk lukewarm. Nothing cold or hot should be taken. No solid food should be eaten for about 120 days. (Raw meat juice heals ulcers more quickly than any other food. It should be fresh, from a young, healthy steer and should be kept lukewarm and sipped slowly.)
Throat trouble: Salty water gargles. Liquid chlorophyll.

We will be exploring further into the realm of foods and diet in *The Essence of Man*, to extend and develop the material presented here. An in-depth knowledge of foods, body chemistry and nutrition is essential to the new day health care professional.

Children and Food

First of all, most children are not allowed to nurse enough to get the right start. The bowels of the child are dependent upon a bacterial activity which helps to start the natural peristaltic action and the contractions of the bowel wall. To start this bacterial activity the child is depending upon the colostrum which comes from the mother's breast the first three days after the child is born. It is very difficult for the child to have the proper start with its bowel movements and to have continued normal activity, without the colostrum feeding the acidophilus bacteria, which is natural in every child's bowel. To give artificial formulas is to give the child an artificial start. There is a direct relation between the acids of the child and the acids of the mother. There is the right relation between the acidophilus bacteria of the bowel and the strength of the colostrum to get the bowel started properly. There are very few mothers who are so weak, so chemically depleted, so bad off physically that they cannot nurse their children, at least for those first few days when the child gets its start.

On the other hand, it is a known fact that when animals lack the chemical element manganese, they refuse to nurse their young. When this chemical element has been put in their diet again, the mother love seems to return. This chemical element is called the "mother-love" element. For a mother to deliberately refuse to nurse the child is probably due to the lack of this chemical, and can be attributed to a faulty diet.

Another contributing factor is smoking in excess, as seen by statistics issued by insurance companies, which tell us that many children die before they are a year old due to the fact that mothers have smoked excessively. While we are talking about smoking, I might mention that it has its direct effect on the child so long as it is attached to the mother, before it is born and while it is nursing. Milk can be polluted by cigarette smoking, as the nicotine can be determined in 30 seconds in the mother's milk after the mother smokes a cigarette. The child's body is dependent on the mother's habits of living.

If the acidophilus bacteria is lacking in the bowel, which happens if the child is not fed properly in the beginning, it may be added to our daily routine, over a couple of months, to build up the acidophilus bacteria in the bowel. There is an acidophilus culture we can buy in the health food stores. This, if supplied regularly and with the proper food, helps to build this bacteria, and

the intestinal flora can be normalized. Any whey product will feed the acidophilus best and sweeten the bowel. Without the proper bowel movements, without the proper bacterial activity in the bowel, then we have gas disturbances, a dry bowel, and many children's complaints can develop from this malfunctioning bowel.

In the very young child, a little sugar of milk added to the raw milk may help to feed this acidophilus bacteria that you are implanting in the bowel. Goat or cow whey, either fresh or powdered, can be added to the diet to help feed this bacteria also. If the child cannot take this acidophilus culture by mouth, it can be given by rectum, through use of a baby enema syringe. This procedure is the first step in establishing good health in the child.

Weaning the Baby

The first thought in taking care of the baby is to take care of the mother. See that the mother has as perfect a body as possible. See that her milk comes from a perfect body. If she is not able to give enough milk, add greens to her diet. The tops of vegetables will furnish that which the body needs. Add two to three pints of vegetable juices a day to the mother's diet.

There are times when the mother does not give much milk, and there must be a definite reason. Probably the baby shouldn't have very much. The baby and mother are one; as the mother is, so is the baby for some time. If you want to add a formula along with the mother's milk, I suggest this formula:

1 oz. raw goat or certified raw milk
1/2 oz. pure cream
3 oz. distilled or spring water
1 tsp sugar of milk

You may make changes by cutting down on the certified milk and substituting soybean milk powder mixed with water to the consistency of milk. This formula may be used in weaning the baby. When the time arrives, it is best to start adding a little barley gruel, and gradually, raw vegetable juices.

When weaning the baby, you may add a little broth made of carrots, onion and parsley, finely cut. This is to be strained and only the broth given. A little prune juice or fig juice can be made from unsulphured dried fruits and can be used very well.

As the baby gets older and becomes used to the formula given previously, the amount of water may be gradually cut down.

As the baby grows, we can add a little bit of hard food to the diet to help toughen the gums. Steel-cut oat meal, cooked for two or three hours in a double boiler and allowed to stand overnight before eating is marvelous for building a strong body.

Never use sugar for children. To sweeten, use fruits. For example, mix a few raisins, prunes, figs or dates into the oats before serving. It is best not to use any meat with children. Let their protein be derived from milk and egg yolks up to the age of seven. Greens are best for building strength and bones. Juices are marvelous for supplying the necessary vitamins.

Do not be afraid to fast the children or skip a meal or two. Children seem to know when it is best to eat and when not to. Do not force them to eat fruit but do not allow them to eat anything between meals, except fruit or fruit juice. When they do not grow properly, or have abnormal growths on their bodies, are cold-blooded, have eye trouble, throat ailments or running sores, it is a sign they are lacking silicon. Add steel-cut oat meal or oat straw tea to the diet. Discover the best natural foods for keeping the body in good health.

Start your children on natural foods and they will want only natural foods during their lives. They will be opposed to anything that is too sweet or too salty. A natural body will want natural food.

Goat's Milk for Children

In early childhood and up to the age of seven, milk in greater proportion in the diet is very necessary. And we should know the necessity of supplements, for milk is deficient in iron. The baby in the beginning of life has been given enough iron to more or less take care of his body's needs for about a year after birth, but after that time, milk has to be supplemented to give the growing body the necessary iron. These supplements should be vegetables, especially green vegetables and the tops of vegetables.

Goat's milk compares favorably to mother's milk, while cow's milk contains elements in proportion suited to the building of heavier bones. The cow also has a much larger liver in proportion to its body than the human baby and for this reason can take care of the larger fat globules found in cow's milk. Cow's milk is being homogenized for easier digestion, but it still does not compare to goat milk in the matter of assimilation. The fat globules in goat's milk are five times smaller than in cow's milk, making it much easier for the liver to aid in the digestive processes. Also, the alkaline properties of goat's milk are higher than those of cow's milk.

The goat is a very active animal, very limber, and we find goat milk much higher in sodium than cow's milk. This joint element, sodium, is one of the necessary elements to start the baby off right, for sodium is the element that keeps the stomach sweet, clean and capable of producing hydrochloric acid that will digest the protein in the milk that is yet to come. There is usually a little less cream in goat's milk than in cow's milk, but after all, we don't want to build too fat a baby and we don't want to overload the liver with an excess of fat to take care of. It is better to raise a healthy baby, and a healthy baby is not necessarily a fat one.

Milk is more easily digested and taken care of if it is mixed with other foods. In a heavy acid stomach milk should definitely be mixed with other foods and, many times, diluted, so it doesn't curdle in the stomach too fast. If the milk does not agree, have the child sip it slowly or take it through a straw, so the stomach can handle it more easily. The child should not drink milk rapidly and in large amounts at one time.

For the child, the best foods to combine with goat milk are vegetables or fruits, and the best fruit can be liquefied, if desired, with the milk. All stewed dried fruits are good with milk, and should be used if fresh fruits are not obtainable.

All digestion of the milk does not take place in the stomach, but the coagulation of the milk begins there, and if milk is taken too fast and without the mixture of other foods, coagulation is very difficult and, after it leaves the stomach, the milk cannot be completely digested by the other gastric juices along the intestinal tract.

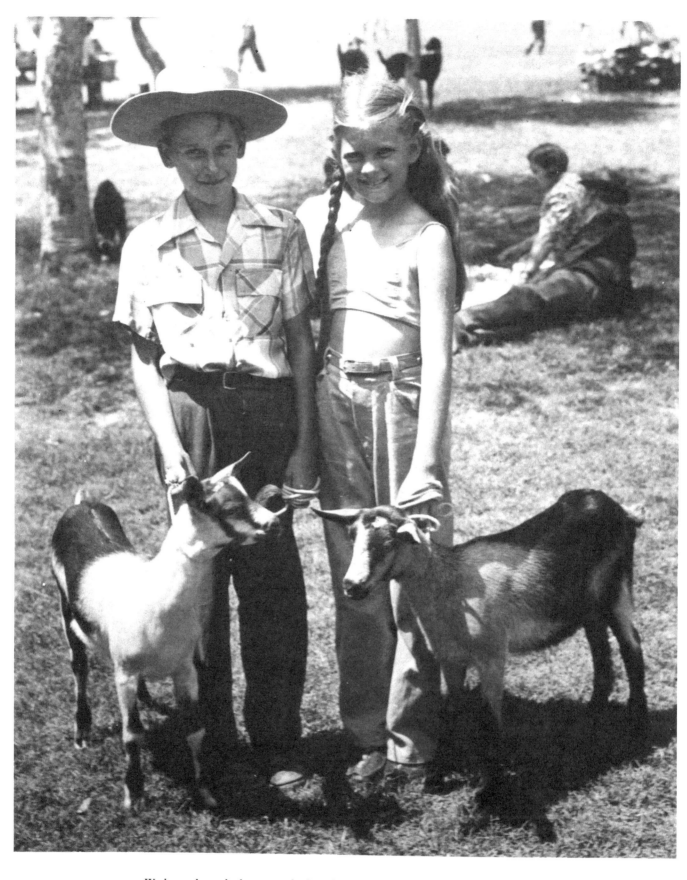

We have always had goats at the Ranch. They are nimble, friendly, curious and intelligent—sodium animals with great limberness of the joints. For getting the greatest life force, the milk should be taken as soon as possible after milking.

Most children who take goat's milk have better bowel movements, and they seem to thrive better than those given cow's milk. We have found, in many cases, that eczema and allergic conditions, asthma and many catarrhal ailments of children have responded by merely using goat's milk instead of cow's milk.

Of course, I believe in raw goat's milk entirely, but there are times when one cannot get the raw milk and will have to use substitutes. There is a dehydrated goat milk on the market which I think is probably better than the dehydrated cow milk, but I do not consider it an entire substitute for the fresh raw milk. When weaning, a little milk sugar or sugar of milk will help in changing over from the mother's milk to the goat's milk.

It is my belief that there is nothing that means more to our intestinal tract, to every cell in our body, to our health and longevity, our beauty and even our happiness, than having lots of salads in our diet. Many children are neglected in this respect because they do not care for salads and we like to please them. You can do a great deal for your children by making half their meals salads. We have had considerable trouble in our home, but we cured this by serving the salad first. Most children are out playing hard, and they come to the table truly hungry. If we start the meal with a big salad it will be easier to train the children in the habit of taking the right foods later in life.

Many chronic ailments are started when we are children. Because raw vegetables contain the natural chemical elements, the use of salads is one way of preventing these chronic ailments that may affect us later in life, such as arthritis, rheumatism, tuberculosis, cancer and diabetes. Starches and proteins are necessary for growing children, but they cannot be built into tissues properly without being combined with vegetables.

We should find ways and means of getting certain vegetables in the child's diet. There are ways of mixing raisins with salads, puffed-up raisins that have been steamed for ten or fifteen minutes, and these add a delightful taste to any green salad. Chlorophyll brings extra oxygen into the blood and children need oxygen to burn up the waste they produce through extreme activities. Extra iron and oxygen are also necessary when tissues are changing so fast and

developing by growing. It is necessary to have the finest material with which to build this structure, for it is in this structure that we have our reserves on which we may call in years to come for any sickness that may develop.

Some greens are slightly bitter, but we sweeten them with raisins or dates, stewed prunes, apricots or peaches. Finely shredded carrot or celery and some of the sweeter vegetables can be mixed with the greens to take away this bitter taste. A salad dressing with cheese flavor or an avocado, improves the taste. There are many ways of changing the taste, and it is important to find ways and means of getting our children to enjoy salads.

In my opinion, people who say, "My children will not eat salads," are not starting the meal correctly. It is a rule in our house that we cannot have the things we like until we have eaten some of the things we MUST eat for our health. It meant a great deal to me to hear my eldest son say that he was so glad that he was taught to eat salads and was shown their value when he was young.

Salads in the diet will keep the child from being constipated. It will produce a strong call to have a bowel movement, which will bring him to the bathroom much quicker than the starch diet of the average American meal. We must teach the child that he should have this natural call, and that he must answer. Vegetables carry a water cellulose that keeps starches from becoming hard and will keep the bowel movements soft, making it easier for the waste material to travel through the intestinal tract. Meals that are overbalanced with starches, sweets and proteins are usually putrefactive, spoil very quickly, and are the basis for many children's diseases.

Problems with the teeth lessen as gum tissues become more firm by the use of more salads in the diet. Colds will occur less often and catarrhal discharges will begin to leave, as we use more of the greens found in the tops of vegetables.

When you have to take lunches to school, use vegetable fillings, chopped pepper and egg, date paste sandwiches, chopped celery and nut butter sandwiches. Remember that the cellulose of vegetables will keep starches from becoming constipating in the body. Be sure that the child has sticks of celery, carrots and slices of green bell peppers along with the starches. One lady was telling me how hard it was to get her children to eat vegetables. All her children are susceptible to colds. She does not have colds as she is the only one who eats salads in her home. We must so discipline our children that they learn to like salads, for their own good.

Confusion Over Foods

It is wonderful to discover all the things we can accomplish with foods when we have the correct information. The problem is in getting the correct information. Food manufacturers and processors, in competing for the greatest possible share of profits, present advertising for their products that goes to the limits of the law in exaggerating the benefits, merits, beauty and taste of their products. At the same time, any disadvantageous features are not mentioned.

So, we are constantly bombarded with advertising propaganda about the merits of foods that actually have little or no food value or that are actually harmful to us.

The average consumer is unaware that there is a great deal of difference between the nutritional value of "live" foods and "dead" foods. Moreover, most shoppers do not know how to interpret the list of ingredients on food labels. Moreover, he or she is greatly influenced by advertising which insists that products filled with additives are "wholesome," "nutritious" and "naturally delicious." It is little wonder that Americans buy according to what is advertised rather than on the basis of sound nutritional knowledge.

Even water is chemically treated. Most city water supplies contain many chemical additives—some 47 in all, although no one city is likely to use all 47. These chemicals are added so as to disinfect, soften, fluoridate, coagulate, chlorinate, oxidate, condition, neutralize, control odor and color, control algae and scale, remove iron and manganese and so forth. This water is not only drunk plain but is the primary ingredient in tea, coffee and many other beverages, in addition to being used for cooking, canning and preserving. We do well to be suspicious of what comes out of our water taps.

Inorganic chemicals are in widespread use as soil fertilizers. These chemicals not only upset the soil balance and bacterial content as described in a previous chapter, but also affect the plants which grow in that soil. James A. Shields, MD, is of the opinion that people who eat food from such fertilized soils are more prone to degenerative and vascular diseases. And a German, Dr. Evers, believes that such degenerative diseases as multiple sclerosis are caused, in part, by the refining and processing of foods and by chemical additives. Incidentally, tests have shown that it takes at least 10 years for the effects of many chemical pesticides and fertilizers to disappear from the soil so that they no longer affect crops.

Food processors and manufacturers have developed some three thousand additives which are used in our foods, and these additives are mostly chemical (not biochemical) in composition. They have not been transformed and evolved by plant life so that we can assimilate them properly. Thus, they act as an accumulative material in the body, an irritant to the tissues. A patient with three thousand eye ulcers was sent to me from an allergy specialist in Chicago. The ulcers would appear mostly after the man had eaten but they left after he came to Hidden Valley Health Ranch, where we were growing foods free of any chemical fertilizers and pesticides. Living on our organically-produced foods cured him, and as long as he stayed with organic produce he had no more trouble. Finally, he got a place of his own and started growing his own food on naturally composted and cultivated soil.

What is in the soil is tremendously important. Even a raw food diet may not be adequate if the chemical composition of the soil is inadequate. The soil may be lacking lime (calcium), iron or chlorine and, consequently, the body will be short of these elements when using food grown in it. Not only the body but the spirit will suffer also from this kind of deprivation. Success, happiness and morality depend on our state of health which depends, in turn, on the chemical elements of the dust of the earth. If we feed our plants properly and eat the food elements needed for our blood, nerves, brain and the various secretions of our glands, we will find that the body will right itself and give harmony throughout its being.

Chemicals in Soils, Plants and Man

As we go up the ladder from soils to plants to animals to man, we find not only an evolving of the vibratory level of the chemical elements but an increasing concentration of some elements as well. Consider the following chart showing the increased amounts of three elements important in human nutrition:

Approximate Ratios of Chemical Elements in Soil, Plants and Man*

Element	Soil	Plants	Man
Calcium	1	8	40
Phosphorus	1	140	200
Sulphur	1	30	130

*Taken from data in *Mineral Nutrition of Plants and Animals* by Frank A. Gilbert (University of Oklahoma Press).

Interestingly, silicon and aluminum, two elements most abundant everywhere on earth, are found only in small amounts in the bodies of animals and man. There are other interesting peculiarities. Animals and men need large amounts of sodium and chlorine, and traces of iodine and cobalt, but none of these appears to be necessary to plant life. However, plants take them in when they are present in the boil. Boron, essential to plants, is not known to be needed by animals. In general, we can't judge the importance of an element by its quantity in the body. There is only about one-sixth ounce of iron in the human system, but without it, we would die.

The dry weight of a plant is approximately 95% composed of carbon, oxygen, hydrogen and nitrogen, all of which are involved in energy production, exchange and storage in the human body. When the soil is high in potassium and low in calcium and a few other elements, starch production increases and protein diminishes. If calcium and sulphur are added, protein content goes up. Elements not included among the main chemicals plants are made of still have a profound effect on their growth and development.

With people and animals, potassium is required to buffer acids produced in working muscle tissue. Lack of potassium foods can slow growth and delay sexual maturity in children, while in adults it is associated with heart and kidney problems. More potassium than sodium is found in the body, despite the fact that sodium in the blood is 18 times the amount of potassium, and this ratio doesn't change when potassium foods and supplements are taken in large quantities. Usually our intake of sodium to potassium should be 2 to 1.

Calcium and phosphorus work very closely together in the human body, with a 2-1/2 to 1 ratio required for optimum health. Calcium in the form of lime has most often been used to sweeten acid soils, yet since the mid-20th century, soil scientists have begun to recognize calcium as a necessary ingredient in fertilizers. Although phosphorus deficiency in soils is the primary cause of low crop yields, calcium deficiency also reduces harvests, and the importance of the relationship between these two elements in the soil may have been underestimated by scientists. Even when a soil is adequately buffered or sweetened, for example, adding more calcium still improved crop yields, probably by assisting in phosphorus and nitrogen utilization. Phosphorus deficiency in cattle has been found on every continent in the world. Phosphorus distribution in the body is 70-80% in the skeleton, 10% in the muscles and 10% in the nerves and brain. Some phosphorus and calcium are needed in all the cells of the body. Studies have shown that unless sufficient calcium is taken, phosphorus can't be used and is excreted. Calcium-poor soils may be as much to blame for phosphorus deficiency in cattle as a lack of phosphorus. In 1968, the U.S. Department of Agriculture released a study showing 30% of the American people were low in calcium. Of course, vitamin D is needed for calcium absorption, and magnesium is an essential element in bones and teeth as well.

Iron is known to be essential to plants and is involved in the production of chlorophyll, although it is not a constituent of chlorophyll. Lack of iron in the soil, or a soil pH which makes iron unavailable, causes yellowing of plant leaves and leads to anemia in livestock. With humans, anemia caused by inadequate iron is sometimes caused by lack of iron in the diet and sometimes by inability to assimilate enough iron. In the latter case, taking copper and cobalt with the iron can improve assimilation of iron. Vitamin B-12, needed for iron assimilation in the bowel, has cobalt in its molecular structure. The best sources of iron in foods are liver, dandelions, parsley, watercress and spinach. Dandelion powder capsules found in the herb departments of natural food stores are a good source of iron.

As in man, chemical deficiencies cause severe problems in plants. These range from chlorosis, leaf-curl, underdeveloped roots and other physiological problems to simply weakening the plant to the point where it is consumed by insects or overcome by disease or parasites. Lack of zinc, like lack of iron, inhibits chlorophyll formation, but also causes scanty foliage and poor fruit. Zinc is needed in all human tissues in about half the amount of iron. It helps in the intestinal assimilation of protein and starch and is found in the pancreas and in insulin. The amount of zinc in a diabetic's pancreas has been found to be about half of that in the same organ in a nondiabetic. Lack of copper in plants leads to stunted growth and disease. In humans, copper assists in iron utilization, but when it is too high, zinc is excreted. My intention is not to cover all problems caused by all deficiencies, but simply to demonstrate that *any* deficiency of *any needed chemical* leads to physiological malfunction in plants, animals and man, often followed by disease.

The art and science of human nutrition is a complex subject, but at its foundation is a simple truth: man must learn to work in harmony with Nature and not in conflict with her in preventing disease conditions and in achieving high-level well-being. Today, depleted soils, toxic sprays and inorganic chemical fertilizers are a fact of life, and it takes a great deal of wisdom and discretion to select foods that will work in the body the way Nature intended.

Deficiencies from One-Sided Diets

When even one of the 16 vital biochemical elements we need for well-being is missing, we cannot remain healthy or do justice to ourselves and our fellow humans. Sometimes, unfortunately, even carefully thought about diets are one-sided or incomplete. For example, we may have a diet lacking in phosphorus and leading to brain inefficiency, nervousness, feeble-mindedness, amnesia, blindness and stupidity. If a diet is made up of all green salads and salad oils, dressings, nuts, fruits and vegetables, it leads to dechlorination of the blood, bacterial infection, colitis, super-hydration, watery bladder or dropsy of some kind. Man dies on a diet limited to processed rice. And if a person lives on a phosphorus-free diet for at least 150 days, the fingertips begin to tingle, the eyesight will weaken, beauty declines and memory fails.

Not only are there deficient diets but some foods, excellent in combination with others, will cause deficiencies if eaten excessively without regard to balance. From quantitative food chemistry, we learn that nuts are low in chlorine, one of the sixteen vital chemical elements. Fruits are lacking in four of the sixteen. Beans are low or lacking in five of the sixteen. Beets are deficient in five; all varieties of cabbage are low in five and high in six of the sixteen; vegetables generally are low or deficient in five; wheat is excessive in sugar and starch and nearly deficient elements.

Cow's milk is low in one and nearly lacking in four of the sixteen chemical elements. Kale is overly high in three and equally low in four. Halibut is deficient in five; nearly all fish is deficient in five. Nearly all sweets are very low in eight and excessive in three chemical elements, and honey is very low in fourteen of the sixteen and excessively high in sugar. The orange is nearly deficient in eight of the sixteen. White bread is deficient in nearly nine. Berries are very low in eight. Potatoes are low in five of the elements and mashed potatoes are almost entirely water and starch.

Koenig's Analysis of Elements in the Body

In the body, there are, of course, more than sixteen chemical elements as we know today, but our concern is with the sixteen major elements needed for human health. Indeed, if we were to concern ourselves with all the chemicals in human systems today we would hear much about lead, arsenic and other toxic metals coming from underground water, from gases and from liquors, including copper from vaccination materials. No wonder we have so many metal mix-ups in our bodies today. Nevertheless, our focus is on the sixteen elements more necessary to our bodies than anything else. Koenig, the outstanding German chemist, has analyzed a man weighing 160 pounds to find the following chemical elements and quantities:

Element	Weight
Oxygen	90 pounds
Carbon	36 pounds
Hydrogen	14 pounds
Calcium	3 pounds
Nitrogen	3 pound-12 oz.
Phosphorus	3 pound-8 oz.
Chlorine	1 pound-4 oz.
Sulphur	4 oz.
Potassium	3-1/2 oz.
Sodium	3 oz.
Fluorine	2-1/2 oz.
Magnesium	2 oz.
Silicon	1-1/2 oz.
Iron	1-1/4 oz.
Iodine	1/6 oz.
Manganese	Trace

Some people have a predominance of one element in their structure over others. There is what is called the heavy calcium, bony type. There is the light-boned silicon type. And there is the heavy, muscular, potassium type. We do not find iodine types or types corresponding to other trace minerals. Because bone metabolism predominates in a man, his temperament, physiology and physique all reflect this condition. Another man whose water absorption is great, is almost nothing but organized similar to a watermelon. Thus the body chemistry is different in each type of person, so that metabolism of the elements and compounds differs considerably among people.

Choosing Foods Properly is Important

The heavy calcium type should have certain foods to maintain his particular kind of body. Because a harmonious or corrective diet is necessary for each type, diets must be studied carefully. We hear of liquid diets, milk diets, vegetable diets, raw food diets, the grape diet and the carrot juice diet. But these diets are not always appropriately corrective or curative. If the blood and tissues lack iron and chlorine, these deficiencies must be supplied at each meal. If some found a compound such as fat, carbohydrates, protein or water, is in excess and then adjusted, progress will occur. We are talking about scientifically responding to the nutritional demands of the body and that is what the word "diet" should imply. To starve one part of the body, say the brain, and to overfeed another part such as the vital system, is not a diet. A raw food diet is not necessarily corrective unless it has the proper biochemical structure or materials in it to suit a particular body trying to normalize itself.

Thus, because foods have particular effects upon the chemistry of the body, the mechanical makeup of one man can handle a given food better than another's. Goat milk is the closest to human milk and a good food for some people, but it does not agree with everyone. Cow's milk and mare's milk build a hairy hide, big bones and solid ligaments for those who have this type of body.

Foods need to be chosen properly, according to chemical type and to the appropriate occasion in one's life. When we are elderly, there are some foods that are very difficult to handle and should be avoided. There are foods that we eat in the winter to heat the blood, such as barley and beans, and there are cooling foods, such as cucumbers, which should be eaten in the summer. We need to know what foods are acid forming and which are constipating. We need to know that some foods are alkaline; some are laxative; some are tonics; some are strength-building.

Iron tonics are alkaline to the blood, whereas potassium tonics are alkaline to the muscles and the urinary system. Sodium drinks are alkaline to the gastro-intestinal system. Silicon tonics are magnetic and preservative. Chlorine is antiseptic, cleansing and germicidal. Water is neutral but tends to wash the alkaline elements out of the body. Coconut cream favors bust development and goat milk is high in fluorine. Fluorine and phosphorus foods are brain builders, whereas chlorine, cholesterol and iron foods are life building.

Food is Our Best Medicine

Blackberries, dewberries and wild cherries are high in tartaric, tannic and malic acids in which we find iron and other salts which favor the blood and the urinary system. Blackberries are also constipating because of the amounts of tannin and iron. Cranberries promote the formation of hipuric acid in the kidneys and liver. Cherries contain a gum that favors the blood and are very high in iron, good cleaners for the liver. Blueberries are excellent for the bowel and elimination. They contain tartaric acid, potassium, sodalite, sodium and iron. Rhubarb favors the bowel but is bad for rheumatism and gallstones because of its oxalic acid. Apples can be very good because of their malic acid and glucose. They are good for nervous people and growing children but in some acid stomachs, apples cannot be handled properly.

oxygen, papain and crayden and are excellent for the bowels, especially if eaten exlusively for one to three days. A diet of figs and goat milk is wonderfully helpful to the gouty or rheumatic person. Peppermint contains pimenthol which is a gas driver. Peaches are very high in magnesium, potassium, phosphorus, oxygen, sugar and distilled water, as well as a sprinkling of hydrocyanic acid, and they are laxative. Cucumbers are good for the blood, for pus tendencies, for summer heat and they are cooling and antiseptic. Lettuce can be alkaline to some people and acid to others. Eucalyptus honey combined with garlic juice favors swollen tonsils. This particular honey contains eucalyptol, cynol, terpene and formic acid.

Onions contain allysulphide and many elements that go deep into cells and send impurities to the surface. Onions have been considered a great germicide and are used in external packs to help with catarrhal problems. Mulberries contain moraxytic acid and favor fevers, because their juice reduces heat without causing perspiration. When the temper is up, with the blood "boiling" and the brain overheated, mulberry juice with the juice of a lime makes a soothing drink. Additionally, mulberry juice is good for stomach disturbances. The lemon has no equal for scurvy.

When we look at a disease, we can always see what biochemical elements are lacking. If the bones do not knit, calcium is lacking. If our foods lack in these two elements, generally, healing will be incomplete. Each fruit and vegetable has its own chemistry, its own metabolism. Each has its unique effects upon the animal or man who takes it into his diet. Thus each element can be used not only as a food but as a medicine. Such knowledge is growing among doctors and patients who constitute a new breed emerging to put our society on a healthier path for the future.

One of the most pressing problems today is the presence in the body of excessive acids, due to improper diet. A heavy carbohydrate diet, for example, will be much too hard for some bodies to handle. Gluten is the master acid-maker in the body, and acids are, of course, the "grim reapers of death." Salt and baking soda similarly cause problems, being irritants to the stomach wall. Salty and spicy diets overstimulate the stomach and lead to excessive secretion of hydrochloric acid. The results are hypochloric ulcer, burning in the stomach, excessive gas and even gloom and melancholia.

When such problems occur, we should know our foods and adjust them so as to live on a dry, chlorine-free diet. Eat small meals often and stop drinking water. Live on the much-beaten egg white and eat fruit and egg-white floats, or the hydrochloric acid will eat into the stomach in the same way rust eats into iron. And we must chew our food well for the stomach's sake. It is not a meat grinder nor a mill and it has no teeth.

Intelligent Vegetarianism

A vegetable diet needs to be studied carefully because strictness here will not supply all the sixteen elements necessary for a balanced diet. Tofu (soybean curd cheese) is desirable for the lacto-vegetarian (no eggs included). The lacto-vegetarian should also have raw milk and raw cheese. Goat milk is the finest dairy product available in this category.

A vegetarian usually needs two proteins in the daily diet because body heat is not derived from cold proteins. Body heat is needed to digest cold vegetarian proteins, and so the circle goes. If the vegetarian uses nuts and seeds, these should be prepared in nut and seed butters, because nuts are not very digestible. All nuts should be acquired in hard shells.

V. G. Rocine wrote that those who include the fish kingdom in the diet (which technically is not vegetarianism), cod fish roe is a wonderful protein source for the brain and nervous system. Prepare it by adding one tablespoon pressed cod roe to a glass of tomato juice, vegetable juice or vegetable broth. Liquefy in the blender. If fish is included in the diet, the best is the kind with fins, scales and white flesh.

Foods which are Easily Digested, Neutral or Laxative

Not only are the following foods easily digested and tolerated by even the weakest of stomachs, but they also have a laxative effect on the intestines and are helpful to the blood. Many of these are foods which promote health and beauty and many are alkaline. The alkaline foods supply the salts essential for the heart, blood and nerves and for oxidation and general secretion and for nourishing the brain and the internal glands.

Easily Digested Foods

Alfalfa sprouts
Almond oil
Almond butter
Anchovies
Apples, baked
Apples, dried, cooked
Apples
Apricots, cooked
Apricots sauce
Artichokes
Asparagus tops
Avocado
Banana
Banana pudding
Beets, well cooked
Beet greens
Bergamot
Blackberry juice sherbet
Black cherries
Black currants
Blueberries
Blueberry juice
Blueberry sauce

Blue Damson plums
Bone broth with milk
Brambleberries
Brambleberry juice
Bread fruit
Broccoli
Cabbage, curly, red, steamed with milk or savoy
Cabbage sprouts
Cardoons
Carrots, young
Castor oil, sparingly
Catnip tea
Celery juice and raw milk
Cauliflower
Celery heart
Celery juice
Celery, crisp, raw
Celery cabbage
Cherries, light
Chicken bone broth w/whole rice and parsley
Chard, young
Clam broth and hop tea
Clam broth and sage tea
Clover blossoms in salads
Coconut cream
Cod, steamed
Cod liver oil
Collards, young
Corn on the cob
Cucumber
Custard
Dates
Dandelion
Eggshell broth with milk and anglefood cake
Elderberries
Fig tea
Figs, black mission, sundried
Fish broth
Fish roe
Flaxseed meal
Flounder, steamed
Fowl, young, broiled
Fruit, jam
Fruit-peel jelly, alkalinized
Hop tea
Kohlrabi
Kumquats
Leeks
Lettuce, young

Lima beans, fresh with beaten egg white
Loquats
Mangoes
Marmalade
Melons
Mulberry juice
Mullet
Mustard greens
Nectarines
Nettle salad
New Zealand spinach
Oatmeal, steel cut, steamed
Okra and tomatoes
Olive oil, virgin
Olives, sundried
Onions, steamed
Oyster broth
Pawpaw
Papaya
Parsnips, young
Peaches, cooked
Fruit pudding with whole rice
Goat butter
Goat buttermilk
Goat buttermilk with angelfood cake
Goat milk cheese, brown or roquefort
Goose, lean, tender
Gooseberries
Grapes, green
Green beans with beaten egg white
Green onions
Green peas, sugar, tender
Herring, smoked
Honey, raw, unfiltered
Prunes, stewed, sundried
Prune tea
Pumpkin
Pursland
Quail, steamed
Raisins, in food, sundried
Red currants
Rice bran muffins
Rice pudding with fruit
Roe, baked
Romaine, youing
Rye, bran muffins
Pears, home preserved
Pears, fresh
Pears, sundried, cooked
Perch, youing, broiled

Pepsin
Persimmons
Pickerel
Pigeon, young
Pike, baked
Pineapple
Pineapple sauce
Pleurisy-root tea
Plover, steamed
Plums, satsuma or sebesten or tamarind
Plumcots
Pomano, steamed
Prune juice
Porgy, steamed
Poultry, young, broiled
Prune sauce
Sago fruit pudding
Salads made of buds, blossoms
Sapota
Sardines
Sauerkraut
Senna, in salads
Senna tea
Shad, steamed
Shallots, young
Smelt, steamed
Snipe
Sole
Spinach, wilted
Squab, broiled
Squash
Strawberries, ripe
Strawberry sherbet
Swiss chard, young
Tamarinds
Tomato sauce
Tuna fish, broiled
Turnips, young
Veal joint broth with rice
Waldorf salad
Watermelon, ripe
Weakfish, broiled
Whey, goat
Whitefish, smoked
Whiting, baked or broiled
Wild duck, broiled
Wild strawberry sherbet
Wild strawberry sauce
Woodcock, broiled
Winter melon

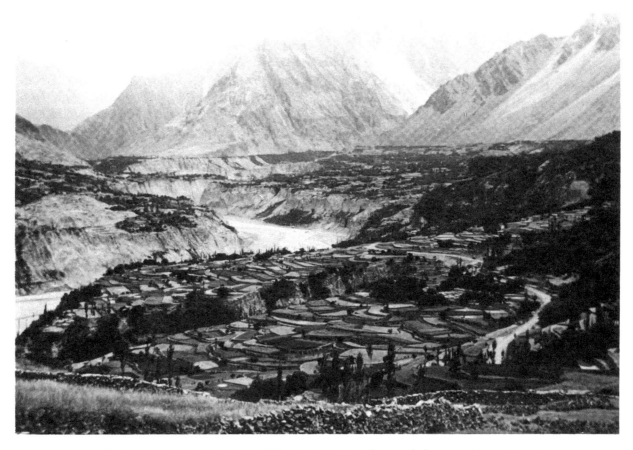

During my visit to the Hunza Valley, I found that the people knew nothing of vitamins, minerals, RNA, amino acids or food combining. Yet they were wonderfully healthy because they had a right way of living. A right way of living is the key to good health.

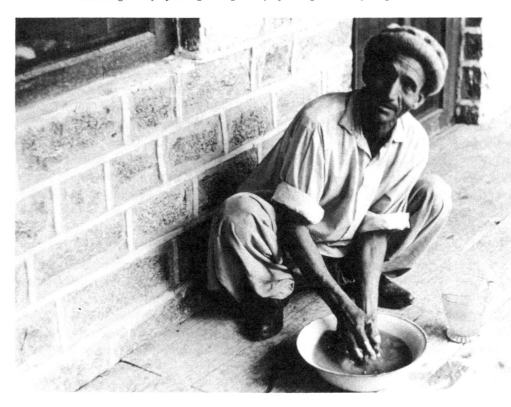

The Hunza people make a delicious drink by rubbing dried apricots together in water.

Basic Food Law

The most fundamental principle I've discovered in over 50 years of experience with patients is that all our food should be natural, pure and whole. So I emphasize the primary law of foods and nutrition: NATURAL—PURE—WHOLE.

This is the basis for my work.

Now the average person doesn't know what pure food is. Can chemical sprays and fertilizers give us pure food? Are hybrid grains and fruits natural? Are packaged foods natural? What about whole foods? When the bran and germ of the wheat kernel are thrown away, is that whole? Stop and think about it. What can we find in the supermarket that is natural, pure and whole these days?

Try and find the purest foods you possibly can, foods organically grown without chemical fertilizers. Try to have those. It is to your advantage to get these things as much as possible. When you get a nice peach that has been colored by the sun, tree ripened, it is so much better than a pickled peach. And, we find that a fresh, natural cucumber is so much better than a waxed one. Let's try to keep away from food products beautified and preserved by man-made cosmetics. This waxing business is really terrible these days. We need to insist on whole grains. Grains with the bran—whole brown rice, whole rye, whole millet and unpearled barley. We're eating with just half of our brains these days. When we have white bread, they claim there is about 27% less calcium in the white flour than in the whole grain flour. You get only half a loaf of bread when you take a white bread instead of the whole wheat. To assure colon health, it is necessary to have adequate bulk and fiber in the diet. These days it is advisable to have a teaspoon or two of bran with each meal to make sure we are getting enough bulk.

So here is what we have to have. We have to have whole foods; we have to have pure foods and we have to have natural foods. This whole food idea is realtively recent and many do not yet understand its importance.

In China and the Philippine Islands, many people will not eat brown rice. They call it "dirty rice."

The preference for white rice over brown (whole) rice in the Far East is only one example of how civilization and technology have corrupted the "food morality" of modern man. I have visited over 52 countries—and many have some crazy food ideas. When you go to Germany, they offer you pickled pig's feet. When you visit Denmark, the custom is beer every morning. England, a nation of tea drinkers, has more rheumatism than any other country in the world. They have to have their tea all day long. We need to understand that tradition can destroy the human body.

My Visit with the King of Hunza

Even the people of Hunza in Nepal, long celebrated for their wonderful health and astonishing longevity have their problems.

My wife Marie and I stayed with the late King of Hunza as guests for 10 days. He told me he had sciatica and bowel problems as we sat drinking tea, in which he'd put four teaspoons of sugar. "I've been to one hospital in Austria and another in England," the King said, "but no one there could help me."

"How many cups of tea do you drink in a day?" I asked.

"About 14," he said. "I have tea with my visitors as a matter of hospitality."

"Well, 14 cups of tea with 4 teaspoons of sugar in each one is the best way I know to get sciatica and bowel troubles," I told him. "You're going to have to do something about that."

"What can I do?" He asked.

I told him I'd try to think of something. Then, Marie and I went out and found some wild peppermint and picked some alfalfa growing in a field. We came back, mixed the peppermint and alfalfa and brewed him a nice pot of herb tea. We watched him try the first cup.

The king put the cup up to his nose and said, "I've never smelled anything so wonderful. I don't believe it needs any sugar in it." He tasted it, smiled and drink the whole thing—without sugar. In a week's time, his sciatica was gone and his bowel troubles were much improved. It was most likely the sugar—56 teaspoons a day—that caused the sciatica and bowel problems, while the caffeine and tannic acid from the tea aggravated his nerves, stomach and bowel.

"By the way," the king said, "a number of my people are suffering from eye disease. Do you know of anything that could help?"

Again, Marie and I went out on a scouting expedition. There is an old saying that beside every problem there lies a solution. If the eyes don't get enough vitamin A, they become susceptible to disease. The people of Hunza had plenty of apricots, in season, but they needed another supplement. Before long, we spotted malva growing right beside the road. There was our solution. Malva is an herb so common around the world that many people regard it as a weed. Yet it is high in vitamin A and chlorophyll, one of the best natural cleansers for the body. We picked some to show the king and told him to tell his people to eat it raw, right from the field or roadside, wherever they happened to be.

Since our visit, a new road has been built to the Hunza Valley, and the people have begun picking up more civilized habits—alcohol, smoking. coffee, soft drinks, white sugar and processed foods. They say the king of Hunza died of a broken heart when he saw the old healthy way of life dying out in his people. Under the old way of life there were no policemen, jails, drugstores, doctors, dentists or hopsitals. For the most part, they didn't need them.

Variety is Essential

Just as nations tend to develop some unhealthy food customs and patterns, so do families. Many families depend on a very limited selection of foods to serve at mealtimes, when nature's garden offers a wide selection. For a balanced, wholesome diet, variety and the correct proportions of foods are essential. The proportions should be: 6 vegetables, 2 fruits, 1 starch and 1 protein. You have to have these every day. Such a varied food regimen frees you from having to worry about calcium, silicon and other needed biochemicals because it's all there. I want to make it easy for you.

What we eat, digest and assimilate should be selected with an eye to providing the blood with all the biochemicals needed by the nerves, glands, organs and tissues. Our blood nutrients should come from about 80% alkaline foods and about 20% acid foods. Everyone's talking about an alkaline diet these days. Many people realize they are too acid—so they are going for the alkaline diets. Vegetarianism is an extreme alkaline diet. But that doesn't mean it is for everyone. Until we have brought our philosophy and lifestyle under the umbrella of the peace and harmony way, we cannot be good vegetarians.

Try vegetables and fruits you haven't tried before. Give some creative thought to making salads as varied, beautiful and taste-appealing as possible. Play around with combinations of fruit, nuts, seeds and honey to find new and healthy snack or dessert ideas.

Variety can be achieved in other ways. It isn't necessary to get into the kind of health food rut where you always have fruit for breakfast, protein for lunch and starch for dinner. Switch around.

I would include variety as one of the food laws. With sufficient variety in the food intake over a period of time, every cell in the body will have access to the nutrients it needs. In fact, to lead fulfilling lives requires that we fulfill the metabolic needs of our bodies at the cellular level. This is why variety is so important.

"Working hard when you are young and earning a competence on which you can retire and enjoy yourself...will bring you little happiness if you are not well enough to enjoy those years. Most of the diseases we associate with this period (retirement) are the direct results of an improper diet in youth."

—Victor Heiser, MD

---

seven

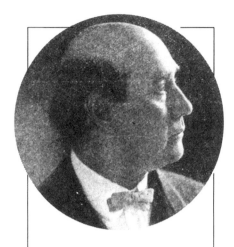

Dr. V. G. Rocine— The man

There is probably no one more qualified to write about Dr. V. G. Rocilne than I. I studied with Dr. Rocine, lectured with him and lived in his home. We discussed my difficult cases as well as my own health problems.

I based my successful sanitarium work on Rocine's teachings, and I will be eternally grateful to him for the legacy of his knowledge

A Giant of Knowledge

I first met Dr. Rocine when he was in his 70s. He was an Isogenetic type, calcium/mental, an individual with perseverance. He could sit and write for 8 to 10 hours at a time.

Until several years after his death, I did not realize what an intelligent all-around man he was. In putting my knowledge together, I became aware that he drew from heaven and earth, and even from consciousnesses in between. He understood each faculty of life from the mineral side all the way up to the spiritual/soul sides of life. He was unique in being able to relate one form of consciousness to another, one field of knowledge to another.

When he held a discussion, whether spiritual, mental or physical, he saw the relationships among the different facets and how they worked together. His comments were music to my ears, and I believe his work was a forerunner of what is called, today, the wholistic healing arts.

I engaged in many studies with Dr. Rocine before finding out what kind of person he was. I realized what he stood for eventually, and that realization took a great deal of thought on my part, together with my patient and sanitarium experiences. Because of the impetus I got from him which was due to the motivation, knowledge and complete study he coordinated for me, I would say I have lived five lifetimes in one.

Many people misunderstood him and many criticized him. Some plagiarized his work, but no one could take anything away from him. He built a profession all his own, a unique path which included chemical types, races, dietetic procedures, and how to look at diets and the chemical elements as they relate to the human body, its vital organs and other structural components. All of this was Rocine's work. He was most unusual.

He was the man who taught me the seven faculties of the brain which need developing to increase a person's effectiveness and power. These faculties are symnoia (fraternity), precinoia (business ability), autonomia (self government), suamanos (suaveness or politeness), techomanas (constructiveness or building skill), philnoia (love) and cheronoia (joy). This learning has meant much to me. I have been able to help many people see that developing these faculties brings success throughout one's life.

Rocine took me as a child and gave me the opportunity to get well—to go from sickness to health or from rags to riches, mentally speaking. I owe him my life. Any credit I can give to him for all I have been able to accomplish in helping other people is certainly warranted. In other words, I want people to know that if I never developed anything original myself, using only what Rocine taught would have allowed me to help more people than anything else I have learned.

Most Complete Teachings

My training and learning came from many specialists. I have had the opportunity to work with colonic specialists Dr. Shellberg of New York City and Dr. John Harvey Kellogg of Battle Creek. I have gone through the hygienic work of Herbert Shelton, Dr. John Tilden of Denver and Dr. Benedict Lust. I have been associated with (and have a good friendship with) Dr. Robert Jackson of Canada. I was a personal friend of St. Lewis Estes, who taught me much about juices. I have gone through the Bircher-Benner Sanitarium in Zurich, Switzerland. I was a student of George Weger, a medical doctor who taught me about fasting. Even though I have trained with many fine men, no one's teachings were as complete as those of Dr. V. G. Rocine.

I believe my success came from developing one particular aspect of life under Dr. Rocine's guidance—the faculty of business sense. The business ideas he taught me were not those that involved money. The great thrust of business is to take all parts, put them together and make a whole project. It is this ability to take all parts and see the relation of one to another that I have absorbed from Dr. Rocine.

While I pursued the study of iridology, which Dr. Rocine knew of but never wrote about, we had many discussions about it. We talked about how iridology deals with the relation of organs to one another and to the body as a whole. We talked about the relation of the brain and its control centers to the tissue structures and functions of the body. Dr. Rocine told me he believed that every aspect of the environment—from noise to air pollution, from scenery to altitude—affects every cell of the body. The air we breathe has an effect on the medulla of the brain, the animation in life center and the sex-life center. All have their related effects and can stimulate any and all organs of the body. The depletion of one organ affects every other organ.

Rocine taught the unity of activity of the body and the differing relationships of the chemical elements to different organs. He taught me that the dust of the earth has everything man needs chemically when coordinated with the proper environment, thinking and goals.

Emphasis on Wholeness

Rocine gave me a sense of putting a team of workers together. In this respect, the iris helped me to see more of the good in Rocine's work than anything, due to the fact that the body must be working together, part-for-part, in order to conduct itself properly and optimally. The thyroid cannot work by itself without iodine. The thyroid and iodine working together help the metabolism of the functions that are found in the bowel, skin, hair and even the mind. They also assist us in being able to stand heights and to have the confidence to go up in elevators. Of course, to correct these problems, we must take care of not only the thyroid but the whole body. Ultimate health, again, depends on wholeness. It is only physically, mentally and spiritually that a good human being can be put together.

Rocine showed that each human is responsible for the next generation. On top of that, he made it clear that good thinking cannot come when a person does not have a good body to nourish the brain. When the diet lacks the materials earmarked to develop faculties of mind and organs in the body, the whole person is not working "on all cylinders," as it were.

Rocine was Inspirational

There was great inspiration from Dr. Rocine to take on more in your life to bring greater happiness, happier marriage, better harmony—and to find one's weaknesses. But, above all things, he had the answer for those weaknesses. While many people say, "You're weak," or "Don't do this" or "Don't do that," very few people ever tell you what to do about it. He showed you a way out.

He taught me to "mind my own mind." He taught also during the time I was so ill that there was a way to do things; there was a way of elevation. He taught me how to enhance mental faculties with certain foods and certain thinking. For example, I became the leader of my body; I led my body out of sickness to something else. I had considerable lung trouble. I also had speech problems, being unable to talk before a group of people. I had nerve depletion from overwork; because I felt I couldn't satisfy everyone. My path was completely nerve depleting. But Rocine turned me around from a stuttering, stammering kid—a sick person—to one who began to see strength come back more and more. After 50 years of following his advice, I've been able to accomplish things that very few people have been able to do.

Rocine gave me the ability to see that the spiritual precedes the physical, but it could not precede the body unless the body was capable of matching the spiritual in all activities. That is why I say that the spirit, power, vitality, energy, light and vibration are things to work with and through. In other words, he taught me that there is a physical-mental relationship when we jump for joy. He also brought out much of this when he said, "You can't expect much brain development from pickles and ice cream"; and, "You can't expect a good bloodstream from 'spooked' flour." He had ways of saying things that really made you think; sometimes I have followed in his exaggerations. You can see the Rocine influence in me; when I lecture, I give the extreme.

Mind, Spirit, Body

I have studied with Dr. Ernest Holmes; studied Fowler's work in Unity; and studied Emmett Foxes' work. I have gone through metaphysical study; I have been with Sai Baba and Sri Aurobindo; I have followed the Eastern and Western philosophies as well as the spiritual, going all the way from the church which I was born into, to the many other philosophies of looking for answers to life's questions. I've found that each of them is incomplete for me because they don't recognize that we have mental faculties and inherent weaknesses. We've got to strengthen them and we can only do so by putting all things together—physical, mental and spiritual.

I remember an illustration I was given years ago. In a group of 17 wayward girls living in England, every one came from a divorced home; every one had been living on fish and chips; every one had a sinful mind; every one had no goals. Their personalities changed in one year's time to the point where people did not recognize these girls. They had lost their boredom and destructive ways; they became new people entirely—through good eating and proper counseling. This is putting together the physical, mental and the spiritual. When sickness produces a depleted mind, naturally a person cannot think properly. We could improve lives if V. G. Rocine's work was more widely practiced.

We Cannot Be One Dimensional

Rocine's contribution to the wholistic movement is that he tells us we cannot be one-sided and one-direction minded. Some people now believe that when they have sex problems, the first thing to do is take zinc—that will solve their problems. They don't think about the mental, soul and memory processes—the goal and ideal processes—each of which has influence on the sex life. Narrowness is revealed by the current emphasis on sex for its own sake,

"Each human is responsible for the next generation."

—V. G. Rocine

82

as shown by pornography which is popular these days. Many factors contribute to this emphasis, such as poor foods, distasteful situations, bad marriages and unhappy job situations.

Dr. Rocine showed me how to get homeopathic principles out of nature, as nature created them for us, without having to put them into triturated amounts, concentrates or extracts. This was possible to do right in your own home through broths, tonics and essences he taught us to use. One great lesson I had from Rocine was that life really begins in the kitchen. It goes back still farther to the soil and the farm. There is a greater doctor in the soil—a greater doctor in the plant—than any doctor who ever sat in an office. These are the doctors we should go to. These are the doctors we should know more about, because foods doctor us. Foods heal and cure us.

Rocine's study of foods was comprehensive and in-depth compared to the knowledge of the average person today. I don't mean to criticize, but being a seeker myself, I just can't say that anyone comes close to him in understanding the deeper truths in food. For instance, take corn. The best corn is yellow. Why is this? Dr. Rocine taught that the highest concentration of phosphates was in yellow cornmeal. Phosphates are excellent brain and nerve builders. There is 4% phosphorus in yellow cornmeal as compared to 2% in the white.

As I continued my studies into Bishop Leadbeater's color work and the works of Annie Besant and Harriet Blavatsky, which Dr. Rocine also investigated, I learned that yellow corn has a specific vibratory rate associated with the highest foods in magnesium. I began to see where magnesium and the yellow color and the phosphates helped to give a person relaxation, especially in the brain and nervous system. When there is hyperactivity or when a person is driving himself mentally, he needs magnesium for control, to settle down and cool off, so to speak.

From Rocine, I could begin to see the relationships of color, phosphates, magnesium, the brain and relaxation. I owe much to Rocine for his coordination of all these stages of consciousness defined in his studies. I wanted to know more about what he gave me; but you see, it's just like a neophyte or a youngster trying to interpret the Bible—you have to have a certain knowledge beforehand to do this. And it wasn't until after I traveled a good deal, seeing people of different countries living on certain foods (certain healthy elderly people lived on calcium foods; they naturally went to the gelatins, the joint materials that kept them free of any joint problems), after all this I began to see life through Rocine's eyes. These are things that very few people ever see. I was able to see copper reflections from the mountains in the Hunza Valley that no one has ever talked about in their work on the Hunza people, yet these copper reflections were having a subtle influence on these people.

I was aware of these things because of what Rocine taught me. He told me there were certain meats that shouldn't be used if persons were mentally inclined toward destructiveness, because they would make such persons more destructive than ever. When he first said that I didn't see where it could have any connection. There seemed to be no sense in it. But I understood what he said only as a youngster. Twenty years later, I recalled and understood his words.

Dr. Jensen's Application

Now I can say that where I fit into all of this is the fact that I have had over 50 year's experience in sanitarium work. I have encountered people who had to be touched mentally before physical things did them any good. I have come to the place now where I realize it isn't what you eat that counts—it's what you digest. It is possible that the mental processes have more to do with digestion than the food itself. We have to have the mind and body working together for good digestion. It is only through Dr. Rocine's works that I can see the relationship of these things. I believe this accounts for the success of my work.

Rocine told much about different races who developed various characteristics because of their specific diet patterns, and I saw this in my world travels. The old men of the Russian Caucasus live in the mountains—the calcium, angular type, not the inventive type, but the plowing, persevering, slow-moving types, which we call calcium types. They were having the calcium foods of the mountains. Then in other countries, I saw people more on the mental side, motivated through the vitality and the force of the brain. I could really see the influence of food in China with the chlorine type of people—those interested in cleanliness; people who are interested in water. They always have their hands in water; they work and live around water.

I've spent considerable time trying to get some of Rocine's work out to the public, and in doing so have talked to his wife, who is also a doctor. She was very much in harmony with the wonderful things we have been doing at the Health Ranch. I'm sure that Dr. Rocine realized that I was not able to be a completely dedicated student, being as busy as I was with many matters. He probably knew there wasn't another Rocine embodied within me. However, in having over 3,000 students, he considered me one of his best. I have tried to represent his work as well as I can.

So, in giving the work of Dr. Rocine, I want it understood he is to have full credit for it. The work I have done has come from my travels, my sanitarium experiences, the 350,000 patients I have treated, the evolution and development of my own life, the sickness I overcame, the mental problems of childhood I had to overcome. I want this book to give deserved credit to Dr. V. G. Rocine. I feel that the accomplishments, whatever they may be from a knowledge standpoint came from the "mother" faculties which have given me the "doctor" ideas and the heart sentiment I have for humanity. These faculties have combined with Rocine's ideas and teaching to help me strive for the good of mankind both in individual treatments and in writing books.

I would have to live several more lifetimes to learn all Rocine had to give. He deserves much more recognition. He has inspired me to help people attain what they need to move one step above where they have been in this world's affairs.

Correspondence with V. G. Rocine

The following correspondence with V. G. Rocine from 1938 through 1943, represents part of a more extensive correspondence between us that lasted until shortly before his death.

July 12, 1938

Dear Dr. Jensen:

It was very interesting and pleasing to us to receive your recent letter, in which we understand that you are now in Los Angeles, California.

We did not have time to go to San Diego, nor to Los Angeles, while we were in California. Our time is never our own.

Go on with your work, Dr. Jensen. Men like you are needed by the millions in this world. People, as a general rule, even doctors, fail to study diets, just as they fail to study types.

You say that there are questions you would like answered, and you say that you think probably I am the man to answer those questions. I do not know whether I could answer your questions satisfactorily or not, nevertheless, I believe that I have brass enough to try it.

We thank you very much for giving us your address so that we may write to you occasionally.

By the way, Dr. Jensen, that new book which I worked on for two years and a half, is now published, and ready for the public. We know that no one else but a student will buy this book; nor will he even understand this book, unless he is a student; neither would we want to sell the book to anyone else but a student. This book sells for $25. We do not know whether you have concluded to get a copy or not; but we want you to know that it is now ready.

Yours very truly,

July 19, 1938

Dear Dr. Jensen:

We received your telegram, in which you ordered two copies of "Building a New Heart," to be sent COD. We are sending two copies.

You ask what the title is of the new book which we mentioned in our letter last time we wrote to you. The title is "The Soul's Functions." It is a very large book. It contains about 700 pages. Because it treats all the faculties of the soul; it covers all humanity. We believe that this is the book for you, and that you are the man for this book. No one else than a *real student would buy a book of this kind. It sells for $25. We only printed 200 copies. It will be used as a textbook in our coming college, if we can get ready for that great work. We need textbooks, and we need teachers, in case we were to start with a college.*

Hoping to hear from you again, and wishing you success and health, we are

Yours truly,

February 11, 1942

Dear Dr. Rocine:

I am enclosing a check to cover the cost of publications I have ordered.

I am seriously planning to take a few days off and would like to come to Portland and spend a few hours with you. There are so many questions I would like to have ironed out and, of course, you know how each person thinks. The channels through which I come to conclusions may be helped tremendously if a few questions I have in mind are answered first. My future studies would probably be a little easier than if I went at it haphazardly.

With very best wishes, I remain

Sincerely yours,

AUTHOR'S NOTE

In October 1942, V. G. Rocine sent copies of the following letter to friends and students about his intended move from Portland, Oregon to Los Angeles, California. Because of wartime rationing of gasoline and unavailability of tires, he didn't go ahead with the planned move, as the sequence of following letters show.

October 1942

Dear Friend:

Having had a wide experience and being more or less retired from public life, and having seen almost unbelievable cures accomplished by nature, by a recuperative climate, by corrective blood-building food, by well adjusted heliotherapy (sun-cure regime), by a corrective regimen of life, by a philosophic psychology or attitude of mind, and by a well adjusted work

according to our own temperament, type talent aptitude and physique; also having given counsel, instruction, perhaps deliberation plussed, helpless, destitute, perhaps ready to commit crazy acts, even suicide, because of their forlorn state of mind, empty purse, puzzled chaotic mind, tired brain, exhausted nerves, and crippled health, then on crutches—having witnessed all such bitter experiences, I am prepared to state that it is possible for anyone of us to turn the course of the **ship of life** *and steer it into the* **harbor of safety**, *as many of us have done by timely prudent council. So long as we live* **there is hope!** *So long as we can eat, drink and digest food, there is no need of despondency. So long as our blood flows in our arteries, we have nothing to fear; so long as our lungs supply us with the revivifying oxygen,* **we need not despair**, *even when we cannot be cured by water-gruel specialists, or by a self-imposed starvation regime. We may be sure that when our doctors cannot cure us; that when we are friendless, loveless, fundless, hopeless, there is something wrong with our psychology, or with our diet, or with our work, or with our habits, or with our regime, or with all combined.*

After Nov. 1st, my **new permanent address** *will be V. G. Rocine, 4727 1-3d, West 18th St., Los Angeles, California. The address on the envelope is only a vacation address.*

Very truly yours,

V. G. Rocine

December 29, 1942

Dear Dr. Jensen:

I am still in Portland, because of that gas rationing, tire scarcity, and other conditions which no one can help except Hitler, and God and those two do not seem to do anything to the war, except to let us poor human beings waddle through the best we can, or in any way we can. I am glad to receive your card. You seem to hunt us up again and again. You seem to remember us, even in our old age.

And do you know I am now starting to write a new book, in which I intend to give something to the public that I never gave before?

And by the way, it will be nothing but chemistry, chemistry, chemistry, in **APPLICATION**, in **DIETS**, in **TREATMENTS**, in **SYMPTOMS**. I have only one student that I am writing this for and that student is going to pay me $600 for that manuscript. He is the only one in the whole world that will get the contents of the Rocine brain and all his discoveries and experiments. I do not yet know whether I will live long enough to complete the book. It will take me at least three years to complete this manuscript. I have now 136 pages written and I am writing at the rate of two pages a day up to 15, even 20 pages some days. Anyone who gets this book will be Rocine No. 2.

What are you doing now, Dr. Jensen? Are you a success? Are you healthy? Do you feel young and vigorous? Or are you drafted? If you ever receive this letter kindly answer me, so that I may know where you are. This reminds me of an Irishman who came to America from Ireland. When he came here he wrote to his girl thus: Now Honey, when you get this letter write to me at once; and if you do not get it, write anyway. Your old lover, Pat.

Yours truly,
V. G. Rocine

December 31, 1942

Dear Dr. Rocine:

Well, I thought you were in Los Angeles by this time at your new permanent address, and you would be surprised if I told you that the very day I received your letter I was going to go to the address 4727-1/3 W. 18th Street to pay you a visit. I was very happy to hear from you. Rest assured I owe a lot to you and your teachings for the success in my work.

You ask if I am a success. I might say that financially I don't amount to an awful lot; however, as a student of the natural healing arts I am getting better results than the average doctor. I have established a sanitarium here in the foothills above the fog belt and outside the city limits; it is truly a retreat from all that is wearisome to the human body. I am enclosing a folder which you may like to look over.

You ask if I am healthy. I could say that if I was not so busy I could be in much better health.

However, I am so interested in serving, that it is difficult for me to say: "Stop," or to get all the rest that I need. At the present time, I am feeling very good. Many of my activities have been curbed since the declaration of war, but in this period now I feel like I want to study this next year, using all my spare time to better myself for the day when there will be plenty of people needing my service. I am unable to lecture or travel, so it may be for everyone's good that I take care of myself and spend a little time studying.

I was quite interested in hearing that you are beginning to write again and you know I am always interested in the work you are doing. At the present time, I could not afford to pay $600 for the manuscript you mention in the letter. However, I am extremely interested in chemistry and its applications in diet treatments and in symptoms. I have been taking a class in agricultural chemistry, trying to work out a way in which I may serve the patients with the proper chemical elements in some form or another along with their regular diet. The foods grown today are so depleted that everyone who comes to me seems to be tissue-starved. It is difficult to tell them how to get the proper elements even though you know what they need.

Another question in my mind is why scientists say that we have some 152 chemical elements in our body and yet we have only the 18 elements listed as the body's need. I know that the addition of many of the elements found in drugs, when added to the body, are only disease-forming, and I am wondering, through the depletion of our soil and the addition of abnormal and unnecessary chemical elements, if we are producing the many different diseases that are coming forth today?

We are especially confronted with occupational diseases as formed from the absorption of the dye from certain kinds of cloth, the radium from clocks and I wonder if the aluminum dust that is floating around in these airplane factories is not responsible for a lot of the lung conditions that are coming to me now; or will this aluminum dust cause trouble only two years after its absorption?

I am so glad to hear you are still active. There are so many things that I would like to talk to you about, as there seem to be no books written on the questions I would like to ask.

I received the letter from the Moore's, Bend, Oregon, in regard to your special announcement, and I am enclosing check for $4.30 for the following:

1. "The Best Food for Man,"—10 cents

2. "Goat Milk as a Body Builder,"—10 cents

3. "Youth-Building Course,"—$3.00

4. "Students' Questions and Recipes,"—$1.00

5. "U.S. Patriotic Defense League,"—10 cents.

He also mentions having a personal interview, and I would appreciate having this one of these days, and when you write me, please let me know if this is possible.

Have you any work on soil chemistry and the preparation of the soil for producing perfect plant life? There are so many people using fertilizers and artificial means of growing plants that I would like to know the real way of producing perfect plant life.

I would be willing to make a special trip to Portland just to see you again, and in the meantime, let me wish you the finest in the New Year.

Sincerely yours,

January 12, 1943

Dear Doctor Jensen:

You have the right idea of having a Health Home in Nature, where nature cures, when a cure is possible. Let us say just one word here, that nature does not cure where it is impossible to cure. There are some people whom no doctor could cure, no medicine reach, even God Himself would not cure them, because they are incurable.

There are certain people who suffer from that kind of diseases that are known as and described as eponymic diseases, and that kind of disease or people no one can cure. We can help them just a little but not very much. We can give them such herbs that nature has made for them and their benefit, and that is all we can do. They will not be cured, but they can live on and on perhaps fifty to a hundred years and not suffer so much, in spite of their diseases.

Remember that there are a great many people who pretend to be prominent scientists, investigators and philosophers, who are in reality nothing but dreamers or advertisers.

You probably did not understand that letter I sent from Bend. I agreed to answer any question that anyone would ask, if they would send $1, and I have done so, thus far, but that did not mean a personal interview. If I were to permit personal interviews, I would not be able to write one single page a year. We have so much work that we cannot do one-tenth of it. But there are some letters that we answer, when we consider them important. All other letters go into the wastebasket.

Soil chemistry is a very interesting subject, and a subject that will be taken up after Dr. Jensen and V. G. Rocine are gone to Vallhalla. People are studying soil chemistry right and left, just as they have been studying human chemistry and food chemistry and got nowhere. It is not soil chemistry that we should study so much as we study geoponics; or in other words, we must **supply** the elements to the soil that are needed by the soil, namely the sixteen chemical elements, the primary elements that man is made of.

You are perfectly right, Dr. Jensen, that there are no books written on those very subjects and questions in which you, yourself and we, ourselves, are interested. This is also why I have started to write such a book. I can assure you that if you ever read this book you will say, after you shall have read it, from cover to cover, you will say, "Here is the book for Dr. Jensen, the book that I have been looking for all my life."

I have already written about 200 pages.

We do not know whether these new books will be written or not, because I do not know how long it pleases the Divine Forces to let me live. But these books will be written if I live long enough, or whether I sell two or three or ten. The idea is that, even if I could sell ten of those books it would not pay for the writing anyway, nor even for the stenographic work and other helpers. I will never make one single dollar by writing these books, but they will be written anyway, because I have made up my mind to write them, if only for my students. And, by the way, there are not very many students in this world. I have had 3000 and all of them were nibblers only.

Hoping to hear from you again and thanking for that letter you wrote. It is an **inspiration.**

Yours truly,
V. G. Rocine

March 2, 1943

Dear Doctor Rocine:

Received your kind letter and was truly glad to hear from you.

I am enclosing $10 to pay for a few of the questions we are asking. I am sorry we can't have our personal interview. I have been most interested in getting to the bottom and dealing with the cause of disease more than treating and diagnosing symptoms. I am recognizing the great need for the chemical properties in soil, plant and man more every day. In our little place in the hills we are working with a few experimental gardens trying to formulate some ideas how to improve our agricultural methods. I do not particularly like farming, but I see such a need in caring for our soil and plants. Truly, our farmers should have more knowledge in the care of their soil.

We are sending under separate cover an article I wrote in the last issue of my magazine called, "Wanted: Soil Doctors." I do not feel it is necessary to use fertilizers, manures, etc., to raise the proper plant life, if the balanced chemicals are in the soil.

Now I want to know if there is such a thing as a formula for the perfect soil and what percentages of the elements should be there? Does the soil have to be different according to the plant life that has to be grown? If you know what the perfect soil is how do you come to that conclusion? Why should there only be 16 chemical elements to make up the human body and not 152 as they have discovered? If there are only 16 chemical elements in the human body, it sounds logical that there should only be 16 in the soil.

We have our own water supply on the place and only a couple of acres, but the health department is demanding that our water be chlorinated. I am positive that this is a poison to our bodies. I am positive that it is bad for my plants and my garden. Is there any way to overcome this to neutralize this condition, or what suggestions have you? Have you any information on where I may find out about the effects of chlorine on the body and on plants? Have you written anything in regard to herbs and their properties, what ones to grow in your garden, etc.? Where can I get something on the study of geoponics?

I am so wound up in this civilized commercial mess, that I am too tied down financially to do all the things that I would like to. Shame on me! However, I am working the same as everyone else, but thinking as I go, hoping that I can leave something of value that my fellowmen may use.

I am unable to pay you $600 in one lump for the book mentioned in your letter. However, I am enclosing a check for $200 and will pay $200 in two months and another $200 two months after that. I am interested in anything you write. While I probably haven't been a close student of yours, you will recognize that a man taking a broadminded viewpoint must try to segregate and refine a lot of the loose knowledge and loose talk that goes around in regard to the healing art.

I am finally getting to the place where I am tired of practicing, but want to know what I am doing.

With best wishes, I remain

Sincerely yours,
Bernard Jensen

eight

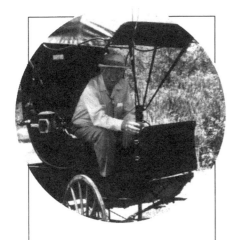

We see others as we see ourselves. Understand yourself, it is better that you may know your brother better.

Great trials are often necessary to prepare us for great responsibilities.

"I am not bound to win, but I am bound to be true. I am not bound to succeed, but I am bound to live up to what lights I have. I must stand with anybody that stands right, stand with him while he is right, and part with him when he goes wrong."

—Abraham Lincoln

Dr. Bruce R. Zimmerman of the Mayo Clinic says, "Patients indeed have played a strong role in choosing the diseases (cancer, heart disease, diabetes, back disease, arthritis and chronic respiratory illness)...by smoking, over-eating and not exercising, which aggravate the diseases." Dr. Jensen says they acquire these conditions as the chemical elements are depleted from their bodies.

V. G. Rocine's analysis of Dr. Jensen

Introduction

Dr. Rocine offered me many insights (affecting proper health) with regard to diet, vocation, marriage, financial difficulties and the chemical shortages we develop in our daily physical and mental activities. Furthermore, he gave me an examination, the results of which I am now going to include in their entirety. This is what led me into a deep study of Rocine's works.

With Dr. Rocine, I studied the foods and chemical brain functioning; secrets of longevity; making over the different organs of the body, especially the heart and stomach; the facts and wonder of the climate; kitchen chemistry; the mind training courses—Menticulture; and, lastly, exalting the great within. From there, I went on to other teachers and other studies.

The report which follows, "To Bernard Jensen," is an example of the kind of analysis issued in response to the requests of Rocine's clients. It contains only one reference which might puzzle the reader, and that is the recommendation to take New Life Food Blend, a nutriment Dr. Rocine developed himself.

Being from Norway, Rocine was well acquainted with concentrating cheese, whey, etc. He knew, of course, that whey was the food highest in sodium, and he was able to concentrate it by boiling it down for some 9 hours. He added a concentrate of Avina Sativa or oatstraw tea. People short of sodium and silicon could best replenish themselves with this product.

Analysis of Dr. Jensen

To Dr. Bernard Jensen, January 1955

You are a strong man in a motor sense and in a mental sense, but you are weaker, vitally speaking. You know this, but you have been driving your strong motor temperament about to the limit. Yes, you are weak in your stomach and power of digestion, mainly because your faculty alimentiveness in the frontal lower brain is weak and therefore you are not and have not been prompted to sensible and careful habits regarding your eating. You eat because you are hungry, but you do not think about eating. People with this active faculty think about the food and like it. Their mind is in this function of digesting; they are very particular about the quality of the food and subconsciously they taste and savor every mouthful. They promise themselves good digestive results from the meal. This you do not do—you cannot do—because your mind is elsewhere, and your digestion is a hit-or-miss matter, without any conscious enjoyment and pleasure in the digestive function (**Mind**—do not read while eating.) This is caused by your lack of action in the mental power of digestion.

But this isn't all of your vital weakness. Your chest brain, the medulla oblongata that takes care of all the chest functions—the lungs and the breathing apparata, the heart, as well as the stomach—are not strong enough to support your tremendous thinking, working and talking activities and your positive ambition to succeed in your undertakings. You are top-heavy, lopsided and unbalanced in this respect.

A severe cold struck you in the chest and weakened a part of your lungs and stopped your tired voice, temporarily. All in all, it is your medulla that has to be rebuilt. Doing so takes time, rest, God and Nature working with your willing mind. What man can do it? What doctor can do it? What pills or vitamins can do it? Even food of the best kind cannot do it alone, but can help. Complete rest of mind and soul can do it, together with right food, quiet and seclusion, and, above all, right air. The greatest food and strength for the medulla is fresh air, pure air, charged with life and ozone—this recharges the medulla as nothing else does.

It will pay you to lay off—put your ambition "on ice" for a season and learn how to develop your medulla. Live a simple life, away from all excitement and especially away from people.

People draw you out and absorb you. They eat up your very life forces and leave you exhausted, even permanently exhausted, if you let them. If you can take yourself in hand now (and it will take courage to do it), give yourself two years to be by yourself (or longer, if necessary), where no one knows you or can see you and hibernate. Go to the high hills and live by yourself. Let someone else sell your books and take care of your obligations. Forget the obligations. Learn to be alone and rest your soul. Your knowledge and wisdom will increase, without any more cramming. You have enough knowledge stored up in your mind now to last a lifetime. In two years' time, more or less, you can return and appear a new man in health and mental capacity.

I think you can realize that as you are now, you cannot go on and depend upon anyone to cure you. You must do it yourself by taking drastic measures to develop your tired medulla. Two or three years' rest in the wilderness of silence and mental peace will do it. Give yourself an abundance of fresh air and a moderate supply of fresh foods. Go to the mountains and go to a height where it is comfortable to breathe, have plenty of blankets and perhaps a sleeping bag to sleep in when it is too cold. Sit in the sunshine each day or walk about until you are tired and sleep and sleep. You know so much about the country in the West that you will know where to go, perhaps near Medford, Oregon, if the altitude is high enough, or to the hills along the Columbia River in Oregon, or the mountaineous region in California near Yosemite Valley. The location is very important. Be sure to keep your chest warm at all times, with wool covering, so that no draft strikes your chest at any time, It would be well, to go up a little higher, from time to time as you find that it is comfortable to breathe when you are higher, for there the lungs are compelled to exercise more.

Live on a one-sided diet, not mixing too many different foods at the same time. You need sodium-chloride foods, which are important for you. Does goat milk agree with you? We think it does or should. Then take with you dehydrated goat milk, and mix it with soft water, if you can get soft water and make this a main part of your daily diet. Then use also New Life Food Blend, dissolved in soft hot water, or you can let it melt slowly in your mouth and drink a little water when necessary, but do not drink much water. Eat wild dark berries, if you can get them, or buy canned black berries and blueberries without sugar and keep on hand. You need little or no bread but can use some whole wheat crackers.

Then Nature will do the building of your vitality and all you need to pay for it will be a few month's time. It may be that Nature will do the job for you in a year, but stay as long as necessary.

If you will not do this for yourself, then we will tell you what to do otherwise that will cure you. This cure will come more slowly and you will have to be constantly on your guard to watch yourself so that you do not go too hard nor wear yourself out to the point of getting too tired. Taking this way you are not so likely to live the full allotment of your years, though you can keep well and work. Whenever any part of the body becomes worn out to the point of partial collapse, that part is never the same again, whether it be stomach, lungs, heart, medulla or cerebellum. That part has to be nurtured and cared for especially and never overworked again. The medulla is the chest brain, and takes care of the organs in the chest, the throat, lungs and breathing apparata, the heart, the stomach and the nerves associated with these organs and parts. It is most important to life and health, and has more to do with sudden death, as has also the cerebellum. The cerebellum belongs more to the muscular system, and is not seemingly weak, in your case, because your activity and overwork are more associated with the nerves and brain. You have studied too long and hard, and have worried, no doubt, because of responsibilities.

You must take it easier, in any case. These trips of yours, lasting nearly a year at a time, put you constantly under high strain. Tension is really killing to almost any type, and especially to one who is naturally tense as you are, with a tendency to do your utmost at every step of the way.

You have a choking sensation in your chest at times, an indication that you are greatly in need of oxygen, iron and sodium. You should begin to take New Life Food Blend regularly and quite liberally. Take it three times a day, a tablespoonful at a time; dissolve it in a cup of hot broth or in simmering water and drink it hot, or sip it. Take it before breakfast, before your evening meal, and again at bedtime—three times a day. It is charged with sodium, chlorine, calcium and iron and balanced also in the other elements. It is a very good food for the cerebellum, medulla and bloodstream, containing as it does the elements most needed by these parts. This is especially true for you

since these are the very elements you mostly use up because of your type.

Keep this food on hand and use it liberally until you are well and strong again. Then you can stop using it for a time, and begin again to take it, but not so much as right now. If you were to take a tablespoon of the Blend during the day, letting a small piece dissolve in your mouth, without the hot water or drink, you would succeed in supplying the elements that your system is constantly using up, or you could use pure concentrated goat whey cheese in the same way, later on, as it is also high in sodium, chlorine, calcium and iron. But right now, and for at least six months, you should use the New Life Food Blend three times a day until you are charged with these elements. Table salt is not so good for the sodium chloride elements, because it is not organized as it is in the goat milk.

You must make it a habit to keep your chest covered with pure wool or wool and silk covering. It is better that you use a small vest made of this material or a piece of folded cloth to size, and not just depend on warm underwear because the chest should be warmer than the rest of your body. This is important, and it should be kept on all year, not only in the colder weather. It will also prevent a chill draft from striking the chest at any time, summer or winter. It should be worn at night also, for the same reason.

Cod liver oil is high in vitamin D, and for this reason, you should take this every day. It will build up your general vitality as well as helping your lung to heal itself. Take a tablespoonful at bedtime, with a few tablespoonsful of orange juice. Get the kind from the drugstore that is flavored with peppermint.

Cod roe is something that will do much for your nerves, canned or fresh, or any kind of fresh roe, such as shad or herring, if you can get them. But canned cod roe is always available in any produce store, and you can keep it on hand. Use a tablespoonful or two, at least each day. You have it baked or heated in an oven with a little butter, and eat it as it is. Or take a tablespoonful of roe and add it to a cup of hot broth or New Life Food Blend drink and take it this way.

Raw egg yolk beaten up in fresh goat milk, and a drop or two of first class vanilla extract, and a teaspoonful of eucalyptus honey added, with the egg whites beaten stiff and folded in is excellent for the nerves. It is alkaline and feeds the nerves and brain. Take this eggnog at least three times every week regularly, whether you feel you need it or not.

Remember that these things taken *regularly* do the work—not just now and then at intervals. You need formic acid food to strengthen your throat. You use your throat a great deal and it is well to take care of it, so that it does not give way at any time.

Formic acid foods and fruits are excellent for you to remember. Fruit is high in formic acid. It is well for you to remember and order other foods instead of just fruit. We will list the best formic acid foods and fruit in your Diet List. For a throat gargle, use unsweetened pineapple juice, fresh or canned, and add a half teaspoonful of eucalyptus honey. This is a healing and strengthening gargle treatment for the throat. Use it when needed or anytime. For a troublesome cough, whenever you are bothered with it, use a tea made of ginger root. Simmer a good piece of ginger root in a cup of water for half an hour or so, and then add a little eucalyptus honey. Sip it, warm, several times if troubled with a cough.

A cup of hot New Life Food Blend taken before meals will strengthen your stomach and aid digestion, improving digestive juices and making digestion more perfect. You then get more strength from your foods and vitality increases.

Eat iron foods religiously and right along, for the purpose of attracting oxygen from the air you breathe—get out and breathe moving air. Inhale rather slowly and smoothly and evenly, without jerking the diaphragm. Then inhale again and keep it up 10 minutes at a time, whenever you can keep your mind on breathing and the air is fresh and pure. Make it a habit and in time you will breathe this way all the time. Food Blend has more iron than liver; calves liver rightly prepared or broiled with an onion, for flavor; take it whenever you can. Dark berries, as blueberries, blackberries or loganberries are high in iron.

Raw meat juice, from lean beefsteak, is another high iron food. If you have a meat juicer, put some raw roundsteak, cut in one-inch pieces, press and add some raw parsley. When you get a half cup or a quarter cup of juice, put the cup in a pan of hot water until it gets to body temperature, and then drink it. You will get the iron and the vitamins that are natural; no food or drink is more vitalizing. *Perhaps you would not be able to do this, but as a last resort, we would advise you to procure it.* You will be surprised at the rapid and wonderful results to your nerves, brain and general vitality. You will feel like a new man almost at once, after taking half a glass of this vitality giver, once a day for a time. It will do you good at all times and give you vitality to endure hard work and hardships, nervous prostration or severe physical and mental exhaustion. It builds vitality quickly. If you care to, you can buy an Enterprise press, No. 34, clean it and pour hot water through it to warm up the iron, and then feed it with pieces of roundsteak that have been heated in a pan but not cooked, so the red meat is unchanged. Sip it while it is lukewarm, but never heat it to change the meat.

You mentioned having some trouble with urination but I did not get it clearly, so do not know the cause. It may be prostate trouble. If so, there are modern methods of surgery for the gland that are bloodless; this should be the best thing to do under necessary circumstances.

Parsley tea is excellent for urinary difficulty. This is to be made of a handful of raw parsley in water to barely cover, simmer for 20 minutes, strain a cup and drink from time to time. Or make the raw parsley juice and take it by the teaspoonful. These are urination promoting.

Hop tea for bitters is something that you should remember to take occasionally. Take a cupful of this tea about once a week or every ten days. Hop tea is good for the nerves as well as for the liver.

A mixture of juniper berries and sarsaparilla in a tea is excellent for painful urination. Simmer a teaspoonful of each in a cup of water, strain and drink it any time needed.

Here is a diet that *feeds the brain and soothes the nerves:*

2 tablespoons of cod roe
2 tablespoons of beaten (stiff) eggwhite
2 tablespoons black cherries, strawberries, plums or persimmon pulp
2 tablespoons well-beaten baked banana
1 teaspoon Upjohn's sodium phosphate

Mix well and freeze. Take this any time you like. Do not forget to use cod roe as we have mentioned elsewhere as food for nerves and brain. Nerve food and brain food *must* come from an animal source such as fish roe or other eggs and egg preparations, necessarily *raw*.

You are a strong man in a muscular and motive sense, but weaker in the vital makeup. This is where you have to watch yourself. Your brain is a master driver, pushed to the limit by your very strong ambition to be recognized as a mental worker, a seeker after knowledge and wisdom. To watch your body and its functions and to improve yourself in this direction is your most important duty—not only now or temporarily, but all the time and permanently.

Your vitality is not so good because your blood is defective in sodium chloride, but you are wiry and enduring and keep going, mostly to your vital detriment. You are subject to congestion of the blood, especially when chilled. The best help for this is the New Life Food Blend as needed. We have named the special and outstanding foods and combination for you to watch and provide for yourself right along, so that you are not bothered or burdened by thinking about too many things, especially when you are too busy and perhaps away from home. But when you leave home, you should pack your grip with such things of these that you need to take along with you. Keep them on hand and you are safe.

In your general diet, you always need organized sodium chloride foods; they are the most important. You need also potassium foods, together with sodium and at times bitter tea and tonic. You need iron foods and tonics. You need alkaline broths that are high in the elements needed for easy digestion, especially when hot or warm. The broths that we mentioned are the best foods to carry the cartilaginous elements, gelatine, ligamentous structures that you need. The alkaline, sodium, potassium, magnesium and calcium elements must not be forgotten. Eggs and goat milk foods (cheese) are an antiuratin. You should use Food Blend, Squibbs bicarbonate of soda, spices (salt with your food) and tonics. The following broths are very valuable for you:

Broths

Bone broth—veal bone, chicken bones or fish bones should be used *in all your* broths. Veal bone broth, cooked slowly, with meat cut off, cooked slowly with carrots, celery, parsley, onions and other vegetables just covered with water. Strained after about three hours. Keep broth in refrigerator and use a cupful heated and New Life Food Blend dissolved in the hot broth, sipped hot before meals or between meals.

Apple peeling in a bone broth, cooked together, strained.
Celery broth with goat milk added when ready.
Chicken bone broth cooked with celery and parsley.
Fish bone broth, cooked with half a lemon.
Crabmeat broth.
Oyster broth with goat milk.

New Life Food Blend was a concentrated dried goat whey, now sold as Whex by Briar Hill Dairies, 279 S.W. 9th St., Chehalis, WA 98532.

Meat and Fish

Rare tender beefsteak, cut thick; cooked rare so the juice is free.
Gizzard of fowl, steamed until tender.
Smoked whitefish, steamed.
Steamed smelt
Steamed, tender young fish, eaten with lemon juice added.
Any tender broiled meat.
Lean lamb chops
Leg of lamb roast
Fresh, tender broiled, baked or steamed fish.
Fresh herring, broiled
Butterfish, broiled or steamed
Cheese, butter, cream, eggs
New Life Food Blend
Broth, goat whey cheese.
Fresh goat milk—a little cream.
Butter, as needed, not too much.
Egg, prepared in any way you like.
Raw eggnogs.

Vegetables

Crisp, raw celery
Steamed celery
Raw, grated carrots
Steamed carrots
Crisp, fresh celery and cabbage, as a salad
Radishes eaten with salt
Boiled beets
Red cabbage, boiled 7 to 10 minutes

Desserts

Fresh fruits or melon
Baked apples with goat cream
Strawberries
Pineapple, fresh or canned, without sugar
Blackberries or blueberries
Few blanched, grated almonds over other foods.
Persimmons
Bananas
Papaya sauce

Drinks

You should not drink much water, and the water that you do drink should be soft, clean, but never mineral water.

Wild cherry juice, mixed with a little water.
Plain fruit juices, blueberry, strawberry, etc.
Celery juice
Fresh goat buttermilk, if you can get it.
Goat buttermilk, mixed with French vichy water.
Gingerale and buttermilk, mixed.
Gingerale and grapefruit juice, mixed.
Distilled warm water
Milk of Magnesia mixed in milk for acidity.
Oat water or tea
Carbonated drinks occasaionally, for gas.
Bitter drinks, such as hop tea
Sage tea, hot, with lemon, for colds.
Parsley, alfalfa or red clover tea

Flavorings

Peppermint
Sage
Eucalyptus honey, sparingly
Beet sugar, sparingly

Dressings

Roquefort cheese
Sour cream
Oyster

Salads

Fish roe
Crabmeat
Celery and pineapple
Banana salad
Tomato with cucumber

Breads

You do not need much bread, and, in fact, you should avoid all kinds of food made of flour and carbohydrates.

Eat a little bread, but not much, and avoid sweetbreads, cakes, etc.
Brown rice bread or muffins.
Brown rice cereal, occasionally.
Rye bread with caraway seeds.
Swedish rye krisp.
Russian rye bread.

Sandwiches

Veal joint jelly slices on rye bread
Lamb roast and raw spinach leaves or lettuce
Roquefort cheese and slice of pineapple
Pineapple and cottage cheese
Crabmeat and celery
Boiled lean ham and celery
Ham and carrot
Baked fish roe and tomato
Sliced chicken and lettuce

Nutrient Losses in Foods
Three washings of rice in water cause the following losses: calcium—10%, iron—21%, phosphorus—5%, riboflavin—17% and niacin—9%. Cooking destroys enzymes, vitamins and some minerals; the longer and hotter food is cooked, the greater the losses. Waterless stainless-steel cookware keeps the most nutrients when properly used. Steaming is second best. Boiling is least preferred. In cooking meats, roasting and broiling cause the least losses of nutrients.

nine

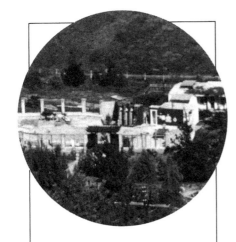

My sanitarium experience

Remember that when you help one organ—every other organ benefits also.

Biochemical remedies do not cover all aspects of wholistic treatment. For mechanical, mental or spiritual disorders, the appropriate disciplines should be utilized.

Americans ate better 200 years ago, according to nutritionists. "Their food was naturally fresh," says Dr. E. Cheraskin. "It had none of the preservatives and coloring agents which we now know are harmful." Dr. Jean Mayer of Harvard University pointed out that the early Americans would never have dreamed of having coffee and donuts for breakfast.

Drinking coffee reduces the body's ability to absorb iron, according to Timothy Morck, a researcher with the Veteran's Administration Hospital in Hampton, Virginia. Drinking coffee an hour before a meal cuts iron absorption by 22%.

My sanitarium experience has been the greatest work I've done. It proved to be the best experimental mode and the best way to give attention to patients, because I lived with them day after day. Such opportunity to help people simply cannot be matched in a doctor's office. Working with nutrition, I saw thousands of my sanitarium patients recover. We had people who came to us on stretchers, many having made reservations for the other side. They had to be brought back to life, one teaspoon at a time. I literally *lived* this work, and that is why I believe in it.

My sanitarium experiences have led me to believe that bodies are servants of the mind and spirit. I have seen how all disease is cured from within—out, from the head down, and in the reverse order that it has been built into the tissues. In no other way could I have come to realize how important it is to know that only from foods can we get the chemicals necessary to rebuild and rejuvenate every organ, or how the chemical story is the most neglected one in the average doctor's procedures for healing. Nutrition must be considered in rebuilding every tissue in the body.

In over 50 years of sanitarium care, my staff and I worked to improve the vital energies of our patients through rest, exercise and nutrition. Rest is very important, because bodies repair best in quietude. Further, we gave our patients the opportunity to get away from negative thoughts and action patterns from the past and to start down a new road so that their bodies could work toward wellness.

Remarkably, some patients who seemed to have very little left to work with in their bodies, possessed a vital force—or survival force—that helped to pull them through. This demonstrates that, although feeding the proper biochemicals is tremendously important, so is that vital force or soul force, which must accompany physical treatment. Both of these work together and both must be present.

In our many years of work, proof of the rightness of our methods was repeatedly demonstrated. Depression and gloom would be left behind. We would see glands

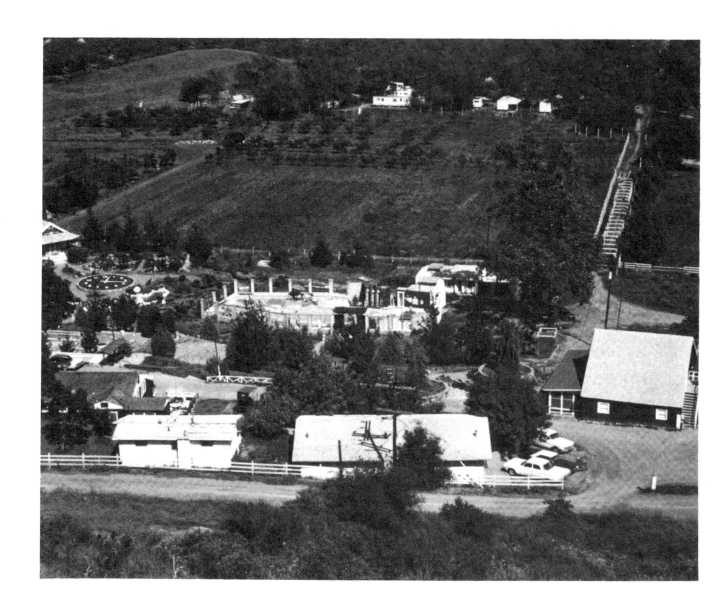

This is my Hidden Valley Health Ranch, Escondido, California. I selected this particular location because of the altitude, climate, clean air, rich black soil and beautiful natural surroundings. We grew a good deal of our own fruits and vegetables, and kept chickens and goats for the fresh eggs and fresh raw milk. I feel the whole environment of a sanitarium should be oriented toward getting and staying well. This constant contact with patients is much different from an office practice where the doctor has little opportunity to get to know a patient as a person, a real human being. If a patient was not improving at my sanitarium, I could see it immediately and take corrective steps. There is no way a sanitarium doctor can get away from his mistakes, so he has to take care of them.

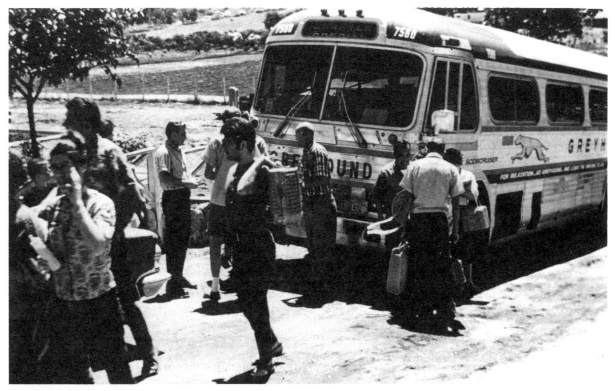

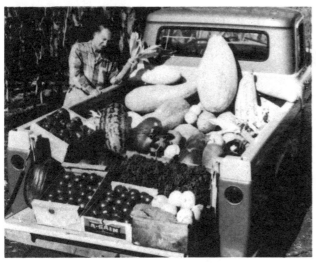

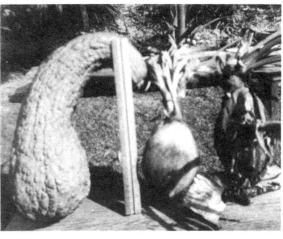

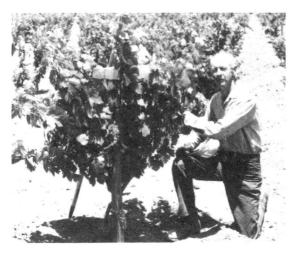

People from all over the world came to my Ranch to learn the principles of right living. We grew many wonderful fruits and vegetables at the Ranch, including grapes. A climate in which grapes thrive is a healthy climate for man. I found many of the oldest people in the world living in the grape areas.

97

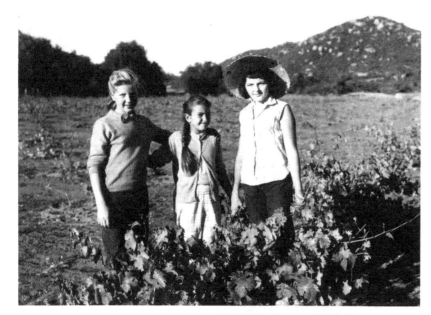

Fresh air, sunshine, nutritious food and a positive attitude toward life are the building blocks of well-being. My sanitariums were always found in beautiful locations.

There is a peace and healthy vitality to Ranch living that few manage to find in the city.

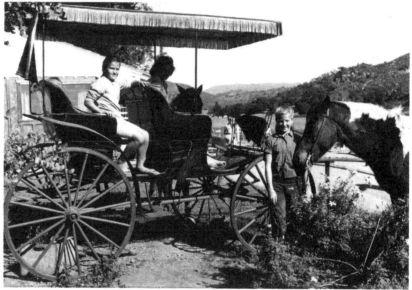

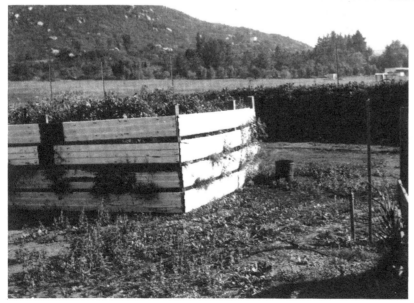

Our compost pile. We used no artificial sprays or chemical fertilizers at the Ranch.

change and the nervous system pick up. New tissues developed. The Pap test would change its findings. I began to see changes in the skin as pimples left. At times, in accordance with Hering's law of cure, I saw emerging more serious problems than those about which the patient originally complained.

For example, one man came and within three weeks he broke out in 90 boils. He blamed the diet, but the truth was that the boils broke out on him as a way of discharging materials that he brought with him. He needed to see that the life force was driving that material out through chemical changes in his body. The life force was doing its job well.

Blood circulated to the organs must be clean, toxin-free, drug-free and chemically balanced. To build a clean bloodstream, the bowel must be clean. In an excellent experiment with barium meal, we found that one week later it was still settled in the diverticula and various pockets in the bowel. This fact led us to conclusions about putrified foodstuff, fermentation problems and low-grade infections in the bowel.

In this sanitarium work, we were also able to see the ptosis in the abdominal organs in "before" and "after" stages. Using barium meal helped us to find the exact position of the transverse colon in cases of prolapsus. We found that gravity was a destructive force to a tired body due to its effect on the transverse colon. By taking pictures of a patient standing up rather than lying down, we were able to determine how the prolapsed colon was creating pressure symptoms and trouble in other organs, especially the prostate gland, the rectum, bladder, uterus, ovaries—all lower abdominal organs. When blood circulation is impaired, organ function is impaired, and tissues begin to starve to death. I began to see why we suffer from hemorrhoids due to ptosis. Through the sanitarium experience, I acquired skills in identifying the sources of many specific troubles.

At the same time, using iridology, I would see the tissue change according to the feeding administered to our patients. It was wonderful that in spite of the genetic pattern in the bones, glands and nervous system, we were able to fortify a patient with a greater vital and spiritual force. Through chemical balance, the patient began working at a higher level, being toxin-free and in good health. After years of troubles, patients began functioning normally.

The chemistry of man is affected by physical, mental and spiritual attributes and when these are working in harmony, the life force lifts our health level and brings us back to a state of wellness.

The Beginnings of My Sanitarium Work

Many of my ideas for sanitarium work were inspired by Dr. V. G. Rocine. As one of his students, I often wondered why he didn't have a big sanitarium of his own, because he believed in this work so deeply. He recommended having a place where mind, body and soul could be cultivated, individually for patients. He often talked about how limiting it was to give a person a lecture once a week when the patient was too weak in the intervening time to recognize what was necessary in order to care for himself.

Sometimes, it takes years before a person learns good health habits. Once determined to do so, it would help (as Dr. Rocine suggested) if we turned our homes into sanitariums. It is difficult, however, for most people to change their habits and homes in order to make a clean sweep and start anew. Most of the people I treated, when I started out, had been to hospitals and felt discouraged or hopeless. They had spent all their money on operations and then lost their trust in doctors. With such problems, I eventually had to turn to the most ideal way of treating patients wherein I could live with them and hope to inspire them.

Before that, when just out of college, I had decided that the ideal way was to have an office with a table to do massage, reflex therapy and chiropractic adjustments. Here, too, I would do my diet counseling and after treatment, I would send the patient home. Then, however, I became very busy, and the busier I became, the more I went downhill. It was not unusual for me to work 16 hours a day so that in time I came to be sick of sickness. I was sick of listening to complaints and nothing else.

The sanitarium experience was entirely different. People came to live in the country with me, giving me a chance to train them. We had lectures three times a week in the evenings. In the morning, we started out with physical activities and exercises. On our walks, I taught them about herbs. We would pick sage along the way, rub it into our hands and breathe it in for stimulation of the olfactory nerves and nasal membranes. For those with sinus problems, we would pick bay leaves in the orchard, also rubbing the leaves into our hands and breathing. In some of the extreme cases, I was able to teach them about salt nasal douches and chlorophyll nasal douches.

I also told them how to put powdered horseradish on the tip of the tongue and to breathe it. That lifted the tops of their heads right off, but it cleaned out their sinuses! Incidentally, no one can clean the sinuses in less than a year's time. Sometimes it can take as many as five years, living a good life.

Dr. George Weger's Inspiration

George Weger, MD, of Redding, California, was probably the one who prompted me to take up sanitarium work seriously. Too, I learned much of my fasting work from him.

One of the first patients in my Oakland office was an 18-year-old boy. Doctors wanted to remove his legs because of poor circulation. It overwhelmed me that a boy so young would have to have both legs amputated. However, the circulation was terrible, and the veins were so swollen that the legs themselves were an ulcerous mess. He was scheduled for surgery on a Monday and I was seeing him on the prior Friday night.

I had been reading *The Genesis and Control of Disease* by Dr. Weger, so I called the boy into my office and asked him if he would consider taking another path if there was a way to go without surgery. He said, "I sure would! You know, I can't believe this is going to happen to me." I called Dr. Weger and he said, "Why don't you bring the boy here and let me see what can be done?"

Of course, you can't merely start feeding a person carrot juice when he has been run over with an automobile. Because there were extreme measures here to be considered, I drove all night and took the boy to Redding. After checking him over for about an hour, Dr. Weger said, "Dr. Jensen, you're a pretty young man yourself. Would you like to see something nice happen to this boy? He doesn't need this operation, but it

will take a little time to see what we can do." I told him I would do anything to see the boy get well. It would mean as much to me to keep his legs as it would to him. Amputation just did not seem the way to go.

The first step was to put the boy on a fast, and the results were amazing! He was climbing trees in 30 days, which he hadn't done in years. He had shoes on for the first time in three years. In short, there was an incredible change. My prayer was a cry as much as a prayer, a cry of thankfulness for what had happened to this boy.

Since Dr. Weger did his work through fasting, I began to think about how I could better care for a boy like this coming into my office. Clearly his case was beyond the capabililties of the usual office practice. There had to be a sanitarium means of taking care of such a patient. With this realization, and in combination with Dr. Rocine's work, I decided to put these concepts into practice.

It was not long before I opened my first sanitarium south of Oakland, California, in the little town of Ben Lomond up in the coastal mountains near Santa Cruz.

But, I had more to learn.

In Philadelphia, I learned more about fasting and running a sanitarium from Dr. Fox, who was operating one of his own.

Then I went to Dr. Tilden's and Dr. Lust's sanitariums in Butler, New Jersey.

I traveled widely visiting many other spots, including milk sanitariums and Nevidick's nature-cure sanitarium in Wisconsin, where they used baths and many other therapies.

The excellent work I observed convinced me that sanitarium work was the proper way to practice. About that time, I wrote a short, inspirational story that came to me during the night. It concerned a doctor who lived on a hill and was extremely busy. Before people could see him, they had to work on his ranch—farming, pruning, digging and so forth. By the time he spoke to them, their troubles had receded. Half of his work was done before the patient ever appeared before him!

This story was a reflection of my belief that, first of all, a doctor should be living in the right place for his own health. Secondly, he should be able to bring people to him to live correctly, to consider what is right and then to live close to nature afterwards.

A Case of Eczema

Additional inspiration came from a boy just back from the war who had gone to high school with me. He had an extreme case of eczema, with skin troubles and fungus on his nails and fingers, under his arms and between his legs. He spent over a year in a foreign country hospital, but had been handled by our own doctors with no results. He believed that if he could "...just get to Bernard, and be with him for awhile, I'm positive I could get out of my troubles."

For months, they would not release him from the hospital in Asia where he was stationed. After a year's time, he prevailed on them to admit him to a hospital in this country. Finally, he was able to get fairly close to me in the Veterans' Hospital at Olive View in California. Once under my care, his skin troubles disappeared in about three or four months.

The Master of the Inn

This patient gave me a book which he said reminded him of me, and which reminded me of the story I had written. It was called *The Master of the Inn* by Robert Herrick, a story about a doctor who had gone up into the hills. He had lost his wife—and I had just lost my first wife. We seemed to have something in common. The book described the hills, pathways, flowers, greenery and the inspiration of breathing for a person out among the trees in the hills. The description stuck in my mind. I was plagued, driven with a desire to find that place. When I wrote to the publishers of this book, they told me it was purely fictional. They also told me they had received over 16,000 inquiries with the same question.

The story tells about a young man who regains his health with the *Master of the Inn* by living in the country and doing things that were good for the recuperation of mind and t rain. Feeling better, this fellow goes back to the city where a friend says, "You look wonderful— where have you been?" Upon learning the answer the friend decides to go there also. When meeting him, the doctor, "master of the inn," says, "Let's take a little walk." During the walk, the doctor tells him he should dig and hoe potatoes, then swim for awhile, and in a few days they will talk again.

Astonished, the fellow goes to his room, calls his friend who had sent him there, and demands to know what kind of place it is. "He wants me to dig potatoes and go swimming!" His friend in the city replies, "If the Master of the Inn told you to dig potatoes and go swimming— dig and swim, boy, dig and swim!" This story moved me tremendously because of what it said about truth and real life. Dig and swim, indeed!

The Hidden Valley Health Ranch became the culmination of my long search for a glorious place to promote health for the thousands of people who have, over the years, been students of my "how-to-live" philosophy.

Most people are willing to dig and swim, but if they do not do so in the country (where nature is) they probably will take two steps forward and two-and-a-half steps back. The best progress will be made in natural surroundings. All these influences and notions led me to set up my first sanitarium at Ben Lomond, California, in 1934-35. I went on to establish the Altadena sanitarium about 1940 and then the Escondido sanitarium in 1952.

I selected Escondido in Southern California because of its wonderful climate, pure clean air, rich soil and its isolation from the noise and turmoil of urban life. Escondido is in a valley surrounded by hills and low mountains.

The following are the basic ingredients in my view, for a successful sanitarium:

Restful moments; quiet; contentment
Peace of mind; healthful programs
Scientifically prepared; skillfully served food
Clear, smog-free, invigorating air
Pure water; nature's choicest vegetables
Wholesome, nutritional dairy products
Ideally superb environment
New, clean, stimulating swimming pool
Musical and variety radio and television programs
Horseback riding over miles of mountain trails
Fishing and boating
Spacious beautiful views
Complete and comfortable rooms
Large, airy dining room

Sheltering trees surrounded by flowers
Ideal elevation for comfort day and night
The "just-right" temperature

We found that patients need to be taught how to live, and I spent more time teaching than treating. People who know the right way to live outgrow the need for a doctor. Here are some of the principles I insisted patients learn:

1. That every disease is the result of wrong living habits.

2. That when a person knows the "art of living correctly" disease automatically leaves.

3. That nature is forever working toward perfect health.

4. That each individual can be sick or well depending upon the way he obeys or disobeys nature's laws.

5. That in order to get well, there must be a complete physical, physiological rest.

6. That the high tension of civilized methods demands more from the average human body than it is able to healthfully sustain.

7. That absolute quiet, natural foods, sleep, rest, air, sunshine, natural water, controlled exercises and playful recreation are an absolute necessity for regaining health.

8. That people should not be "treated" just for their ailments, but should be taught "how to live" to build a perfectly healthy body.

9. That to serve properly, a person must be balanced, physically, mentally and spiritually.

The belief in, and application of these tenets is a patient's assurance of full enjoyment of life's abundant blessings.

Create Beauty Around You—Your Home—Your Sanitarium

Anyone concerned with health ought to establish his or her home as a sanitarium in its own right. In any sanitarium, real sharing and concern are to be found, but the physical surroundings, too, are extremely important. First of all, your home should be beautiful, because beauty, itself, heals. Beauty comes in decorations and colors chosen in the presence of air, sunshine and flowers. In and around our homes, we need greenery. We need inspiration

that plants give. Observing them, we will train our minds as we conclude that everything has its purpose, whether flower or thorn. In time, we will learn that wherever there is disease, there is a cure right beside it.

We must be cautious, however, with the color red in decorations, because red suggests viciousness and is like having an ill-tempered dog around. Red, being strictly an arterial stimulant, is not conducive to relaxation because constant exposure to it hampers getting well. In fact, experiments have been made with various colors, and red has been shown to stimulate people to work harder for two or three hours, but after that short time, they want to fight. They become so aggressive they can't keep their minds under control as their impatience and irritability grow.

Goats Are Important, Too

Animals, too, should be part of our sanitariums, particularly goats. I became acquainted with goats through Dr. Rocine and included them in all my sanitariums. What can be done with goats is unbelievable, because the goat is a profitable animal. It is the poor man's cow and dairy. "With the same expense required to keep one cow or a horse," said Dr. Rocine, "you can keep ten goats." He said further, "Goats can live and thrive where a cow would starve to death." Indeed, the goat is a browser, living on brush, leaves and tree bark, whereas, the cow is a grazer, necessarily sticking to the ground. The goat can live on many foods unsuitable to the cow because of its digestive system.

For me, the goat is a lovable child. Wherever goats are kept in any number throughout the country, they are there because someone is sick, has tuberculosis, tonsil troubles or ulcers.

I was well aware of all these matters as I prepared for my sanitarium experience. When I did go into it, goats played an important part in our healing programs. I had 100 goats at the Altadena sanitarium. When I sold it, the goats went to the Altadena Dairy. This marked the beginning of the first big, commercial goat dairy in Southern California.

The Natural Gymnasium

Every sanitarium should have a gymnasium. By this, I mean, particularly, a *natural* gymnasium. At my sanitarium, we have been able to ride bicycles and take long walks in the hills so that patients can develop new, invigorating circulation. All organs die if the circulation of blood is impaired, which shows how important exercise is.

Certainly, my experiences with numerous elderly people have shown that one of the secrets of long life is to keep the legs active. In fact, in Germany, it is recommended that people with heart trouble walk as a way of changing their lifestyles and thus, of helping their hearts. They walk up a 3% grade the first week, a 6% grade the second and an 8% grade the third, and a little more each succeeding week, until the heart is strengthened.

In Germany, I also spent time studying the Kneipp water baths. Eventually, I installed a beautiful rock building at the Escondido sanitarium where people would walk in cold water up to their knees for a 30-foot distance. They didn't walk slowly but really moved along because the water was cold. Once out of the water, they would walk through grass and sand. This is the best way to develop good circulation in the legs. At about the fourth day of this treatment, people would tell me they were going to bed for the first time in years with warm feet. Natural health was returning to them because they were living healthfully.

The Proper Kitchen

It is extremely important to have the proper kitchen. We are used to thinking that we should have a kitchen designed to do a lot of cooking. This is nonsense, because 60% of one's food should be consumed raw. Here is where the training comes in as you learn how to make vegetable juices and mix vegetable juices with goat's milk. Drinking goat's milk when it is first brought to the kitchen is very healthy. Be sure to make clabbered milk from fresh and note that goat's milk can be sweetened with honey.

The most important gadgets for your kitchen are for making salads and juices. For cooking, we need the proper utensils to use with low heat—stainless steel pots and pans with tight-fitting lids so that no air can reach hot foods and cause oxidation. You can cook wheat into a cereal with this low-heat method. If you place it in the ground, it will still grow even though you have cooked it. This is the proper way to cook grains. We should be trained in food preparing skills so that our home is a health home or a sanitarium, especially including our kitchens.

Moreover, too much cooking in the kitchen, producing smoke and fumes will generate germ life that lives in the walls where fats and oils have permeated. Don't be afraid to paint your kitchen at least once a year to set things right again.

Bathroom Routines

The bathroom must not only reflect the decorative and cleanliness qualities we have already talked about but also be stocked and arranged properly for routines essential to maintaining good health. One has to do skin brushing. Enemas are needed if extra internal cleansing is required. Obviously, teeth and hair must be cleaned properly. We should know what a natural shampoo is for the hair and how to brush it to keep it in good health. We need knowledge of aloe vera for the skin and a supply of epsom salts, especially when there is a tendency toward arthritis.

Any so-called disease can involve several systems simultaneously.

Vegetable juices are an all-around body builder. Best all-around foods are bee pollen, chlorella, spirulina, propoulis, gensing.

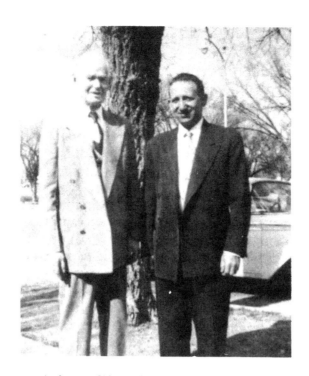

At the age of 93, Dr. George Heard, the famous dentist of "the town without a toothache" (Hereford, Texas—Deaf Smith County) told me, "Nutrition is the foundation of all good health. Because of the calcium-rich soil in Deaf Smith County, Dr. Heard didn't pull a single tooth in 30 years of practice.

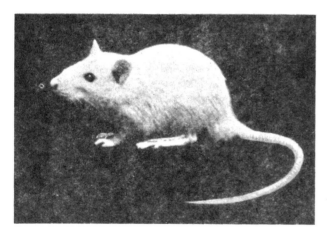

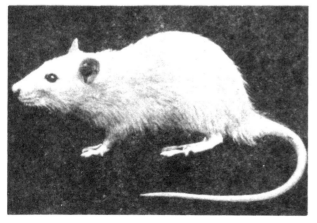

The stunted rat shown at the top of the illustration lacked calcium, another element aside from phosphorus, essential to bone growth. A lack of both calcium and phosphorus has the same effect as the lack of either. The rate of growth is dependent upon the available amount of the scarcest element. In actual practice, in both animal and human nutrition, calcium is much more frequently supplied in insufficient quantities than is phosphorus. The best known food for calcium supply is milk.

Photograph Bureau of Home Economics, U.S. Dept. Agriculture

104

ten

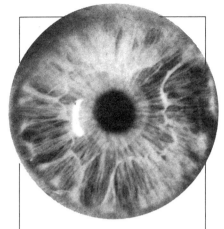

Iridology, nutrition and the chemical elements

In previous chapters, we have described how important nutrition and the right balance of chemical elements in the body are to the well-being of the body. We have discussed how the lack of chemical elements in the soil leads to plant life depleted of nutrients which, in turn, provides depleted foods inadequate for human nutrition. Finally, we have suggested that chemical imbalance in the body is the source of all dis-ease. If we had a way of "seeing" into the tissues of the body, we could then discover which parts of the body are lacking in chemical balance and we could work toward restoring that balance by nutritional means to prevent disease before it occurs or get rid of it after it occurs.

Fortunately, the science of iridology provides us with a means of understanding what is going on in the tissues of the body. Iridology, therefore, compliments nutrition to an extent which allows us to observe whether progress is taking place in rebuilding and rejuvenating tissue in specific parts of the human anatomy.

Iridology is based on the discovery over a century ago by Dr. Ignatz von Peczely that the iris is a kind of "map" of all the organs, tissues and structures of the body. The eye is actually an extension of the brain and is the most sensitive tissue to meet the outside world. The brain, which constantly monitors the condition of all parts of the body, relays that information to the nerves that go to the iris. Changes in the iris fibers and tissue, then, reflexly represent what is going on in the body. Iridology, or iris analysis, has been refined into a fine art and an increasingly reliable tool by generations of iridologists since its discovery.

Iridology reveals tissue inflammation, the stage of inflammation (acute subacute, chronic or degenerative) and its location in the body. It shows inherent strengths and weaknesses, acidity, anemia, lymphatic congestion, condition of the nerves, constitution and health level. We can look into the eye and determine what has been done to the body through incorrect living, improper diet, accidents and injuries.

Iridology's Teamwork with Nutrition

An iridologist, by examining the iris or a photograph of it, can tell what organs or tissues in the body are overactive (acute stage) or underactive (subacute, chronic, degenerative). Since we know what chemical nutrients are needed by each structure and what foods contain those nutrients, we can develop a specific nutritional program to cleanse the bloodstream, raise the general health level and supply the right biochemicals for organs and structures lacking them. Overactive organs require more of specific biochemicals to meet their needs, while underactive organs suffer from more long-term deprivation. In both cases, nutrients are needed.

Iridology shows where the chemical shortages are; nutrition tells how to meet their needs. It's a perfect symbiotic relationship. When healing begins to take place, white healing lines come into the areas of the iris where problems were formerly revealed. Iridology proves that nutrition works.

Iridology and Depletion

As we have said before, chemically-depleted foods cannot build a good body, and iridology can demonstrate that. When tissues lack key nutrients—even one—inflammation results initially in hyperactivity, later in hypoactivity. Hyperactivity is an increase in metabolic rate, possibly directed toward gathering more of the nutrient or nutrients needed by the tissue. Goiter may be a case in point. When the thyroid lacks the iodine so necessary to its functioning, it enlarges to increase its efficiency in gathering what little iodine may be available in the blood. After a period of time in the acute hyperactive state, the tissue lapses into hypoactivity, a lower metabolic state. An underactive organ or tissue cannot assimilate nutrients or get rid of wastes as well as normal or overactive tissue. This is a danger point because toxic wastes, drug residues or pollutants such as heavy metals may begin to settle in the underactive tissue, causing a deepening state of inflammation and hypoactivity. This is the vicious circle stage. Unless the chemicals needed by the tissue are supplied, it grows even weaker, less active and

more toxic laden. Iridology reveals this deteriorization.

The ultimate consequence of chemical depletion, toxic settlements and inflammation is dis-ease. Germ life and viruses feed on underactive, depleted tissue in which cells are dying and catarrh and toxins are gathering. In the words of Dr. W. Albrecht, Department of Agriculture, University of Missouri, "Disease preys on an undernourished body." The particular disease that emerges and the particular set of symptoms that manifests depend upon the constitution, inherent strengths and weaknesses and the lifestyle of the individual. Like a chain, the body is only as strong as its weakest link. The links that "break" first determine the disease that manifests.

For example, a lack of silicon may bring problems with the skin, a silicon organ. Pimples, boils, acne and roughness appear. The fingernails and toenails peel, crack and break. Likewise, every disease is associated with a lack of one or more essential chemical elements.

Drugs cannot get rid of disease because they cannot build or rejuvenate tissue as foods can. Drugs have their place, but only food can replace old worn-out tissue with new. Toxic settlements and drug deposits can also often be seen in the iris. By means of various types of iris signs, the iridologist knows which organs have become depleted.

Iridology can show when tissue is getting more and more depleted, and it can show when a nutritional program is working well.

We find that wholesome, natural foods do not destroy cells, unless wrongly prepared or eaten in excess. (An excess of almost anything can have destructive effects on the body.) Junk foods, fried foods, devitalized "foodless" foods can harm the body in two ways: by failing to provide chemicals needed in the diet and by introducing toxins (additives, biochemicals altered by processing or cooking) into the system.

In iridology we can tell from the area surrounding the pupil (the stomach ring) whether there is hyperchlorhydria or hypochlorhydria, too much or too little hydrochloric acid. We need hydrochloric acid to digest proteins, but too much of it can lead to ulcers or other conditions. Whether tissue is

CHART TO IRIDOLOGY

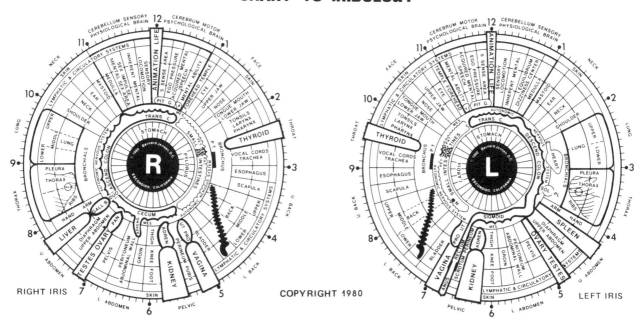

RIGHT IRIS 7

COPYRIGHT 1980

LEFT IRIS

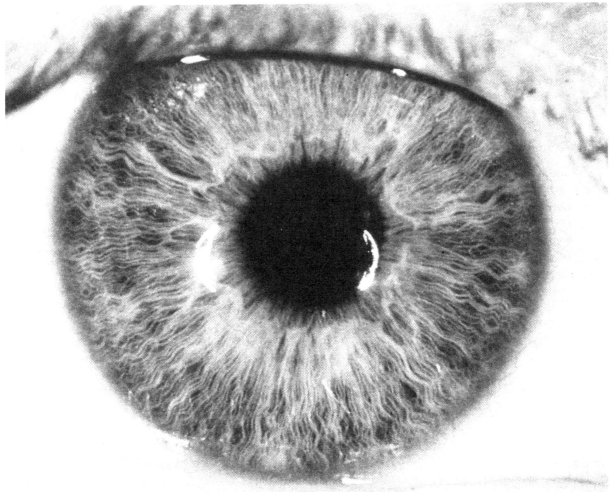

Iris analysis is the simplest, fastest and most reliable way to tell whether the body is responding to the nutrition program we are following. When the white healing lines come into the dark lesions, we know that internal tissue is responding to our nutritional regimen.

overactive or underactive, it needs to be fed more of the proper chemical elements.

Iridology analyzes tissue conditions. Nutrition corrects tissue conditions by restoring chemical balance. This is how iridology and nutrition work together, hand in glove.

As a change in the diet is made, its effects are seen in the eyes. Healing is signaled by the appearance of white healing lines. When dark areas of the iris lighten, or when white acute areas return to normal, healing is taking place. New tissue is coming in to replace the old. We know that the right foods have been taken because we see the evidence in the iris.

Chemical Elements and Human Body Structures

According to Dr. Koenig, the chemical elements that make up a 160 pound man or woman are as follows:

90 lb oxygen	3 oz potassium
36 lb carbon	2-1/2 oz sodium
14 lb hydrogen	2 oz fluorine
3 lb 12 oz calcium	1-12 oz magnesium
3 lb 8 oz nitrogen	1/4 oz silicon
1 lb 4 oz phosphorus	1/6 oz iron
4 oz chlorine	Trace of iodine
3-1/2 oz sulphur	Trace of manganese

The Body and The Chemical Elements

Body proteins: Carbon, hydrogen, oxygen, nitrogen plus phosphorus, sulphur and iron in many cases.

Body fat: Carbon, hydrogen, oxygen.

Required for cell metabolism: Iron, phosphorus, sodium, potassium, calcium, magnesium, sulphur, manganese, copper.

Percentage of water in tissues: Fat—20%, blood—80%, bone—25%, kidneys—80%, liver—70%, muscle—75%, skin—70%, brain—85%, nerves—70%.

Muscle: Potassium, magnesium, chlorine, manganese, calcium, phosphorus, selenium.

Bones and teeth: Calcium, phosphorus, magnesium, fluorine, silicon, copper, manganese.

Joints and ligaments: Sodium, iron, manganese.

Hair and nails: Silicon, iron, sulphur, zinc, chlorine.

Skin: Silicon, sulphur, sodium, manganese, copper.

Brain and nervous system: Phosphorus, magnesium, potassium, sodium, iodine, sulphur, silicon, calcium, manganese.

Heart: Magnesium, iron, potassium, calcium, phosphorus.

Blood: Iron, copper, zinc, sodium, potassium, calcium.

Blood vessels: Magnesium, silicon, sulphur.

Spleen: Iron, copper, fluorine, sodium, potassium, magnesium.

Liver: Zinc, selenium, sulphur, iron, potassium, magnesium.

Kidneys: Potassium, chlorine, fluorine, manganese, magnesium, calcium, iron, silicon.

Lungs: Phosphorus, manganese, silicon.

Gastrointestinal system: Sodium, potassium, chlorine, fluorine, iodine, calcium, iron.

Anus: Silicon.

Bladder: Silicon, fluorine.

Inner ear: Magnesium, fluorine, iron, chlorine.

Eyes: Sulphur, fluorine.

Pituitary: Iodine, phosphorus, sulphur, manganese, bromine.

Pineal: Phosphorus, sulphur, manganese.

Adrenal medulla: Phosphorus, sulphur, manganese, iodine.

Adrenal cortex: Calcium, fluorine, iron, silicon.

Thyroid, parathyroids, thymus: Sodium, potassium, chlorine, magnesium, iodine.

Pancreas, Islets of Langerhans: Zinc, manganese, potassium, chromium.

Prostate: Zinc, silicon, magnesium.

Testes, ovaries: Silicon, manganese, magnesium, phosphorus, zinc.

Introduction to the Chemical Elements

These are the sixteen chemical elements found in man, as presented in the work of Dr. V. G. Rocine with whom I studied. In his words, "A well-chemically balanced body is a healthy body." Additionally, there are traces of other elements. For complete coverage, we will be going into the chemical elements in depth in the next section of the book. For now, listed below are brief summaries of the sixteen elements.

Oxygen. Oxygen is needed by each individual cell in the body, for building, energizing and burning up waste. It affects each individual differently, according to the other chemical elements in the body. An ample supply of oxygen is needed in order to supply the lungs, blood and tissues, keep the arteries elastic, eyes glowing, heart active and agile. Some of the high oxygen foods are: liquid chlorophyll, iron tonics, red juicy meats, beets, grapes, tomatoes, onions, leeks, wild cherry juice and so forth. The best oxygen "foods" for the respiratory system are fresh mountain air, clean air and the higher altitudes.

Carbon. Carbon is the principal element of growth. Wherever carbon and oxygen are at work, one upon the other, there is heat generation, growth and generation of carbonic acid gas. Carbon is the basic element of cell birth and cell life and mainly supports the vital systems. An excess results in obesity, boils, fatty degeneration, anemia, high blood pressure. Carbon, or its compounds, occur mainly in starches, sweets, fats and also in most proteins. To counteract excess, avoid greasy foods such as fatty game, meats, oily fish, goose, fatty sausage and gravies. Foods low in fat are bass, bone broth, buttermilk, skimmed milk, goat milk cheese and cottage cheese, cauliflower, young carrots, tender cabbage, chard, string beans, blueberries, blackberries.

Hydrogen. Hydrogen is present in bodily secretions, soft tissue, lymph, brain, lungs, glands, liver, kidneys, spleen, pancreas. Hydrogen foods are the moisture-carrying foods, such as apricots, cherries, all berries, fruit juices, cabbage, tomatoes, leaf lettuce, Swiss chard, watercress. The nerves must be bathed in fresh moisture. Without hydrogen, the blood could not flow and waste and toxic materials could not be washed out of the body. An excess of water in the body, however, causes pressure and enlargement of body organs.

Calcium. Calcium gives vitality, endurance, heals wounds, counteracts acids, is tone-building in the body, and, of course, builds and maintains bone structure and teeth, where needed mostly. Calcium is the knitting element. Blood-clotting problems indicate a calcium deficiency. The metabolism of calcium needs vitamin F. Principal sources are bran and cheese (very high), raw goat cheese, Swiss, Dutch edam or gouda cheeses. Milk, raw egg yolk, figs, prunes, dates, onions, tops of vegetables, kale, cauliflower, bone meal, turnip greens, kidney beans, soy beans and lentils.

Nitrogen. Nitrogen, as found in food or in air, is a restraining element, the opposite of oxygen. Oxygen is like fire. Nitrogen is stillness itself. Without nitrogen, oxygen would burn us up and life would cease to exist. Nitrogen enters human tissue under many different names—in the solid elastic tissue, lymph, muscles, blood plasma, in the crystalline lens of the eyes, connective tissue, mucous membranes, skin, hair, nails. The main supply of nitrogen is found in proteins, the principal muscle builder. Nitrogen yields heat and muscular energy. A deficiency leads to muscular exhaustion, numbness, tired feelings. An excess of nitrogen, however, results in autointoxication, stagnation, swelling, forgetfulness, headache, enlargement of heart, so it is very important to keep nitrogen in proper balance. Nitrogen (or very high protein) foods are almonds, beans, beef, fish, goat cheese, lean veal, liver, quail, Swiss cheese, other cheeses and unleavened breads. Low nitrogen foods are young kale, milk whey, okra, ripe olives, parsley, apricots, artichokes, string beans, young carrots, romaine lettuce, tomatoes, turnips, wild cherry juice and wintergreen.

Phosphorus. Phosphorus is found (and needed mostly) in the nervous system and is a brain and bone element. This is a nerve builder and nourishes the brain, builds power of thought, stimulates growth of hair and bone and helps the thinking processes and intelligence. Indications of phosphorus deficiency are loss of patience, neurosis, craving of excitement, psychosis, fears and anxiety. Phosphorus and sulphur foods should be eaten together and are controlled by iodine. Phosphorus also needs more oxygen. An excess will cause weak kidneys and lungs. Principal sources of phosphorus are sea foods, milk, raw egg yolk, parsnips, whole wheat, barley, yellow corn, nuts, peas, beans and lentils.

Chlorine. Chlorine is found (and needed mostly) in the digestive system and glandular secretions. It is the cleanser in the body, expels waste, freshens, purifies, disinfects. Deficiency contributes to sluggish liver and glandular swellings. Goat's milk provides chlorine and helps effectively in kidney problems because of its germicidal effect. Other principal sources are raw milk, fish, cheese, coconut, beets, radishes, dry figs, endive, watercress, cucumber, carrots, leeks, Roquefort cheese, Danish blue cheese, Swiss cheese, Italian cheese, all green vegetables.

Sulphur. Sulphur is a brain and tissue chemical element, found (and needed mostly) in the nervous system. Sulphur tones the system, purifies and activates the body, intensifies feelings and emotions. Sulphur needs iodine to work properly. Driving force for goals and achievements are stimulated by sulphur foods. Indications of sulphur deficiency are fretting, pouting, retiring late and rising early, poor appetite in the morning, extremes of variety and change. Indication of excess sulphur is face burning. An excess indicates need for chlorine and magnesium foods. Principal sources of sulphur are cabbage, cauliflower, onions, asparagus, carrots, horseradish, shrimp, chestnuts, mustard greens, radish, spinach, leeks, garlic, apples, turnip and beet tops, plums, prunes, apricots, peaches, raw egg yolk and melons.

Potassium. Potassium is a tissue and secretion chemical element. It is found (and needed mostly) in the digestive system. Potassium is a healer in the body, liver activator, makes tissues elastic, muscles supple, creates grace, beauty and a good disposition. Potassium is strongly alkaline. Indications of deficiency are a desire for cold foods, sour foods and acid drinks. Principal sources are potato skins, dandelion, dill, sage, dried olives, parsley, blueberries, peaches, prunes, coconut, gooseberries, cabbage, figs and almonds.

Sodium. Sodium is a gland, ligament and blood builder. It is found (and needed mostly) in the digestive system. Sodium is the youth maintainer in the body. Sodium aids digestion, counteracts acidosis, halts fermentation, purifies the blood, forms saliva, bile and the pancreatic juices. Flexibility of tendons needs high sodium foods. Sodium aids the intestinal flora. Indications of deficiency are restlessness, depression, nervousness, poor concentration, tender abdominal muscles, sore cervical glands, puffiness in face and body and inactive spleen. Principal sources are okra, celery, carrots, beets, cucumbers, asparagus, turnips, strawberries, oatmeal, raw egg yolk, coconut, black figs, spinach, sprouts, peas, goat cheese and goat milk, goat whey, fish, oysters, clams, lobster, milk and lentils.

Fluorine. Fluorine is found (and needed mostly) in the structural system, tooth enamel and for preserving bones. It is a disease resister and a beautifier in the body, strengthening tendons and knitting bones. Fluorine combines with calcium. It is stored in the spleen, eye structure, elastic tissues. Fluorine is destroyed by too high cooking temperature. Raw goat milk contains highest content of fluorine. Other principal sources are cauliflower, cabbage, cheese, cow milk, raw egg yolk, cod liver oil, brussels sprouts, spinach, tomatoes, watercress, salad vegetables and black bass (fish).

Magnesium. Magnesium is nature's laxative, a nerve mineral found (and needed mostly) in the digestive system. It prevents and relieves autointoxication, refreshes the system and is a new cell promoter in the body. Indications of magnesium deficiency are tenderness, excitement problems and excessive emotion. Principal sources are grapefruit, oranges, figs, whole barley, corn, yellow cornmeal, wheat bran, coconut, goat milk and raw egg yolk.

Silicon. Silicon is found (and needed mostly) in the structural system, nails, skin, teeth and hair and in the ligaments. Silicon creates a magnetic quality and is the surgeon in the body, giving keen hearing, sparkling eyes, hard teeth, glossy hair, tones the system and gives resistance to the body. Silicon is especially important for agility in the body for walking and dancing. Indications of silicon deficiency are coordination problems, fungus diseases, parched lips, feeling of approaching death, impotence and sexual disability. Principal sources of silicon are oats, barley, brown rice, rye, corn, peas, beans, lentils, wheat, spinach, asparagus, lettuce, tomatoes, cabbage, figs, strawberries, rice polishings, oat straw tea, watermelon seeds and peelings, coconut, sage, thyme, hops, prunes, bone marrow, raw egg yolk, pecans, cod liver oil and halibut liver oil.

Iron. Iron is essential in the blood as the oxygen carrier, prevents anemia, promotes vitality and ambition. Iron foods attract oxygen. Indications of iron deficiencies are weakness, lassitude, skin eruptions, leukorrhea, tendency for crying, personal magnetism often fails, asthma problems, bronchitis and hemorrhages. Principal sources are all green, leafy vegetables, wild blackberries and black cherries, egg yolk, liver, oysters, potato peeling broth, whole wheat, parsley, parsnips, spinach, Swiss chard, goat brown cheese, artichokes, asparagus, nettle tea, leeks, lamb's lettuce, white onions, rice bran, whole rye meal and salad greens.

Iodine. Iodine is a gland and brain element. It is a metabolism normalizer in the body, prevents goiter, normalizes gland and cell action, ejects and counteracts poisons. Indication of iodine deficiency are claustrophobia, fears, flabby arms, pronunciation difficulties and mental depression. Principal sources of iodine are powdered Nova Scotia dulse, sea lettuce, sea foods, carrots, pears, onions, tomatoes, pineapple, potato skin, cod liver oil, garlic, watercress, green leek soup, clam juice and nettle tea.

Manganese. Manganese is a memory element, tissue strengthener, for linings of body structure, increases resistance, improves memory, coordinates thought and action and is needed mostly in the nervous system. Manganese is dependent on iron and phosphorus. Indications of deficiency are facial neuralgia, angry and silent moods and rectal cramps after meals. Principal sources of manganese are nasturtium leaves, raw egg yolk, almonds, black walnuts, watercress, mint, parsley, wintergreen, endive, pignolia nuts.

Nature has given us hundreds of foods that contain healing elements for our health and well-being. We should study these foods, analyze and understand the natural healing properties they contain. Many hundreds of commercial foods and drinks become slow-acting poisons *by default* because they lack the necessary chemical elements needed to maintain and rebuild the cells and tissues of the body.

Applying the laws of health leads to liveliness, suppleness, strength, youthful freshness and charm, even in middle age and old age.

A genuine food chemist and nutritionist knows that the proper foods cure in one way— they build up the blood and tone the organs, nerve centers, brain centers and the glandular system. When deficient food elements are supplied in the proper balance, the organs take on new strength. A new world opens for the mind and its creativity.

All of these normalizing changes back up good health and can be viewed in the iris. This is the invaluable link iridology has in correlation with nutrition.

"It is estimated that one-half of the fatal cancers in women and one-third in men may be attributed in part to diet habits.
"If the 'dangerous' elements in food could be identified, they then could be avoided, thus preventing many cancers."
—Dr. Paul A. Marks
Cancer Research Center
Columbia University

Who wants a cancer diet? Avoid all food additives and refined foods. They may be carcinogenic. Is it worth the chance and waiting through years of research for inconclusive conclusions?

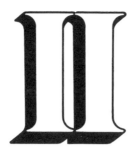

You and Mother Earth

Dr. V. G. Rocine's discovery of the relationship between biochemical deficiencies and the basic human temperament types was ingenious. Very simply, we find there is a calcium type of person, a silicon type of person, and types corresponding to the other 14 elements so important in human nutrition. In the calcium type, there is a greater need for calcium foods in order for that person to express his or her particular temperament, and if a calcium deficiency develops, not only is the body affected but the soul. The same principle follows for each of the chemical types of people.

Deficiencies, Rocine believed, always affect body, soul and spirit. It is said that man is a spirit who lives in a body and has a soul. The spirit encourages the soul to develop its attributes and express them through the activities of the body. Yet, we must remember, the body is made of the dust of the earth. Unless the body has the right chemicals in the right proportions, it cannot express health; it can only express disease.

These are not principles taught in our medical schools. Nevertheless, they must be understood if man expects to learn how to cooperate with nature in the healing process.

The world has no medical schools that can teach their students how to cure disease. No university in the world today, no medical school, no university-trained dietician, no doctor, no professor sufficiently understands quantitative food chemistry, chemical diagnosis, chemical types of people, food materials from the viewpoint of quantitative food chemistry, the proper preparation and combination of food and diet, as required by a sick person, because all of such studies are not taught in universities nor in medical schools, neither are the real causes of diseases known.

Each human chemical type has its own chemistry, its own disease tendencies, its own diathesis and its own diet needs. The mind and the emotions, the climate, the air pressure, the electrical tension of the atmosphere, the altitude, the habits of the man and hundreds of other conditions have their effects on health and disease. Different diets also have their effects on health and

disease. Excess acidity is a most prolific cause of disease. One chemical type is subject to one kind of acidity and gas formation. Fatty foods, when eaten to excess and metabolized, result in a special kind of acidity and disease. A high protein diet leads to ailments and diseases of a different type. An excessive carbohydrate diet terminates in a still different kind of gas generation, acidity and diseases. An excessive salty diet or excessive chlorine diet leads to another kind of acidity and disease.

We find that the soil itself may not contain the right chemical elements required for vigorous plants or for nutritious vegetables, greens, fruits, nuts and grains. Thus the food elements essential for the health of man and animals, may not be contained in the food. This would lead to disease in plants, animals and people. Deficiencies are passed down the food chain along with weaknesses and tendencies to disease.

Canners, millers and cooks, pare, peel, cut, slice, grind and cook away from 4 to 12 essential food elements in their processing of the food most people eat. Our government ignores such activities for the most part. We cannot rely on our political representatives, universities or doctors to make sure we are getting nutritious food or a balanced diet.

It is up to us to take responsibility for our own food, meal preparation and health knowledge. If doctors did more educating they would do less medicating, but unless we are prepared to learn, the availability of a teacher of right living does no good.

Each of the chemical elements has its own story to tell. Although each of us is more dependent on some chemical elements than others, we all need the 16 major elements plus a number of vital trace elements to stay healthy and to experience high level well-being. Any person can become deficient in any of the chemical elements, and some deficiencies can be very difficult to identify.

These days we find many people relying on mineral supplements from the health food store, and although these have their place, I must emphasize that we should get most of our minerals from foods. No chemical exists in isolation, except when prepared by laboratories. In nature, chemicals occur in groups—and we need these more complex forms in our bodies to ensure proper utilization and to avoid deficiencies. For example, without sufficient iodine and vitamin D, calcium cannot be properly used in the body; without vitamin B-12, iron cannot be assimilated. It is much more efficient and safe to get our minerals, vitamins and other nutrients from foods.

V. G. Rocine was a homeopathist who emphasized that the cell salts needed for health were naturally triturated and potentized by plants in the process of photosynthesis. This, he believed, raised the vibratory level of biochemicals to the point where they could be assimilated best by man. No human laboratory has yet learned to make foods better than Nature, or to improve upon Nature's methods. Foods bring in a sufficient variety of nutrients that the body can pick and choose what it needs, provided that we have sufficient variety in the diet.

Rocine believed that when we understand the chemical elements and temperament types, we have the basic knowledge necessary to take care of ourselves. I believe this is the kind of thing both doctors and patients must know to bring on the new day in the healing arts.

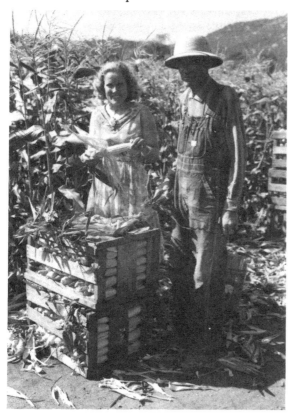 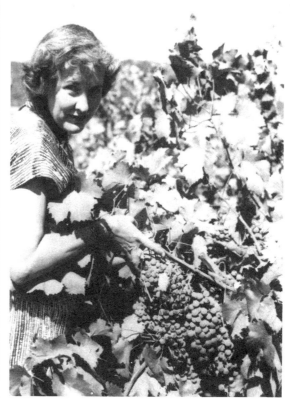

Foods from Mother Earth, properly grown on good soil, are man's best medicine. The woman on the right healed herself of cancer using a grape diet.

one

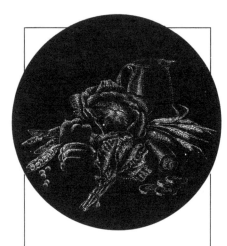

Calcium, the "knitter"

Many years ago, when I was the foreman of a creamery, I had an experience which showed me the great value of calcium. We had to purchase eggs, butter, cheese and so forth, and I was in charge of the truck drivers who delivered these products. Because they were not usually gentle when they handled the egg crates, the truck drivers were responsible for breaking a tremendous number of eggs when they delivered them.

So, I set about researching eggshells. I became intrigued with Petaluma, California, known as the egg capital of the world, because eggs were shipped from there to all parts of the globe, arriving in excellent condition. Why? The eggshells were tough.

The egg farmers revealed to me the small, but significant, secret responsible for those hard eggshells. They were feeding their hens green kale.

I rushed home to look up the nutritional value of green kale and found it to be one of the highest of all calcium greens—one of the highest of all calcium foods. Was it really possible to produce hard eggshells by feeding the chickens properly? It was.

I found, too, that by feeding the hens alfalfa, a light-colored yolk could be changed to a dark color in a matter of three days. I found that cayenne produced a dark red yolk.

It became evident to me that foods were responsible for the composition of eggshells as well as the color of the yolk and, in fact, the entire biochemical composition of those eggs. This experience prompted me to begin seeking more knowledge about biochemical elements and their influence on the physical body. I wanted to know how and what biochemical elements were needed by various tissues to change the body to build the best health expression.

In the research of Dr. Weston A. Price, author of *Nutrition and Physical Disease*, I discovered why calcium is so important in health. Dr. Price traveled all over the world to study health and nutrition in primitive and isolated cultures. Repeatedly he found that natives whose diets consisted largely of whole, raw natural fruits and vegetables, and fresh meat or fish, were free of those diseases common in civilized countries. They had healthy straight teeth and symmetrical dental arches. In contrast, natives of those same tribes and groups who moved to the cities and ate "civilized" food—packaged, processed, preserved and so on—quickly degenerated. The teeth deteriorated first. Second generation children had narrower facial bone structures, poorly-formed dental arches and soft teeth that decayed rapidly. In other words, calcium is one of the first elements in the body to go out of balance when the diet is inadequate, opening the door to a host of diseases and degenerative conditions.

During my search, I studied with Dr. Melvin E. Page, a dental surgeon from Florida, who had discovered that the endocrine glands exert a great deal of control over calcium in the body. He discovered that sugar is one of the main villains in throwing off endocrine system balance and calcium balance. Dr. Page found that elderly patients experiencing loss of calcium from the jawbone could be successfully treated with small doses of glandular substance and a change in diet. He found cavities in teeth could be almost eliminated by balancing the endocrine system and by eating wholesome, natural foods. The first sign of calcium imbalance, then, is dental cavities.

I went to see Dr. George Heard, a dentist in Deaf Smith County, Texas in 1959, when he was 93. They had nicknamed his home town "the town without a toothache" because of his remarkable work. More than any other person, Dr. Heard persuaded me that calcium was the most important element in the body. The soil in Deaf Smith County is high in calcium, and the healthy white teeth of so many who live there is attributed to diets including raw milk, plenty of raw fresh fruits and vegetables and a sparing amount of meat with little or no white sugar, white flour products or processed foods. The people of Deaf Smith County had far fewer health problems than the national average.

Evidence that calcium imbalance is one of the keys to understanding the beginning of chronic disease continues to pile up.

Following his trip to Hunza Valley in West Pakistan in the late 1970s, Dr. Robert J. Jensen wrote to me about the hardy Hunzans I had visited some years ago:

"The Hunzans' health is still exemplary in spite of many negative factors that are relatively new to them since the advent of the new road.

"Tooth decay, tooth crowding and dental plaque in the young people are all indications of more severe metabolic and systematic health problems yet to be experienced by the Hunzans.

"Although the Hunzans are experiencing their first exposure to and conditions of tuberculosis, they have not yet succumbed to their first case of cancer. However, the Hunzans are selling more and more of their apricot crop for rupees and replacing the apricot oil with imported vegetable oils. They are consuming more and more sugar, salt, black tea and tobacco and have now begun to use artificial fertilizer. I cannot see how they can possibly continue to resist all forms of cancer for very long.

"I was surprised to find as many lesions (dark spots) on the irides as I did and I can only conclude that in spite of some organic and/or functional weaknesses that much of their good health is due to their continuous exercise as well as a fairly consistent whole food diet."

Calcium Deficiencies

Calcium, I am certain, is one of the most important of the 16 major biochemical elements needed in human nutrition. I concentrate on 4 elements, particularly, with greatest success—calcium, silicon, sodium and iodine—and find that there are often deficiencies in each of them.

A calcium deficiency is generally associated with blood impurities due to the eliminative tract not functioning properly. Then we experience lowered tone in the entire body accompanied by a lack of drive to overcome adversities.

I can find signs of calcium deficiency by examining the fingers. If they are not straight, it is generally a sign that the person did not have sufficient calcium at birth. No matter how much calcium we put into the body, an inherently weak organ cannot hold and store much of this element. Often the fingernails are mottled with white spots, indicating that calcium is in short supply. If a patient is not getting enough calcium, a history of tooth decay is usually the case, and the teeth may be blotched with patches. Healing in any department is slow.

A pregnant woman is in need of extra calcium and iron, the two most important elements to supply during pregnancy. If there is

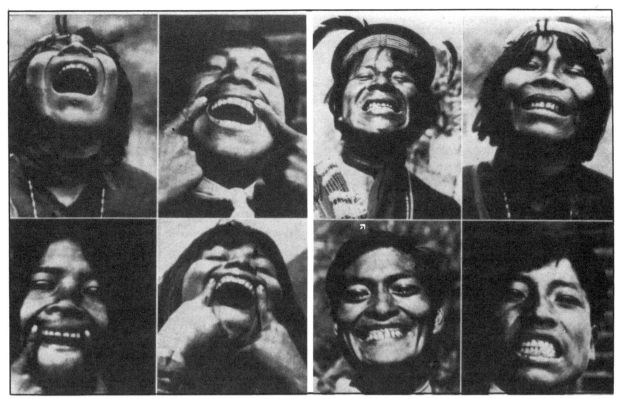

Dr. Price found the dental arches, teeth and facial features of Peruvian jungle Indians to be fully developed. The teeth were free of dental caries. I use Dr. Price's methods in my work.

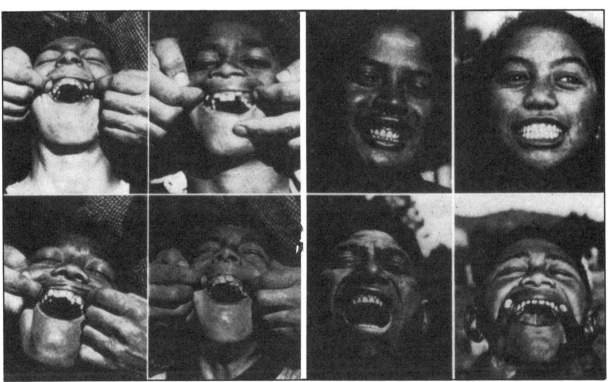

Rural Maoris of New Zealand on their native diet had beautiful teeth and bodies (left). Those from the cities, however, eating "civilized food," developed narrow dental arches, poor facial structure and crowded teeth.

Courtesy of The Price-Pottenger Foundation, 5622 Dartford Way, San Diego, CA 92120.

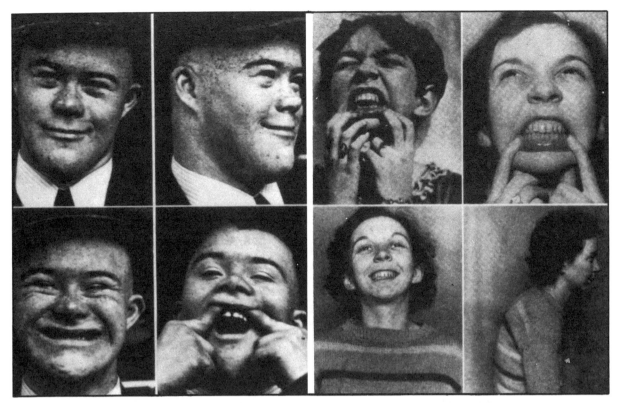

*The young Mongoloid at left shows lack of development in the middle third of the face. The upper dental arch is too small for the lower. Right: This girl hald a deformity of the facial features and also a contracted pelvic arch. She nearly lost her life with the birth of her first child. **(Courtesy of The Price-Pottenger Foundation, 5622 Dartford Way, San Diego, CA 92120.)***

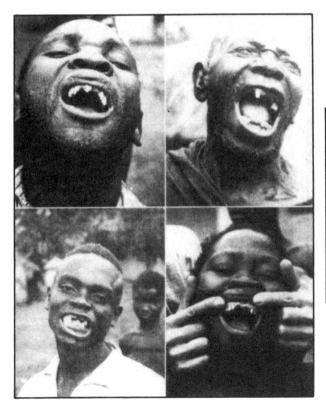

*Where native Africans have adopted modern foods, cavities develop, teeth deteriorate and serious health problems begin to arise. **(Courtesy of The Price-Pottenger Foundation.)***

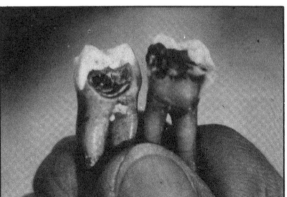

These teeth were taken from one of my patients.

117

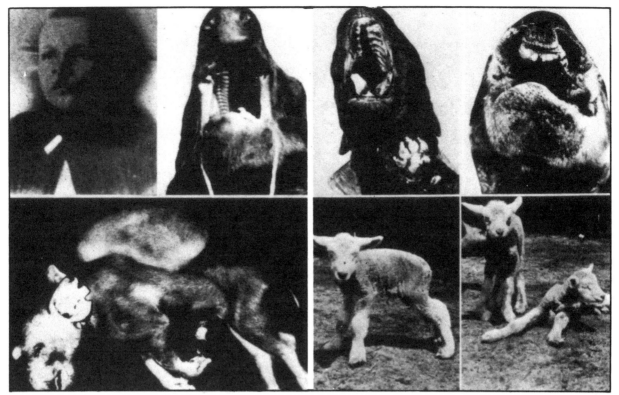

Upper left series: Boy with cleft palate and harelip; pig and cleft palate; pig with club feet, ear deformities, tumors and no eyeballs due to lack of vitamin A in mother's diet. *(Courtesy of The Price-Pottenger Foundation, Professor Hale.)*

Upper right series: Young domestic animals with birth defects. Pup with cleft palate. In two previous litters, all the pups were born deformed and soon died. Upper right, one of Professor Hale's pigs with double harelip. Below, two blind lambs and one with a club foot.

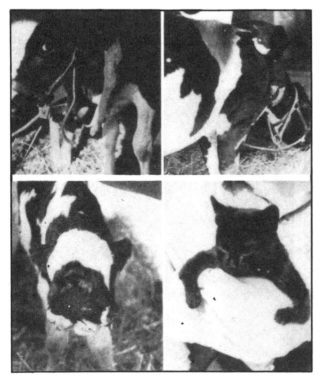

Typical deformities in domestic animals. Upper left: Two cows with extra foreleg hanging from shoulder. Lower left: Double-faced calf. Lower right: Cat with deformed legs. *(Courtesy of The Price-Pottenger Foundation)*

Dr. Weston Price, a dentist, traveled all over the world in search of native groups in excellent health. He found a direct correlation between good teeth and good health, poor teeth and poor health, and concluded that calcium metabolism was one of the basic keys to health.

Teeth with cavities, rotten teeth and poorly-formed dental arches indicate inadequate nutrition, according to Dr. Price. Native groups that ate whole, pure, natural foods were healthy. Those that began eating the refined, packaged foods of civilization soon showed a variety of ailments and diseases.

When the calcium metabolism is thrown into imbalance due to improper eating habits, the endocrine system also becomes imbalanced. (Animals are not immune to malnutrition and its consequences. If proper eating habits are restored, the endocrine glands follow the return of calcium balance. If junk foods and refined foods (very little difference) remain prominent in the diet, the health further degenerates and chronic diseases of various kinds appear.

**MINERALS SUPPLIED BY NATIVE DIETS
AS COMPARED TO AMERICAN DIET***

(Quantities are *multiples* of amounts in U.S. daily diet)

	Eskimos	Swiss	Gaelics	Canadian Indians	Australian Aborigines	Maoris New Zealand	Central Africa	Peruvian Indians
Calcium	5.4	3.7	2.1	5.8	4.6	6.2	3.5	6.6
Phosphorus	5.0	2.2	2.3	5.8	6.2	6.9	4.1	5.5
Iron	1.5	3.1	1.0	2.7	50.6	58.3	16.6	5.1
Magnesium	7.9	2.5	1.3	4.3	17.0	23.4	5.4	13.6
Copper	1.8	-	-	1.5	-	-	-	-
Iodine	49.0	-	-	8.8	-	-	-	-
Fat-soluble vitamins	10.0	10.0	10.0	10.0	10.0	10.0	10.0	10.0

*From *Nutrition and Physical Degeneration* by Weston A. Price.

a calcium shortage, the child will not be a "finished child." Nature does the best she can with the materials she has to work with, but the fingers are often crooked in children of mothers who gave birth to them in rapid succession without allowing their bodies to recuperate between pregnancies.

At one time in the recent past, scientists were trying to disprove that the fetus draws all sustenance from the mother. They were saying that calcium for the new baby was not taken directly from the mother. I remember that they alleged it was an "old wives' tale" to say a mother lost a tooth for each baby she bore. They might as well have tried to prove that black is white too!

The baby in the womb is actually drawing on the mother's supply of calcium and silicon especially. Insufficient calcium and silicon will lead a mother to lose her hair due to what her child is taking from her. The importance of calcium is shown in a case that came to Dr. Rocine. As I sat beside him, I listened to a young woman patient say, "I'm five months pregnant and I would like to have a perfect child."

Dr. Rocine leaned over, examined her hands and fingers and said, "You're lacking calcium and other necessary minerals. You know, darling, you should have started preparing five years ago to have that 'perfect' child."

By using liquid chlorophyll and greens in my sanitarium work, we cared for many women suffering from menstrual disorders, especially those with cramps and hemorrhaging during their periods. We fed them calcium in foods and supplements. As a result, many of them overcame the hemorrhaging. Keep in mind that menstrual blood contains forty times the calcium of regular blood, so excessive flow heavily depletes this element and iron as well. If not checked, calcium deficiency can trigger many other symptoms in the body and its organs, preparing for the later emergence of serious diseases.

At one time, we had a twelve-year-old boy with forty-eight pinhole cavities in his teeth. By changing his diet and adding calcium foods and calcium broth, as well as salads and greens, all the cavities in his teeth repaired themselves within a year. His mother took the lesson to heart and fixed him healthy lunches to take to school. She didn't want him eating regular school lunches heavy in refined sugar—the greatest leacher of calcium in the body.

Indeed, calcium is one of the "champion" elements needed by growing children. Most of us are familiar with the expression "growing pains," which may refer to cramps in the legs, "stitches" in the side or lack of concentration in school. But, if we add calcium foods and supplements to the growing child's diet and make sure he or she has a correct balance of calcium, all these symptoms begin to leave.

One of my most impressive cases was that of a girl who came to me with thirteen leg ulcers. She had spent three years in sanitariums and doctors' offices unsuccessfully trying to stop the discharge of yellow-green pus from ulcers the size of silver dollars. I had just been reading about the people in the Hunza Valley of West Pakistan, where 65% of their foods are grown in the sunshine, whereas, according to the U.S. Government, Americans have only 16% edible vegetation grown in the sunshine. I placed this girl on green tops of vegetables—nine tops of vegetables and water each day. In three weeks, the leg ulcers were completely healed. The case was diagnosed as pellagra—a calcium deficiency—and she responded beautifully to the green vegetable juice. Using iridology, I watched delicate white healing lines fill in the dark (and apparently toxic) inherent weaknesses in the leg area.

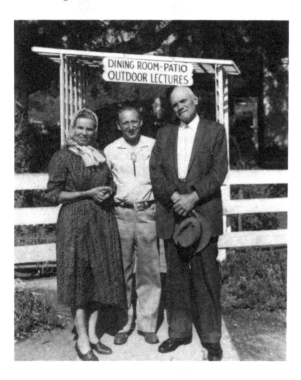

Peter Maloff and his wife, Lucy, of the Doukobors of Canada stayed at our Ranch for a Rejuvenation Seminar. The Doukobors are a community of Russian Christians who fled persecution in their native land to settle in North America. They are vegetarians, a strong and healthy people—calcium types.

On another occasion, a girl came to us because the doctors wanted to operate on her knees. She was only 15 years of age, but the cartilage had not developed properly, which resulted in difficulty in walking. So I said, "Let's allow one year and see what we can do." With a persistent regimen of adding the calcium foods and the veal joint broth Dr. Rocine talked about so much in developing the proper joint

structure, we saw wonderful results. In one year, she was able to overcome the knee problem to the extent that X-rays showed she did not need the operation.

When we don't get enough calcium, osteoporosis develops, weakening the bones and allowing easy breakage. An estimated 600,000 bone fractures per year in this country are due to osteoporosis. Over 50% of Caucasian women are known to have spinal fractures.

Calcium as a "Knitter"

Calcium is the leading element in promoting healing or knitting anywhere it is necessary; whether it is in the bones, tissues or any part of the body. Blood produces healing by transporting calcium to the needed area. Dr. Nils Liljequist, the Swedish homeopath who is credited as being one of the discoverers of iridology, called the healing lines in the iris "calcium luteum" lines. When calcium is carried sufficiently in the blood, the fibrinogen knits ulcers and bones, just as mother used to darn holes in a sock. This is the way healing lines look in the iris, indicating the new fiber structure, like new timber we put under a house. It also represents another knitting process—the filling in of an inherent weakness. Calcium is more important to healing than any other element.

Thus, for the rebuilding or regeneration of any patient I've ever treated, I always consider calcium first. Calcium is needed in every organ of the body, even in the brain. A sick person is in a recessive, negative state. To bring about a positive state, calcium is necessary.

Some people are mentally highstrung and sometimes thought to be off on "Cloud Nine" or to be "flighty." Calcium, a rock-hard physical element, is one of the greatest elements to "ground" these highstrung individuals. However, the calcium that is found in the brain is entirely different from that found in the bones, and must be a soluble calcium. Without the presence of soluble highly-evolved calcium for the mind, we find not only the problems of the highstrung person, but also those of inferiority complex and lack of will. The faculties of the mind cannot work without calcium. Indeed, the tone of a man physically, mentally and even spiritually is dependent upon the calcium in his body.

Facts About Calcium

There are facts about calcium that everyone should know. Cooking, for example, breaks down many elements, including calcium. Forty percent less calcium is found in white sugar than in raw; and blackstrap molasses, a healthful, nutritious sweetener, contains 258 times as much calcium as white sugar. There is 40% more calcium in the outer leaves of cabbage. Seeds are a good calcium source because they build the whole man, not merely part of him. Cereals, prepared by slow cooking or steaming, are also excellent calcium sources as is cheese or raw milk. However, foods high in oxalic acid—such as spinach, cranberries and rhubarb increase the body's excretion of calcium.

Calcium Types

Many of the people of Europe are what we might call calcium-type people. They are angular and slow going. They develop bones well in their bodies. In contrast, the mental and fast person often does not develop bones easily and is inclined more toward tuberculosis. But tuberculosis never develops in one who is a calcium type. Russia is primarily a calcium nation. The women and men are calcium types generally. Where there is heavy calcium expressing itself through people, you find a lot of plodders—physical people. They want to work with the plow and soil. This type of person is not very inventive, as a rule.

Appropriate Calcium Sources

In my studies of calcium, I have come to the conclusion that eggshells are not a good source for getting our calcium content. I believe in the protomorphogen work of Royal Lee who suggests we can use joint materials to rebuild joints; prostate extract to rebuild prostates; thyroid extract to rebuild thyroids; and, ovarian extract to rebuild ovaries. We do not have calcium structures in our bodies to compare with the eggshell's proportion of chemical elements. Thus, it is better to get calcium out of cod roe or fish eggs that do not have the hard calcium shell. Here the calcium is interspersed and yet still in balance with other important elements. Calcium in seed form, as in cod roe, is still in a soluble form, but when it gets into an eggshell, it has gone beyond our specific needs. The body has to break that eggshell down to use it and it doesn't suit our nature to eat it.

Bone meal is a more appropriate source of calcium because it has a gelatin quality to it—gelatin is 40% calcium. Bone meal definitely gives us good material to feed people who have been short on calcium and are suffering, for instance, from arthritis. I also use Rocine's veal joint broth because it is a high calcium broth with a balanced proportion of sodium and calcium, assuring that the calcium is not hardened. Gelatin is the dominant quality of the broth, in which neither calcium nor sodium has the upper hand so that we do not build hard joints, nor do we become like the jellyfish. I turn to the soluble calcium and sodium in this gelatin form as much as possible. Man has been trying to obtain results from an eggshell calcium made into a calcium citrate, a calcium combined with citric acid, but this is inferior to the protomorphogen from nature itself.

Another important source of calcium turned up in the work of Dr. Goldstein, who in 1915, won an award for what he did for the people of the South. In this case, people were growing cotton right up to the edge of their houses, leaving them little space to grow vegetables. As a result, they developed a calcium deficiency and pellagra, caused by a lack of calcium. Dr. Goldstein reintroduced the importance of growing turnip greens. Turnip greens and bacon or turnip greens and beans are two of the foods used by the people of the South to overcome pellagra and develop wonderful teeth through effective calcium control. When they reduced the quantity and variety of their vegetables, in order to grow cotton, their health deteriorated.

Elsewhere in the South, where natural cane sugar was a regular part of the diet, there was good calcium control to regulate the balance of minerals. If raw, unprocessed cane was used, pellagra and tooth decay were effectively controlled.

As with Dr. Goldstein and the turnip greens, we find that in Japan, a mother who doesn't have enough milk will take extra greens. Green vegetables make milk in the mother just the way they do in animals who eat grass and the greens help to stabilize calcium. We should note here that it is important to take the milk or the meat of the young animal, not the old, to avoid acquiring hard calcium. I only take milk from the youngest goats possible, not from ones where the joints are beginning to get stiff and hard, where they are losing their teeth and where calcium is beginning to drain from the body. When these animals get old, they don't have the correct sodium balance in the body, so you must make sure to take milk from only the young and active animals.

Calcium Highlights

In summary, we find that calcium, the hard element in the body—the knitter— is contained in the hard tissues of the body. It gives us courage and the power to carry through. It makes the will stronger and builds strength and endurance. We find that calcium is necessary for the teeth, bones and all healing. It is essential in forming hemoglobin in the blood and especially for the clotting of blood and maintaining the alkalinity of the blood. It is necessary to keep calcium in soluble form and not allow it to settle in the joints, which occurs when it is out of balance and falls out of solution. We find that if calcium salts are lacking in the blood, the nutritional balance of the whole body is upset. The bones and joints ache, the lungs deteriorate and the digestion becomes underactive.

If there is an excess of calcium and not enough sodium in the system, there is danger of hardening of the different tissues. One function of sodium in the body is to keep calcium in soluble form. Even when calcium is comparatively low, there can be too much of it in the body if there is a shortage of sodium and chlorine. Symptoms of imbalance, therefore, are the result.

Having too much potassium salt, on the other hand, draws out the sodium salts and leads to calcium deposits which may cause bony growths, calcariferous deposits, arterial hardening, arthritis and cataracts.

Finally, we find that sugar draws calcium out of the system. An excess of concentrated carbohydrates, especially refined sweets, has a harmful impact upon the endocrine glands, controlling the amount of calcium in solution in the blood. People who live on high carbohydrates will generally have dental caries, joint problems and mental difficulties.

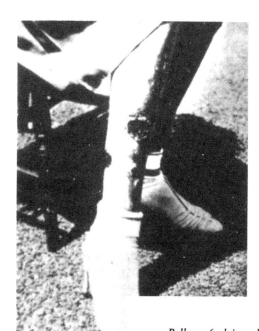

BEFORE

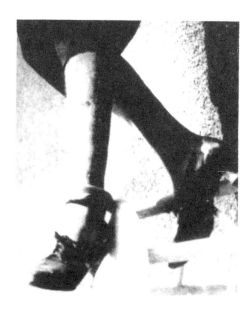

AFTER

Pellagra (calcium deficiency) preceded the appearance of these leg ulcers. They healed when the calcium balance was restored. Adults need from 1000 to 1500 mg of calcium in the diet per day and half that amount of magnesium, but this woman didn't respond to the chemical calcium her doctors gave her. We brought in the healing by giving her green vegetable leaf juices. (Story, pp. 119-120.)

CALCIUM
"The Knitter"

GENERAL CHARACTERISTICS

Calcium, the "knitter" element, is an alkaline, positive mineral, grayish or pale yellow in hue. Its atomic weight is 40.09; its specific gravity is 1.576 (1.5 times heavier than water). Calcium has a powerful attraction for oxygen; other elements with which it readily associates are sulphur, silicon and carbon. Some of the common calcium compounds are oxides, fluorides, hydroxides, chlorides, sulphates, nitrates, carbonates, phosphates and silicates. Common colloids are calcium phosphate and calcium fluoride.

Calcium is an abundant element found in water, in the ash of plants and in all soils. Its carbonate form is integral to marble, limestone, chalk, lime (calcium is often referred to as lime). Pure limestone contains 57 parts lime and 43 parts carbonic acid. Lime is a valuable soil fertilizer because it liberates the soil alkalies necessary to plant nourishment and growth. In addition, it decomposes vegetable matter and facilitates the release of vitality in plants.

Proven Value of Calcium

Calcium is a proven aid in egg production; it is known to result in eggs with harder shells and to increase egg production in general. When poultry is fed ground bones or cracked oyster shells and other calcium foods such as green kale, the quantity and quality of eggs improve noticeably.

Lime is valuable in metallurgy, the leather industry, the manufacture of soap, as an acid neutralizer, and in mortar and cement. Medicine uses lime in antacid preparations for the purpose of destroying inert, noxious vegetable matter. Heavy clay soils are decomposed with the aid of lime for ease in fertilizing.

Mineral to Vegetable to Animal

Calcium must undergo evolution to travel from the rock form to a form assimilable by the human body. It is taken up by the soil for plants, then passes into seeds and vegetables and thence to animals. In the vegetable as well as the animal product form it is assimilable by the human body, which is able to convert it to blood and bone.

CALCIUM: ITS ROLE IN THE HUMAN BODY

A man weighing 150 pounds contains approximately 3 pounds, 12 ounces of calcium in his body. This calcium joins forces with magnesium, phosphorus, fluorine and silicon in bones and teeth. Berzelius, a well-known Swedish chemist in the early nineteenth century (1779-1848), analyzed bone composition as follows:

Phosphate of lime	51.04%
Gelatin	32.17%
Carbonate of lime	11.30%
Fluoride of calcium	2.00%
Chloride of sodium	1.20%
Phosphate of magnesium	1.16%
Blood vessels	1.13%

Calcium Responsible for Solidity

Calcium is responsible for solidity as well as movement of the body. It is essential to walking and to mental and physical activities of all descriptions; without calcium the body would be like a jellyfish. One experiment conducted by Cornell University fed a chicken a calcium-deficient diet; at the time of the chicken's maturity it would not stand upright and its legs were twisted knots.

"Calcium must undergo evolution to travel from the rock form to a form assimilable by the human body. It is taken up by the soil for plants, then passes into seeds and vegetables and thence to animals. In the vegetable as well as the animal product form it is assimilable by the human body, which is able to convert it to blood and bone."

Lack of Calcium Causes Many Problems

Lack of calcium in the body results in defective teeth, defective bone metabolism and eventually chronic diseases. To a lesser extent, the same is true when there is deficiency of silicon, magnesium, fluorine, chlorine, sodium, phosphorus or manganese. Calcium phosphate and carbonate are integral to proper bone and teeth solidity; lack of these salts encourages rickets. Calcium fluoride is a constituent of bones and teeth, as is calcium carbonate, which is held in solution by carbonic acid in the fluids of the body.

Calcium's Role in the Body

The role of calcium in the body is similar to that in soil. It aids digestion, nutrition and neutralization, promotes good growth, vitality and vigor by helping to regulate metabolism properly.

When the body is cut or wounded, calcium in the blood causes coagulation to prevent hemorrhaging; if not for sufficient calcium, excessive bleeding would ensue. Wounds heal slowly and poorly if calcium is lacking at the time of an injury; scars remain to commemorate the event.

Conditions Prevented by Calcium

Nervous prostration, stomach acidity and anemia are a few of the ailments attributed to lack of calcium. It is a soother of nerves, notably the vegetative and automatic. Asthma, hay fever, tuberculosis and blood disorders are prevented by calcium; germs instrumental in pneumonia, consumption, scrofula, pyrogenic and necrotic diseases are combatted by calcium; many species of germ life and various diseases are warded off by calcium. It inhibits oxalic acid poisoning. It lends strength to the walls of arteries and veins. Nearly all muscular movements require calcium, and every cell must have calcium for proper nutrition. Food yields its vitality as a result of calcium. Tissue salts and elements such as phosphorus, potassium, fluorine, sodium, silicon, magnesium, manganese, iron and the colloids and vitamins work in conjunction with calcium for physical and mental well-being.

Calcium is responsible for solidity as well as movement of the body. It is essential to walking and to mental and physical activities of all descriptions; without calcium the body would be like a jellyfish."

Importance of Calcium Reserve

If calcium salts are lacking in the diet, the calcium reserve in the body is depleted trying to maintain proper calcium balance for metabolism. Teeth and bones must yield their supply of calcium, weakening their integrity; when calcium reserve in teeth is exhausted, germ life penetrates the protective enamel coating and decay sets in.

Sugar Intake Depletes Calcium Supply

Calcium and sugar have a powerful affinity for one another; the more sugar consumed, the more calcium precipitated. Excessive sugar consumption therefore erodes teeth and also contributes to stomach acidity. Plain water takes up approximately one part calcium per one thousand parts; the addition of a liberal amount of sugar increases the uptake 35 or 40 times. Thus, the more sugar available to the system, the more calcium will be robbed; a carbohydrate diet precipitates calcium from the body at a rapid rate. A diet high in glucose and sugar preparations which lack calcium also robs the body of essential calcium. If calcium salts in the blood are depleted, digestive and nutritive disturbances result.

The role of calcium in the body is similar to that in soil. It aids digestion, nutrition and neutralization, promotes good growth, solidity and vigor by helping to regulate metabolism properly."

Children Need Calcium

Teeth and bones of growing children require considerable calcium in the form of organic phosphate of calcium and calcium carbonate. If the diet during these years is rich in calcium, they will not suffer bone and teeth disturbances (growing pains, tooth decay, etc.). Foods rich in calcium include raw milk, raw goat milk, nuts, raw dairy products, egg yolks, seeds, cabbage, lentils, beans, millet, rye, yellow cornmeal, rice.

The mother should ensure a diet rich in calcium while carrying a child—and twenty years prior. Children deficient in calcium manifest hip troubles; difficulties with tendons of the feet, arteries, skull bones, sutures and other solid matter; scurvy, bone softening, poor teeth, rickets and varied catarrhal and tubercular complications.

Adults and the Elderly Need Calcium

A normal adult requires about one and one-half grams of calcium per day. One quart of raw milk furnishes that quota, but a milk diet is not recommended. An elderly person requires not only calcium-containing foods, but also foods rich in sodium and chlorine in order for calcium to be properly utilized. Deficiency of sodium and chlorine salts results in arteriosclerosis and hardenings in many parts of the body.

In situations due to abnormal blood coagulation, such as bleeding, hemorrhages, urticaria and chilblains, calcium is indicated.

"A diet high in glucose and sugar preparations which lack calcium also robs the body of essential calcium."

Role of Calcium Salts

Calcium salts remove phosphates through the intestines, reducing the work of the kidneys by reducing phosphates in the urine. The diabetic patient is helped by calcium salts and other salts which prevent demineralization of the tissues.

Role of Calcium Phosphate

Calcium phosphate, an odorless, tasteless white powder which withstands absorption, is used by the body for bone functions. The blood corpuscles contain about 0.114 parts per thousand; cartilage, fluids and certain tissues contain smaller percentages. Calcium phosphate combines with organic material; it is held in solution in the urine by sodium phosphate. Milk contains 0.27% calcium phosphate.

Food Sources of Calcium Preferable

Calcium concoctions have been used by physicians for centuries. It is preferable, however, to obtain calcium from food sources for greater assimilability and health benefits. Nature organizes salts (or elements) in a way in which the human body can easily assimilate or utilize them; they come from organic (biochemic) sources.

Benefits of Veal Joint Broth

Veal joint broth, prepared by slow simmering to extract the gelatinous substances from the animal product, is beneficial in such maladies as purpura, hemophilia, oozing wounds, bleeding hemorrhoids, hemorrhage-related ailments. The same broth is beneficial when applied externally as a wash in cases of indolent ulcers and chronic eczema, due to its gelatinous and calcium makeup. Milk may be added to the broth, as milk has a curative property for swellings, stiff and blood-charged areas, injuries or contusions.

Some Individuals Do Not Digest Calcium

Some types of individuals have systems which refuse calcium, even in organic food form; about one half the calcium consumed by them is excreted through the feces. The colon requires calcium, chlorine, sodium, fluorine and magnesium for maintaining the proper percentage of "friendly bacteria" or bacillus acidophilus to guard against invasion by germ life and bacillus coli.

Assimilation of Calcium and Its Salts

Calcium chloride is easily assimilated by the human organism; acid calcium phosphate and lactate are assimilated moderately well; sulphate and carbonate are more insoluble, except in waters

"An elderly person requires not only calcium-containing foods... but also foods rich in sodium and chlorine in order for calcium to be properly utilized."

with a high carbonic acid content. Sulphate in waters is not absorbed by the body. The health of the stomach and intestines determines the extent to which calcium is absorbed; other factors influencing calcium assimilation are climate, occupation and temperament of the patient. Calcium is more readily assimilated in mountainous, windy climates.

The Calciferic Type

The calcium-type individual, called Calciferic, is characterized by a solid, compact frame and tissues; he is dense in construction with considerable brain and bone to the square foot, as compared with other men. The bones require such huge quantities of calcium that the body fluid, blood and secretions are deprived of it.

"Nature organizes salts (or elements) in a way in which the human body can easily assimilate or utilize them; they come from organic (biochemic) sources."

The Power of Calcium

Calcium has a good effect upon the brain, producing qualities of oratory proficiency, love, compassion, expansion, intellect bordering on genius and tremendous powers of concentration.

The power of calcium is latent but has great potential when aroused. The calcium type is calm, quiet and unemotional, even apathetic. He is like the Rock of Gibraltar, granite and steel combined and like the silent Indian who sees all. His actions appear awkward, ungainly, incomplete, dull; he is slow to comprehend, but there are wonderful powers within his soul waiting for birth. He comes into his own in his own due time, never rushed.

Editor's Note: Some individuals absorb or assimilate larger quantities of certain biochemical elements. Their affinity for particular elements creates physical, mental and spiritual characteristics which express and reflect the properties of those dominant biochemical elements. This individuality creates the chemical types.

CALCIUM: SIGNS OF EXCESS

Characteristics of the Calciferic Type

The calcium-excess patient, like the calcium type, has tremendous latent power slumbering within. Love sentiments, poetry, theater life, society conventionality, music are of little interest to him; tender lovemaking is not important; cultivated behavior and courtesy are not part of his makeup. His language may be offensive to many; he is earthy, interested only in hard facts; his manner is blunt, hard, direct, sometimes tactless; his feelings are steel clad, his manners unpolished, his speech blunt. He is serene until crossed, at which time he may become argumentative, sullen, melancholy, revengeful. When aroused to anger, he is hypercritical, stubborn, chastizing, complaining, disagreeable. He is almost never the one to start a quarrel, but he ends one in his favor; a wife particularly should consider the nature of the calcium type when contemplating a quarrel with him. He is grouchy in the early morning and even tempered in the evening.

Inclinations of the Calcium Type (Calciferic)

A predominance of calcium in the body inclines an individual toward heaviness of mind, temperament, head; he is steady and unyielding, unchanging in animosity, steady in love, hard-working in vocation, powerful, somber, revengeful, heavy handed in action and writing, industrious in aims, perpetually inventive, patient in regard to goals. He leans toward the earthy, tangible things in life—facts, intellect and reasoning that can be verified. He is averse to revolutionary movements, systems, lifestyles, beliefs, and is apt to censure such things. His maladies, customs, inclinations, infirmities are extensive and lengthy; they are apt to be chronic, steadfast, unceasing. This type is constructed to endure indefinitely—the most endurable of all types. He is more likely to die at work than in a hospital ward.

Talents and Behaviors of the Calcium Type (Calciferic)

Thomas Edison is an example of the calcium inventory. The calcium type persists at an invention, scientific investigation or laboratory experimentation indefinitely, to the detriment of personal care

and good nutrition. He begins slowly but finishes well; he makes a good executive, attorney or contractor. He is interested in such down-to-earth occupations as stone work, real estate, construction.

When calcium is excessive, literary faculties are undermined, but not so reason, understanding, power. (However, if calcium deficiency becomes chronic, the above faculties are weakened and perception becomes difficult.) The calcium-excess type is unyielding, conscientious, rigid, refusing to brook profanity or principle. Inappropriate action and behavior of others drives him to distraction because ethics, integrity and morals have great meaning to him.

Typical Traits of the Calcium Type

The body of the calcium man is slow moving, slow to manifest tissue changes or building or decay; his brain is late in developing. He learns little from written instruction; observation is his best teacher. His likes and aversions are definite and pronounced. Indecision is not one of his faults.

Calcium Type Not Afraid of Battle

Warfare and conflicts are to the liking of the Calciferic type. He is at home on the battlefield, in the military camp. He is undaunted by and unafraid of threats, warfare, conflict, guns, swords or knives.

Calcium Children Can be Willful

Calcium children are willful, strong and rebellious if parents try to use force and extreme punishment.

Strength of Calcium Type (Calciferic)

The calcium man or woman is powerful, deliberate and patient. Abraham Lincoln is an example of the indestructible, powerful Calciferic type. When opposed, persons of this type show their true strength.

Excess Calcium in the Body

In times when calcium is oversupplied and sodium is deficient in the body, there is a tendency to hardening in the body, calcification and ossification. Actually, excess calcium is not the cause of hardening; shortage of sodium, which keeps calcium in solution, and chlorine make calcium content seem higher. A patient exhibiting these characteristics is generally thin, bony, emaciated.

A disorder similar to epilepsy may result from excess calcium in the bloodstream. To remedy the condition, calcium must be reduced in the dietary intake and sodium and chlorine increased.

"...excess calcium is not the cause of hardening; shortage of sodium, which keeps calcium in solution and chlorine make calcium content seem higher."

Vegetarian Diet May Reduce Mineral Reserve

A strict vegetarian diet, adding milk, eggs and other calcium foods, actually precipitates the reserve of sodium and chlorine from the body; this is a result of excess potassium in the dietary intake; potassium, as it is excreted, carries with it 50 to 60 ounces of sodium per ounce of potassium. Potassium intake must therefore be balanced by the intake of other biochemical elements. Manganese, silicon, fluorine and chlorine are important to the body's metabolism and general health; sufficient quantities of each must be provided as food supplements.

Excess Calcium Leads to Growths

The calcium type commonly exhibits bony growths, external or internal, due to excess calcium in the blood or bones. A bony growth in the cranium, if it grows downward, may eventually produce insanity from pressure on brain matter. Many body regions are prone to bony growths; calcium deposits may lead to hardening of the arteries, defective eyesight, impaired hearing. Osteomata, bone calcification, calciferous tubules, hardening of canal walls anywhere in the body are likely, as are gouty or calcic concretions and some forms of calculus, such as vesical, prostatic, fusible, bronchial, uterine, salivary, renal, lacteal, nasal or urinary. Cartilagenous tumors or hardening of hip bones are possible; these may interfere with nerve action of sciatic nerves and result in sciatica or other very painful ailments. Ossifying myolitis, bone

enlargement, bone tumors, bone sarcoma, carcinoma or hardening may occur in joints or in other solid parts; such growths may manifest in the gall bladder or urinary tubules; hardening in the ovaries, testicles or uterine tubes may also take place.

Excess calcium may lead to stony growths in the bilary passage. Uric acid calculi may develop, or phosphatic calculi, or stones composed of calcium oxalate, or cataracts—all from calcium excess and/or sodium deficiency.

Ailments of Calcium Excess

Prolonged conditions of excess calcium and sodium shortage result in gout symptoms, ultimately in chronic gout. These and other hardening processes occurring in the body have distinctive symptoms, sensations, disorders, each with its attendant aches and pains. The cerebellum may develop tension and pressure; ears become congested; lips crack; the sacrum becomes sore; there is ripping, burning, tingling, penetrating pain in the loins and hips. Ligaments, shoulder bones, forearms, toes, hips, ankles, fingers, clavicles, joints, even kidneys or heart may demonstrate rheumatic symptoms. The patella becomes sore; walking is troublesome. Perspiration is chaotic; gouty concretions form; ankles or knee joints crack when moved.

Aches, Fevers and Swellings

There may be dry joints, due to drying of synovia (joint oil) or due to its not being secreted properly because of excess calcium, urates, acids and sodium deficiency. The skin may develop cold sweats; metatarsal joints and tendoachilles may ache. Urine is strong and phosphate and carbonate of lime are found in it. Uric and lithic acid and basic salts form compounds in joints. The individual favors dry heat, as well as pressure and vigorous massage if bones are not too tender. His face may become moist on one side and hot on the other, or tender and numb; the posterior section of the tophead is painful. Reading and study induce sleep. Shivers play up and down the spine. There are crawling body sensations; vertigo from movement; cracking in ears; stinging pain in teeth; stabbing jawbone pains; tender and sore bones from lying on them; aversion to physical labor; restless sleep; swelling of joints; a bloated feeling in the abdomen;

cold localized in small areas of the body; rapid and oppressed breathing, due to excessive carbonic acid, lack of sodium, chlorine and oxygen. There may be complaints of ringing ears; rushing, rustling sounds in the body; feverish body and cold extremities; a shrunken feeling in the brain.

Calcium Patient Avoids People

The calcium-excess patient has an aversion to people; he feels dull and dazed; the world seems too close to him. He finds sitting in one position for any length of time intolerable because of soreness of the coccyx. He suffers anal itch, left ear itch; the urethra may close suddenly, resulting in sudden stoppage of urination and excruciating pain. The chest frame may be painful, bones, joints and tendons stiff; tendons may manifest gouty nodes, which may also appear in joints and bones, accompanied by contractive, drawing, painful feelings. At a given time, one area of the body is more affected. Rheumatic areas are always chilled; ankles may swell; tenderness may occur in popliteal spaces; cords, tendons, motor nerves, ligaments and periosteal structures contract, develop knots, sting, twist or develop pains due to presence of rheumatic or gouty acids and deposits.

Moisture Affects Calcium Type (Calciferic)

Moisture has considerable influence on the calcium-excess patient; baths, cold air, drafts, moisture are unpleasant and intensify his condition. Conditions of body heat, dampness and sweating may alternate. Cold, damp air results in stiff, cold, unpleasant feelings and painful joints. Oxidation is low due to sodium deficiency and overabundance of carbonic acid, which is the reason for chills; feet alternate between burning fever and icy coldness. Conditions worsen prior to a storm because the air's electrical tension is changed and the air transports gases and ferments to which the blood is susceptible.

More Symptoms of Calcium Excess

Breathing often manifests a whistling sound in the nose. Teeth become extremely sensitive and may darken in color. The patient's body may develop such tenderness that the pressure of clothes, shoes or socks is intolerable. Any vibratory motion or jarring causes pain. Synovitis, paralytic stiffness in motor nerves, tendons, bones and joints, is likely. The stomach and digestive system produce gas; flatus is troublesome. Fingers turn inward as disorders become more serious; toes turn downward. Ankles develop dropsy; the white of the eyes turns blue and shiny; pains seem to dart and fly over and through the body, due to acids found in calcium parts of the body; throat becomes scratchy; neck and extremities develop stiffness; joints and parts of skin surface become glossy.

Complaints of Female Calcium Type

Female patients have complaints similar to those of males. Daytime and dry sunny weather are more tolerable, even if the temperature is low. Nighttime brings aches upon retiring. There may be drowsiness during daytime hours.

Relationship of Sodium to Calcium

It is important to emphasize that calcium excess demands more sodium salts. Sodium is important to carbonic acid elimination and is also an important constituent of the blood. Deficiency of sodium salts in the blood or other parts of the body results in less than proper expelling of carbon dioxide and numerous carbon dioxide symptoms when calcium is oversupplied and sodium deficient. Many odd symptoms result in the calcium patient.

Symptoms of Calcium Excess/Sodium Deficiency

Specific bone spots, chilling to touch, may be extremely painful for a short time. Urination by drops is painful and scalding; leucorrhea is yellow, itching and burning; tiny pea-like tumors may form. Blood vessels throb; gums and peridental membranes develop calcic inflammation; calciferous bone tubules harden. There may be lithic, lithofelic and uratic concretions; lithemia; kidney inflammation; intestinal concretions; hundreds of assorted ailments and much suffering.

Calcium-Sodium Balance Always Necessary

Dietary discretion in younger years ensures against hardening processes in later years—hardening of arteries, joint stiffness, tendon stiffness—and against pain in periosteal parts and hardening of the pleural wall. Unnecessary calcium would be eliminated rather than staying in the body to form arterial and venous wall deposits. Of course, if sodium is lacking, calcium may be excessive by comparison. Advancing years raise requirements for sodium, potassium, chlorine, fluorine, manganese, magnesium and iodine; at the same time, calcium requirements are reduced.

Treatment of Calcium Excess

A diet should supply the above elements generously, as well as plenty of vitamins and sodium from vegetative sources. A dry, windy climate is beneficial. Foods such as wild strawberries, goat milk, raw egg yolk tonics, okra and celery; rest; warmth; nutritional training in proper meal planning; sufficient exercises—all are in demand when calcium is excessive.

CALCIUM: SIGNS OF DEFICIENCY

Mental Symptoms of Calcium Deficiency

Calcium deficiency reduces memory ability—for names, dates, cities, locations, times, vocations. Recall is difficult; thinking is a strain. Small details are observed, but not major happenings. Writing is preferable to talking; brain fatigue and boredom set in; speaking is incoherent and word usage improper; meanings are vague. There is lack of patience, fatigue, indifference, disgust for life in general.

Other Qualities of Calcium-Deficient Patient

Other qualities of the calcium-short patient are selfishness, ill temper, heedlessness of others' needs, antisocial conduct, lack of warmth for people, lack of personality. He is adverse to interaction with people, impatient with personal and business functions, easily offended; he dwells on unfortunate happenings and thinks he has bad luck. He wanders around the house without a purpose or not knowing what is desired; is subject to sighing, pouting, sulking, silent moods; cannot carry out plans for lack of vitality and power; is rooted to home but unsatisfied there because travel is fancied—but travel is not satisfying because of longing for home and hearth; refuses recreation and pleasurable pastimes; takes a job for which he is overqualified, preferring it to one with superior opportunities. Nightfall brings on fears; this patient is inundated by apprehensions; adverse mental states focus in the epigastric plexus (pit of stomach). Bad luck, failures, personal damages, maladies, accidents, complaints are uppermost in his mind. The past is more important than the future; he falls into a rut and is unable to climb out again.

130

Calcium Lack Brings on Fears

The calcium-impoverished patient is anguished and sorrowful, and these mental states manifest at the slightest opportunity; sorrow may be outwardly visible or bottled up inside, but it is powerful and painful. The present and future are worrisome and formidable; he fears for his own condition and is very apprehensive about death. The patient is suspicious and distrustful of everyone. He is negative and fearful of the worst results and consequences. He shows pessimism toward people, systems and plans. Emotions of fear, courage, will power are strongly affected. Power and valor are most lacking. When calcium—synonymous with bravery, hope and strength—is lacking, so are these qualities.

> *When calcium—synonymous with bravery, hope and strength—is lacking, so are these qualities.*

Lungs Affected by Calcium Lack

Afflictions of nutritional origin manifest when calcium is deficient. Lack of sodium, chlorine and calcium contribute to development of tuberculosis if a patient has a weak lung structure, weak vital functions, poor circulation. Oxygenation is affected by the calcium metabolism in the body—knotty lung tubercules can imprison calcium; calcium may be deposited or precipitated to excess or disintegrated by diseases so that blood, functions and tissues are divested of their share. Thus insufficient oxygen is imbibed, resulting in malnutrition, low energy, softening of bones, emaciation, wasting, abnormal functions and premature demise.

Tuberculosis

Tuberculosis is due in part to calcium, chlorine, fluorine, sodium, silicon, oxygen, manganese, iodine, iron deficiencies. This malady manifests many peculiarities: the chest rises and falls involuntarily; hands shake; the diaphragm is unsteady, the nose bleeds; after noon the head aches dully, probably due to increased carbonic acid in the air. Sunlight diminishes carbonic acid in the air and thus improves the patient's condition; but bright artificial lights adversely affect the eyes and eyeballs. Sunlight enhances calcium assimilation and helps control calcium in the body. The tuberculosis patient is thus benefitted by sunbaths and fresh air.

Weather Affects Calcium-Deficient Patient

The calcium-deficient patient craves more air and his lungs feel congested. Dry, balmy weather improves his condition, as do dry heat and sunshine in midday at a high altitude; wind is unpleasant for nerves and increases irritation. Drafts and dampness cause colds. Approaching storms, humidity, air pressure, temperature changes, electrical air tension alterations, overcast skies or chilling winds are keenly felt by this patient; crisp, cold night air is intolerable; fresh air causes dizziness, staggering upon rising, night sweats; the chest is oppressed and feels weighted in damp weather. There is a heavy feeling in the head, as if it were clamped inside a vise.

Symptoms of Calcium Lack

Drowsiness overcomes the patient near sundown; he goes to bed early and sleeps soundly until about midnight; after midnight his sleep is disturbed, and he rises early. Comfort during sleep depends upon his head being raised and his reclining on his back. The approach of evening causes decrease in body temperature; it rises again near morning. The spine and lower limbs chill easily and fever sets in. Skin evaporation is augmented because a cool, moist skin acts as a magnet for body heat. Palms are damp, skin dark, chilled and clammy; feet are cold; face flushed and feverish. There is a flush underneath eyebones; shrunken flesh; lack of muscle tone; wrinkled skin; thinness in spite of dietary intake; sunken side of face; weak vital centers; aged look beyond years.

Appetite of Calcium-Deprived Patient

The patient suffering from calcium lack— specifically from tuberculosis—has a voracious appetite but little is digested. Meat, fish, poultry, stimulants, spices, condiments, potatoes, fatty gravy and sauces, salt, carbonated and alcoholic drinks are favored. As morning approaches, appetite increases.

Further Symptoms

The left side of upper abdomen or back of neck has pounding sensations (similar to symptoms of iron deficiency). Other signs of calcium poverty are poor circulation, diminished sense of smell, oppressed breathing, low oxidation, spells of exhaustion, stabbing pains, cold regions of the body, pain in kidney area, heightened sexual desire, fatigued limbs, coughing, catarrhal problems, nagging cold, sharp pains under lower ribs, sore sternum, tender shoulder joints, weak and crippled arms, bone pains, flexor lameness, stiffness, partial paralysis, numbness. Eventually the upper spine curves forward with increasing severity; central vertebrae bend inward or outward or laterally; hemorrhages are likely, as are convulsions of the lower chest and a hoarse, raspy voice. Small blood vessels of the brain are so congested that minimal motion or shaking—even walking—adversely affects the brain; work, running, jogging, exercise are extremely fatiguing and cause loss of breath.

Calcium Deficiency in Children

Calcium deficiency in infants and children has serious results. Walking and talking come late; feeblemindedness is possible; bones are small, narrow and fragile, even soft; the brain, intellect, nerves and bone metabolism suffer.

Carbon Type Manifests Calcium Deficiency

The carbon type of individual, or one who consumes excessive carbohydrate foods, manifests calcium deficiency (though not necessarily tuberculosis). Many obese carbon patients exude an odor resembling vinegar, indicating that calcium is in demand; when it is supplied, the odor vanishes, because calcium has deodorant, disinfectant, purifying properties as well as nutritional benefits.

Calcium Vital to Health

Calcium is vital to bone construction and repair, body strength and soundness, fertilization and purification. Good health is simply not possible without a calcium reserve in the body.

Ailments Due to Calcium Lack

Growths, tumors, sores, abscesses, fevers, inflammations, discharges plague the calcium-deficient patient. There may be misshapen or deformed fingers, ankles, nose bones, hips, jaws, cranial bones; missing teeth, tooth decay and complications; undersized organs or limbs;

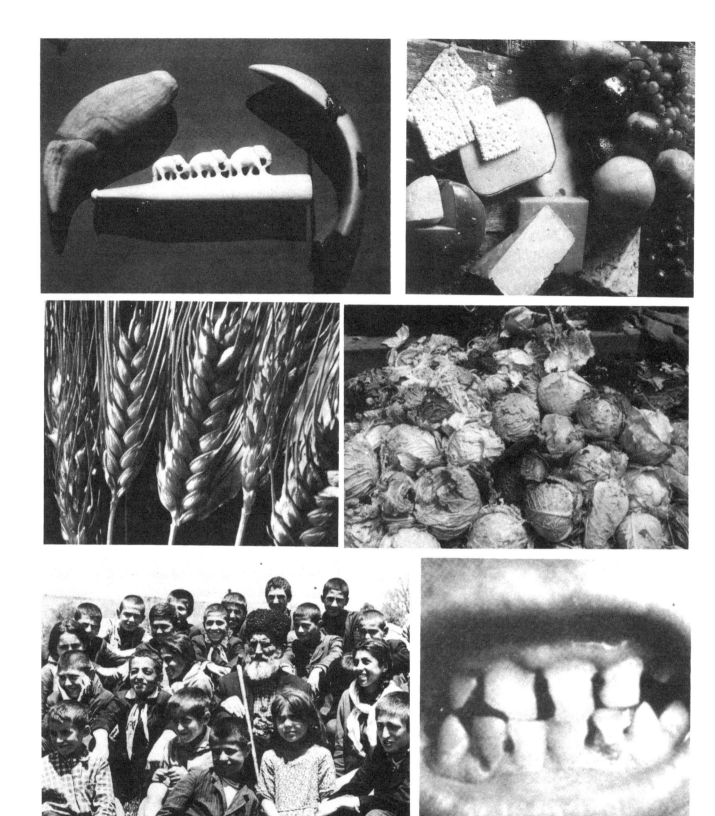

Calcium is the foundation element in teeth, tusks and bones in all animals. Calcium foods build strong bodies, endurance, patience and steady nerves. Cheese, wheat and cabbage are three of the best calcium foods. S. Mislimov, 168 years old, is shown with some of his 220 relatives. He is a calcium type. The teeth shown above are those of a 12-year-ol boy sent to me by a dentist because his tooth decay came from poor nutrition.

paranormal structures and organs; closures, gaps, divisions, separations, dislocations, implantations, auxiliary parts, transformations, gargantuan growth, flaws in build and form. Many of these are of hereditary origin, as well as being linked to nutrition and cell-building material in the mother during pregnancy and lactation. The early development of the child is crucial.

Complications Due to Calcium Lack

Lack of calcium and other elements contributes to such complications as tooth decay; malnutrition; blood deficiencies; vomiting; urticaria; chilblains; nauseating headache; faulty blood coagulation facilitating hemorrhaging; tuberculosis; slow convalescence; phosphaturia; exophthalmic goiter; epistaxis; liver sluggishness causing bleeding hemorrhoids; discharging wounds; hemoptysis; hemorrhagic purpura; enterorrhagia; hemophilia; chronic digestive catarrh; profuse mucus discharge; propensity to fibrinous bronchitis, urethritis. Burns, sores, scalds, scars heal poorly when calcium is lacking. Calcium deficiency may cause shortening of arms or legs or thickening of some diaphysis. It may form the groundwork for a pathologic diathesis and slowly induce such afflictions as swelling submaxillary glands; chronic slimy salivation; craving for salt, tobacco, smoking or stimulants; inunguinal gland swelling; smarting pains in genitals; bone softening; swelling knuckles; sluggish activity of red blood corpuscles; dull headache; enlarged mesenteric glands; bronchial congestion; claylike complexion; sour stomach; wrinkled skin; cystic goiter; lame flexor muscles; goiters; cyst formation; ulcerous cicatrices; bone ulceration; tuberculosis; pus generation (suppuration); polypi or growths in various parts of the body; earaches; bloating and obesity in stout people; extreme emaciation in slender people; rickets; pelvic discharges; nervous problems; bladder catarrh; prostatitis; cystinuria; vesical catarrh; delayed teething or intrauterine rachitis.

Other Indications of Calcium Shortage

Other indications of calcium shortage are disintegrating tissues, deficient blood, agonizing headaches, sciatic neuralgia, fevers, inflammations, skin ailments, bone decay, germ resident maladies, discharges, congestion, ruptures, sprains, strains, displacements, venous dilation, paramychia, tabes

coxaria, mesentereitis, parenchymatous deterioration; degenerating transformations in bones, tissues and organs; suppuration everywhere; prolapsed organs. The will is soft, strength and endurance lacking; there are inferiority complexes, extreme emotions, negative and pessimistic behavior, poor memory, hermit-like tendencies, thinking difficulties, sorrow, shyness, unfounded fears and apprehensions, melancholy and morbid moods, indecision.

Physical Symptoms of Calcium Shortage

Identifiable physical symptoms depicting lack of calcium are numerous. They include aches in bones and joints, lung disintegration, faulty digestion, catarrhal congestion, nasal and sinus trouble, bronchitis, colds, osteoporosis, ulcers, necrosis, insomnia, nervousness, scrofula, muscle aches, excessive tooth decay, pyorrhea, finger tremors, shortness of breath, nervous breakdowns, convulsions, itching pimples, cold extremities, hoarseness, chronic cough, stunted growth (in children), hardening of canal walls, calcium deposits in lungs, bone tumors, hardening of ear bones, joint hardening, sciatica, gall bladder or kidney stones, feeble hands, pain in nerves, shifting pains, cracked skin on hands, rheumatic pains and tension, jawbone pains, toothaches, cold spots, alternating hot and cold perspiration. Calcium lack is also implicated in such disorders as eczema, asthma, cramps, freckles, painful and delayed childbirth, dim vision, boring pains through the eyes, poor appetite, earache, frequent colds, hemorrhoids, varicose veins, muscular fatigue, anemia, goiter, tender stomach region, pain following meals, pain in forearm muscles (often involving only one side), painful biceps, pain and pressure or stiffness in various parts of the body, arthritis, heart conditions (angina pectoris and tachycardia), rheumatism. A calcium diet is often beneficial to these conditions and may also aid in conditions of rosacea, acne, psoriasis, lichen impetigo, prurigo, fish skin disease (ichthyosis).

Brain Throbbing and Melancholy

Other calcium-deficiency symptoms visible to the trained physician or nutritionist are strabismus, depression, melancholy, boredom, mental confusion, congested and dull feeling in head, abnormally large head growth in children, foreboding of approaching night, remorse, suspicion, distrust, preference for solitude; heart atria may develop unexplainable hypertrophic conditions; inner brain centrum throbs; patient refuses to believe what he anticipates and is fearful, emotional, easily disturbed; his courage and will are nearly negated; fears are mainly vocal.

Further Physical Symptoms of Calcium Shortage

If cranial sutures grow and ossify improperly, calcium is needed, the same is true when bones are undersized and soft in pudgy children or infants having an idiotic expression and drooling foamy saliva. Calcium is also indicated in times of bone diseases or tooth decay; when there is soft, flabby obesity along with massive cystic goiters and perhaps dropsy; when eyelids are itchy; when germ life invades tissues and lungs; when glands swell, harden and suppurate; when there is scrofula of lymph glands, fractures heal poorly, bones are fragile; when the face appears bloated, wrinkled and aged; when there is soreness in various parts of the body, fever, extreme perspiration of face and neck; when bones and spine are arched and curved; when junctions of epiphyseal shafts thicken or become hypertrophic, developing growths that signify rickets; when pea-like lumps form in submaxillary glands, under lower jaw.

Bones Soften, Blood Thins

A calcium-rich diet is also in demand when the following symptoms are present: a strange crackling, vibrating, whistling sound in the ears while eating, talking, singing or moving the lower jaw; a displeasing odor from the skin, like vinegar, offal, mustiness or carbonic acid in a closed room; shortening of a limb, heralding the onset of rachitis, or thickening of the end of a bone near a joint; growth to other bones forming an epiphysis and indicating epiphysitis; bone softening in adults, particularly in mothers who were divested of bone material for the new infant; osteomalacia in graying men and women; soreness of the tip or sides of the tongue; strong craving for narcotics, tobacco, stimulants, salt, spices and condiments, milk, meat, eggs and chlorine foods; liver pressure; thin blood resulting in easy bleeding; morning cough; severe, dull headaches; earaches with discharge; sensitivity to dampness; swelling of knuckles; claylike complexion; overconcern for self—fears, desires, health.

Weather Intensifies Ailments

If the inguinal glands swell, calcium is indicated, as is it when there is a creeping sensation in the arms or in the rectum; when wet feet, damp, cold weather, a cold room or a cold shower intensify ailments; when there is a smarting sensation in the genitals or os uteri; when the throat is raw and scratchy and the voice hoarse; when suppuration or catarrh and phlegm are generated, demanding an abundance of chlorine foods (the body has been divested of chlorine reserves, indicated by early symptoms of a salty taste in the mouth, then a sweet taste and ultimately a bloody taste when the reserve is completely exhausted).

Other Conditions Requiring Calcium

Calcium foods are demanded when the lungs or other body parts develop abscesses; when the thyroid gland enlarges due to iodine deficiency; when pus is generated in body tissue due to an alarming rate of fluorine, chlorine, oxygen and iron consumption; when knees swell; when clammy perspiration forms on legs; when night sweats are a frequent problem; when pressure produces numbness; when skin turns yellowish and wrinkles; when scars are painful or ulcerated; when eyeballs are sore, tip of nose cold, upper lip swollen; when cold wind produces toothache; when actions are awkward, slow and deliberate; when malnutrition develops, tissues and urine become overacidic; when blood coagulation is poor, resulting in hemorrhaging; when stomach is sour, throat mucus-congested, sexual desire increased, groin region painful, arms and legs fatigued; breathing short and difficult; when expectorations are yellow and foamy with black specks; when the back of the neck and base of the throat vibrate, pulse is shaky, some blood vessels vibrate in unison with the heart; when upper dorsal region of the spine is curved forward; when arms bruise and cramp easily; when sternum and clavicle are sensitive when the individual leans forward or lifts heavy objects; when roots of nails are swollen and level with the skin; when nails turn blue, develop white spots, curve outward and the top has a convex shape; when sides of the chest cave in (auxiliary borders); when thighs, sacral bones and knees ache; when nose is congested; when bones are chilled in certain spots; when joints are rheumatic, mesenteric glands enlarged, bronchials congested. All above symptoms call for a liberal calcium diet.

Patients Manifest Different Combinations of Symptoms

Each patient manifests different symptoms, and not all of the above symptoms appear in any one patient. Other elements influence the symptoms according to the body chemistry at a given time. The calcium reserve must be totally defunct for all or the majority of the symptoms described to manifest. Symptoms develop periodically and the extremely chronic state goes beyond all symptoms. The doctor or nutritionist must be aware of the many contributing factors unique to each individual.

A calcium-rich diet is the obvious treatment for calcium deficiency.

HIGHEST CALCIUM FOODS

It is important to note at the beginning that up to 32% of available calcium is destroyed when food is heated above 150 degrees Fahrenheit (boiling point is 212 degrees). Consequently, pasteurized milk is a limited source of calcium, as are canned foods, which are processed using excessively high heat.

One of the highest calcium broths, especially for growing children, is made from barley and green kale. This is an old Danish soup very good for growing children. Cereals and grains are also excellent calcium sources. A concentrated supplemental form of calcium is bone meal or, for vegetarians, calcium lactate. Natural calcium supplements (in food form) will not cause hardening of the arteries or calcium deposits, affect blood pressure or produce other adverse symptoms. Dolomite is an inferior calcium source because the body's ability to assimilate it is questionable.

High sources of food calcium are sesame seeds, dulse, Irish moss, kelp, greens. Seeds, nuts and cereal grains (unrefined) are all excellent sources of calcium. High calcium foods are listed below. * denotes highest sources.

Agar	Cauliflower	Kohlrabi
Almonds	*Cheeses (hard & cottage; raw)	Lentils
Avocados	Chia seeds	*Milk: goat & cow; raw
Barley	Coconut	Millet
Beet greens	Cornmeal, yellow	Oats
Beans	Cream, raw	Onions
Blackstrap molasses	Dandelion greens	Parsnips
Bran	*Dulse	Prunes
Brazilnuts	Egg yolk	Rice polish
Broccoli	Figs	Rye
Brown rice	Filberts	*Sesame seeds
Brussels sprouts	Fish	Soy milk
Buckwheat	Gelatin	Veal joint jelly or broth
Butter, raw	*Greens	Walnuts
Cabbage	*Irish moss	Watercress
Carrots	*Kelp	Wheat (whole)

CALCIUM MENUS

Raw cottage cheese; steamed green kale; green salad made from parsley, watercress, spinach and other assorted greens; celery stuffed with raw almond or sesame seed butter; glass of half raw goat milk and half carrot juice.

Broiled halibut or red snapper, cole slaw, steamed kohlrabi, brussels sprouts, gelatin mold made with strawberries, bananas and pecans; glass of raw milk or clabbered milk.

Veal joint broth, brown rice (steamed), steamed parsnips, steamed beet or collard greens, leafy green salad, sun-dried black olives, three-bean salad, comfrey tea, bleu cheese or roquefort dressing.

Steamed rye or millet, revived Black Mission figs, dates, revived raisins, nut butter, raw cream, butter, soft-boiled eggs, glass of raw goat milk or dwarf nettle tea.

Chef's salad made of natural Swiss cheese, raw Monterey Jack cheese, raw cheddar cheese, avocados, ripe olives, celery, parsley, tomatoes, green onions, shredded beets and carrots, leaf lettuce, dandelion greens, anchovies or sardines (optional), sprinkling of raw sunflower seeds; barley and green kale soup; soy milk; tofu dressing.

SUMMARY OF CALCIUM

GENERAL CHARACTERISTICS

"Knitter" element   Found in water, ash, soils (lime)
Alkaline   Calcium type = Calciferic type

CALCIUM IN THE HUMAN BODY

Responsible for solidity
Essential during pregnancy for growth of baby
Helps scars heal
Fights germs, scurvy
Present in cartilage, fluids, certain tissues
Soothes nerves
Prevents asthma, hay fever, tuberculosis, rickets
Facilitates curdling processes

SIGNS OF CALCIUM EXCESS (CHARACTERISTICS OF CALCIFERIC TYPE)

Earthy, blunt, hard, slow, indestructible
Danger of hardening diseases, gout, growths
Problems with ears, eyes, tendons
Adversely affected by moisture

SIGNS OF CALCIUM DEFICIENCY

Lack of strength   Cramps in calves
Fear, indecision   Boredom, brain fatigue
Aches, pain, fatigue   Digestive problems
Profuse perspiration   Bone softening
Catarrh   Rickets or scurvy
Lack of willpower   Tuberculosis and other lung ailments
Hemorrhaging   Fevers, abscesses

HIGHEST CALCIUM FOODS

Dulse, kelp, Irish moss   Calf's foot jelly
Sesame seeds, other seeds   Meat next to the bone
All greens   Cauliflower
Nuts and unrefined grains   Celery cabbage
Eggshell tea   Celery
Bone broth   Egg yolk
Veal joint jelly   Fish
Cow milk   Gelatin dishes
Goat milk   Cottage cheese
Skimmed milk   Lemons
All kinds of cheese   Nettles
  except brown   Shredded wheat biscuits
Black radishes   Whole wheat bread
Curly cabbage   Rhubarb

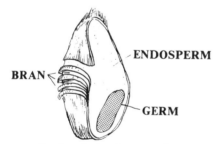

In the whole wheat are the minerals, germ life and bran necessary as food for the body.

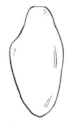

Refined and demineralized flour products are void of the proper vitamin and mineral content.

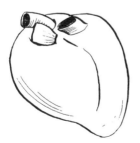

Sound heart tissues develop best from whole natural foods.

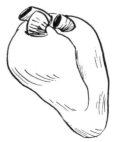

Poor functioning heart tissues can develop from refined demineralized foods.

137

two

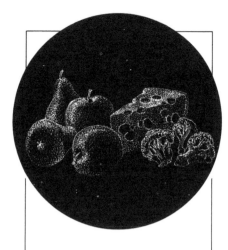

Carbon the "builder"

Carbon is an elusive element to observe or study because its impact on the body is so subtle. In contrast, calcium is an element that produces hardness, power and tone in the body, but it must be balanced by the soft and subtle elements such as carbon—a vital element. The other vital elements are hydrogen, nitrogen and oxygen, called air elements. No particular element should be allowed to manifest more strength than any other, so we must consider balancing each biochemical element. Many times we can balance excessive elements by adding a counteracting element, because doing so helps to reduce the overabundant condition.

In discussing various elements, we should realize that thinking ability goes with the elements in the body, according to the properties of that element. When we speak of the vital temperament (heavy in hydrogen, carbon, nitrogen or oxygen), we recognize many traits in mental activities and characteristics. *Indeed, many mental traits absorb and attract chemical elements that make a person what he is.* Although no two people are exactly alike, it is possible to change mental faculties with biochemical elements. We may influence, for instance, fondness for sleep, disinclination for the proper foods or lethargy. It is fascinating to see how the physical, mental and spiritual attributes are integrated by the influence of various biochemical elements and how each affects the other.

Identifying Features of Carbon

To summarize, carbon or its compounds in food form, occur mainly in sugar, starch, sweets, fats and in most proteins. Carbon is the basic element of cell birth and cell life, the "cradle of creation," and the principal element in growth. Wherever carbon and oxygen are at work, one upon the other, there is heat generation, growth and generation of carbonic acid. Carbon supports the vital system. When there is an excess of carbon in the system, it leads to some form of obesity. In fact, almost all people eat an excess of carbohydrates, fats or proteins, or all of them combined. An excess of fat in the body results in boils, fatty obesity, fatty degeneration, anemia, high blood pressure and many other ailments that can only be cured through correcting the diet and living habits. Finally, when there is an excess of carbon in the body, we dislike work and want to lie down. We can become simple-minded. Keep in mind that all sugar and starch foods in excess lead to too much carbon.

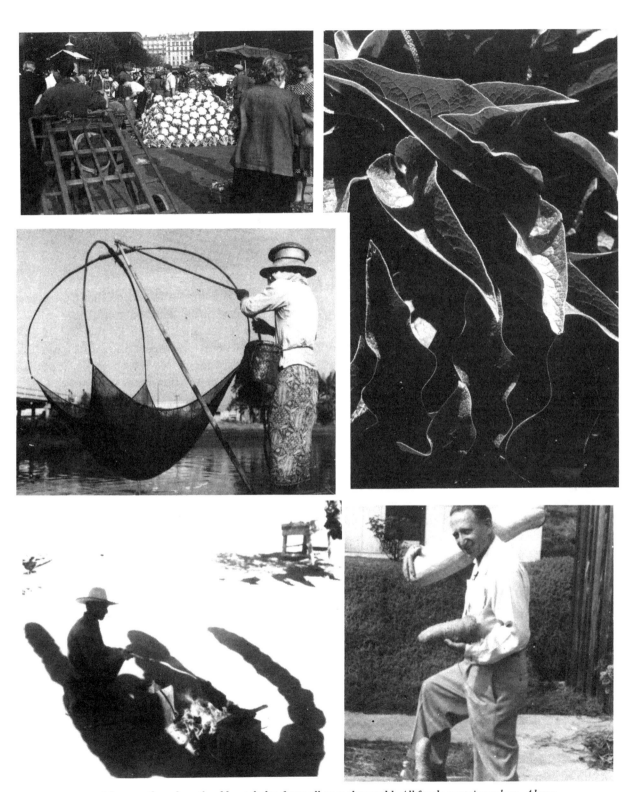

I have gathered my food knowledge from all over the world. All foods contain carbon. Along with nitrogen and oxygen, carbon is one of the mainstays of life.

CARBON
"The Builder"

GENERAL CHARACTERISTICS

Carbon, a negative, tasteless, odorless element, is unique in its ability to become hard, as in diamonds or soft, as in graphite. Its molecular structure is complex; it enters the composition of all carbohydrates: glucoses, disaccharides, trisaccharides and polysaccharides. Carbon is the most creative or prolific of elements, followed by hydrogen, oxygen and nitrogen, with each of which it easily combines. Carbon is an integral part of many minerals such as dolomite, chalk, coal and coal beds, diamonds and graphite. It has the capacity to split and reform into a range of composite animal, vegetable and mineral structures. Its atomic weight is 12; specific gravity, 2.35. This negative element is so profuse that it makes up approximately one half of the vegetable kingdom alone.

Carbon Unites and Absorbs

The constructive principle of carbon operates according to the creative impulse which acts as a catalyst, be it in the mineral, vegetable or animal kingdom. Agents of heat, sunlight and various organic elements transform carbon into its organic form. Carbon, known as the builder, possesses many unique properties, two of which are (1) union of carbon atoms with carbon atoms to almost infinite capacity, and (2) union of carbon atoms with hydrogen atoms to form a variety of molecules. This creative element is affected neither by water nor by air; furthermore, neither acids nor alkalis can corrode it. Carbon is well known for its ability to absorb ferments, moisture and gases from liquids or from the atmosphere; for example, carbon in its charcoal form purifies water run through a charcoal filter.

"A creative, conceptive, birth element...carbon."

CARBON: ITS ROLE IN THE HUMAN BODY

The Carboferic Type

A man weighing 160 pounds contains approximately forty-five pounds of carbon in his body. Certain types of individuals absorb more carbon—fleshy, vital, stout, powerful people; this carbon type of body is called Carboferic or vital.

A creative, conceptive, birth element, carbon is responsible for the conception or beginning of life, although it must be in the presence of tranquillity, harmony and warmth in order for the life principle to spark. The vital body of man and his mental faculties are influenced greatly by carbon. The more carbon consumed, the greater the demand for oxygen to generate body warmth; low heat production is a consequence of low oxygen and high carbon content in the body. Principal carbon food sources include grains, fats, oils, sugars, fibers and starches.

Carbon, Sugars and Carbohydrates

As carbon is the major constituent of sugars, we refer to them as carbohydrates. A variety of sugars enter the human body: fructose (fruit sugar), lactose (milk sugar), glucose (starch sugar or grape sugar), saccharose (cane sugar), refined sugar and so forth. Sugars are often referred to as saccharides.

Sugar Metabolism

The liver produces a sugar called glycogen which is comparable to starch sugar. Muscle metabolism is highly dependent upon carbon, as muscles demand sugar for warmth and energy; with about a one percent glycogen content, they account for some forty percent of body weight. Under heavy muscular exertion, the glycogen content of muscles is reduced; during rest periods, this sugar level rises. The hepatic veins (drainage ducts of the liver which transport blood to the vena cava and then to the heart) contain more sugar than does any other part of the body, and arterial blood contains more sugar than does venous blood. In the event liver cells are unable to extract sugar, the general circulatory system receives it and passes it on to the kidneys for excretion. Normally glycogen is transported to the muscles where it is oxidized, stored, organized into living material, converted into heat and energy (fuel). If muscle tissues lack vitality, the normal process is disrupted and incomplete. Tissues are unable to use glycogen properly when tissue oxidation is incomplete or potassium deficient. In such cases, tissues refuse the glycogen and it is excreted excessively in the urine. This condition is known as diabetes mellitus or glycosuria.

Carbon lack Contributes to Many Ailments

Sugars, fats and proteins, all containing carbon, have other functions in the body as well. If the system is unable to utilize sugars, fats and fibrins, emaciation results, along with muscular, blood, nerve and disposition coldness. Carbon deficiency is a contributory factor to many ailments.

Cell Organization Depends on Carbon

Cell organization, whether in vegetables, animals or man, is dependent upon carbon. This creative, building element is integral in all protoplasmic functions. Cell birth is influenced by carbon in conjunction with hydrogen, oxygen and nitrogen, in the presence of heat, light and tranquility.

SIGNS OF CARBON EXCESS

Characteristics of the Carboferic Type

The characteristics of the Carboferic type are distinctive—be it in appearance, disposition, moods, actions or aspirations. The properties of carbon are exhibited in such an individual: inert, sleepy, tranquil, immobile. The body is fleshy and tissues flabby; functions and metabolism are lethargic; the mind is sluggish, dazed, slow; auto-fermentation results in a drunken-like stupor; the individual evidences shyness, lack of motivation, laziness, adverseness to work and effort; he becomes stout, heavy, unhappy, feeble, sickly. Other manifestations include gluttonous appetite, gourmet tendencies; fondness for sleep, pleasure, inactivity, peacefulness, warmth, luxury and abundance. Clothing must be in style, tailored to fit; social interaction is important; pompous, splendid, luxurious surroundings are preferred; flippant behavior and idle pleasures are attractive. This type longs for sunshine and light, spring and summer seasons, the singing of birds, profuse vegetation. Although the appetite is powerful, there is a disinclination to prepare food for oneself; appetite runs to wines, cakes, candy, desserts, starchy foods, fats, oils, honey, rich fruit juices and sugary drinks. Appearance may be attractive but grace is lacking; dancing, singing, conversation and athletics are difficult due to incoordination. Bravery is deficient as is executive ability; emotions are unsteady and susceptible to panic when unforeseen circumstances arise; depression, melancholy moods, worry, fears, illness, fatigue appear often. High aspirations are not realized; good intentions not carried out; resolutions are lost. Muscles are poorly coordinated; finger dexterity is lacking; hands are awkward and objects are easily dropped.

The Female Carbon Type

The female carbon type is frail in activity, fearful and cowardly in manner; her pulse is weak; the will is weak and saying "no" is difficult or impossible; the mind is cloudy and thoughts are unstructured; harsh circumstances may provoke suicide; wants are not known; pleasure, eating, clothes, sleep are favorite pastimes. She has little or no concept of money or budgeting and bookkeeping; she finds kitchen work or farm living to be drudgery.

The Male Carbon Type

The carboferic man is more a money-spender than a money-maker. The mind tends to be empty; mathematical problems are difficult or impossible, as is thought in general; sciences are not adequately grasped. He is uncommunicative, shy and reticent; acts as if in a dream state. He has a terror of insanity; loathing for himself; chilled and miserable feelings; a tendency toward accidents. His bones are fragile; eyelids and head are heavy; finger and foot muscles grow numb, seemingly for no reason. He is kind and well-meaning but clumsy; trivial incidents are grievous. There are choking and shivering body sensations; uneasy mental fears. Fleeing or suicide are preferable to standing and fighting or quarreling. Extremely hot or cold drinks and food are unfavorable; warm foods and drinks are beneficial.

Disease Predispositions of the Carbon Type (Carboferic)

Disease predispositions are to congestive, anemic, diabetic, paralytic, nervous and gastro-intestinal ailments. Disorders include fatty degeneration, faulty oxidation, dropsy, feeblemindedness suffocating spells, asthma due to internal gases, lack of blood fibrin, nephritic complications, physical incapacity, fatty obesity, unsteady nerves, iliosacral ailments, cystic goiter, boils, paresis of motor nerves. Fractures, bruises, dislocations are likely. Symptoms may be excessive drowsiness, carbonemia, arterial degeneration, mumps, pyemia, weakness, paralysis, edema, albuminuria, dizziness, sunstroke, apoplexy, lockjaw, pyogenic pyemia, erysipelas due to incubation of streptococci and similar infirmities. If carbon assimilation is excessive, the assimilation and utilization of calcium, iron, fluorine, silicon and potassium are reduced; heart muscle weakness is a consequence. Men may turn to alcohol, but women are less likely to do so. An over amount of carbon causes further craving for carbohydrates, especially sugars. Glycosuria (diabetes) may manifest as a

result of deficiency of certain elements because excessive assimilation of carbohydrates and excessive conversion of foods into sugars creates the deficiency. Motor areas of the brain and locomotor system become enfeebled because these elements are deficient.

Problems of Those Who Overabsorb Carbohydrates

Some individuals have an abnormal craving for sugar and starch. As their bodies absorb an overamount of these substances, carbohydrate metabolism becomes superfluous, contributing to a saccharine or amylic plethora and autointoxication from carbon by-products. Consequently, vital tissue salts necessary for oxidation of the blood and tissue oxidation are inadequately assimilated, and this facilitates lack of oxygen in the body. Thus carbon dioxide waste products cause suffering. The patient may appear healthy but is weak and ill; ambition is lacking; fatigue is great; the stomach feels prolapsed and food may taste greasy; mucus colitis and gas may be troublesome; constitutional resistance is low, as vital alkaline salts are insufficiently assimilated; paralysis is possible; there is susceptibility to sunstroke and heat stroke; powerful heat, summer heat and sunshine may melt myolin cells in the brain and spinal marrow, facilitating paralysis; spinal weakness makes one subject to injury. The nervous system seems incapacitated; there may be congestive headaches, gallstones, liver problems, heart leakage, fatiguing neuritis, brain fever, swelling of limbs, aversion to acid foods. Animal products are aggravating to ailments; vegetable products are better accepted as they are higher in carbon and vegetable salts. Potassium, sodium, iron, calcium, silicon, chlorine and fluorine are poorly assimilated if available.

Too Much Carbon Diminishes Sex Drive

Flesh on hips and abdomen may look like tallow; mucous membranes are rough and irritated; sweat is acid and scorching; liver is enlarged; walls of colon are rough, raw and sore; whole body may be sore; abdomen or peritoneum is sore; periosteum is painful due to acids; feet are tender; tissues become waterlogged; water is excessively retained in the body; watery fluids may deposit in joints. Breath is short and patient yawns profusely. Complaints of neuritis in arms; ache in lower back head due to acid; corrosive, stinging autointoxication aggravating nerves; dry gums; sore mouth; full throat; acid stomach from excess of waste products, carbon and other agents present in the system. During surgery, tissues tear easily and their decomposition is likely. Physical sex drive is diminished by mental sex impulse is normal. Mental or physical work is difficult. Patient is distressed over problems which never materialize; evil is imagined all around him. Sultry, humid weather causes more oppression because of more carbon dioxide in the air; cool, clear days allow the intake of more oxygen; mercury and barometric changes are keenly felt.

Nervous Problems

This patient believes trouble to be in the nervous system; he feels like screaming or exploding over trivial problems; his natural proclivity for sociable behavior, kindness, good-heartedness is upset by unsteady, restless nerves. Excessive carbon dioxide and other products are generated; internal processes of carbon decomposition are overactive day and night, causing difficulty in burning up or expelling autointoxication products; oxidation is low. Overconsumption of carbon foods (starches) causes carbon plethora or carbohydrate gluttony; autointoxication causes a kind of food inebriation.

Carbon Dioxide

Combustion and respiration produce carbon dioxide, CO_2. A small quantity of carbon dioxide, generated by the soil and organic decay, is found in the air. Stagnant or still air, such as in insufficiently ventilated rooms and public halls, is higher in CO_2. If present in two- to five-percent proportions, carbon dioxide causes dangerous symptoms and possible death. (If a candle will not burn, carbon dioxide in the air is excessive.)

Carbon Dioxide in the Body

When carbon dioxide is in the blood, oxygen is excluded and proper oxidation in blood and tissues is prohibited. If great quantities of carbohydrates are consumed, more oxygen and tissue salts are required; there is greater decomposition, gas production and acid formation; and there results, as well, a disinclination to work and exercise necessary for maximum combustion and elimination. The patient may describe symptoms of dull senses, fatigue, mental confusion, lack of perception of

what he is doing or where he is, stupidity; breathing is difficult or incomplete; throat seems blocked, preventing proper respiration; if excess CO_2 is present, the throat contracts and respiration is spasmodic; nose and throat evidence vibrating and irritating feelings. Further symptoms include lack of concentration; heavy head; vertigo; noises in the ears; tendency to remain immobile; drowsiness; inability to motivate the body. If sufficient fresh air for adequate combustion and metabolism is not available and if tissue salts are deficient (to work with oxygen), autointoxication may reach dangerous proportions. Yet even limited quantities of carbon dioxide depress the brain circulation center, heart action, blood flow, respiration and pulse rate.

Results of Too Much Carbon in the Body

A superfluous amount of carbon (sweets, fat, starch, fibrin) in the body causes internal acid generation and flatulence or gas; tissues become acidic; acid nerve matter causes crampy, crawling neuritis; scorbutic rheumatism may result, as may retention of fatigue products—especially phosphoric acid, carbonic acid, glycerin-phosphoric acid, phosphates—which produce greater predisposition to body gases and/or acids. Tissue waste, tissue water and fluids and impurities are not removed efficiently. Growths or water cysts are possible somewhere in the body, and operations for such afford only temporary relief and are dangerous because the patient suffers from low vitality. Other indications of carbon intemperance include intestinal stasis favorable to toxin-forming bacterial flora which intensify the trouble; development of nervous disorders due to acidity in tissues and nerves, spinal material, bone marrow, periosteum, pericranium, peritoneum and nerve matter throughout the body; spinal weakness, especially in small of back; great sensitivity to cold; pain in cords of arms and hands; aches in more solid fibrous matter; aching elbow joints, especially during cold, damp or windy weather.

The carbon patient is not vigorous or hardy when in the best of health; intervals of rest are necessary. He suffers from constant drowsy feelings; lack of ambition; pains in heart or shoulders or other body regions. Heart murmur signals regurgitation of blood; chaotic heart alternates from feverish to weak to palpitating. Ailments are numerous.

Carbon-Excess Patients' Needs

The patient needs hills, mountain air and a diet consisting of liberal quantities of potassium, iron, calcium, silicon and sodium foods to heighten oxidation and burn up excessive carbon by-products. This diet also improves bowel evacuation and elimination by other excretory channels; general elimination of carbon dioxide can be improved accordingly.

Acids Cause Suffering

Acids are the basic cause of the carbon-excess patient's suffering. Acids produced by the body must be neutralized; carbon by-products must be eliminated; body gases must be expelled. Oxygen in the blood and tissues must be increased; foods rich in necessary tissue salts must be provided. Autointoxication is due to many causes and acids, toxins, gases, ferments in different types of patients require different treatments. If the body is inundated by excessive acids and metabolic end-products; when certain organic tissue salt reserves are exhausted and those elements not resupplied; when consumption of carbohydrates is excessive—the maladies and infirmities resulting are difficult to correct. Years of correct scientific eating are required.

Conditions of the Female Carbon Type (Carboferic)

The female carbon-excess patient develops anemia, becomes bloated, feeble in feet, numb in arms, fingers and hands; muscular coordination is deficient; motion and muscular control is lacking; finger tendons lack strength; tendons, cords, muscles and nerves in feet and lower legs fail to coordinate properly for work or exercise. She has difficulty in walking and controlling movements; experiences feebleness in nerves and locomotive structures of the body. Her head feels tired and a tired sensation prevails throughout her body; her brain feels enlarged; her mental functions are stupified and confused; her cerebellum is adversely affected by acids; cerebellum circulation is disrupted causing faulty memory. She is unable to follow the conversation of others or herself. Hemorrhage somewhere in the body is likely because heart salts are deficient. The brain, cerebellum, nerves, muscles are malnourished though she looks healthy. She feels better when standing but is perpetually feeble;

she experiences a stretching tendency of lower legs, arms, neck and body, due to restlessness, especially when she is with others; her lower bowel becomes distended; some vital organs are dispositioned due to internal carbon plethora or gases, fluids or cysts developing in some parts of the body. There is a tendency to fainting; sensitivity to electrical storms; fear of electricity, bright light, the dark, ghosts, lawsuits, snakes, mice, etc.; nerves are unsteady; grotesque dreams are disturbing to sleep.

She is Nervous and Restless

She suffers from generation of gas in the digestive track; feelings of suffocation, which she tends to blame on the air; intimidation by others; restlessness after retiring for the night; craving for coffee because it seems to bring temporary relief (men crave stimulants to an even greater extent); deficiency in resistive ability; inability to tolerate cold, heat or temperature alterations; soreness and stiffness in the back; lumbago pain; crawling, stinging, tingling and chilly sensations in the spine or elsewhere; nervous ailments, neurotic sensations, uncomfortable feelings, swelling. She believes she has every disease in the medical books and refuses to listen to a doctor or nutritionist who disagrees with her diet and lack of exercise.

She Craves Harmful Foods

The female patient often lacks will power to adhere to the corrective diet; her resolutions are often discarded in favor of her fondness for starches, fats, meats and sugary foods, resulting in continued overconsumption of these foods. Her taste tends toward pastries, cakes, refined rice, potatoes, pies, cornmeal dishes, doughnuts, crullers, butter, cream, ice cream, dumplings, spaghetti, bananas, coffee, common tea, pancakes and syrup, foods fried in fat, sugary fruit syrups, puddings, custard, chocolate, yeast breads, soda crackers, white bread, jelly, hashes, chocolate creams, oily nuts, peanut butter, foaming beverages, sweetened preserves and fermented foods. Her cravings for foods that magnify her condition are powerful; they are a result of the excess of those foods already in the body. (So the alcoholic craves alcohol because her whole body is saturated with it.)

Treatment of Carbon-Excess Patient

Appetite is a symptom; it is not a gauge of what one should have. The appetite should be strictly supervised. These patients need the supervision available in a sanitarium in the open country and hills where the air is pure and clean.

SIGNS OF CARBON DEFICIENCY

When Carbon is Lacking, Other Elements are Lacking

When carbon is deficient, other (bio)chemical elements are also lacking for various reasons. If one of the vital impulses is hypoactive, carbon may not be digested and assimilated properly. Poor appetite (controlled by mental faculty) may hinder carbon assimilation. One patient may lack sodium and chlorine needed for digestion; another may be short of nerve and brain force; another may have a deluge of waste products in the body which are not sufficiently eliminated; in still another, gases and acids may have broken down chemical elements in the body, thus disrupting metabolic functions. White blood corpuscles may be deficient; emaciation is severe; protoplasm is deficient, having a disastrous effect upon the body, mind, functions and temperament when carbon is lacking. Carbon and other chemical elements are not digested or assimilated properly in patients lacking social tendencies and emotions of love, joy, happiness, laughter, hope and compassion.

Emotional Characteristics of the Carbon-Deficient Patient

The mind is usually unfeeling; the soul icy; the personality bitter; the digestive and salivary secretions inefficient or poisoned; the vital impulse in the brain that controls carbon metabolism (notably sugar) inflamed, diseased or somewhat deficient from birth in the carbon-impoverished patient. This patient's manner is remote, conduct unyielding and unfriendly, judgment odd, business interactions strained, wit biting; humanitarian tendencies are largely absent. He ignores people generally; complains of fancied injustices or persecution; dislikes strong light and disdains social interaction; whines, mutters, rants about the behavior of others; has an aversion to what people are doing, their speech, teachings, education, deportment, organizations; is hypersensitive, nervous, malevolent in actions, overcritical and fault-finding, obstinate, antisocial, hermit-like, overly sensitive to the comments of others, easily offended.

Tendencies Resulting from Emotions and Diet

If this patient does not change his outlook, develop healthy emotions or alter his dietary errors, dyspepsia, diabetes or hypochondria are likely. He is prone to acquiring eccentricities common to the dyspeptic patient; difficult to please, argumentative, dissenting, disspirited, melancholy, worrisome, indifferent, distorted in outlook, gruesome. This individual is prone to eat and drink or use harmful items such as spices, alcohol, condiments, drugs, narcotics, chemical preparations, tannic acid tea, coffee and other indigestible substances. His cells and tissues are deficient in protoplasmic function powers. He may be abnormally obsessed with his work; experience fitful and chaotic brain impulses during illness; exhibit frenzied, jerky movements; and appear aged beyond his years.

Carbon Lack Produces Emaciation

If the carbon element is lacking in the body, hunger vanishes; gastric secretions are diminished or lacking; intestinal and digestive juices are absent; salivary glands do not produce; digestion and absorption of carbon is dysfunctional. As the disorder progresses the patient becomes increasingly emaciated, thin, dyspeptic; he eventually shrivels and withers away.

Antidotes for Carbon Deficiency

An emaciated individual must cultivate sociability, happiness, compassion, hope, love, laughter, joviality, friendliness, concern for others and their activities, sentimentality, affection, love of innocent pastimes, contentment, a positive mental attitude, optimism and similar happy states of mind. He must develop a genuine interest in foods, food preparations, nutrition, the culinary arts; he must acquire a liking for dining and its pleasures and anything related to food and food preparation. If these aspirations are realized the patient will gain weight and well-being; digestion will improve, as will assimilation and utilization of nutrients.

Gradually the brain impulses that regulate carbon metabolism (notably for sweets and fats) will improve.

Optimism is Essential

Optimism is enhanced by certain elements—silicon, oxygen, iron, carbon, manganese, magnesium; other favorable agents are joy, hope, laughter, ideals, goals, love, social tendencies, emotions. These qualities contribute to increasing trust in humanity, eagerness for the future, a hopeful outlook on life, positive mental attitudes and an active participation in living. Conversely, if the above-mentioned agents are not operative or operate only minimally; if the will faculties, higher reasoning power, commercial and self-preservation instincts are strong; if there is strong influence of nitrogen, calcium, fluorine, chlorine and phosphorus in the mental and physical makeup, the mind runs toward pessimism and the disposition is pessimistic. Memory is more retrospective; mind views are remote; reason is more contemplative; the entire mental activity is regressive, so the patient dwells in the past.

Carbon Lack Causes Disharmony

Carbon deficiency results in disharmony among other elements, especially when oxygen and hydrogen are also deficient. The mind dwells in the past when such corroding elements as chlorine are strong; there is little concern for the present or the future. One is inclined toward extreme pessimism, melancholy, worry, ill temper, apprehension, excitability, disheartenment and high imagination.

Carbon Shortage is Rare

It is rare that carbon is lacking in the body. (When it is excessive, it is generally because 1. assimilation of carbon is excessive and patient is overweight; and 2. intake of sweets, fats and proteins is excessive, causing emaciation and food intoxication.) When carbon is lacking, the patient is extremely emaciated, gaunt, malnourished, lacking organic force and action in the protoplasmic function of cells. Generally speaking, tissue salts are more commonly deficient, and as a result the body is unable to use sweets and fats.

Deficiency of Carbonates and Salts

Each chemical element has a specific influence in the body, and its lack or deficiency causes specific effects. For instance, lack of sodium carbonate causes malfunction of the digestive system and gas is generated. If potassium carbonate is deficient, fatty constituents are not assimilated and tissue oxidation is undermined. Lack of iron salts precipitates anemia. Acid formation is the result of lack of tissue salts and a preponderance of organic elements (carbon, hydrogen, nitrogen, oxygen). Many body functions are damaged due to excessive gases, acids, metabolism products; nerves, kidneys, liver, spleen, pancreas, sexual organs, circulation, brain, heart and other functions are adversely affected.

Emaciated Patients Lack Tissue Salts

In the majority of cases of emaciation, malnutrition and neuresthenia, patients lack tissue salts rather than carbon. As a result of these shortages, sweets, fats, starches and proteins are not digested or assimilated properly. Foods rich in the organic elements should be minimized at such times. In most instances an emaciated patient requires a diet rich in chemical elements (tissue salts) at first, in order to facilitate digestion of organic elements. This patient demands foods rich in iron, calcium, silicon, sodium chloride, sodium carbonate and potassium carbonate for proper digestion of carbohydrates, fats and proteins. A diet consisting of fats, carbohydrates or proteins causes further emaciation, illness and suffering; digestive ability for desired fats, sweets or proteins is further reduced.

"When carbon is lacking... vitality, vim, power, flesh and looks suffer."

Carbon and Salts Vital to Cell Functions

Carbon and other organic elements enter strongly into the protoplasmic functions of cells of plants, animals or humans. The properties of protoplasm are the foundation for all vital functions of nutrition, secretion, growth, reproduction, motility in all living organisms. But the tissue or organo-metallic salts are also vital to cell functions.

146

Carbon Metabolism Difficulties

When carbon is lacking, for whatever reason or if carbon and other organic elements are not properly digested, vitality, vim, power, flesh and looks suffer. Several reasons underlie carbon hunger or carbon metabolism difficulties: (1) low vital energy and nerve force, causing inability to digest and assimilate organic elements; (2) depletion of brain and nerve force; (3) deficiency of tissue salts; (4) acids, gases, toxins, poisons in the body affecting metabolism of fats, sugars and proteins; (5) excess of carbohydrates, fats and proteins in the system, causing food intoxication.

Interrelationship of Elements

The organic elements (carbon, hydrogen, oxygen, nitrogen) are cooperative in body functions. If assimilation of certain elements is too great, others are excluded almost entirely. For example, fats may be over-assimilated or nearly excluded from the body; so with sugars or proteins. Brain impulses regulate metabolism of various elements such as fats, sugars, phosphates, proteins, lecithin or iron. If the brain faculty and physical metabolism are weakened, partially destroyed, ill, paralyzed or inflamed, the specific metabolic function (digestion, assimilation, repair or elimination) becomes abnormal. Paranormal habits, feelings, preferences and aversions develop; specific ailments manifest; and, ultimately, chronic diseases appear.

Some Bodies Do Not Digest Carbon (Sugars)

Patients unable to digest and assimilate carbon, notably as sweets, adequately for muscles and other constituents of the body are tall, gaunt, thin, melancholy, slight of bone structure. They are susceptible to maladies of the kidneys, pancreas and glycogenic brain faculty. Foods high in sugar content have an adverse effect in their bodies. Diabetes (glycosuria) is likely if sugar foods are consumed excessively.

Low Sugar Tolerance

If tissue oxidation is defective, and when sugar tolerance is low in elderly, fleshy patients, the intolerance for sweets is due to a dietary deficiency of certain tissue salts necessary for normal sugar metabolism. As a result of these tissue salt deficiencies, sugar is excreted through the kidneys; the patients may develop dropsy, albuminuria, glycosuria, even when obese (indicating that they have large quantities of organic elements in their tissues). Potassium, potassium carbonate, sodium carbonate and iron are deficient in the diet or have not been assimilated by the system, often for a number of years. Diet is the cause of low sugar tolerance in many obese individuals.

Results of Inability to Digest Sugars

A patient who is hereditarily tall, thin, gaunt, melancholy, absent-minded, pessimistic, adverse to social interaction and irascible, exhibits hereditary deficiency in carbon (sweets, sugars) assimilation. Digestive ability is feeble and the muscular system inferior; low muscular oxidation is apparent. He is hereditarily susceptible not only to poor muscle oxidation but also to diabetes. His appetite ranges from ravenous to nil. Digestion is poor and nutrients are not sufficiently assimilated. Sugar and starch metabolism is faulty or fluctuating; sugar is found in large quantities in the urine almost continually; tissues are starving for sugar but cannot assimilate it unless it contains liberal quantities of tissue salts; diabetes is a possibility from birth to death. This patient is withered in appearance and lives a short life.

Symptoms of Carbon Deficiency

Carbon is deficient when a patient is extremely emaciated, acutely thirsty, feverish and irritable, melancholy and hypochondriacal; when the body rejects sweets and they are evacuated through the kidneys; when the appearance is tall, lean, gaunt; when urine is inconsistent and has a low specific gravity; when a sugar diet is intolerable or sickening, indicating that sugar supply and acceptance is dangerously low; when there is a predisposition to muscular prostration, stomach ulcers, vomiting and flatulence; when the patient is extremely depressed, distrustful, imagining persecution, poisoning or wrath of the deity, apathetic, despondent, preoccupied, fearful of imaginary foes or beasts; when he craves iced, watery beverages and consumes chilled water by the gallon; when his leg and foot muscles are weak, his scalp dry and itchy, his hair dry and brittle; when his appetite for liquors and artificial "foods" increases; when his disposition becomes cynical and pessimistic.

Treatment of the Carbon-Deficient Patient

The carbon-deficient patient requires a balmy climate, hills, and warmth, where vegetation is luxuriant. He must develop faculties of joy, happiness, social and love emotions, feelings of compassion, humanitarian characteristics, kindness and other warm soul qualities; he must also receive foods rich in potassium, potassium carbonate, sodium carbonate, in order to assimilate and utilize carbon in the form of sweets for muscles and vital organs. It is important to remember that the diabetic constitution can handle sweets (sugars) organized into tissue salts. For example, oats are rich in sugar (57.8%) and salts or ash (2 to 5%). Oats possess a muscle and nerve tonic valuable to the tissues of the diabetic. Similar sugars are tolerated by the diabetic and are beneficial to his condition.

HIGHEST CARBON FOODS

Carbon and its compounds are found largely in sugars, starches, sweets, fats and in most proteins. Carbon is often oversupplied in the body, especially due to refining of grains. Foods high in fat include:

Almonds	Olive and peanut oils
Avocados	Peanuts
Butter (cow, goat)	Pinons
Cheese (cream, goat, roquefort, Swiss)	Pistachios
Cream (coconut, goat, cow)	Popcorn
Egg yolk	Turkey
Fatty meat, fowl, fish, gravy	Walnuts

Foods high in carbohydrate (sugars and starches) include:

Acorns	Lentils
Almonds	Molasses
Apricots	Oats
Apples, fresh or dried	Pears, dried
Barley	Peas
Beans	Prunes
Breads	Raisins
Buckwheat	Raspberries, dried
Chestnuts	Rice and wild rice
Corn, yellow	Rice bran and polishings
Cornmeal (yellow is best)	Rye
Dates, dried	Sorghum
Figs	Sugars
Grapes and grape juice	Wheat bran and wheat germ

CARBON MENUS

Steamed rye cereal, poached eggs, butter, cream, rice polishings and wheat germ, revived raisins in cereal, grapes, sweet apples, cardamom tea.

Lentil casserole, corn on the cob, green salad with roquefort cheese dressing, butter, goat milk, steamed carrots and turnips.

Steamed cornmeal cereal, revived dried pears and figs and prunes, butter, cream, egg souffle, grape juice.

Barley and green kale soup, green peppers stuffed with wild rice, green salad with nut butter and egg yolk dressing, goat milk and carrot juice (half and half).

Salmon loaf, celery stuffed with nut butter, green salad with sour cream and avocado dressing, steamed beets and parsnips, milk.

SUMMARY OF CARBON

GENERAL CHARACTERISTICS

"Builder" element

Most creative, prolific element

Found in all carbohydrates

Carbon type = Carboferic type

CARBON IN THE HUMAN BODY

Supports vital systems

Essential to muscle metabolism

Basic to cell birth and life

Integral to protoplasmic functions

SIGNS OF CARBON EXCESS (CHARACTERISTICS OF CARBOFERIC TYPE)

Fatty obesity	High blood pressure	Boils
Anemia	Flabby tissues	Diabetes
Laziness	Drowsiness	Low resistance
Low sex drive	Carbohydrate gluttony	Nervous problems
Acid generation	Water cysts	Restlessness

SIGNS OF CARBON DEFICIENCY

Lack of feeling

Negativity

Remoteness, distance

Emaciation

Criticism

Melancholy

HIGHEST CARBON FOODS

Sugars

Sweet fruits

Starches

Grains, breads

Fats

Cheeses

Most proteins

Meats, fish

three

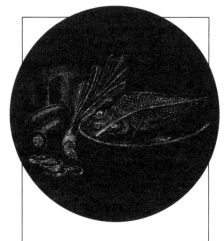

The electrical current in the system depends mostly on chlorine, sodium and iron.

Universal medicine in the future will use all the constructive principles from the wholistic healing arts.

Chlorine acts as the "laundry man" in the body.

Catarrh of the stomach and bowel is washed away if sodium chloride is in good supply.

Chlorine is an analgesic agent to the nervous system, expecially in hysterical patients.

Boston Red Sox shortstop, Stan Papi, was sent to a mental hospital, drugged, given electric shock therapy and driven to the edge of suicide because doctors did not recognize the symptoms of low blood sugar—hypoglycemia. After beginning a strict diet, he was back to normal in two months.

Chlorine, the "cleanser"

The first job I ever had was in a chlorine factory. In this factory, people were coughing all day long. They had an irritation of the throat and lungs—in the bronchial tubes. Then after I had worked there about six months, another employee told me that no one ever lived more than five years after getting a job in that factory. Chlorine in a factory is a killer. But it has the opposite effect when we find it in our food. It is the most wonderful cleanser in the body we can use.

What Chlorine Does

Chlorine is usually found where sodium is very high and is usually in the form of sodium chloride. Elements are not always found singly, because they "get married" to other elements, as in the case of sodium phosphate, sodium sulphate and sodium chlorate. Chlorine expels waste matter, helps to clean the blood and keeps the joints and tendons supple. Catarrh, phlegm, heavy limbs, water-logged tissues, distended stomachs, fever dropsy, neuralgia, chlorosis, hysteria, Bright's disease, torpid liver, phyorrhea, costive bowels—all of these conditions call for the proper chlorine balance through natural foods. Chlorine is one of the finest elements for helping the hydrochloric acid balance in the body and ending stomach troubles. It gets rid of gas in the body and the intestinal tract. In fact, sodium and chlorine were the two favorites of Dr. Rocine when he wanted to take care of flatulence in the intestinal tract or to get rid of any toxic material in the body.

Chlorine is one of the chemical elements needed in the intestinal wall for peristaltic action, along with sodium, magnesium, calcium and potassium. Also, it aids in tissue construction and makes nerves better conductors. Electrical current in the system depends upon the presence of sodium, chlorine and potassium. Additionally, chlorine and sodium help with the distribution of water throughout the organism. Chlorine is water soluble, meaning that it reaches all the organs and cells in the body. Thus, chlorine, a water cleanser, gets into the tissues of all parts of the body better than anything else, since all the fluids in the body have to carry chlorine. Furthermore, it is probably one of the finest elements for rejuvenation, working well with calcium in this respect, in the form of calcium chloride.

Chlorine Foods

Chlorine is to be found, particularly, in celery and celery juice. We use it along with carrot juice and also combine the two to create perhaps our greatest cleansing tonic. It is also found in raw goat milk or even in higher concentration, in goat whey. Goat milk helps in treating colitis and any colic condition or fermentation and putrefaction of any kind. It is found in all greens and salad vegetables. Thus, chlorine, the great cleanser, is usually found in vegetable juices and vegetables, and in the fruits which are cleansers. If it wasn't for chlorine in the body, we would not have a clean body.

Chlorine, in Sum

Chlorine and its compounds are important for efficient digestion. Chlorine has powerful disinfecting and germicidal properties, and increases the warmth in the stomach and increases bowel action. It is, in effect, the laundry man in the body and an enemy to germs, pus, moisture, disease and obesity. In fact, it extracts moisture from the body so rapidly that it is possible to reduce a waterlogged man six pounds in one day on a chlorine diet. Chlorine, however, should always be organized by Nature. Common table salt is not a food and actually creates chlorine imbalance. We can trace stomach burning and acidity to the overconsumption of table salt.

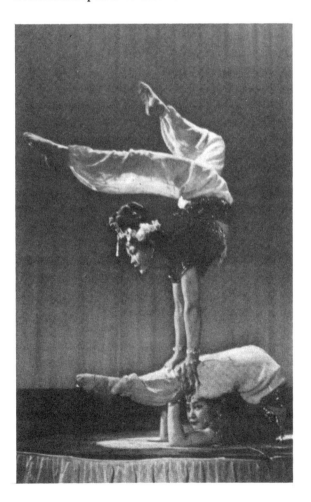

The flexibililty, precision, balance and coordination of these Chinese acrobats is wonderful to see. This is a 2500-year-old art in China. The Chinese have a lot of chlorine in their makeup that gives them limber, acrobatic bodies.

CHLORINE
"The Cleanser"

GENERAL CHARACTERISTICS

Chlorine, known as the "cleanser" in the body, expels waste, freshens, purifies and disinfects. Chlorine is a gaseous element highly susceptible to disintegration by heat. Its atomic weight is 35.5, specific gravity is 2.435 and electrical charge is negative. The "cleanser" has a yellowish-green color and is caustic with an offensive odor which produces choking sensations. Chlorine has powerful disinfecting powers and is water soluble. It unites readily with hydrogen, forming hydrochloric acid essential to proper digestion. It also forms the colloidal compound potassium chloride. When we refer here to sodium chloride, we mean its food form rather than common table salt, which is not a colloidal compound and is not readily assimilable by the body.

Commercial Use of Chlorine

As a commercial product, a chlorine compound is used as a valuable deodorizer, germicide and disinfectant. It is used mainly on surfaces such as walls and woodwork or paneling to destroy bacteria and germs. It is also a bleaching agent used extensively on white fabrics but not on colors or colored wallpaper. It is used as a disinfectant in swimming pools.

Uses of Chloroform

Another chlorine compound is chloroform, a product of the chemical reaction of chlorine on alcohol. Chloroform has long been used as an analgesic, anesthetic and hypnotic agent fostering in the body such symptoms as pupil dilation, rigidity, loss of consciousness, low blood pressure, temperature drop, shallow breathing, brain paralysis; paralysis of spinal cord, medulla and heart; and depression of respiratory departments, blood vessels and muscles. It has been found that prolonged usage of chloroform raises the excretion of phosphate, sulphate and nitrogen, causing fatty degeneration of heart, cardiac ganglia, kidneys and liver. It also helps the passing of flatus (gas) and peristaltic action in general.

CHLORINE: ITS ROLE IN THE HUMAN BODY

Chlorine is found and needed mostly in the digestive system and secretions. The human body contains only about three fourths of an ounce of chlorine; however, the chlorine type of person draws much more of this element into his body. The Chinese, often associated with the laundry business and cleansing, may be termed a chlorine race.

Chlorine Aids Muscles, Digestion, Osmosis

Metabolism and health, in general, are favorably affected by the "cleanser" when the balance is normal—neither too high nor too low. An excess of chlorine in the system has the potential for throat, sinus, lung and alimentary canal irritation and constriction; an excess irritates membrane surfaces in general. When supplied in optimal quantities, it warms the stomach and bowel by raising peristaltic function and freeing internal muscular heat. Chlorine unites with potassium to work within the muscular system and indirectly gives tone to the motor centers in general. The sexual system is excited, but not reinforced, by chlorine; tetanus, inebriation and intestinal colic are hindered. Fermentation and infections in the intestines are counteracted by chlorine and, in times of bloating and gas formation, it is needed in food form. Hydrochloric acid in correct balance ensures good digestion. When chlorine is balanced in the blood, osmosis performs the function of cell nutrition; union of sodium and chlorine in food form improve this osmotic process by distributing the nutritive solution.

Balance of Elements Necessary

For each ounce of potassium eliminated from the body, 55 ounces of sodium and chlorine are expelled, necessitating a diet high in sodium and chlorine foods to maintain the ratio. Goat milk is high in both sodium and chlorine. Chlorine is present in high amounts in fish and goat milk, as mentioned, but in low amounts in fruits and vegetables. Potassium is found largely in bitter greens, sundried black olives, potato peelings, dulse and kelp. The results of a diet overbalanced with potassium are bloating, gas generation, poor digestion, flatus and other ailments. It is important to keep a balance of all the biochemical elements in the body.

"...chlorine acts as the 'laundry man' in the body...."

The Chlorine Type

The chlorine type is solid, compact and strong for his size and weight. His muscles, ligaments, tendons are well-formed and efficient; they do not hold water, and excess fat and starch do not build in the system. The body chemistry consists largely of chlorine, fluorine, gelatin, sodium, potassium and phosphates. Organic chlorine promotes activity in the fibrous tissues and cells, making them dense yet elastic.

Cleansing Power of Chlorine

The purifying powers of chlorine, when it is well supplied in the blood, fight germs and bacteria in wounds, injuries and burns. Disease odors (even of contagious diseases), noxious effluvia and harmful germ life are combatted by the "cleanser." Germs and impurities are removed via fluids in the body which reach each cell; chlorine acts as the "laundryman" in the body, having a detergent effect upon cells and tissues.

Water Suspends Chlorine and Other Elements in Solution

A person weighing 165 pounds carries about 115 pounds of water, mostly in organic form although some is free. Water is found in saliva to 99%, in blood to 80% and to 75% in muscles. The amount of watery humidity determines the degree of fluidity. Organic and inorganic compounds (both chemical and biochemical) are suspended in water solution, enhancing assimilation of building material into the blood; then worn-out material is expelled through the same medium. Tissue fluidity, elasticity, pliability and consistency are in direct proportion to the amount of water contained in that tissue.

Distilled Water Not Advisable

In an average-sized man's body, about six and one-half pounds of water are eliminated daily from the tissues through the skin, kidneys and lungs. It is due to chlorine's process of purging osmosis that impurities, germs, pus and used materials are removed from the body, preventing autointoxication or self poisoning. Water is the medium used by chlorine in its "laundering" of the body. Consumption of distilled water in large quantities washes waste products and toxins from the body, destroys germs and cleanses the organism with the aid of chlorine; but prolonged usage of distilled water is not advised because it also draws mineral salts from the body. It is more indicated in cases of arthritis, hardening and deposits in the body.

Chlorine Affects Urine

The presence of inorganic-free chlorine in the system increases urination in direct proportion to the amount of cold water consumed. Urea is momentarily increased, as is the action with chloride of sodium, with sulphate and with phosphate. Solid particles appearing in the urine are temporarily increased, but their relative quantity is actually less.

Vegetarians Need Chlorine Salts

During hot, dry weather, those who consume great amounts of cold water precipitate sodium and chlorine rapidly. Excess water drinking leaches chlorine and other biochemic salts. A diet largely of vegetables draws chlorine from the body, often with the effects of flatus and diarrhea in hot and humid areas; constipation is more common in cold, dry regions. Vegetable acids and juices increase kidney activity and, along with potassium, extract sodium and chlorine in great quantities. A vegetable diet must be accompanied by foods containing liberal supplies of chlorine and sodium salts. If vegetable salts are deficient, scurvy is a result; chlorine salt deficiency leads to another form of scurvy.

Action of Sodium Chloride

The compound of sodium and chlorine (sodium chloride) is active in cartilage. This compound aids internal lavation and distribution of water in the body, ensures proper balance of humidity and exchange of watery fluids, and prevents precipitation of certain other biochemic salts due to reduced tissue metabolism, notably of albumin. Albuminuria and dropsy can be consequences.

Effects of Sodium Chloride in the Body

Approximately 200 grams of sodium chloride are present in tissues of the average-sized man. It is most concentrated in blood, lymph fluid and pancreatic secretion, but is found in other tissues and fluids as well. This organic chlorine compound controls diffusion and the exchange of new and worn-out material in the cells. The blood fails to take in the proper amount of water if sodium chloride is lacking in the blood or in the water. Red blood corpuscles hold the proper shape when sodium chloride is in correct balance, because the water balance or humidity ratio is thereby maintained. Red blood corpuscles are weakened and devitalized when sodium chloride is deficient.

Benefit of Raw Goat Milk

Good nutrition is influenced by the sodium chloride content in the body; it affects disintegration of proteins as shown by increased urea elimination with a diet high in sodium chloride. Raw goat milk provides chlorine effective in kidney problems because of its germicidal effect.

Sodium Chloride Reduces Acidity

Food sodium chloride is absorbed by the blood where it replaces that which is worn out in the metabolic process. Chlorine is vital to the formation of hydrochloric acid for good digestion. In the presence of sodium chloride, potassium-rich vegetable foods are transformed by chemical processes forming other compounds. If these compounds are overabundant, the kidneys must expel them and so sodium chloride is precipitated from the bloodstream. The vegetarian diet of man or of animals requires foods high in sodium and chlorine. Some acidity in the digestive tract is reduced by sodium chloride; however, there are several different acids in the stomach and various types of people do react differently to sodium chloride.

Cleansing Action of Sodium Chloride Salt

Albumin is partly diffused with the aid of sodium chloride through its attraction for water and its solvency. Sodium chloride, the major tissue worker in the body, diffuses throughout tissues and holds to them firmly. As tissue water is drawn from cells, it must be replenished from fresh sources; worn-out tissue fluid must be exchanged efficiently for new, pure fluids containing building material. The proper balance of assimilation and elimination cannot be overemphasized. Salt creates thirst for water by washing out the old fluids.

Sodium Chloride Enhances Peristalsis, Circulation

Catarrh of the stomach and bowel is washed away if sodium chloride is in good supply, preventing decomposition and fermentation. If mucus membranes become inflamed, diarrhea and constipation alternate. These conditions also arise from increased peristaltic activity due to increased secretions. The result is that food is speeded through the digestive system without being fully digested.

Peristalsis is increased, circulation improved, catarrh, phlegm and mucus removed, stomach regenerated and intestines strengthened when a diet high in sodium chloride is provided to flush the system with healing fluid.

Chlorine Improves Many Conditions

Blood diseases, heart dilation or palpitation, nervous disorders, poor digestion, hysteria, neuralgia, improper metabolism, muscle incapacity, skin inflammation, lymphatic system problems, joint troubles and torpid liver are all improved when chlorine is provided in proper amounts as a sodium chloride compound.

Gastric Secretions and Hydrochloric Acid

Chlorides are important constituents of gastric secretions: the gastric secretion is composed of 0.55% potassium chloride, 0.06% calcium chloride, 1.46% sodium chloride, 0.2% hydrochloric acid. Water represents 994.4 parts (per 1000) and salts make up 3.19 parts; the salts include magnesium phosphate, calcium phosphate and iron phosphate, in addition to lactic, phosphoric and acetic acids produced through food fermentation or bacterial growth. Hydrochloric acid encourages action of gastric ferments and prevents or stops putrifaction and fermentation activity, chiefly through destroying microorganisms. It prevents hardening of connective tissue, improves digestion of proteins and calcium, and aids pepsin activity. Indigestion results when chlorides are deficient in the gastric secretion. No two people have the same amount of hydrochloric acid; each person's balance must be maintained.

Chlorides in Blood Plasma

Blood plasma salts consist principally of sodium and potassium chloride, sulphate and phosphate, and calcium and magnesium phosphate. Chlorides predominate in the ratio of 5.5 parts per thousand; calcium phosphate makes up 2.0 parts. Some of these salts help maintain blood alkalinity.

Salts in Milk

Cow's milk, goat milk and human milk differ greatly in chemical balance. Cow's milk contains a larger percentage of salts, for the purpose of forming horns, hooves, hide, large bones and fibrous structures, as indicated by the predominance of calcium phosphate. Human milk is made up of more sulphur, chlorine and potassium. Goat milk is higher in potassium chloride, fluorine and potassium phosphate than are the other milks.

Salts in Perspiration

Perspiration is made up largely of sodium chloride and an alkaline phosphate, carbonic acid in free form and specific alkaline bases.

Sodium Chloride Affects Heartbeat

The heartbeat is quickened and sustained by sodium chloride, calcium phosphate and potassium chloride. Dr. Alexis Carrel kept a chicken heart alive for twenty years with a solution of the proper balance of organic salts and efficient removal of waste products; thus we see that there is a specific ratio of biochemic salts required for heart activity. If these salts are deficient in the blood, heart complications may result; cardiac centers of the brain and spinal cord may also be affected. It is important to remember that each person is different in the amount of biochemical elements required.

Chlorine is Analgesic

Chlorine is an analgesic agent to the nervous system, nerve centers and brain neurons, especially in hysterical patients. It decreases intense nerve pain by reducing excess conduction of nerve messages; its effect is similar to chloroform but to a lesser degree. Worms in the large intestine are combatted by chlorine as are intestinal parasites, germs and spores. Chlorine also fights pneumonia. Hydric obesity indicates lack of chlorine, as this element would extract hydrogen (water) from the body. Some forms of chlorine are hypnotic—i.e., chloroform, chloretone, chloral—when overly supplied in the body.

Sodium Chloride in Food Form is NOT Common Table Salt

All metallic elements which enter the human body should be in the biochemic form as organized and evolved through plant life; this is true of any of the sixteen biochemical elements. Throughout this chapter we refer to sodium chloride as the food form of that compound, not as common table salt.

SIGNS OF CHLORINE EXCESS

The Chlorine Type (Marasmic)

Individuals who absorb great quantities of free chlorine are known as the Marasmic type. They tend to be serious to the point of melancholy and depression. Temperamental, caustic and mischievous, they may both cause and take offense easily. Their dismal, gloomy outlook on life is caused in part by their chlorine-related acidity, biliousness and attendant discomfort.

Marasmic Type Believes the Worst

Although pessimism and suspicion cloud the personality of the Marasmic, he may also exhibit moments of humor, good nature, teasing, even hilarity. He may fight one minute and embrace the next. Cynicism, jealousy and gloating are some of his less attractive traits. His religion tends to be one of fear—fear of punishment and evil. His imagination is vivid, and he is apt to believe the worst of any situation or person.

Chlorine Type Prone to Alcoholism

If a chlorine type takes to drinking, he is likely to become an alcoholic; drinkers aggravate their conditions by consumption of alcohol, which essentially chloroforms the brain. Chlorine types keep to themselves or to their "own kind;" they are undyingly loyal to their family and native land.

Evil Fascinates the Chlorine Type (Marasmic)

The Marasmic type finds evil fascinating. He may himself become malicious, cruel, selfish and mean, or he may experience such negativity vicariously, through newspapers, television and others' stories. Idleness is anathema to the chlorine man; he must stay busy in order to avoid succumbing to his facinations and apprehensions.

The Marasmic is a Nonconformist

Sudden changes are not uncommon among Marasmics: they may suddenly disappear for hours or days, returning without explanation or apology; they may spend money lavishly for a short time, then return to their more characteristic seriousness and industry. Neither a leader nor a true follower, the chlorine type needs a job which offers variety but does not demand politeness and sociability. Like Will Rogers, other chlorine types are nonconformists.

The Female Chlorine Type (Marasmic)

Women of the chlorine type have similar traits. Like men, they crave salt, tea, coffee, even alcohol and other drugs. They are careless about their appearance, listless, indifferent, seemingly confused. They are afraid of thunderstorms and are easily frightened in the dark. They often act as though they are alone, muttering to themselves and paying no attention to others. Traits such as dislike, animosity, radicalism, caustic humor, fitfulness, dislike for study or reading, preference for seclusion characterize the chlorine female and signify chlorine excess.

Chlorine-Free Climate Helps Marasmic Regain Health

Fortunately, the Marasmic type is instinctively attracted to a humid, watery, relatively chlorine-free climate. In such an atmosphere he is able to regain his health and decrease his negativity and unhappiness.

Chlorine Excess Causes Emaciation

Overconsumption of chlorine escalates output of nitrogen, hydrogen, oxygen, carbon, sulphur, phosphorus, fats and sweets, preventing normal retention of these elements by the body. Great emaciation is the result, along with varied disease symptoms. Children do not grow properly; health in maturity and long life are endangered. Digestion becomes unbalanced and oxidation is reduced. Hyperchlorhydria (excess hydrochloric acid) contributes to chronic salivation and stomach ulcers. Inorganic chlorine amplifies these manifestations and adversely affects the lymphatic system; motor function is crippled, as are cerebral vitality, muscular force, overall vitality and tendon function. Bone sheaths are injured; so are periosteal structures, facial, gastric and esophageal tissues. The result is akin to neurasthenia and as difficult to correct; actually it is asthenia and lowered vitality of the motor faculties. Lower limbs may be curved inward or outward or even backcurved.

Self-Hypnosis A Danger

A patient consuming too much chlorine is subject to self hypnosis, sporadic functions, vasomotor disturbances, atonic disorders, enteric difficulties, respiratory and pulmonary problems, extreme prostration, ulcers, fiery sensations, periodic collapses. The muscular system may atrophy as may the glandular system. Throat and heart symptoms appear, as do narcotic neurosis, reproductive system malfunctions, manias, fears, narcotic and morphine dependencies and bluish, painful hemorrhoids. Glands produce sporadic secretions—are either overproductive or too dry and sluggish. Brain, heart nerves, motor nerves and motor centers are encumbered.

Patient Craves Salty Foods

Such a patient can eat all day and still remain hungry or eat a heavy meal and become ravenous in a short time. Poor digestion and nutrition are the causes. He or she craves salty meals, salty drinks, salted fish; nuts, pickles, sausage, cheese; salty pork, bacon; butter, carrots, cocoa drinks; sauerkraut, lentils and codfish and other foods which are salted heavily.

Salty Foods Cause Complications

All high chlorine foods are contraindicated, although the patient is drawn to them. He devours them readily and then suffers from ulcers inside the mouth; a red and thickened tongue; dry skin, heated and fevered; sunken facial planes; dilated pupils; weak and wiry pulse; swollen anus; blue and painful piles; poor digestion or indigestion; sparse saliva secretion; stomach ulcers; muscular prostration; inner walls and membranes scorched by excess chlorine or hydrochloric acid; thin urine and stools, even involuntary passing because these tissues have lost their resiliency, are dried up or have been scorched by hydrochloric acid; sour, scorching tears; face which is beet red, purple or colorless; mesmerized soul; distorted features; lack of love; odd habits. The throat closes and voice becomes high pitched and squeaky; throat causes yawning and spitting inclinations; anger produces thirst for ice water which only aggravates the condition.

Patients Need Warm, Moist Climate

Body extremities of chlorine-excess patients are chilly and blue tinged; there is quick respiration; the mouth froths when patient is angered; nerves convulse; tendons jerk; arms and legs cramp and tingle; calves, heels and toes cramp; joints feel bruised. The right side of the body succumbs more readily to cold, moisture, wind and arthritis or rheumatism. Sneezing plagues the person because nasal passages are dry and acrid. The chest is sore, elbows tender, small of back sore and aching, breastbone sensitive; membranes burn and sting, and pains are fleeting. These patients complain of outer coldness and internal fever, such as in joints and membranes. A warm, moist atmosphere is called for.

Problems of the Chlorine Female (Marasmic)

Females having an overbalance of chlorine in the body have headaches; breathing oppression; coughs; digestion and stomach problems; skin eruptions on arms and around mouth, even chest, showing disturbed digestion; eyes sting; heart muscles become atonic and weakened, with women being more prone to heart complications. The woman may also suffer subnormal temperature, lax muscular system, encumbered central nervous system, numb extremities, cold perspiration, dull senses and brain, weak muscles, poor circulation, defective protein metabolism, incoherent speech, erratic actions, waxy skin, semi-translucent fingers, congested vasomotor system, dry membranes, painful facial nerves, muscle tremors, ulcerated stomach wall.

Female Subject to Fainting

In times of anger, the chlorine-excess woman has a high-strung appearance with a high-pitched voice due to throat stricture. Lack of air produces choking sensations; face turns bluish because the blood leaves the cerebellum and medulla; fainting may result.

Further Symptoms of Chlorine Excess

Those suffering from chlorine overabundance bolt their food. Large quantities of water are necessary because water runs through the body as if it were a sieve, and is not utilized or retained. This offsets hydrogen and moisture assimilation. If venereal diseases are contracted, the body chemistry is further damaged. Alcoholism and drug addiction weaken functions even further; there is a tendency toward such dependencies. If excess hydrochloric acid is formed, indigestion and ulcers may result. Hyperchlorhydria (excess hydrochloric acid) is characterized by burning in the stomach; acidic saliva; mucus membrane strings in urine or regurgitations; extreme thirst; feverish skin; restlessness; slow digestion; discomfort in digestion; exhausted-looking features; tired eyes; melancholy moods; sensuality alternating with impotence; headaches; offensive breath; muttering and moaning; fermentation of food; poor protein metabolism, inconsistent urine. All such symptoms signify too much chlorine in body tissues and fluids.

Long-Range Effects of Chlorine Excess

Long-range effects of overindulgence in chlorine foods include lowered brain activity, depressed spinal cord reflexes; the medulla and the circulatory system are robbed of their power and effectiveness; blood pressure is lowered; cutaneous vessels are paralyzed, motor nerves weakened; fatty degeneration may result from defective protein metabolism; lower lobes of lungs are weakened by inward pressure, causing dyspnea (labored or difficult breathing); vocal chords are distorted, skin function below normal, degenerative changes occur in the epidermis, damaging complexion with a rash; feet lose control of balance; fingers are uncoordinated; breathing is short and shallow; some women eventually suffer a form of anemia due to defective breathing, but those who spend much time outdoors are not so susceptible because they breathe more deeply.

Treatment of Chlorine Excess

Chlorine foods should be temporarily eliminated from the diet, for sixty to ninety days. Egg white should be the main staple in the diet, along with albumin water cooked with egg white, milk products (not goat milk), egg shakes made from egg whites. Cold water should be avoided. The diet should be high in albumin and calcium.

SIGNS OF CHLORINE DEFICIENCY

Mental Indications of Deficiency

When chlorine is deficient the mind is filled with gloom; the patient has little or no self-esteem or confidence. Indications are morbidity, languor, inner unrest, lack of spirit, self preoccupation, sense of doom, sentimentality, acute physical sensitivity, restlessness, fluttering and long-range anxiety. Unpleasant and deplorable happenings assume astronomical proportions and the patient dwells unnecessarily upon them. He thinks the whole cosmos is out of balance due to his ill humor and sickness. Sympathy is hungered for but not accepted if offered; it provokes tears in a woman and exasperates a man. Both take offense readily, become dismayed or displeased, startle easily; hunger for love, understanding and comradeship but rebuke it when given, creating enemies, due to the condition of the brain, nervous system and spleen. There is great fear of hell and punishment. The future seems black with failure, poverty, disease, pain, ruin; these fears cannot be quieted even though the patient is not convinced of their truth.

The Opposite Sex is A Target for Anger

The opposite sex is a focal point of dislike, be it spouse, lover or parent. Temper is peevish and quick, moods restless and personality provokable, argumentative, critical, angry, sulky and antisocial, even though such moods are unintentional. Nerves are so irritated that the patient is not himself.

Early Signs of Deficiency

Early chlorine-deficiency signs are hyperactivity, quick movements, speediness; as acuteness of condition increases, the patient exhibits weakness, drowsiness, mental dullness, lackluster and laziness while in a state of constant irritation. Between three and seven a.m., the patient feels worse but is better when attention can be focused. Work improves feelings, but trivial matters are harassing.

Morning A Difficult Time

By-products of autointoxication attack nerves, organic functions and the brain, making mental concentration difficult, particularly in the morning, adding to a heavy feeling in the head. After the individual begins to function mentally and physically in the morning, toxins and acids are eliminated and a feeling of greater well-being results. But, brain work is still difficult; the cobwebs need to be swept out completely. Roaring in the ears is produced by extreme mental concentration, exerting debates, diligent study; dizziness may also be a complaint. There is difficulty in retaining thoughts and centering them.

Behavior is Unorthodox

Good manners are neglected and the opinions of society disregarded; world affairs are of little concern. Higher senses are partially paralyzed and perversions are possible. People who knew this patient in the past may have trouble fathoming his moods. Sex drive is heightened, but a muscle force is lowered. Orthodox behavior is shunned; study no longer interests, nor do love commitments, responsibilities, courtesy, chivalry, knowledge or life itself. Anxiety is a constant companion.

Moods and Fears Are Many

As chlorine hunger increases, the mind is plagued with apprehensions and solitude is feared. Dreams and visions are frightening during the night and the imagination during the day is childish. Responses are overly quick or slow. Direct or too-sharp questions are disdained. Extreme modesty, clumsiness and excitement may manifest. The spleen is besieged, producing hypochondria: multiple afflictions and illnesses are imagined. Moods swing from depressed to excited. A heavy protein meal aggravates symptoms as do temper, passion, wind and trivialities. Symptoms are more intense in the morning, less so in evening. Listlessness is a constant state; recreation is disliked; intoxicants are desired; senses of taste, touch, heat and pain are amplified while those of sight, smell and hearing are dulled; mucus membranes are fevered and arid; all things are disquieting; vague fears about one's own condition hang on; sulking moods have no explanation; depression and apprehension cling to the mind.

Physical Indications of Deficiency

The head may fall backward and the body fall to the side. Balance is precarious though one may not actually fall down. Frigid weather or humid cold is unpleasant. There is a sensation of head pressure and a weight; one may roll the head from side to side in an attempt to clear it; top of head may be grasped and eyes closed.

Ailments Due to Chlorine Lack

Deficiency of chlorine contributes to sluggish liver and glandular swelling. If chlorine is absent, appetite wanes, metabolism suffers; secretions become abnormal, skin heated, bowels inactive, moods unpredictable, mouth tender, breath bad and eyelids heavy. Hydrochloric acid is deficient, which harms albumin metabolism and causes flatus to develop in the digestive tract from fermented food. The scalp convulses, skin surfaces are very sensitive and fibrous structures of the body are tender. Other manifestations are appendicitis; a specific form of dyspepsia; intestinal putrefaction; heart complications in obese patients; gout in lean patients and ligamentous types; tension and tightness in joints and tendons; susceptibility to pneumonia; proneness to inflammation of spleen due to shortage of blood salts; tendency toward diseases of germ-life origin, bacteria or toxins; nervous indigestion; alternating diarrhea and constipation; tendon afflictions, also cartilage and joint afflictions; atrophy of albumin absorption process (albuminuria); eventual digestive weakness; bowel stasis; rectal and anal complications; chronic skin ailments; St. Vitus' dance; intense pain; spinal pain; neuralgic toothache; scrofula; paralyzed bowel; and portal vein system depletion.

Mucus and Catarrh Develop

The chlorine-short patient may complain of catarrh and pus, but this is dependent upon his chemical type. Mucus of the ear, adenoids or other areas may form; there is mucus in the urine (blennuria), vaginal or urethral catarrh, adenoma, ptosis, mucousy eyelids, stuttering, lung and bronchial catarrh, glandular stasis, splenic problems or hypochondriacal tendencies.

Chlorine Lack Intensifies Pain

For years, painful urination may plague the patient, even after chlorine is reinforced in the diet. There is a morbid fear of and aversion to pain, because lack of chlorine intensifies pain. Asthenopia, erythemia, ciliary muscle debility and eyesight disturbances such as hysterical amblyopia may develop.

Digestion is Delayed

Other indications for which the doctor, nutritionist or nurse should watch are purple extremities, blue lips, yellowish-blue or greenish-blue skin tone, gray nail roots. Stomach may bloat or spleen, liver and lower lung may swell; there may be painful contractions of the periosteum. Facial muscles jerk and lower lip twitches; limbs feel weighted down. Transverse colon is ballooned; liver and spleen have vague, sharp pains; urine has red, sandy sediment; stomach and esophagus are inflamed; tissues refuse albumin. Inside of mouth is raw, sore, scorched; tongue is heavy with white coating; inflamed and thickened taste buds result in popillary eminences like little points at posterior side of root of tongue; gums swell and teeth become loose. Nose picking is common due to ticklish feeling in nose; digestion of fats, albumin, starches and sugars is delayed; there is throbbing in gums and teeth; saliva and urine may appear bloody. Hunger is intense and then disappears; an empty stomach is more tolerable than a full one. Suffocating sensations attack one periodically.

Head and Spinal Pains

Further signs include epigastric pressure; acrid breath; spine tenderness, especially in the sacral region; sweaty palms; muscle spasms; convulsing motor nerves; contracting tendons; prostration with aversion to movement; difficulty in arising early; weak eyesight; sour and fetid perspiration; moaning, muttering, snoring; restless sleep; frontal headache moving to backhead; throbbing in temple region; irritation from noise; flickers, flashes before the eyes; dizziness and nausea produced by motion of cars, trains, buses, planes, boats; aching bones; groin pains; fleeting chest pains; fondness for acid and subacid foods and drinks; tongue paralysis; much sneezing; itch behind ears, on top of head, in anus or perineal area; bulging eyes, albumin excess or shortage or urea, phosphates, epithelial cells, spermotozoa, calcium oxalate, indican in the urine; specific gravity of urine below 1018.

Cramps, Fatigue—Even Deafness

The symptoms continue: pain in spermatic cords or orchis; catamenial intermission; toothache without cavities; light inflammation of sexual parts; throat contortions; partially blocked and narrowed channels and ducts; atonic blood vessels; low blood pressure; heart action reduced by chilly winds; one leg appearing shorter than the other; fingers fumbling; rheumatic-like pains; lumbar region (spinal) pains; splenic cramps; shortened upper chest action; burning in kidneys; sore hip joints, also buttocks and sacrum; frequent urination; inclination to abortion and uterine hemorrhage; flaking and falling of epidermis; dislike of exertion; foot numbness following short rest; burning, aching muscles; shiny nose; oily-appearing face; dropsy; fatigue from alleged overwork or in cases of no work at all; heat waves shooting from epigastric plexus to surface of the body; sluggish liver; swollen glands; warts; cysts; breast lumps; mumps; mouth ulcers and deafness due to catarrh; bunions; swollen legs and feet; skin itch and rashes. All of these signs point to chlorine starvation and demand a high-chlorine diet.

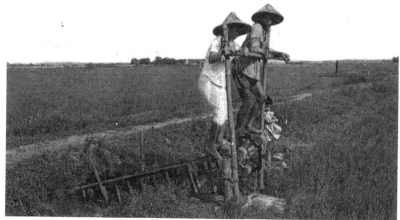

The Chinese are a "water people," always working with or around water. These two are irrigating fields.

160

HIGHEST CHLORINE FOODS

Fish are the richest source of chlorine, followed by raw goat milk. Chlorine-carrying foods are listed below. * denotes highest foods in chlorine.

Asparagus
Avocados
Bananas
Beans
Beechnuts
Beets
Blackberries
Brazilnuts
Breadfruit
Brussels sprouts
Cabbage, red, common, savoy
Carrots
Cauliflower
Celery
Cheeses (Danish bleu, Italian, Roquefort, Swiss)
Chickory
Chickpeas, dried
Chives
Coconut
Corn
Cowpeas, dried
Cucumbers

Dandelion greens
Dates
Dock (sorrel)
Eggplant
Endive
Figs
Filberts
*Fish
Fowl
*Goat milk, raw
Guava
Horseradish, raw
Jerusalem artichoke
Kale
Kelp

Kohlrabi
Lean meat
Leeks
Lentils
Lettuce, leaf & sea
Mangoes
Oats

Onions, dry
Parsnips
Peaches
Peas
Pineapple
Potatoes with skins
Radishes
Raisins
Red raspberries
Rutabaga
Salsify
Sauerkraut
Spinach
Strawberries
Sunflower seeds

Sweet potatoes
Tomatoes
Turnips
Veal joint broth
Watercress
Watermelon
White beans, dried

CHLORINE MENUS

Broiled halibut; cole slaw; leafy green salad made with cucumbers; radishes; fresh sweet peas, shredded carrots and beets; steamed raisin pudding; tomato juice or clam cocktail.

Chef's salad made of raw cheese sticks, sardine and anchovy bits, red and savoy cabbage, greens (dandelion, watercress, etc.); coconut milk flavored with revived figs or dates; veal joint broth.

Steamed yellow cornmeal; lentil sprout omelet with avocado, topped with sunflower seeds; clabbered raw goat milk; watermelon or blackberries and raspberries or fruit in juice form.

Raw cottage cheese, raw goat cheese, pineapple, guavas, mangos, fresh peaches, breadfruit, bananas on bed of greens, pineapple kefir.

Baked potato with skin, cornbread, steamed asparagus, steamed parsnips, fish broth, sour cream and chives; green salad made with lentil sprouts, radishes, ripe tomatoes, leaf lettuce, eggplant, cauliflower, sauerkraut; carrot juice and goat milk half and half.

SUMMARY OF CHLORINE

GENERAL CHARACTERISTICS

"Cleanser" element

Powerful disinfectant

Essential in hydrochloric acid, chloroform, sodium chloride compounds

Chlorine type = Marasmic type

CHLORINE IN THE HUMAN BODY

Sodium chloride reduces acidity, enhances circulation

Increases osmosis

Important for efficient digestion

Liberates muscle heat

Decreases nerve pain (analgesic)

Most concentrated in blood, lymph and pancreatic fluids

Fights germs and bacteria

Combats odors

Removes impurities

SIGNS OF CHLORINE EXCESS (CHARACTERISTICS OF MARASMIC TYPE)

Marasmic exhibits characteristics of chlorine-deficient patient, as well: pessimism, suspicion, melancholy, apprehension, fear

Nonconformity; unorthodox behavior

Craving for salty foods

Poor digestion

Numbness, poor circulation

Inconsistent urine

Jerking, cramping muscles

Emaciation

Muscular weakness

Tendency toward drug dependencies

Muscular weakness

Dryness of skin and tissues

SIGNS OF CHLORINE DEFICIENCY

Depression, morbidity

Peevishness, sulkiness

Sensation of head pressure and weight

Glandular swelling

Catarrh

Inflammation and pain

Restlessness, anxiety

Difficulty concentrating

Sluggish liver

Poor appetite, metabolism

Painful urination

Muscular spasms and cramps

HIGHEST CHLORINE FOODS

Fish

Raw goat milk

four

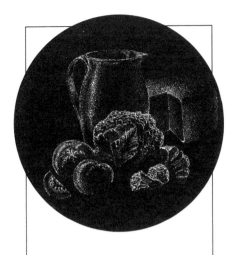

Fluorine, the "decay resistance" element

Fluorine is especially important today because so much food is cooked, thereby destroying this element. Like iodine, fluorine is an elusive element. It is water soluble but easily lost. Fluorine is what we call an unstable element. The moment that heat hits the fluorine food, it is lost into the air.

The highest source of fluorine is black bass, but who is going to eat raw, black bass? Who is going to eat green quince, the second highest source, unless it is prepared as a cooked marmalade with so much white sugar that all the value is destroyed?

The third highest source of fluorine is raw goat milk, and very few people are interested in it. Pasteurized milk, on the other hand, does not contain fluorine because it has been heated, and, in fact, the lack of fluorine then allows epidemics of colds and flu. I am not saying that the milk itself produces the disease, but when milk or any food is deficient in the elements it should have, then the animal, the plant or the human being that has to live from that food is deficient. That deficiency encourages disease.

Again, we must emphasize that the fluorine spoken of here is not the unevolved chemical that is added to water but an important element evolved to a higher level of vibration through the fruit and vegetable kingdom. It is available to us in raw foods, and raw foods should be 60% of our diet. If food must be cooked, use low heat, stainless steel cookware, and cook by steaming, not by quick cooking with high heat. Unfortunately, today, far too many of our foods are either baked, boiled, charred, barbecued or roasted excessively. Bread is baked at very high heat, as are pastries, and all canned fruits and vegetables are processed with extremely high heat. All these foods lack fluorine. Although we should take in fluorine foods to help prevent disease, eating so much cooked food actually promotes weakened natural defenses in the body because of the fluorine deficiency that is left.

The point here is one of natural law; that is, we can derive nourishment and good health directly from the earth. When you take a whole food and disrupt its chemical bonds, changing and destroying some of the elements intended to be there, you are creating a food that, when eaten, welcomes disease. Every disease represents a shortage of a certain chemical element. That is the basic philosophy that we have come to understand from our work. In other words, if you are eating a food that once was a whole food, but after cooking lacks a specific element, then you are creating a subtle imbalance. If you do not take care of the mineral deficiency, you're going to have the flu again—and again—and again.

We are surely speaking now of the profession of the future, which will be to understand how to unravel the mystery of these imbalances.

Recently the head of the Health Department of San Diego suggested that people who are susceptible to the flu get their shots early. But I almost wanted to say, "Shame on you if you are subject to the flu! You have not been getting enough fluorine for resistance. You have neglected the foods that keep you well."

I am convinced that proper nutrition would make it unnecessary to get shots, vaccinations and immunizations of all kinds. Indeed, we should live on foods that prevent viruses and "contagious" diseases.

In this country, however, we are free to do whatever we wish. People are free to have diseases. But disease is not free after you get it! It becomes very expensive. Too many doctors are making a living from ignorant people.

Now, it is a terrible thing to tell a sick person he is ignorant. We are all ignorant in some way, but to be ignorant of our bodily needs is a shame that doctors must take some responsibility for, because they should know better. No doctoring should go on without treating the body from a mineral, biochemical standpoint—from a wholistic viewpoint. No acupuncturist, chiropractor or any healing arts practitioner can get a body well without diet awareness.

A person who lives on coffee and doughnuts or on pickles and ice cream will never really get well in the long run. Without using nutritional and chemical principles, such a person's treatment is only a charade that doesn't provide a long-term cure.

Calcium Has Affinity for Fluorine

Calcium has an affinity for fluorine. Calcium fluoride is a long life element; the long-lived people of Europe are people who have a high proportion of active calcium and fluorine working together. This is why we can dig up skeletons that have been in the ground for a thousand years and find them still preserved if there is a lot of fluorine. It is fluorine on the outside of the teeth in combination with the calcium that hardens and protects teeth from cavities. We find that goat's milk has both calcium and a high fluorine content.

Problems Due to Fluorine Deficiency

To begin with, when teeth decay, we know that the fluorine is not there. It has diminished in the body. You cannot make good hard teeth without fluorine. Fluorine is the element that brings the beauty to bones and teeth by creating a hard surface on the outside of the calcium, so that no germ life can attack and no acids can get in and break it down. Without the fluorine, the acids and germ life can dig in and cause trouble. In fact, there are claims that we have more germ life in the mouth than in the rectum. We find that germ life lives in the mouth because we have the material there for it to grow. Ninety percent of all people have tubercular germs in the mouth and throat, but that doesn't mean all these people will develop tuberculosis. If you don't get enough calcium and fluorine however, you may be open to it.

In cases of osteomyelitis, for example, a person comes in with a running sore from the bone. We find that a discharge settles at that spot then, and there is no healing. Healing should come from the inside out, but we find that the person doesn't have the fluorine to keep away the discharge. He or she is suffering a lack of the fluorine and calcium mixture in the body. I see many such imbalances.

A person goes out on a little ski jaunt and gets the littlest bang in a bone structure in the thigh or calf. Then he can't repair or rebuild that structure effectively. Again, the chemical balance for repair and healing is missing.

A person who has an ulcer of the leg lacks silicon, calcium and fluorine. If we get to the place where we have a leg ulcer and a low-grade virus affecting it, there is a lack of fluorine. Fluorine is lacking wherever there is a virus in the body—wherever germ life can attack the body.

Sources of Fluorine

The raw food faddist probably has a better chance of overcoming germ life in the body than the person who eats mostly cooked foods. So again, remember that the diet should have at least 60% raw foods. We find fluorine in most raw foods. There is a good deal of it in salads, but also in nuts, seeds and raw milk products. We can find a good deal of fluorine where there is high calcium in a food, as in milk and grains.

Fluorine is found in fish and bones and, of course, in quince. There are ways of assuring the presence of fluorine by having it in a tonic, dessert—as Dr. Rocine would suggest—or in a marmalade. My wife and I have developed a recipe where we add pineapple to quince and put it in the liquefier. Also, we make a raw marmalade (instead of having it cooked) so that all the fluorine is left in.

The price we pay for fluorine deficiency makes it very much worth our while to see that we get enough of this vital protective element in our diet.

Calcium Is Needed Throughout Adult Years.
"Bones are 'highly dynamic tissue,' maintained by a balance of bone formation and bone resorption going on all the time, regardless of age," says G. Donald Whedon, MD, Senior Science Adviser of the National Institute of Arthritis, Diabetes, Digestive and Kidney Diseases. An estimated half of the nation's girls between 12 and 14 are getting only 2/3 of the RDA of calcium, while from 15 to 17 they are getting only 50% and from 19 to 74 only 60% of the RDA. Women have twice as many problems from osteoporosis as men. Presently, the calcium RDA is 800 mg per day for adults and young children, but some experts believe that 1000-1200 mg would be more realistic.

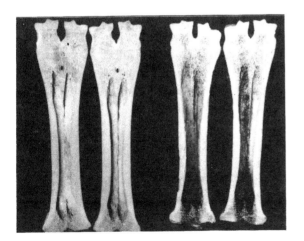 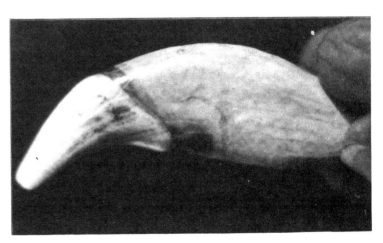

Fluorine hardens and protects bones and teeth. These bones are from animals raised on calcium-rich soil at Mineral Gardens Farm, Kentucky. Bones at left from a 29-month-old animal weighed 560 gm before halving. Bones on right from a 36-month-old animal weighed 380 gm.

FLUORINE
"The Anti-Resistant Element"

GENERAL CHARACTERISTICS

Fluorine, the "anti-resistant" element, is a colorless, emerald green gas. Its atomic weight is 19.0; specific gravity is 1.31. It carries a negative electrical charge. Its most outstanding property is that it is the one element which withstands unity with oxygen as a compound. Fluorine combines readily with many other elements, especially with calcium to form calcium fluoride or calcic fluoride, a fluor-spar. The pure form of calcic fluoride is made up of almost 49% fluorine and the remainder calcium. Fluor-spar is present in metal-bearing rock housing silver, lead and cobalt ores. Generally it manifests as amber, green, azure or red, though occasionally it is transparent. Additionally, fluorine enters cryolite rocks, slate, gneiss, sandstone, limestone, coal beds and numerous volcanic derivatives. The term "fluorine" comes from the Latin *fluere*, meaning "to flow."

Commercial Uses of Fluorine

In combination with hydrogen, fluorine forms hydrofluoric acid, a volatile corrosive agent used for etching glass products; the acid eats away the silicon (sand) in glass. Sodium aluminum fluoride, a crystal form called cryolite, contains albumin as well as fluorine. Cryolite is valuable in glaze and soda manufacture. Fluorine was used in Egyptian embalming, the actual process of which is no longer known.

166

FLUORINE: ITS ROLE IN THE HUMAN BODY

The "resistant" element is active in the bony structure and other hard tissues of the body. In conjunction with calcium, it forms strong bones, tough tooth enamel and healthy hair and nails; it also reinforces blood vessels. Amazingly, all this is done with only about three to four ounces of fluorine in normal reserve in the human body. Calcium is reinforced by fluorine—preventing tooth decay, ulceration, calcification, suppuration, induration, infiltration and excessive calcium buildup. Oxygen is prevented from permeating strong, polished surfaces of bones and teeth by the presence of fluorine in their construction. Extreme heat generation and centralization in osseous (bony) tissues is prevented by fluorine.

Fluorine Builds and Disinfects

The deepest internal tissues are subject to the influence of fluorine. Bone cell cementation, hair construction, tooth formation, meninges (pia-arachnoid and dura mater) construction require fluorine; without sufficient fluorine these structures are damaged. Certain glands are dependent upon fluorine for proper function. Construction of nails, canal walls, bone linings, sinus walls requires fluorine. Few hard, polished tissues or structures are exempt from fluorine influence. It is a purifier, disinfectant, germicide, resistant agent and building block throughout the entire body.

Fluorine Helps Preserve Youthfulness

In a sense, fluorine is a beauty and youth element capable of ensuring a long and youthful life when provided in ample quantities in the diet. Individuals who have an adequate fluorine reserve for normal body functions remain youthful; they are able to resist old age and preserve their bodies.

Fluorine Vital to Solid Tissue

The spleen is strongly affected by and must have fluorine in order to function properly. Even the eyes must have fluorine. Muscular tissue depends on fluorine and calcium for its hard, shiny protective surface. Solid membranes, integuments (the natural covering of the body), arterial and venous walls, hair, nails and teeth must have fluorine and calcium. Without fluorine, solid tissue cannot function adequately; it cannot be properly constructed, maintained or repaired. Fluorine keeps solid tissue purified and prevents fermentation. It acts as a disinfectant, germicidal, antiseptic, antipyic (preventing suppuration), antiparasitic, antisyphilitic and antipyretic (effective against fever) agent. Germs, oxygen, toxins, impurities, bacterial gases, acids and calcic and other toxins are combatted by fluorine. Dental cavities are prevented so long as the enamel is hard and complete.

"The 'resistant' element is active in the bony structure and other hard tissues of the body. In conjunction with calcium, it forms strong bones, tough tooth enamel and healthy hair and nails; it also reinforces blood vessels."

Some Diseases Destroy Fluorine Reserve

Fluorine is not invincible to certain diseases, germ life, poisons, toxins or pus; these cripple the fluorine reserve. Some agents disasterous to fluorine are mumps, tuberculosis germs, syphilis germs, erysipelas, specific bacterial toxins and vaccines. If the fluorine supply is exhausted, bones, solid tissues, skin, teeth, membranes, periosteum, pericranium are adversely affected. If tooth enamel is undermined, oxygen, bacteria and ferments cause decay.

Bones Require Fluorine

It is interesting to note that the skull of a corpse is like plaster if fluorine was not abundant during life. But if fluorine was well supplied, the skull remains hard and durable. Bone cells are cemented into a solid structure by fluorine, silicon, calcium and certain other elements; the result is a polished, shiny veneer resisting corrosion and decomposition by oxygen. If fluorine is deficient, bone processes are faulty. The ideal balance of fluorine in the body heightens calcium assimilation, osteogenesis and keratinization (keratin is the basis for bones, horns, nails, etc.). Fluorine improves absorption of gelatin, magnesium phosphate, sodium chloride, calcium carbonate and other vital tissue salts which the body requires in organic form. Remember that fluorine must be supplied in the organic form as provided by nature's garden. Inorganic or drug forms are not suitable.

Fluorine—Oxygen Balance Important

Tissues such as ligaments made up of hard, fibrous material require fluorine as does connective tissue. Cartilage in the joints depends on fluorine for durability. Broken bones need fluorine, as well as calcium, for knitting rapidly. Oxygen would destroy bones and other hard, fibrous tissues if fluorine were not present.

SIGNS OF FLUORINE EXCESS

Patient is Hungry but Not Thirsty

Indirectly fluorine excess affects the brain, emotions, personality and disposition. It increases sexual drive and encourages extreme sensuality and overindulgence in sexual activity, possibly due to fluorine's unfavorable action on cerebral and spinal meninges. These structures are assaulted, as are additional inner osseous tissues. Reproductive ability is destroyed, and protective membranes and linings are irritated and inflamed. Food appetite is also increased, causing the patient to eat and drink too much; the result is obesity and a coarse appearance. Wines, liquors, coffee, sweets and fatty foods are preferred. Hunger pangs are incessant; but the patient is never thirsty, even when skin is bloated, fiery, arid and feverish.

Fluorine Excess Rare but Serious

It must be emphasized that fluorine excess in the average person is rare because of our refined diet and the absence of raw foods. If it is ever in excess, however, the signs are pronounced. Certain areas of the body are inundated with excess blood and other parts are anemic. Blood rushes to the brain. Recall is almost nullified. Pericranium, periosteum, dura mater are affected resulting in brain disturbance. Corpus callosum, falx cerebri, tentorium cerebelli, falx cerebelli and Pacchionian glands (at the inner surface of the skull vertex) which contain "brain sand" (calcareous concretions) are undermined; the result is ulceration, inflammation or hardening of some of these membranes, the Pacchionian glands or some other area in the head—even the pineal gland, putuitary body, peduncles, venous sinuses. The outcome may be deranged brain function. Religious insanity may manifest; the patient may ask for prayers to save his unworthy and damned soul; the cause may simply be the too-strong effect of fluorine on the deeper and more rigid tissues and glands.

The Fluorine Excess Patient is Fearful

If fluorine is over supplied in the system, the patient worries about his profession, his family, loved ones and responsibilities. He moves like a tornado to get work done, but in many instances, work is impossible. Death is longed for. Hell and damnation are constant fears, contemplation of the future fosters apprehension. Status in the community seems precarious; business seems unstable. Self confidence is nil. Mirth alternates with depression; worry and laughter are magnified. Morning brings optimism; evening brings pessimism and despondency. Symptoms mount and intensify in the evening. Hot weather, moisture, humidity or motion are unpleasant. Contradiction is not accepted, even from those who were previously respected and revered. Sorrow exaggerates symptoms; disappointments are very stressful and deeply felt.

Pains and Aches are Numerous

Sensory cortical centers are pathologically stimulated, resulting in negative, unilateral and visual hallucinations. Imaginary objects seem real; an object may be viewed as having one side only. More dense eye structures are affected; perceptions of senses are altered or destroyed—especially taste, smell and hearing. The fluorine-excess patient has a nasal twang in the voice. He or she may prefer invalidism. Moaning, crying and screaming may take place during sleep; pains and aches are numerous. There is a tendency to grin while conversing. The mental image of pain produces physical manifestation.

Ailments are Varied

In the rare event of fluorine excess, there is a predisposition to ulcers, scabs, suppurations, indurations in the deeper tissues, which are achy; layers are shed like dead skin. Cavities and bone decay are prevalent. There may be bone complications or problems in membranes and canal walls; eyesight problems; dizziness when moving; tendency to fall to left side; violent cranial and meningeal headache that disappears when the patient enters the open air and sunshine; crust formation on the nose, frontal sinuses and other places; easily-bleeding gums and teeth with odor of decay; ulcers, nodes, hard lumps in membranes; fatty deposits around the heart; intolerable itching in the afternoon; excruciating pains; dry catarrh; enlarged, feverish, red nose tip; mastoiditis; pressure from inside outward to the surface of the body or head; swollen face; hair falling out; other hair and scalp ailments; shiny eyes; contracted pupils; bulging eyeballs; tender eye bones; eyelashes falling out; eyelids becoming red; objects appearing distorted, double or only partly visible; forehead throbbing on one side; bones feeling bruised or broken; itching, smarting, drilling pains.

Motion Causes Discomfort

Feet itch near evening, never in the morning. Skin itches when confined indoors but not in sunlight and open air. Nails look rough. Scalp develops scabs; skin may become scabby in places. Body temperature alternates between chill and overheating; cold affects patient most when he retires for the night. Condition worsens periodically, such as every third day, every third week or every afternoon. Motion is nauseating or irritating. Transportation in autos, trains, buses, planes, causes anxiety, pain or discomfort. Physical stress shoots waves of blood to the heart and brain resulting in pains resembling gout. Exercise and movement cause apprehension about the heart or palpitation and sensations simulating heart failure. Rest augments tendon tension. Reclining on parts of the body produces numbness. Jumping downward several feet, energetic dancing or other sudden jarring of body or head makes blood rush to lower extremities which suddenly swell and turn scarlet. Bone linings thicken and become tender, sore, stiff and painful. A short walk dispels blood from limbs and moves it into internal organs and the brain. Blood is not circulated evenly but is oversupplied in certain areas while others are impoverished. Arms seem partially paralyzed and are difficult to lift; neck muscles feel too short, rigid and stiff. All these symptoms indicate oversaturation of fluorine.

Coughing and Dry Catarrh are Symptomatic

Chronic overconsumption or overbalance of fluorine produces coughing at night, not in the daytime. Dry, sticky catarrh and phlegm congest the throat; voice sounds croupy. A patient may lose consciousness briefly. He breathes deeply but complains that it is impossible to get enough air. Sexual organs may harden; piles are inflexible and bleed. Urine decomposes after standing a few minutes; it contains excessive sediment of decomposed, whitish, muddled, foul-smelling material indicating tissue decay. Young mothers have a diminished flow of milk during lactation; the infant does not receive sufficient milk. Calcium function is disrupted, and the bony structure is adversely affected.

Innermost Body Parts Decay

The fluorine-excess patient suffers from an inflamed and enlarged splenic artery. Sudden death is possible. Gas is continually generated and gas pressure is noted on the left side as if under the heart. Palpitation may result. Caustic belching and an offensive, rotting odor from hair and breath indicate that the innermost body parts are decaying.

Fluorine Deficiency Not Uncommon

Fluorine hunger is a very real possibility with our highly refined, boiled, fried, baked diets. However, there is a second type of fluorine hunger characteristic of patients inheriting disease tendencies such as syphilitic pathogenesis. In these conditions, the fluorine balance is broken down until fluorine starvation is the result. Patients subject to inherited pathology are distinctive in appearance, physique and personality. If fluorine hunger is of a nutritional origin, the general appearance and temperament are unaffected. A certain pathology alters body chemistry and allows diseases to be transmitted to offspring. Any disease alters body chemistry and reaches chronic stages where it remains until the missing biochemical elements are supplied or the condition degenerates. Heredity-based fluorine deficiency indicates that patients have a pathogenic tendency in the blood and cells; patients with this trait are called "pargenic" types.

The Pargenic Type

The pargenic type is heavy with bloated cheeks, greasy or oily skin, thick neck, protruding lower abdomen, full axillary (armpit) expanse, weak and cracked lower lip, big chest, large lower back of head, gloomy disposition, brittle bones, large hips, heavy shoulders, large feet, swollen and red lower lip, wide head, heavy chin, greasy neck, thick lower eyelids, granulated eyelids, guarded and secretive temperament, large extremities. This type tends to be clumsy, inept, heavy, unwieldy, stupid. Moods are fixed and he may act sullen for weeks. Listening is difficult for him, but when his attention is secured, he is cynical, malevolent, acid and sarcastic. Pleasing people is never a trait; wishes of others are not considered. The pargenic type lives and acts according to his whims. His plans are kept secret; he distrusts people. He is never verbal about his beliefs, lifestyle, aspirations, inner conflicts, public confrontations, fears, disillusionments and emotions. Friends and acquaintances cannot determine the source of his moodiness. His temperament is solemn and melancholy; he ponders imaginary misfortunes. Ideas, plans, knowledge, thoughts often escape him; but he never loses sight of hates, animosity, fears, suspicions, false assumptions. Reasoning is strong, but the pargenic learns little from books. Things read and studied are cast aside, but reasoning is powerful for general principles. Mental effort is taxing, but reasoning ability once stirred is thorough; mental ability is strong but not easily accessible. This type is obtuse, eccentric and absent minded. The complexion ranges from fiery red to ashen; skin has a dirty cast, more so in hot weather. Pargenic types are plagued by inflamed complexion, warts, puffiness, patchy baldness, tubercles, fallen eyelashes and eyebrows, inflamed roots of nails, birttle and swollen bones, croupy throat, cracked and ridged nails, crooked legs, granulated eyelids, depression and chaotic habits. Hands are feverish, feet sore, face swollen and breathing difficult. Delusions of persecution haunt at times. One may think that police or detectives are in pursuit, perhaps that he is the victim of evil plots or demonic intentions. Darkness is frightening. His writing is sloppy and awkward. Typing, dentistry, piano-playing are not his talents. People are less interesting than nature and animals. The authenticity and credibility of others is doubted; human nature is considered evil in general and not worthy of trust.

Manifestations of Fluorine Deficiency

A patient manifesting fluorine hunger has difficulty rising in the morning; great effort is required to arouse the mental faculties and the physical body. His head feels dizzy; regrets are tormenting; memory is faulty and mind clouded. Hunger is absent in the morning, but by the afternoon, the fluorine patient is ravenous for food and drinks. Thirst is also absent in the morning, but the afternoon brings craving for liquids other than pure water. Fatty food is favored but often nauseating. The psychological sex drive is feverish. Nausea is so strong that the patient must often lie down (the magnesium-deficient patient, by contrast, craves motion which improves that condition). Any motion may bring nausea. In the daytime, the patient is cold; he is exceedingly cold—to the point of shivering—when in a warm bed at night.

Fluorine Lack Causes Worry and Indifference

Further ailments include a sense of oppression in the chest with difficulty breathing; morning deafness (not in afternoon); fatty or oily perspiration which is more profuse at night; failure to remember duties, promises, meetings,

engagements; indifference or aversion to wife, husband or children; greater preoccupation with strangers; worry apprehension and fearfulness; bravery and daring; self satisfaction; cantankerous moods; sense of weight in forehead; feeling of paralysis in brain; silent sorrow. All are indications of fluorine hunger.

Patient Subject to Nervous Stress

A distinction of the fluorine hunger patient is that he or she seems rational and, at the same time, exhibits idiosyncracies; intellectual reasoning is keen but disposition is variable. The patient may insist that voices of evil spirits are whispering in his ears. Romantic disappointments are almost unberable; mental distress is more severe than doctors and acquaintances detect. The patient may present shivers in brain and nerves; powerful headaches; nervous stress; fainting; nearly unconscious states; obtuse, unstable brain sensations that burn and jerk and are localized in epigastric plexus and stomach; increased energy during thunder and lightning storms. Head swells, tissues puff up. Vision may be double or distorted. Visions manifest in daylight.

Voices and Whispers Are Heard

The fluorine-hunger patient experiences many dreams of sexual activities. He may have unrealistic belief that he is ingenious, dexterous, adroit. Everything is preferred on a grand scale; subordinates are looked down on, as are superiors and employers. There is a tendency to become "clairvoyant" or "clairaudient" believing that voices and visions are advising on business and personal matters. The patient may insist that voices, whispers and sounds are involved when religion is considered. Religion may be viewed with terror and doctrines misinterpreted. Moods swing from ecstacy to deep despondency. At one time, valor and power are felt; at another, cowardice and weakness. Cursing may be resorted to. When eyes are closed there may be hallucinations—alligators, snakes, frogs, lizards, gutters, rivers, seas, devils, witches.

Patients Often Considered "Odd"

Observers note that the fluorine patient is awkward and vulgar; but the patient is convinced he is polished, dashing, graceful and irresistible to women. False confidence may foster wild speculation and unjustified investments. It may appear to others that this patient is mentally deranged. Some individuals either abhor God and religion or become religious maniacs; others suffer religious melancholia. At times obsession for riches, fame, power, command is great, sometimes almost insane. Men and women may seek marriage for financial gain. Men are crass, unpolished, rustic, rude, uncivil. Excessive sexual desire is evident; puberty comes early in girls and boys with hereditary syphilitic infection in blood and nervous system. Fluorine patients are often considered "odd" or peculiar. They may feel they have psychic premonitions of the future of the universe. Their voices are husky, faces red and feverish, and appetites gigantic. Heavy meals are indulged in and appetites are unrestrainable.

Disorganization Manifests

Other fluorine-deficiency symptoms may be noted. Speech is broken and stuttering likely; nerves, vocal cords, tongue and brain are not coordinated. Study, concentration, recall, memorizing are difficult. The brain may be feverish while the body is cold. Deception and treachery are attractive. Study brings on drowsiness. Insanity is feared; suicide is contemplated. Avid interest is cultivated in occult subjects (astrology, demonology, spiritualism, mysticism, magic, mediumship), weather, wind, pathology, etc. The patient is unable to keep track of possessions; desk is disorganized; belongings are in piles. Trances may be readily induced. Speech is poor with incorrect pronunciations, bad grammar and improper word usage. Reflexes are slow. Fumes and gases are disturbing; water and bathing are disliked. Irritation and inflammation of the cerebral meninges may intensify sexual, psychic and mystical powers, as may irritation of cranial bones and specific cephalic glands. Pus, acids, toxins have an irritating effect resulting in moodiness, strange activity and behavior.

Hair May Fall Out

In cases of fluorine poverty, the hair, spleen, corneal structures, nails, beard, glossy surface of structures, skin, rigid membranes, are adversely influenced. Hair may fall out. Spleen may become enlarged. Veins may become distended. There is a tendency toward diphtheria. There may be decay of teeth and bones; bone metabolism may be

unfinished. Conjunctiva may harden. Sclerosis manifests in brain tissue or arterial walls. Eyesight is weakened. Patient takes on an aged and wrinkled appearance. Solid parts are indurated. Tumors may grow in the liver, spleen, bones or skin. Kidney stones form. Parotid gland tumors develop. Calcifying tumors form in female organs. Tubules of the body develop hard nodules. Bladder may form calcium stones; calcium nodules may block mammary canals. Hard, fleshy tumors may appear on skin, gums. Sizable bone tumors may grow in vertebral bones; outer skull may develop bony growths. Growths may appear in the ears and reduce hearing ability. Calcification may begin in or around cerebellar areas damaging the coordination and culminating in irreversible paralysis.

Tissues May Harden

There is danger of sclerosis in the body; tissues may develop hyperplasia. Prostate may shrink, harden and diminish in function; sterility is a possibility. Meninges of brain may harden and irreparable insanity result. Dura mater may harden and cause complications. Larynx may develop neoplasm; voice may take on a rasping and hoarse quality because throat tissue is damaged.

Total Fluorine Depletion Results in Abnormalities

In the event fluorine is utterly depleted, the consequences are serious. Atrophy of cells manifests. Bone marrow function is unfavorably changed by alterations in periosteal and osseous structures; these changes impede red blood cell production (erythrocytogenesis). Other complications in the pargenic patient are nervous system degeneration, mesenteric degeneration, scrofulous lymphatic degeneration, pulmonary tuberculosis, atheroma, hardening of the endocardium, locomotor ataxia (because posterior columns of spinal cord become sclerotic), club foot and other prenatal deformities caused by alteration of bone function and tissue structure. The fluorine-starved patient may be characterized by unsightly nails, ingrowing toenails, deformed fingertips, onychia, malformed teeth, osteoma, osteomalacia, deterioration in solid structures, altered or paranormal ossature of bony frame. Broken bones may set incorrectly and grow crooked or poorly. Bone metabolism is altered. Enchondroma in bone cartilage, bone caries, bone granulation, bulb-shaped joint swellings, curvature of bones,

171

curvature of spine, abnormal growth, sarcoma, osteosclerosis, osteosarcoma; nonhealing bone fractures, malignant caries in bone joints, pulsating bone tumors, osseous skin formation, hardening glands, osteides in pulp cavities of teeth, faulty formation of bone cement, ossified organ coverings, bone separation, gouty eyes, carcinoma of the eyes, deterioration of eye tissue, bone disintegration, scaly eyebrows and baldness are all indications of total fluorine depletion.

Expectant Mothers Need Fluorine

The abnormalities continue: bulging eyeballs, psoriasis, alopecia, distorted pelvic bones, degenerating retina, thickening and distension of uterus or cervical glands, mutation in bone formation, corneal degeneration, mucus production in throat tissue, decubitus with cerebral lesions, tuberculosis, other disorders of joints and bony frame, venous and arterial sclerosis. If the expectant mother lacks fluorine, there is grave danger of a deformed infant.

Lack of Fluorine Means Fragile Bones

Fluorine is likened to cement for ceramic tiles. It cements the body's bony structures together and prevents decay deterioration, crumbing or rotting. Bones demand fluorine for strength, durability, elasticity. A glossy, tough tooth enamel is dependent upon a liberal fluorine reserve in the body. Lack of fluorine reserve means brittle, fragile bones. Vaccinations and syphilis are formidable foes of fluorine; they are responsible for breaking down the fluorine supply in the body. As a result, bone and teeth abnormalities manifest.

Fluorine Deficiency Results in Eye Problems

The pargenic, fluorine-deficient patient may exhibit pus diathesis, ulcerations, suppuration and other degenerative processes from birth to death because of hereditary pathology. However, the malnutrition-based fluorine starvation may also manifest suppurative (pus formation) and deteriorative processes. Common conditions observed in fluorine deficiency patients, especially pargenic types, include the following: membranous ruptures, dilation of blood vessels, suppuration in organs, varicose veins, skin ulcers that fail to heal, inflammation of nail roots, deterioration of jaw bones, degeneration in mastoid function, abscesses,

decomposition, liver enlargement, swelling (of spleen, lungs, skull, brain, nails, bones, skin areas) without apparent cause, numerous bunions, calcium deposited in tumors or tubercles, chronic bone pathologies, bone necrosis, bone gangrene, callus, faulty bones and teeth, bone inflammation, watery obesity, bone inflammation, pulsating bone tumors, osseous bone tumors in the brain, osseous cysts, bone ulcers, eyebrow inflammation, swollen eyeballs, ocular muscle paralysis, total blindness, predisposition to parasitic eye diseases, eye discharges, chronic bone aches, renal calculi, nephritic colic, chronic pyelitis from calculi, more serious illnesses from aneurysms (dilation of arterial wall), chronic vesicle catarrh.

Predisposition to Pus Development and Catarrh

Fluorine-deficient patients may have mucus and ammonia in the urine with low specific gravity of urine or blood. Organic heart disease is evident in some. Renal edema, uremia, cardia, otitis, osteoporosis, venous swelling, phlebolithiasis, venous ruptures and hemorrhages occur in such patients. All manifest deterioration, suppuration and ulcerative conditions. A high fluorine diet is necessary in the following conditions, as well: venous stenosis, prostate catarrh, osteophlebitis, dry eczema, scalp sores with odorous discharge, chronic catarrh of nasal bones, cracked wings of nostrils, petechia, ankylosis, tooth ulceration, spleen congestion, sexual organ deterioration, waxy degeneration of various parts, chronic cough during winter but not during warm weather, episodic arthritis that debilitates, predisposition to intertrigo, lachrymal fistula, degeneration and suppuration in various parts of the body.

Three to Twenty Years Necessary to Correct Fluorine Starvation

Other idiosyncracies of fluorine-deficiency patients are urethral catarrh, bilious diarrhea, chronic bone rheumatism identified by numbness. Venous stasis, pleural degeneration, swelling and enlargements in various locations, nose hemorrhages, head and pulmonary congestion, boils, eye catarrh with inflammation, chronic finger neuritis, discharging ulcers, stiffness and pain in joints preceding a storm, knee swelling, itching vesicles discharging yellow pus, bloating, morning sluggishness, motion sickness, ravenous appetite at times, greasy perspiration, chronic laryngitis or bronchitis, throat ulceration, large styes, joint dislocation, danger of injury from minor falls or blows, distorted vision that can develop into total blindness—all such symptoms denote fluorine famine. The fluorine patient develops chronic ailments as the fluorine starvation progresses, and these afflictions are numerous. A form of epilepsy related to fluorine hunger is a possibility. Three to twenty years are required to correct the conditions resulting from fluorine starvation, especially in pargenic patients.

"No patient will exhibit all of the symptoms and diseases at one time. When a few basic symptoms are identified, the fluorine case is no longer an enigma."

Sexual Problems Occur

Oxygenation is faulty in fluorine-hunger patients, as is combustion. Impurities, pus, toxins, germs are at work undermining the health and constitution. Pus and toxins promote diseased function in many body systems. Such disease processes can affect the reproductive organs and sexual centers in the brain. The result may be sexual deviance including nymphomania, overt sensuality, hallucinations, satyriasis and excessive sexual preoccupation. The mental faculty controlling the sex impulse is weakened. The reproductive instinct is corrupted, and polygamous tendencies may be followed.

Female Fluorine-Deficiency Disorders

A female patient lacking fluorine may develop vaginitis, bilious nausea with exhaustion, faucitis, breast swelling (lactiferous), lactic retention facilitated by induration and pus formation, yellow discharges, abnormal metabolism of solid tissue, hydrocele, induration of reproductive organs culminating in sterility, severe mental distress and anguish that remains unknown to others (the fluorine patient is close mouthed, reticent, suspicious), leg cramps, trance states, disturbed equilibrium, motion sickness, susceptibility to sunstroke and heat stroke from ordinary exposure,

poor nervous system nutrition leading to nervous breakdown or depletion. Other disorders of fluorine-deficient women are ovaritis; chronic catarrh in the pelvic bones; cranial pains with acute sensitivity to pressure; sclerosis (hardening) of the liver, ovaries or uterus; frequent menses; sweating in cold air; chronic salivation; melancholia and depression; disturbance by pain, aches and distress at night; perspiration on one side; sandy urinary calculi; eye disturbances such as conjunctivitis, neuralgia, opthalmia, eye catarrh (especially in the pargenic type); retention of urine; scanty urination with severe pains that make limbs feel as if they will explode; nearly unbearable headache or uterine pains.

Prolapsus May Occur

In both men and women there may be calcification in skull bones or vertebral bones (even at an early age). Other fluorine-deficiency symptoms include the following: aches worsening with motion and diminishing when pressure is applied; prolapsus of transverse colon; uterine, anal and rectal prolapsus; study of mysticism; belief in mysterious treatments; faith in miracles; craving for common tea; priapism in males; spinal fluid inflammation caused by infiltration of suppurative process from vertebrae or spinal meninges.

Hallucinations and Delusions

The gamut of symptoms varies and manifests at various times in the patient's life—some transient, some elemental and fixed. No patient will exhibit all of the symptoms and diseases at one time. When a few basic symptoms are identified, the fluorine case is no longer an enigma. A patient may develop all the symptoms, along with thousands of others, during a lifetime; but each individual is different. Vital elemental symptoms are as follows: a sluggish brain; difficulty in beginning thought processes; great energy for general mental activities or for study, once thought processes are functioning; fantasies of sexual scenes; premature sexual impulse in adolescence; terror of insanity; voracious appetite; eyelids appearing granular, gluey, puffed, red and inflamed; imaginary voices believed to be real; hallucinations and delusions; paranoia; intolerable aches and pains; skin pigment dirty, greasy, oily, puffy and yellowish when cold, warm or moist; morning depression and sorrow; difficulty in awakening in morning or starting brain function;

clumsy action and movement; tactless and blunt speech; parts of body puffed or swollen—especially head, neck, skin, flesh of chest, lower abdomen, skin of forehead, thighs; backward, illiterate behavior; extraordinary errors in speech, writing, conversation, pronounciation or word usage; bones fracturing easily from minor blows, falls or accidents; retarded healing of fractures; loose, sore, soft gums; saliva dribbling from mouth when patient talks, sings or whistles; brain and nerves feverish and body chilled; body odor of decay and rotting; ulcerating bones; sensuality; objects seeming to move away when patient fixes his gaze for a short time; intense sensitivity to pressure of heat in torrid weather; intense cerebellar throbbing with inflammation in hot weather; susceptibility to harmful effects of innoculations; tooth decay in childhood; matted hair; scurfy scalp; extreme detestation of nightfall aggravated by superstitious fears.

More Indications of Fluorine Lack

Further indications of deficiency of fluorine include aching eyeballs; momentary blindness from stooping; dense yellow discharges; exhaustion in hot weather or during great exertion; catarrhal eyelids; sticky eyelids and greasy emission from skin on head, face and neck; bilious or nervous episodes brought on by drinking cold water; itch following bathing or perspiration with intensification of symptoms; bunions, ingrown toenails; agitated feeling after sleep; disorders of nails, eyelashes, eyebrows; a yellowish, slimy coating of the tongue; moles and brownish amber spots on the skin; nails growing upward; itching vesicles filled with yellow pus; distress caused by cold compresses; hair, whiskers, eyebrows and eyelashes angling or curving in or out; corners of eyes oozing pus-like material; bloating of lips, head, limbs; eyes bloated in the morning; decayed, rotten taste in mouth; chilly feeling under eyelids; oppressed, labored, deep breathing; anesthesia in hands; red, enlarged nose tip; bulging eyeballs; vile sputum; gums bleeding easily; intensification of thirst as day progresses, but agitation if icy drinks are taken; extraordinary terror of extreme heat and cold; chaotic mind; sore corns and scars; clammy, fetid sweating of feet or other parts; sickly, yellowish complexion with mucus tubercles and eruptions of pus; fits of sneezing; diminished hearing, sight, smell and taste; darker-than-usual blood due to faulty combustion in brain and bones; hair falling out in clumps;

hallucinations caused by irritation; interpenetration or ulceration of the brain peduncles, pineal gland, pituitary gland, tentorium cerebelli, venous sinuses of brain and pericranium, cerebral and spinal meninges. Patients lacking fluorine tend to dispute the doctor when questioned regarding symptoms and illness; they feel that everyone is unworthy of trust.

More Subtle Symptoms of Fluorine Starvation

Other fluorine starvation symptoms are subtle and transient. Energy feels restrained or restricted; moods alternate between joyful and dejected, glad and sad or depressed. There may be consuming interest in psychic phenomena, magic, mysticism, ESP (extra sensory perception). Milk is disagreeable or brings on bilious symptoms or semi nausea. Eyes and vision are defective. Legs cramp. Teeth are irregular. Patient may experience fainting episodes with occasional unconsciousness. Equilibrium may be unsteady. Sleep fails to refresh. There may be craving for common tea, susceptibility to effects of syphilis or vaccinations, syphilitic and vasicular disorders. Boils and corns are numerous and painful. Pulse rate is low. Voice has nasal, tremorous, hoarse quality. Odors, fumes and gases are detected easily. Rumbling sound in intestines is caused by generation of gases. Patient feels loathing for life in general and, especially for bosses. Urine is hot, rusty, vile; urination is painful. Underside of nails thicken. Patient feels that the body is only an empty vessel. Wine, coffee, fatty foods are desired. Fatty, salty, sweet, oily, milky, creamy foods produce nausea, but they are craved. Blood congestion occurs in the base of brain and in the forehead. Pains in mastoid areas are accompanied by aggravated itching of ears. Nose develops crusty deposits; tongue becomes fissured; muscles become stiff; tongue is feverish; hands become chapped and painful; legs, feet and thighs are fatigued; veins are congested; fingers, arms and neck muscles seem stiff and partially deadened. Fatty foods produce hiccoughs. Sundown brings feelings of fatigue with greater generation of catarrh and phlegm. Throat and stomach yield obtuse, tremorous, jerky, heated, putrid sensations. Fluorine-deficient patients may also exhibit a tendency toward chronic throat ailments; hip bone complications; mental pictures when darkness falls or eyes are closed; burning sensations in specific small patches of skin;

spermatorrhea during sleep; predisposition to quarrels, to opposition, denial and scepticism of others' statements; melancholy personality; cynical temperament; secretiveness about plans; undue familiarity with opposite sex.

Treatment Involves Fluorine-Rich Diet

The above symptoms indicate fluorine starvation. In these conditions, a diet rich in fluorine foods is essential.

▬HIGHEST FLUORINE FOODS▬

Most diets are relatively fluorine-free because any cooking destroys fluorine. The best sources of fluorine are raw goat milk and raw green quince. Fluorine is also present in good quantities in sea plants, sea water and raw fish. It is found in measurable quantities in the following:

Avocados	Goat whey
Blackeyed peas	Greens
Brussels sprouts	Juniper berries
Cabbage	Lemon grass
Caraway seed	Licorice
Cauliflower	Mother's milk
Cheese (raw)	New Zealand spinach
Dates	Parsley
Egg yolk, raw	Rice polishings
Endive	Rye bran or meal
Garlic	Sea cabbage
Goat butter (raw)	Sea lettuce
Goat buttermilk (raw)	Spinach
Goat cream (raw)	Tomatoes

FLUORINE MENUS

Goat cottage cheese; salad made of endive, parsley, sea lettuce, sprouted blackeyed peas, greens; garlic and roquefort dressing; goat buttermilk.

Veal joint broth simmered slowly; home-smoked fish marinated in garlic and lemon juice; salad of avocado, endive, parsley, tomatoes, sprouted French kidney beans, chervil and greens; dressing made of egg yolks, caraway seeds, goat sour cream and homemade mayonnaise; raw quince juice sweetened with honey.

Steamed rye topped with raw goat butter, caraway seed meal, rice polishings and rye bran, dates, avocado wedges, goat cream; raw egg yolk in black cherry juice.

Assorted raw cheese sticks (goat and cow cheese); cole slaw; steamed brussels sprouts; steamed spinach; sliced tomatoes; avocado wedges, cauliflowerettes on bed of greens and parsley; goat butter; homemade egg mayonnaise seasoned with dried sea vegetation; juniper berry tea (steeped).

175

SUMMARY OF FLUORINE

GENERAL CHARACTERISTICS

"Resistant" element   Combines readily with calcium
Does not combine with oxygen   No fluorine type

FLUORINE IN THE HUMAN BODY

Found in blood and joints   Protects from germs and infection
Acts upon spleen, tooth enamel,   Prevents decay, softening, ulcers
bones, skin, hair, nails, tendons,   Preserves youthfulness
iris

SIGNS OF FLUORINE EXCESS

Fluorine excess rare   Circulation out of balance
Extreme sensuality   Irritated membranes, linings
Obese, coarse appearance   Fearfulness, worry
Pessimism in evening   Hallucinations
Predisposition to ulcers   Bone decay and cavities
Motion discomfort   Cough and dry catarrh

SIGNS OF FLUORINE DEFICIENCY

Difficulty thinking   Swollen, granular eyelids
Hallucinations   Skin clammy, puffy or scaly
Sadness in morning   Indifference or worry
Crumbling teeth and bones   Nervous stress
Disorganization   Falling hair
Slow healing of fractures   Fondess for fatty foods
Partial or total blindness   Catarrh and pus development

HIGHEST FLUORINE FOODS

Raw goat milk   Sea plants
Raw green quince   Raw fish

Americans lose 56 million teeth every year, and 40% have a minimum of 18 fillings, cavities or missing teeth.

---

five

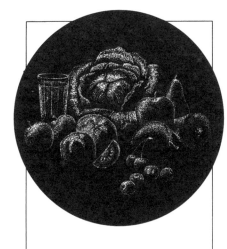

Hydrogen, the "moisturizer"

Without hydrogen, the blood could not flow, nor could waste be washed out of the body, and we would then die in our own impurity. Hydrogen is abundantly present in the secretions, excretions, soft tissue, blood, serum, lymph, brain, lungs, glands, liver, kidneys, spleen, pancreas and muscles. It prevents inflammation, promotes osmosis and moistens lung surfaces for gas diffusion. As a solvent, it helps to regulate body temperature and irrigates the cells and organs.

Excess of Hydrogen

Dr. Rocine called the person who attracts and holds water the hydripheric person. Water is made up, partly, of hydrogen, the "moisturizer." The hydripheric person can gather moisture from the air. I have seen hydripheric types take a sweat or steam bath and gain five pounds, whereas ordinarily these procedures would help a patient lose weight. An excess of water in the body causes pressure and enlargement of all surrounding organs, resulting in disease.

The hydrogen or hydropheric type is characterized by a couple of signs that I watch very carefully. Sometimes the ankles appear heavy and swollen, and sometimes the palms of the hands at the base of the fingers show puffiness. Obesity is also a problem. At one time, we had a patient who told us she had gained and lost nearly 5,000 pounds during her life. Through efforts to eliminate the water from her system, she lost weight, but began to regain it as soon as she started eating, especially watery foods. She was continually on a diet.

In iridology, we call this type lymphatic, noting that these people have sluggish tissues because of the heavy amount of water they contain. Tissue response is subnormal because it is boggy, flabby and bulky. Blood is not circulated properly and metabolism is low. The urine is light-colored and odorless.

The temperamental characteristics of the hydripheric type are the even, flowing, mellow qualities of water itself. Actions are in moderation rather than to extremes. This type can be romantic and soulful and very

Hydrogen is the lightest element in the Periodic Table of Chemical Elements, a gas in its natural state and a partner with oxygen in the commonest liquid on the planet. It is highly explosive in its gaseous form, is valuable as a rocket fuel and has been used to make the most powerful weapon known to man—the hydrogen bomb. Hydrogen is present in our drinking water, in all fruit and vegetable juices and in all three basic types of food—protein, starch and fat.

The natural potato is 100% potato. The packaged potato may contain potato flakes, natural and artificial flavors, sodium bisulfates, ascorbic acid, calcium stearoly-2-lactylate, BHA, BHT, monoglycerides and several other chemicals.

slow to anger. On the other hand, this person cannot keep up with many active people due to sluggishness.

Possibilities for Cures

One of the problems in helping hydripheric patients through diet and nutrition is that we tend to recommend the vegetable and fruit kingdoms, but this person gains weight on these watery foods. Thus, we recommend more solid foods, particularly protein, the fiery element. Fire elements help burn up excess water. Iodine, too, is helpful in burning up excess water by raising the metabolic rates of the body.

Taking 10 or 12 dulse tablets daily can help raise metabolism. Fish, a good iodine source, is excellent protein for the hydripheric type.

Corrective exercises are great for the hydripheric type because they help raise body temperature which, in turn, helps to eliminate water through perspiration. Living in an arid climate would certainly help to burn up excessive moisture and keep weight down.

The hydripheric must understand, however, that water retention is an inherent quality in him or her, *inherited from peoperties of the mother and/or father. In one generation, it is difficult to change such tendencies. The hydripheric type should strive to keep water retention under control and accept never being able to attain thinness. We all must accept the inborn qualities of our bodies.*

"Unless we eat food properly prepared, we suffer from inferior physical development, mental instability, low endurance and lack of resistance to infection."

—Dr. E. V. McCollum
Johns Hopkins Hospital
Baltimore, MD

'The average housewife peels her vegetables, thus throwing away the part directly under the skin containing the most plentiful amount of mineral salts; then the remaining portion is boiled and the water which has also dissolved out more minerals, is thrown away."

—Dr. Charles H. Mayo

"Out of four thousand cases recently examined in a New York hospital, only two were not suffering from a lack of calcium."
—Journal of the American Medical Association

"The new method now much used, of cooking foods in closed vessels without adding water, preserves the minerals and most of the vitamins."
—Dr. Herman H. Bundesen, former chairman,
Chicago Board of Health

HYDROGEN
"The Moisturizer"

GENERAL CHARACTERISTICS

The word hydrogen means "water generator" or "water producer." This nonpoisonous, gaseous element is colorless, odorless and tasteless. Its most common compound is water, H_2O. Hydrogen is nature's lightest element, with an atomic weight of one (1.0); its light weight makes it the standard of atomic weight and volume for the chemist. The specific gravity of hydrogen is 0.069. In combination with nitrogen, carbon and oxygen, hydrogen creates many vital organic compounds; by itself, hydrogen does not support life. Under ideal conditions, combined hydrogen and oxygen produce great heat. Tremendous potential energy sleeps within hydrogen. If conditions are right, it explodes or vibrates powerfully. It is the agent responsible for boiler explosions, clouds, soil fertilizing, steamship power and the cooling of the atmosphere.

Ubiquitous Hydrogen

Hydrogen is present in almost all living things. It is found in animal and vegetable tissues and even in minerals. It is the moisturizer or (in combination with oxygen) water element of vegetable, animal and human life. It is able to permeate or filter through matter and to rise or descend to an amazing degree. Its properties of inflammability, explosiveness, expansion and diffusion are greater than those of any other element. It enters and penetrates vegetable fibers, animal organs, human tissue, stone walls, mortar or cement with almost magical ease.

Hydrogen Characteristics

Hydrogen goes about its work silently, calmly. But like carbon, it is a creator, in soil, rock, vegetation, trees, brain and heart. It is characteristically silent, mysterious, passive, inert, sleepy, secretive. Water, that most common hydrogen compound, is cooling and soothing.

Although water, which is actually a food, is only 11% hydrogen; certain foods, called water-carrying foods, contain a relatively high percentage of hydrogen. For example, pears are 83% water (or 9% hydrogen); watermelon is 93%, pumpkin 97%, celery 95%, lettuce up to 97%, nuts from 2% to 53%, cheese from 20% to 77% water.

HYDROGEN: ITS ROLE IN THE HUMAN BODY

A man weighing 160 pounds has in his body about 15 pounds of hydrogen, the greatest amounts being in the lymphatic glands, liver, blood, kidneys, spleen, pancreas, bladder, secretions, excretions, evaporative matter and perspiration. Hydrogen is essential for the processes of digestion, nutrition, assimilation, elimination. It is vital for transporting nutrients through the arteries to the brain and tissues of all parts of the body. Numerous biochemic processes depend upon hydrogen; it prevents centralized inflammation, guards life, enhances osmosis, moistens lung surfaces for gas dispersion. It promotes consistency of vital tissues and aids in regulation of body temperature. Water and oil (hydrogen compounds) support communication between cells, organs, parts and faculties. Hydrogen, water, moisture and vapors are found even in the brain and in bone and solid material.

Hydrogen Soothes the Nerves

Hydrogen has a soothing, softening effect upon the body, mind and soul. By itself it cannot support life, yet without it, life cannot exist. Hydrogen (water) is essential in nerve matter, the sexual system and all body constituents. Nerve matter must have moisture for proper function. A moist, slightly alkaline medium makes for the most efficient nerve performance. (Nerve aches are due to acidity.) Lack of moisture (water) in the body causes erratic nerve functions and brain activity. Arid atmospheric heat is damaging to nerves and irritating to the brain convolutions. Deficiency of water in the body results in restless nerves; dry air precipitates body heat more rapidly by evaporation and radiation, resulting in water deficiency. On the other hand, a humid, sultry, moist atmosphere contributes to an internal accumulation of heat, which facilitates an aversion to muscular and nervous activity; energy decreases and fatigue increases.

Facts About Water Intake

The solvent ability of water is increased by heat. Warm water quenches thirst better than does cold; cold water quickens the nerves in the stomach and vitalizes the brain. To promote health, water must be thoroughly oxidized; thus even distilled water should be aerated well. The more heat is generated in and by the body, the more moisture is required to maintain the proper body temperature; hydrogen moisture is essential for regulation, especially inasmuch as greater heat generation predisposes one to impulsive behavior.

Importance of Water in the Body

Each organ of the body needs a watery medium. Cells, notably nerve cells, must be immersed in water; water is the avenue of dispersion. Blood flow and transport of nourishment depend upon water. When water is deficient in the body, centralization of heat and congestion are possible. Perspiration bathes the body during physical exertion; discontinuation of heat generation results in a cold,

clammy skin surface. In the event that congestion and acidity invade the body, exercise is crucial to the elimination of such substances.

Elimination of Water

Under normal conditions, 500 to 700 grams of water are expelled from the body of an adult male in 24 hours. Atmospheric temperature regulates the amount of water expelled through the lungs. An arid climate requires more water, as does heavy labor; in fact, all activities, physical or mental, require moisture to one degree or another. Chlorine precipitates great quantities of water, as does a dry, salty diet or a fever. Water is removed by the lungs, skin, kidneys due to evaporation and perspiration. A dry nitrogen diet also uses large quantities of water. When kidney elimination increases, especially during the winter, perspiration and evaporation decrease. A deficiency of water anywhere in the system, but especially in the bowel, results in constipation; oversupply of moisture causes increased bowel activity. Consequently, a dry, cold climate produces more constipation, while a hot, humid climate facilitates more diarrhea. Constipation sufferers benefit from an ocean voyage.

Uses of Water

Contrary to popular assumption, cold water does not reduce body temperature; hot water does, by converting heat into perspiration. Cold water reduces the pulse rate and increases arterial tension. Moderate quantities of hot or cold water augment peristaltic action. Cold water remains in the stomach longer than does hot water, which passes rapidly through. Cold water should not be consumed with a meal because it slows digestion; it does, however, increase the secretion of digestive juices, even more than does hot water. Urine flow is increased by cold water, whereas hot water reduces it but increases perspiration and evaporation. Cold water consumption increases fat oxidation in warm-blooded, stout people, but not in thin people; hot water reduces fat metabolism and leads eventually to leanness. Hot water drinking in sultry, humid weather raises body temperature while cold water reduces it. Cold water is craved in times of fever. Diabetic patients are benefitted by hot water. Hot water consumption reduces weight in a hearty, active, vital patient who has active kidneys. Hot water, providing it is no more than three ounces, drunk during a meal, aids digestion. Large quantities of water consumed at one time overstrain the muscles of the digestive tract.

Distilled Water

Distilled water is beneficial in times of gout, rheumatism or arthritis. It helps dissolve deposits in joints, remove gases, toxins and inorganic minerals foreign to the body. Warm distilled water is preferable to cold. Considerable quantities of distilled water increase urination, helping to remove acids, toxins and other harmful products.

Water Involved in Many Bodily Functions

A large quantity of water in the body raises the level of watery plasma and quickens activity of circulation if absorbed; it encourages elimination of toxins and waste products from normal metabolic functions. Water makes urea more copious and increases bile flow. If hydrogen moisture is liberally supplied to the body, pancreatic secretions are increased; parotid gland secretion is increased; perspiration and evaporation are increased; mineral salts superfluous to the system are washed away; harmful gases are removed. Water bathes tissues and removes inorganic metallic poisons. Nerves and involuntary muscles are soothed by the action of water. Sex desire, but not sexual prowess, is heightened by water. The physical senses, especially hearing, smell and touch, are enhanced by water. The soul is content, the mind calm, the personality soothed by moisture in brain convolutions and nerve cells. Nerve impulses are more efficiently transferred by water. However, an overabundance of water or lymph fluid can lead to edema and disturbed tissue functions. If the quantity of water is too low, lymph function and nerves are disturbed; moisture improves lymphogenesis and cell diffusion. Osmotic pressure, secretion, respiratory pressure, cell vibration, tissue functions, blood flow, cell filtration and reproduction are all favored by water. A liberal supply of moisture increases perspiration and makes taste buds more acute. It aids in regulation of gas pressure in the blood and in the body in general. Certain areas of the skin become more sensitive to the touch. Each drop of blood, lymph fluid, each cell of nerve, bone, muscle, tissue, must have water (hydrogen moisture). Body processes are disrupted when the water balance is distorted (too high or too low). Hydrogen must be properly absorbed and utilized by the body for normal metabolism. A Hydripheric type may be developed if too much water is absorbed, consumed or utilized by a patient; this causes misery, bloated feelings, slowed action.

SIGNS OF HYDROGEN EXCESS

The Hydripheric Type

Because a considerable amount of hydrogen in the body soothes nerves, emotions, mind and temperament, the Hydripheric type is even-tempered, calm, easygoing, tender in action, liberal, condescending, merciful, forgiving, understanding, compassionate, polite, gentle toward people and animals or objects. A Hydripheric judge is more lenient; a Hydripheric doctor is not inclined toward surgery and harsh drugs; a Hydripheric dentist lessens pain for his patients. This type is lymphatic, slow moving, perhaps indolent and adverse to strenuous physical labor or altercations and quarrels. However, the Hydripheric person is a sleeping giant; powerful energy lies slumbering just below the surface.

The personality of the hydrogen type resembles the element and water. Such a person is at home in water or near it; he absorbs water directly from the air; he may become a watery mass of flesh. His dietary habits are pronounced. He prefers juicy dishes, mild drinks, juicy vegetables and meats, tasty liquid dishes; solid food is not favored; delicate flavors are appreciated as are pleasing aromas; bread is broken into small pieces and often consumed in soups.

Hydripheric's Senses are Keen

The senses of the Hydripheric individual are highly attuned. Odors, pleasant or unpleasant, are easily detected. Atmospheric changes are readily detected; an approaching storm is easily anticipated. Bathing and swimming are enjoyed. The study of gases, hydrology, drug concocting, oceanography are commonly pursued by this type. Because the fall season does not provide sufficient oxygen for his tissues and blood, he may develop illnesses at this time; the hills and mountains are beneficial in autumn. A Hydripheric man is attracted to a slender, lithe, flexible-bodied girl.

The Hydripheric Female

The hydrogen woman is characterized by a love of beautiful vegetation and delicate trees, gurgling brooks, calm oceans, tender lovers and doctors, peacefulness, gentle treatment. Her mental faculties are etheric and hazy, as are her soul and spirit. Her complexion is pale, delicate and watery. Emotions and thoughts are often difficult for her to express; her feelings are an enigma, hidden from the observer. On the surface she is cold and remote, but at the same time romantic, unspoiled, yielding, innocent, nearly etheric, soulful. She possesses a mystique that fascinates men, as in the legends of the mermaid.

Hydripheric Woman is Imaginative

This woman cries and suffers in secret, refusing to let her emotions show. Her imagination is vividly at work on soul, mind, emotions. She has few friends besides her husband, lover, children or God. The world is awe inspiring and mysterious to her because of her dreamy, abstract, fantasizing, romantic, apprehensive nature. External factors are very influential; intimidation ruffles her easily. Morning labor is dreaded but once begun, is continued; she prefers to sit like a statue all day doing embroidery or needlepoint. She recalls recent events with difficulty but remembers happenings of the distant past. She mothers her children, plants, animals, trees with great tenderness; thus her children are well tended and healthy.

She is Concerned with the Trivial

The Hydripheric female is plagued by trivial happenings but almost unscathed by major misfortunes. Disappointments cannot be forgotten or forgiven. Her husband's voiced opinion can cut her like a knife if derogatory; what other men say about her has little bearing; her husband or lover's kindness is essential. She prefers the home and hearth to outdoor excursions or travel. She is subject to accidents when away from home. Her love can become possessively jealous at times. In youth her skin is rosy and attractively delicate; in later life it is ravaged by illness; pinches leave angry black and blue marks; sores heal slowly and scars remain visible. Hot summer weather produces an oxygen deficiency, as does the autumn; during these seasons she is benefitted by the hills and mountains.

Her Sense of Smell is Unfailing

The Hydripheric homemaker is an excellent cook, a critical judge of food quality. Her dishes are a delight to the gourmet diner. Her sense of smell is unfailing in her cooking and food selection. She is fastidious, washing her hands a hundred times daily and rinsing each dish or glass before using. Her olfactory sense can detect odors such as gases, fumes, hospital smells, foreigners, tobacco, alcohol, factories, food establishments, drugs, foods—which are barely evident to others.

Symptoms of Hydrogen Excess

Symptoms of excess hydrogen in the system are distinctive. Hydric obesity is the most obvious manifestation; the system is waterlogged and weakened. Symptoms may be described as cystic, herpatic, neurotic, edemic, anemic, hydremic. Illnesses are transient and periodic and exhaustive in nature, but rarely chronic. Enlargement of some vital organ is likely, as are cyst formation and malnutrition in membranes, facilitating atrophy. The patient is susceptible to lymphatic obesity, ruptures, hemorrhages, muscular atrophy, sores, hydric dyspnea, heart murmur, watery asthma, enlargement of spleen, glands, liver, kidneys, extremities or colon; heart palpitation due to fevered chest brain (medulla); protrusion of eyes and eyeballs, chest oppression, lymphatism, sudden diarrhea, organic heart complications, high arterial tension; mucus and epithelial cells in urine, indicative of destructive alterations in the solid tissues. Hemoglobin, fibrin, albumin and leucocytes are often subnormal.

Inflammation, Tenderness and Pain

Patients who overconsume hydrogen are subject to pressing pains in the groin area, nerve stitches and general body aches; to inflammatory skin patches, membranous vesicles, creeping eruptions, herpetic ailments, gastrointestinal malfunctions, angioneurotic edema. Vertebrae of the neck and shoulders are often tender, painful, maybe from cold or congestive fever and pain. Contracting pains in spine, genital contractions, drawing in groin and hip areas or lower extremities, rectal pain and descending colon pain during defecation, scraping sensations, chest cramps, stitches of pain in other parts of the body are all common complaints.

The Heart is Affected

The heart region may manifest explosive pains, as may the chest and upper shoulder areas. There may be swelling of fingers; stinging pains between shoulders, in brachial plexus region or armpits, may cause arm convulsions or nerve twitches; momentary inflammation of brachial plexus nerve matter and spinal ganglia may cause neurotic tendencies. Other symptoms include heavy extremities; high blood pressure; feeble pulse in evening; hoarse voice late in the day; suffocating symptoms upon dropping to sleep; slimy stools; diarrhea followed by cold sweats; faint spells; tumors in iliac fossa; water discharges; urethral aches; itching; painful piles due to lack of tissue salts; smarting pain in pelvic area upon stretching or raising the arms or pressing them downward; involuntary discharges; lassitude.

Disease Tendencies in Hydrogen Type (Hydripheric)

The Hydripheric type is subject to measles, scarlet fever, scarlatina, periodic fevers, circulatory weakness, spreading skin blisters, excessively hot or cold hands, rectal protrusion, fainting spells, abdominal colic, uterine and ovarian cramps, fauces catarrh, vomiting, coughing, throat catarrh and biliousness during oppressive weather. Other possibilities are comatose states of mind, cataleptic day trance, acid perspiration that discolors clothing with yellowish stains, wheezing asthma, flabby muscles, digestive disturbances during childhood dentation, late teething, complications in mesentery glands, hyperactivity of lacteals with attending inflammation and irritation.

Sluggish Metabolism in Hydrogen Type (Hydripheric)

Metabolism is abnormal in the hydrogen type due to excessive tissue moisture. The brain may become sluggish in volitive, motor, executive and intellectual capacities. Hydripheric students have difficulty studying diligently, especially in the areas of science and mathematics, profound reasoning, quick thinking. If any faculty is weak or vital force low, the nutrients that contribute to vitality are not properly assimilated and appropriated. Thus organic complications arise easily.

Appearance is Deceptive

This patient appears healthy and robust but is in actuality ill and lacking in vitality. Resistive and recuperative powers are low. Glands, arteries, veins, membranes break easily, resulting in ruptures and hemorrhages. The superfluous amount of hydrogen in the body makes the assimilation of valuable tissue salts difficult; blood is poor; liver and sensory department are often feverish when heat is lacking in other parts of the body; internal heat may be accompanied by outer chills due to internal fever of nerves and liver; nerve force is deficient, notably in motor nerves.

Constitutional Weaknesses of Hydrogen Type (Hydripheric)

The general constitution of this type is weak. The muscles, cords, tendons, muscular fibers of membranes, arterial and venous walls, canal walls and other fibrous structures are weak; tissues are highly sensitive, joints weak; afflictions of wrists, neck, knees, ankles or joints are common; heart is weak; anemic convulsions due to anemia of chest brain (medulla) and cerebellum can cause sudden heart failure; inability to control eye muscles may arise due to erratic tension in nerves which control muscles of eyeball; tremor and muscular palsy are possibilities.

Hydripheric Conditions

In the Hydripheric type, intemperance in hydrogen consumption contributes to hyperactivity of lymphatic glands and resultant lymphatic obesity, enlargement of lymph glands and excessive hydrogen deposits in tissues. Joint dropsy, excessive hydration, dermatitis, dermal lesion due to profuse perspiration, hydroderma, uterine hypertrophy, uterine tube distension, uterine gland hyperactivity, profuse perspiration, dropsical effusion of ear cavities, venous stagnation and neurotic pains are bothersome. There may be ovarian dropsy, hydrothorax (water settled in chest), anassarca (water settled under skin), edema, peritoneal dropsy, hydrocele, uterine dropsy, false pregnancy; ultimately watery discharges and uterine hemorrhages may be the result, particularly when the reproductive system is weak and hydration excessive.

Problems of the Hydripheric Female

The reproductive system of the Hydripheric type is generally weak; pregnancy is precarious and miscarriages a threat; milkleg and reproductive complications are common; menstrual flow is profuse in youth and middle years; and in later years, subject to stoppage or disruption; minimal excitement may precipitate menstruation and lead to hemorrhages; mothers tend to be overweight; there may be headache with absence of period, frequent stinging pains in lower spine, involuntary nocturnal discharges, diseases of nerve matter in lower spine related to generative organs.

Love-Related Problems

The hydrogen female is subject to jealousy which may lead to female troubles; if she experiences disappointment in love, she may never get over it, as it undermines the heart brain, the heart activity center. Love emotions affect respiration via the medulla (chest brain) center; this weakens the heart, cerebellum and whole cerebral structure, which is the source of love emotion. Weakness in the cerebellum and uterine structures should not be accompanied by a liquid diet during pregnancy. The uterus lacks distention power and this may result in miscarriage. Emissions, hemorrhages, membrane ruptures are possible.

Problems in the Male

Muscular weakness, including reproductive system muscles, may lead to sterility. A diet high in calcium, silicon, protein, chlorine, potassium, phosphates, sodium is indicated. The mental sex centers are not sterile, only the physical function; the above diet will gradually restore potency.

Susceptibility to Heat and Light

The hydrogen patient's nerves absorb sunlight rapidly; it passes equally rapidly into brain cells and nerve substance, creating emotions and sensations. The pulse rises and diminishes quickly and a pulse is felt in the fingertips. When first awakening in the morning, there is a tendency to sneeze when light hits the optic nerves. Strong sunlight produces chills, fever and enfeebling perspiration on occasion. Prostration may occur in the street, in a stifling room, in bright sunlight or while swimming in the ocean if the sun's rays beat down suddenly. This is due to the excessive water in the body, thin skin, active sensory and emotive mechanism, which allow sun to enter the body rapidly. The sensitive nerve matter is affected and motor nerve contractions and cerebral anemia may result. Thus such patients may drown without warning when swimming or even bathing.

Excessive heat, powerful emotions and extreme sunlight can lead to anemia. Sultry summer heat can precipitate sodium as can oppressive rooms, both of which influence the medulla and cerebellum, causing anemic conditions of these brain centers; this may in turn contribute to spasmodic convulsions or sudden death. Powerful emotions cause perspiration over the entire body.

Highly-Developed Senses of the Hydrogen Type (Hydripheric)

This type of patient possesses highly-developed senses of touch, hearing, smell, as mentioned previously. He may hear sounds he is reluctant to admit to others for fear he will be disbelieved. The nerve ends of hearing apparatus are acute and the eardrum is very sensitive. The keen sense of smell is due to secretion of a cerebral fluid from the cerebellum during times of cerebral anemia. Physical senses are most acute in nocturnal hours when intellect, reason, volition, concentration and motor activities are slowed down.

Hydripherics are Sensitive and Reactive

Excessive moisture in the Hydripheric body results in sensations of chilliness; chilling winds penetrate to the marrow of the bones; cold sensations are experienced over the eyes, never under them. The salivary, parotid, gastric, intestinal, skin and lymphatic glands are massive and impressionable. The liver, spleen, lacteals, kidneys, skin pores, tear ducts, white brain fibers, arachnoid membrane are all acutely developed, active and full of moisture, lymph and oily material; hence the activities of these body constituents are highly sensitive and reactive. The sense of direction is weak; but the sense of being touched is acute. Rapid motion of trains or autos produces a sense of dizziness.

Hydrogen Type Unable to Digest Solid Food

Indigestion in the Hydripheric type is due to inability to handle solid food. Digestion of solid food is improved by residence in the hills and mountains, in breezy climates and by exercise after meals. An enlarged or overheated liver produces burning sensations when reclining. Internal gas generation produces abdominal hardening; this gas presses against the lungs, heart, spinal centers causing erratic breathing functions and fever; further effects include inguinal pain, nerve pain, labored breathing, upper chest contractions, throat lumps and contractions, mouth dryness, bladder and kidney pain which influences kidney function and causes retention of body acids which should be eliminated and emission of a vinegar odor from the body. There may be hiccough after meals; heartburn following intake of meat, smoked fish or solid food; general aversion to solid food. Emotions influence digestive ability as they affect all organs.

Symptoms of Hydrogen Excess

The hydrogen excess patient has rosy, attractive skin that is soft and delicate. He is predisposed to watery or rosy eczema and other skin and scalp diseases. Acute manifestations of these afflictions result in itching, discharges, infiltration, redness of skin and scalp. Other indications are eczema of flexor joint surfaces; ear eczema; head eczema; thin crusty eczema in adolescence; eczema due to active congestion of skin with patches resembling erythemia; facial eczema that may simulate erysipelas; eczema that manifests deep, painful cracks and fissures of skin on hands and over joints; irradiating eczema with accuminate papules which may linger long, even for years; groin eczema or eczema on inner nate surfaces or armpits or beneath the mammary glands; lip eczema developing painful fissures; hand eczema and finger eczema showing deep vesicles and extending to palms and knuckles; weeping eczema with large, raw, weeping areas dotted with red points; eczema that looks like ringworm; ear passage eczema; eczema of nostrils or eyebrows; lichen circumscriptus; eczema pedum; eczema vesiculosum that itches and burns, is worse at night and has a crusty, excoriating appearance; eczema squamosum of neck and extremities. These assorted types of eczema, related to overconsumption of hydrogen, may be partly due to overconsumption of certain foods and condiments or sauces which are poisonous to the body.

Symptoms Resemble Gout

Suppurations which exude an offensive odor and cause swelling, pasty skin often occur. Moisture can manifest in certain body areas, possibly behind the ears, resulting in eczema, pus, fissures, scabs, sores or bloody discharges. Proud flesh is a common manifestation of hydrogen-excess patients, as are the following: water collection under skin and between joints, deforming the hands; enlargement of lower face and neck and puffiness of lower face; skin blotches with sticky, doughy fluid; dry, fine, mealy, peeling eruptions, effusions of serous fluid in areolar tissue; exfoliation; eruption between fingers; loose nails; swelling roots of nails; crippled joints; stiff neck; numb thumbs; moist face pimples; nodules; ulcerated corners of mouth and gums; pyorrhea; heat-induced toothache.

Although the hydrogen patient appears healthy, he complains of ailments often considered imaginary by doctors. In actuality this patient is weak, low in vitality, sickly. Such symptoms as exfoliation of the epidermis; swelling of lower extremities and lower abdomen; acrid pus; burning pains in the limbs; extreme tenderness of feet; toe convulsions; numb and stiff fingers, toes, arms, neck and legs due to anerethisia of the cerebellum are real. The physician who is not familiar with chemical types of people often falsely diagnoses the patient as suffering from gout or rheumatism.

Hydripheric Appetite Skirmish

The nutritionist may have difficulty convincing the hydrogen patient to observe the guidelines of a strict diet. The patient desires water, fluids, liquid food, fruit juices, watery vegetables and extracts of other fluid-carrying foods, so an appetite skirmish is often in action.

Treatment of Hydrogen Type (Hydripheric)

The hydrogen-excess or Hydripheric patient is low in vital energy. This must be treated by climates that facilitate dehydration and assimilation of solid nutrients. Chlorine-carrying foods are beneficial in reducing water content of the body; also helpful is a dry, salty diet (organic sodium and chlorine foods) and foods with liberal alkaline content. Fats and carbohydrates should be severely limited, as should foods high in water content. Foods high in protein are recommended; exercise is imperative, as is a vocation that is deeply satisfying.

SIGNS OF HYDROGEN DEFICIENCY

Water and hydrogen are essential to proper activity of the body. If moisture is deficient, nerves become irritated, metabolism chaotic, tissues inflamed; the entire body becomes dehydrated. Since water has a cooling function in the body, lack of it produces excessive heat localized in specific areas, which disrupts nerve impulses and brain cells. Lymph glands, tissues and cells become sluggish; body gases, toxins, acids and waste products are not adequately expelled. The brain's activities are disturbed, which results in extreme actions and conversation; ideas are disjointed, chaotic; the individual is incoherent, adverse to brain labor, rash, unable to hear clearly or grasp what is spoken; schoolwork becomes difficult; the individual becomes antisocial, clumsy in speaking, apathetic, impatient, uncommunicative, revengeful, hateful, anxious, preoccupied, at a loss for words, disheartened, fearful, sleepy, disinterested, suspicious, steeped in a troubled life. In talking with others, he is unable to convey his thoughts or he overstresses what he is saying; he is averse to questions. Extreme dryness and abnormal nerve heat are generated in the body when water's cooling, soothing, pleasing qualities are lacking.

Characteristics of Dehydrated Patient

The patient who is dehydrated develops strange, monotonous, arbitrary, greedy, foolish, sentimental characteristics; these qualities are particularly evident in lean, angular, emaciated elderly people who are cross, antisocial, narrowminded, remote, finicky, intolerant, selfish, arbitrary, stubborn, independent, tyrannical. The dehydrated patient fails to assimilate moisture and fatty nutrients due to the deficiency of moisture and hydrogen and because oil and fatty matter are lacking in the body; thus they are difficult to please. As a result of hydrogen poverty, the brain shrinks, face furrows, habits become odd and temperament becomes greedy. Eventually this patient develops senile or feebleminded characteristics due to lack of moisture, lubrication and fatty matter—not because of old age.

Common Ailments of the Elderly Due to Moisture Deficiency

Symptoms of moisture deficiency in the body include stiff bones and joints, hardening of body canals, sluggish bowel, stiffening and shrinkage of the brain, hardness of hearing apparatus, faulty eyesight, irritated nerves and brain—ailments common to elderly, lean, emaciated, gouty, rheumatic patients.

Complications from Dehydration

In the event that moisture assimilation is faulty, the whole body suffers. Lymphatic glands, lymph fluid, blood, liver, kidneys, spleen, pancreas, bladder, secretory and excretory organs are all dry, sluggish, hardened, stiff; evaporation and perspiration is defective; cells lack moisture; impulse transmission between the brain, nerves and body is undermined; more heat is likely to localize in a certain region of the body. Assorted ailments may trouble the hydrogen-deficient patient, such as: periodic or chronic headaches; gastric pains; rectal and genital pains; hoarseness; knee stiffness; stiffness elsewhere in the body; tendon and motor nerve tension; synovial rheumatism; gouty tendencies; joint swelling; spinal stiffness; extreme nervousness; emaciation; insomnia; convulsions; arm tremor; sero-fibrous pneumonia; sluggish liver; hysterical aphonia; throat constriction; spasmodic jerking of nerves in some part of body; hemorrhoids due to sickened blood; rectal paralysis or other paralysis; enteritis; blindness; fainting spells. A brain concussion is dangerous; strong emotions, fiery passion or agitation have disagreeable side effects. Mucus membranes may become arid and inflamed; glands, skin, nails and more solid tissues become indurated.

Hydrogen Necessary in Youth

Even in youth the hydrogen element may be deficient, giving a patient an aged appearance and other symptoms resembling old age and senility. If a young patient lacks hydrogen, water is not assimilated or utilized; fatty nutrients are not digested and assimilated sufficiently; so the body lacks material which is vital to joints, marrow, nerves, brain, auditory structures and other body parts in need of lubrication for optimum movement.

Hydrogen Vital in Old Age

With advanced years, many person's abilities to absorb moisture and digest and assimilate fatty nutrients are reduced; attendant complications are often mistakenly referred to as "old age ailments." Other persons, however, retain the moisture-assimilating capacities into advanced age, as well as the ability to assimilate fatty nutrients. When the moisture-absorbing capabilities are lost, the proper diet and climate are beneficial; pleasing occupations are likewise needed.

Symptoms of Hydrogen Lack

In the patient lacking moisture in the body, symptoms are pronounced. They include hardness and dryness throughout the body, ossification, dull senses, dry catarrh and mucus, crampy tendons and nerves, gouty joints, rheumatism in muscles, mental confusion, mental inadequacy, neck stiffness, skin itch, sore hip joints, lame or deadened nerves, sleepiness, chaotic heat production, thick and ununiform nails, cramps in calves, irascible temperament, extreme desire for heavy work, powerful desire for narcotics or alcoholic beverages, troublesome holding of urine, weighty sensation in brain, predisposition to epilepsy, emaciation, ringing or buzzing in ears along with deafness, weakened or lost sense of smell, leathery skin tone, hard and fissured tongue.

Talking Causes Fatigue

Further symptoms include brain fatigue from conversing or public speaking; brain shrinkage causing strange feelings when reclining, bending or rising; inclination to vertigo; feeble, weak pulse rate; drowsiness during daytime; claylike complexion and wrinkled face; infrequent flush of small cheek areas; scratchy, rough throat; liver shrinkage and hypochondria constriction; irritation of nerve ends at skin surface; itching, stinging, inflammation of nerve nets, producing feverish skin; stiff, painful, cracking skin; peeling, cracking of lip cuticle; wasting away of soft parts of body; faulty lymphatic system functions; susceptibility to dry consumption, due to lack of lung humidity; stiffness in virtually all body regions after sitting still for brief periods; stiffness and cramping upon rising from sitting position; lack of sweat function even in sultry weather; sense of touch almost lost; weight produced in head by study and thinking; headache; farsightedness; loss of thirst sensation except in heat, feverish or inflammatory states; heavy, milky sediment in urine; frequent urge to urinate with inability or difficulty; contraction of fingers and tendons of feet; feverish nervous system; restlessness and feverish feeling in nocturnal hours; strong preference for salty or chlorine-rich foods.

TREATMENT OF HYDROGEN DEFICIENCY

Once the moisture-assimilating capability of the body is diminished or lost, it is difficult to restore. The patient is in need of water-carrying foods, liquids and fluids, watery tonics and juices— an almost entirely fluid diet; a humid, warm climate; satisfying outdoor work around trees and bushes; development of love emotions; fondness for liquid foods, juices, tonics; development of pleasure in taste, smell, thirst faculties—all of which will revitalize the organism by reactivating the moisture-assimilating capacity, notably in younger patients and partially in elderly individuals.

Americans should eat more poultry and fish and less meat, according to a report issued by the staff of the U.S. Senate Select Committee on Nutrition and Human Needs.

Nutrition and Pregnancy
Water retention, morning sickness, swollen breasts and fatigue during pregnancy are caused by a lack of proper vitamins and minerals.

People who hold water in the system have too much sodium and not enough potassium.

HIGHEST HYDROGEN FOODS

The foods highest in water or moisture are high-hydrogen foods. Liquids are therefore highest in hydrogen: water, fruit and vegetable juices, broths, goat and cow's milk. Citrus fruits contain much water but should be eaten only if tree ripened and in season. The foods and beverages highest in hydrogen include:

Apricots	Muskmelon
Asparagus	Okra
Blackberries & juice	Papaya
Blueberries & juice	Parsley
Broccoli	Peaches
Brussels sprouts	Pineapple
Buttermilk	Prunes
Cabbage (red, common, savoy)	Pumpkin
Carrots & juice	Radishes
Celery & juice	Rutabaga
Chard	Sauerkraut
Cherries & juice	Sorrel
Eggplant	Spinach
Fish, tender	Squash
Guavas	Strawberries
Horseradish	Tomatoes & juice
Juniper tea	Turnips
Kohlrabi	Watercress
Mangos	Watermelon
Milk	Whey (goat, cow)

HYDROGEN MENUS

Mixed vegetable drink, veal joint broth, steamed whitefish; green salad of assorted greens, tomatoes, shredded beets and carrots, celery, leeks, parsley, tomato dressing; steamed okra, steamed squash.

Tomato juice and cod roe, barley and green kale soup, butternut squash; green salad of assorted greens, watercress, tomatoes, cucumbers, celery, green onions, summer squash slices, green pepper, radishes, mushrooms, avocado dressing; steamed asparagus, eggplant and tomato casserole, juniper berry tea.

Fish broth, steamed red snapper, cole slaw, sauerkraut, steamed pumpkin pudding, steamed kale and broccoli, nettle tea.

SUMMARY OF HYDROGEN

GENERAL CHARACTERISTICS

"Moisturizer" element
Present in animals, vegetables, minerals

Water 11% hydrogen
Hydrogen type = Hydripheric type

HYDROGEN IN THE HUMAN BODY

Soothes nerves
Moisturizes tissues
Helps transport nutrients (in water)
Promotes elimination

Prevents inflammation
Promotes osmosis
Helps regulate temperature
Irrigates organs and cells

SIGNS OF HYDROGEN EXCESS (CHARACTERISTICS OF HYDRIPHERIC TYPE)

Even tempered, merciful, compassionate, gentle, tender, forgiving, slow moving
Obesity, swelling ankles
Sluggishness, sleepiness
Loose flesh, puffiness under skin
Susceptibility to heat and light

Preference for juicy foods; aversion to solid foods
Unfailing sense of smell
Enlarged vital organs
Weakness, exhaustion
Symptoms similar to gout

SIGNS OF HYDROGEN DEFICIENCY

Dehydration
Emaciation, leanness
Crampy tendons
Appetite for salty food

Irritability
Dry skin, throat
Wrinkled skin
Perspiration lack

Gout
Arthritis, rheumatism
Shrinkage of liver
Excess body heat

HIGHEST HYDROGEN FOODS

Water
Citrus fruits
Milk
Whey

Fruit & vegetable juices
Drinks & tonics
Broths
Kefir

six

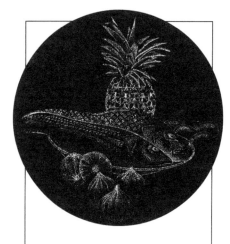

Iodine, the "metabolizer"

At one time, I cared for 19 factory workers who had been overcome with fumes from carbon tetrachloride, used to clean metals, when a reconditioned fan was installed incorrectly.Later, several of the men were divorced and others experienced marital discord due to sexual problems and impotence. Still others found their senses slowed to the point that they could no longer hold a job. Before I began treatment, many remedies were tried to no avail. It was not until iodine was replaced in their bodies that functions returned to normal.

Iodine is one of the most vital of the 16 biochemical elements, keeping us in a quickened state of health. When bodily functions become underactive, it is well to look to the thyroid gland and the proper intake of iodine through foods and food supplements.

One of the most outstanding cases I have had was that of a child with an open sore at the base of the spine.. Doctors had been unable to heal it in the three years following her birth. In checking both mother and child, I found that iodine was lacking, causing extremely low metabolism. I prescribed 30 dulse tablets a day, and in less than three weeks' time, the sore was healed.

Of course, a keen observer would say the little girl lacked calcium. I would say so, also, but I have found that it is the *control* of calcium that is needed mostly, provided by iodine and thereby assisting the repair and building of new tissue in the body. This approach to controlling calcium is supported by Professor Cavanaugh of Cornell University, who found that the general health of white leghorn hens was improved, and their eggs had harder shells, when using iodine.

Another case concerned an 18-year-old girl with a large goiter, with which she had suffered for six months. This case involved family conflict over the girl's boyfriend. Six months earlier, she had been told to drop the boyfriend or face confinement to her room. The mother said she would rather see her daughter dead than dating that boy. I told her she was doing a pretty good job of getting her wish!

About three weeks later, I was called back again to help, and I suggested that the girl be allowed to return to the boyfriend. The girl said that he wouldn't have her now due to the growth on her neck. As I found out, after speaking with him, however, the truth was that he had begun dating another girl. I persuaded him to date two girls for a while, and in another six months, the goiter had disappeared. Today, this couple has a happy marriage and two children.

This case taught me some important lessons. The girl's problems extended beyond the goiter to a family feud involving resentments, frustrated love, loneliness—in short, a long list of mental problems and related physical disorders. Feeding her iodine alone was never going to get the job done. No food could keep up with the iodine she was breaking down emotionally. Similarly, if an ulcer is caused by your boss, you need to do more than take sodium to neutralize the acids causing that ulcer.

Here is where physical problems meet mental and spiritual ones. It is important to be mentally clear, in order to have the inward calm that does not wear out the iodine from stress in the thyroid gland. Every doctor should know where the physical problem ends and when the spirit must take over, utilizing the mind. Above and beyond all the minerals we can replace, we should never forget the curing power of love. No salve will do as much for the human soul.

Nevertheless, the importance of iodine, with one of the highest vibratory rates of all the elements, is very clear. It is one of the four particularly significant elements usually missing in any patient, the others being calcium, silicon and sodium. Western society seems to burn these elements out the most. We live in an uncertain world in which finances and relationships are creating emotional strain. The emotions are mostly handled by the thyroid gland, so that iodine is used in excess during much of the day. Consequently, it is deficient in most people.

Signs of Iodine Deficiency

Generally, people in need of iodine are lethargic, dragging and depressed. Frustrated self expression, lack of emotional control, fear of elevators and extreme discomfort with anything snug around the throat are also indicators. Mongolism and hyperactivity in children suggest iodine may be burned out. Even infertility and impotency are due to a lack of iodine. I've seen many a childless marriage produce children when this element was brought into balance. I have also seen excessively large families as a result of iodine deficiency.

Iodine is one of the first elements consumed by misuse of the mental processes, so whenever we find nerve depletion or unbalanced emotions, we should suspect there is a need for iodine. I am convinced that every criminal is short of it.

Iodine deficiency can be the result of an underactive or an overactive thyroid, calling for what is known as "replacement therapy," in this case, the feeding of iodine. We do need to be careful, however, in overstimulating the body with iodine because it can quicken the heart activity too much. In most cases, the organs are underactive, with the patient leading a very slow life metabolically. As such, we cannot expect the body to be doing its job. Protein is also necessary for this underactivity.

Nearly all of my patients have cold hands and feet, a condition of sick people with low metabolism and poor circulation. Absence of heat in the body means a patient cannot properly digest his food until that heat returns. Iodine restores heat. Other ways to help raise metabolism and bring more heat to the body should also be considered, such as exercise, hot and cold baths and living in a higher altitude where the thyroid is always stimulated. With these measures, all the elements will have a better opportunity to be drawn to their proper tissues to promote a warm body and a good circulation.

We especially see the hypoglycemic patient as deficient in iodine. This patient has produced a good deal of depression and nerve depletion through overanxiety and overuse of the nervous system. Here we need a very carefully studied diet, even beyond the call for iodine, as well as exercise and work to produce more positive mental attitudes.

Draining the Iodine Reserves

The thyroid gland furnishes a secretion which destroys injurious toxins in the blood before the blood enters the brain. In their experiments, Bright and Kishin showed that with insufficient iodine in the thyroid, it becomes overheated, irritated and goitrous.

Those who have plenty of iodine in their foods do not suffer from brain intoxication, nervous ailments and defective bone and brain metabolism nearly as much as those living on a large proportion of meats, starches and chemically preserved foods. These iodine-deficient foods drain the body of iodine reserves.

Even vegetarians—who scorn the foods just mentioned—are often deficient in iodine, because they have cold bodies that cannot digest cold proteins well. Cold proteins such as seeds and nuts are difficult for strict vegetarians to handle. I recommend that nuts and seeds be taken only in the form of milk drinks and butters, because they are thus more easily assimilated. People living on raw foods direct from the refrigerator are putting an extra demand on the thyroid to supply heat for digestion. Animal proteins help provide this heat—goat milk and egg yolks are good, if meat, fowl and fish are avoided. We should be sure to bring to the thyroid gland all the elements it needs.

Iodine is rarely found in cooked foods or any processed foods, such as white flour products. Moreover, since it is water soluble, we have to be careful about boiling our foods and thereby washing the iodine out of the fiber structure.

Cooking at high heat also allows iodine to escape in steam, especially when aluminum utensils with loose-fitting lids are used. Usually, the iodine and other elements not lost in steam are thrown out with the cooking water so that very little is left intact in the food. All cooking should be done by steaming over very low heat, using stainless steel, low-heat cookware with tight-fitting lids.

As indicated by the aforementioned case of the 19 factory workers overcome with tetrachloride gases, the thyroid gland is vital to the respiratory processes. Today, we overuse the thyroid and lose control of proper breathing through exposure to the exhaust fumes on our freeways and in our cities. Pollution exhausts iodine control in the body. In extreme cases, we can become drowsy, doze off and lose control of our mental faculties. In fact, prolonged exposure to concentrated levels of pollutants may result in permanent brain damage or death. Almost all of us are exposed to toxic gases to some extent.

The Properly Functioning Thyroid

Iodine, we might say, is the body's sanitary police force guarding the brain and mind, with its office in the thyroid gland. Iodine guards the brain by destroying harmful toxins and increasing the assimilation of certain salts for normal metabolism. This process oxidizes toxic materials affecting the brain.

Additionally, iodine is water soluble, entering the lymph fluids and thereby traveling to every cell in the body. Carried in this way to every part of the body, it is highly sensitive to the total organism's electrical balance. Due to its solubility, very little iodine is needed, only 0.14 of a grain daily.

Utilizing iodine, the thyroid quickens the metabolism of all the organs of the body. Without it, all organs function slowly. The thyroid secretion thus increases the rate of the pulse, lowers arterial pressure and augments respiration and the demand for oxygen. I have treated many cases of indigestion and constipation by quickening the thyroid metabolism by means of dulse tablets and urging control of the emotions.

Iodine's Relationship to Other Elements

The 16 biochemical elements combine in specific patterns to make tissues perform as they do. Interestingly, different types of people require elements that have evolved in unique ways to suit their special type. Not all people use iodine from the same foods; some receive more iodine from certain foods than from others. Keep in mind that there are those who think faster; those who run faster or jump higher; those who retain facts better. These kinds of differences stem from faculties and tissue made up of a unique biochemical balance in each case, according to the individual's needs for the elements and trace elements. Thus we have thousands of combinations. No two people are alike.

As a rule, when we are balancing the chemical elements in the body and when tissue is worked hard through overuse, we must recognize that we may be wearing out the dominant elements in the organs where they are stored in highest proportions. If an organ isn't working enough or is hyperactive, it is also lacking in elements. To find normalcy is something no chart can tell us because each individual is different in his or her needs. Not too much nor too little is the amount of iodine we need to carry on suitable life expression. In a balanced state, we will be without pains, mental resentments or other quirks.

Usually, we have troubles due to a combination of deficiencies. For instance, the problem of cataracts comes from calcium being out of solution due to a lack of iodine (no iodine to control the calcium). There is also a direct relationship between phosphorus and iodine which creates vigorous oxidation to increase the brain's alertness and reduce toxicity through circulatory activity.

There is one occasion when I do not believe in using iodine—if a patient has tuberculosis. When there are tubercles which have been controlled and calcified, the use of iodine could break up these calcifications and bring back the tuberculosis, even though it is years in the past. It is better to leave this condition alone. Remember that when we use the drugless healing art, according to Hering's law of cure, all illnesses reverse and go through a remission period, in which we pick up again our old troubles. Thus, gradually, we reverse from the chronic stage of disease toward good health by entering healing crises when an acute stage has been reached—often the discharge stage. (Chronic diseases are created in the first place, of course, due to deficiencies in the chemical elements.) Iodine really puts the fire under calcium and "sets" it in the body, so we have to be very careful in caring for tuberculosis.

Administering Iodine

Many of my patients have been helped by iodine (organic or biochemical) painted on the soles of the feet. The body can absorb whatever quantity of iodine it requires from the large pores of the feet. I find this method effective because the body is especially temperamental in taking in iodine, and it is difficult to measure the exact amount a person needs. The soles of the feet absorb just what is needed, raising the body's metabolic rate. We have also used liquid chlorophyll wrapped around the throat so that a patient could absorb iodine through the skin in this way.

The day will come when we will have colloidal minerals in such a form that they can be absorbed by using packs on the skin. The body will be able to use them as needed instead of the doctor's attempting to prescribe the exact amount required, which is often very difficult to predict. We might even some day use the inner soles of our shoes, making them to be high in liquid iodine or chlorophyll, for example. The iodine would help metabolism, as already indicated, and the chlorophyll would contribute to a good blood count. Even elements such as sodium, silicon, calcium and iron could be absorbed in the colloidal form.

Sources of Iodine

Since iodine is one of the most important elements, you should make sure to include high iodine foods in the diet. They include seafoods, fish roe, kelp, eggs, papayas, mangoes, pineapples and foods grown near the ocean. Onions draw iodine from the air to the soil. If iodine supplementation is used, make sure it is from a biochemical or food source. I like to use dulse tablets because dulse is higher in manganese than kelp, and manganese is another important element. Perhaps the simplest way to get iodine is by using Nova Scotia dulse leaves. For wonderful results, place some in a blender and chop until fine, using a small amount of water.

In Switzerland, there is a law requiring people to take iodine. In the County of Bern, Switzerland, for example, people have a lot of goiter trouble. Being water soluble, iodine is washed from the soil into the ocean, causing mountainous areas to be lacking in this element. India, too, has trouble with goiters, as we also do in this country. On the other hand, Japan rarely has a case of goiter. The Japanese markets are stocked with a tremendous variety of seafoods. They make bread, soups, and even candy from what they harvest from the sea.

One of the most important books on the subject of hypothyroidism has been written by Broda O. Barnes, MD, and is titled *Hypothyroidism: The Unsuspected Illness*. It contains hundreds of conditions, symptoms and emotions expressed due to problems in thyroid function and deficiencies in iodine in iodine. In conclusion, I will reproduce a brief synopsis of some of the primary symptoms found in Broda Barnes' test patients.

Reprinted from

HYPOTHYROIDISM: THE UNSUSPECTED ILLNESS
Broda O. Barnes, MD, and Lawrence Galton
Thomas Y. Crowell Company, New York, 1976 (available in health stores)

INCIDENCE OF SYMPTOMS AND SIGNS OF HYPOTHYROIDISM:

	Study A % of 77 Cases	Study B % of 100 Cases
Weakness	99	98
Dry skin	97	79
Coarse skin	97	70
Lethargy	91	85
Slow speech	91	56
Edema (swelling of eyelids)	90	86
Sensation of cold	89	95
Decreased sweating	89	68
Cold skin	83	80
Thick tongue	76	60
Edema of face	68	95
Coarseness of hair	67	75
Heart enlargement	66	-*
Pallor of skin	61	50
Impaired memory	59	65
Constipation	57	54
Gain in weight	57	76
Loss of hair	52	41
Pallor of lips	45	50
Labored/difficult breathing	35	72
Swelling of feet	32	57
Hoarseness	30	74
Loss of appetite	31	40
Nervousness	30	51
Excessive menstruation	25	33
Deafness	24	40
Palpitations	20	23
Poor heart sounds	18	-
Pain over heart	13	16
Poor vision	11	-
Changes in back of eye	9	-
Painful menstruation	9	-
Loss of weight	9	9
Emotional instability	3	-
Choking sensation	-	-
Fineness of hair	-	-
Cyanosis (bluish discoloration of skin)	-	-
Difficulty in swallowing	-	-
Brittle nails	-	41
Depression	-	60
Muscle weakness	-	61
Muscle pain	49	36
Joint pain	-	29
Burning/tingling sensation	-	56
Heat intolerance	-	2
Slowing of mental activity	-	49
Slow movements	-	73

*Dash means not reported found.

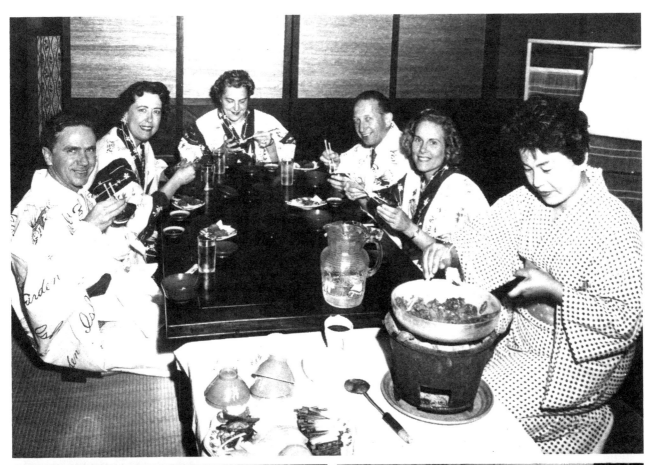

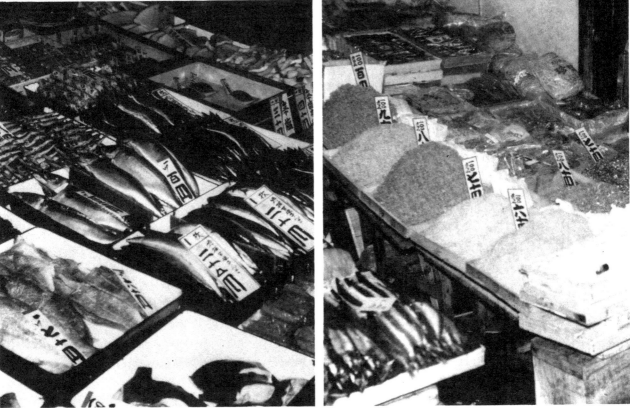

Here we are with friends at a traditional Japanese restaurant. The Japanese, unlike the Swiss and the Hunzas, do not get goiters because so much of their food comes from the sea and is rich in iodine.

195

IODINE
"The Metabolizer"

GENERAL CHARACTERISTICS

From the Greek *ioeides*, meaning violet colored, comes the name iodine. It is a striking, dense, violet vapor whose properties include: acrid taste, nonmetallic, bluish-black to blue-violet color, negative electrical charge, atomic weight 126, water solubility. Oxygen and hydrogen unite readily with the violet element to form iodic acid.

Iodine is most abundant in ocean water, some mineral waters, sea animals and vegetation, land-dwelling plants, waters of some rivers, in thyroid gland secretions and in some food substances. Most ordinary foods do not contain iodine; foods which do, contain only minute amounts.

IODINE: ITS ROLE IN THE HUMAN BODY

Iodine Neutralizes Toxins

Modern science has determined that iodine is present in thyroid gland secretions and is vital to normal brain function. It is also found to be necessary for neutralizing specific toxic substances in the body. Unfortunately, our current modes of milling, refining, manufacturing and processing foods remove iodine as well as many other vital elements. Certain ailments are the direct result of iodine deficiency.

Iodine Vital for Thyroid Function

Goiter is directly attributed to iodine shortage. It is also known that the secretion of the thyroid gland enhances assimilation of calcium, silicon, fluorine, chlorine and other biochemical elements. Calcium destined for bones depends on a good thyroid secretion for proper assimilation; iodine deficiency produces weakened bone metabolism; the nervous system, including the brain, is also weakened. A diet lacking trace iodine weakens the thyroid function; this leads to formation of albuminous toxins which affect the brain and nervous system adversely. When unneutralized albumin toxins enter the brain, the blood, the nervous system and the rest of the body may become intoxicated.

Auto-Intoxicated Animals Pass Toxins on to Humans

Beef shipped in the Fall contain three times as much iodine as that shipped between December and May. Slaughter animals fed an abundance of commercial food preparations are saturated with toxins. The animals suffer from autointoxication which they pass along to the consumer.

Processed Foods Weaken Thyroid Gland

Persons who ensure an adequate supply of iodine in their diet do not develop goiter, scrofula, brain auto-intoxication, nervous ailments, poor bone and brain metabolism, etc. Conversely, those living extensively on meat, starch, refined, manufactured and preserved foods, albumin-rich foods, devitaminized and demineralized foods irritate and weaken or incapacitate the thyroid gland.

Iodine Essential for Children

The thyroid does not normally function until age two or three; but in some children, the function commences between ages five and twelve. Because foods high in albumin can be difficult to handle before the thyroid begins to function, it may be advisable to withhold meat from children until that time. Milk, because it is not highly toxic or albuminous, is the natural food for the young before the thyroid begins to function. Iodine is essential to help protect growing children against toxins in their systems.

"Metabolism is increased by iodine and this is imperative for efficiency of anabolism and catabolism—assimilation and breaking down of foodstuffs for metabolism."

Iodine Aids Metabolism

Iodine, concentrated in the thyroid gland, is the guard against harmful toxins entering the brain and other parts of the body; the blood passes through the thyroid every hour and a half. In addition, iodine aids phosphorus assimilation; phosphorus is essential for an alert and sharp mind. Metabolism is increased by iodine and this is imperative for efficiency of anabolism and catabolism—assimilation and breaking down of foodstuffs for metabolism. Iodine causes pulse rate to be increased, arterial pressure lowered, respiration increased; it increases quantity of urine and utilization of oxygen and improves assimilation of certain mineral salts—especially calcium. Sufficient iodine (thyroid secretion) prevents myxedema, catarrh buildup, flabby and soft tissue, soft bones,

idiocy, dry skin and hair, thick, scaly skin and an ungainly body. Exophthalmic goiter is averted, as are cartical disorders and menstrual complications, and even glandular imbalances and scrofula. (Scrofula is tuberculosis of the lymph nodes of the neck.)

Glands Need Iodine

Any gland concerned with neutralization of toxins depends partly upon the thyroid secretion. Even the spleen needs iodine, as does the liver. Plentiful iodine guarantees that sores and ulcers are rare and easily healed when they do appear. The uterus needs iodine; so do heart linings, mental functions and toxins and acids generated by body processes. Lack of iodine is a possible contributing factor to retarded growth in children, poor bone development, bad teeth, dull mental faculties and poor elimination. Metabolism of calcium, fluorine and other biochemical elements is made more effective by ample thyroid secretion. Though rare, an excessive dose of thyroid extract can produce a cachexia which is commonly known as hyperthyroidism. If the doses are normal (and excess is very uncommon), body weight is reduced, fat and proteins dissolved, more oxygen demanded, assimilation improved, more nitrogen and phosphorus excreted in the urine, more carbon dioxide expelled through the lungs.

SIGNS OF IODINE EXCESS

Iodine Excess A Rarity

There is very little danger of an overamount of iodine from foods, inasmuch as only traces are present in them. In fact, most foods lack iodine completely. Drug iodine and iodine added to drinking water are more likely to be detrimental as they are unorganized forms which are not biochemic and therefore not assimilable by the body. Three grains of crystal or drug iodine can produce iodine poisoning in some individuals; iodine poisoning is characterized by edema of the tongue, mucus membrane collapse, respiratory afflictions, brain intoxication, excessive saliva, throat constriction, albuminuria, anuria and, in extreme cases, death.

Iodine-Excess Patient is Extremely Nervous

One suffering from too much iodine is fearful and concerned about the future—for himself and his friends—to the point of becoming neurotic; he is extremely nervous in temperament and movement; he is anxious about job, health, prosperity, adverse conditions, changes or anything relating to the future. Cardiac neurosis and hypertensive nerves can develop. Such a patient disdains rugged, sharp, pointed, rough, jagged, thorny, toothed representations in animals or tools; even needles, knives, forks, saws bother him. Nerves experience pricks to the surface; eyeballs have a protruding pressure or actually protrude from the sockets; eyeballs seem too large; distance vision is good and near vision poor, with abnormal sensitivity in the retina. Nerve and brain tissues are irritated and on edge.

The Heart is Overly Sensitive

A patient experiencing iodine excess has an overly-sensitive heart—to emotions, movement, everyday happenings—with palpitations and hearing alternately poor and sharp. Thirst and hunger are extreme, then appetite almost disappears. Nerves often twitch in spasms and respiration is speeded up. Vigorous action brings on chills, flushes, heat waves, compressive scalp feelings, thirst, hunger, perspiration, skin dryness, stabbing pains alternating regularly. Nerve tremor is a result of walking as is shortness of breath or breathing difficulty. Insomnia may be a symptom. A sudden jarring of the head produces painful vibration to the nerves, head and eyes, and even temporary partial anemia and paleness, heart palpitation, neck stiffness, pain sensation of the scalp and heart. When lying prone, the right side is preferred because the left side bothers the heart. Sense of touch is acute (hyperaphia). Restlessness and emotional turmoil may manifest. Tingling vibrations shoot through nerves like sonic waves. Changes of weather bring on unpleasant sensations of the eyes and eyelids, especially in the nerves. Morning headaches may plague such a patient in the lower part of the backhead, moving up to the temple region and then stopping in the eyes—usually the left eye.

Certain Types More Sensitive to Iodine

Characteristics distinctive of iodine excess or poisoning are neuralgia, alternating and unilateral, usually settling in the left side. Prime effects are on the heart linings, uterine linings, retina, sensory nerves, some motor nerves and plexuses, the eyes, not to mention the thyroid gland. Persons suffering from anemia, diabetes, old-age symptoms, those who tend toward albuminuria and predominant starch metabolism, emotional and weak-hearted types are overly sensitive to iodine—either in excess or deficiency, whether in drug form or biochemic (as found in food).

"A major indication of iodine hunger is an extremely nervous condition."

Further Signs of Iodine Excess

Other signs of iodine excess are tendency toward exophthalmos, exophthalmic goiter, throat constriction, tongue edema, albumin in urine, increased flow of urine, elevation in body temperature, stomach colic, dizziness, fainting, vomiting, shortness of breath, fast respiration rate, throat swelling, tachycardia, loss of weight due to excess burning of fat and oxidation, prostration, eye neumitis, brain disorders, neurotic habits at night, insomnia, psychotic feelings, intense restlessness, hyperalgesia, endocarditis, cerebrosis, hemialgia, retinitis, presbyopia, migratory neuralgia, hyperorexia, hemidrosis, night toothache, great hunger and thirst alternating with aversion to food and drinks. Nervous heart palpitation along with neck and shoulder rheumatism is common, as is rheumatism of the uterus, heart, eyes or nervous system.

SIGNS OF IODINE DEFICIENCY

Extreme Nervousness A Major Sign

A major indication of iodine hunger is an extremely nervous condition. Dreamlike stupor and weakness of intellectual faculties causing lack of direction and control; tendency to cry easily and excessively; saliva streaming from mouth; parched thirst but little water at a time consumed; gasping occasionally for air as if suffocating; stiffness from motion, especially in neck muscles; arm tension; pounding head; numb fingers; stinging in temples; alternating hot and cold waves over skin; dry palms alternating with sweating or same symptoms in the head; quest for fresh air and abhorrence for closed, warm, stuffy rooms; flashes of sharp pains in the head and nerves; feeling that something has been neglected, forgotten or left unfinished—which prevents contentment and peace; hearing deteriorating; sense of odor missing; worry when stomach is empty; heart palpitation from work, walking or other sensitivity. Sunset, the time when plants and sky become more electrically magnetic, produces feelings of restlessness.

Behavior May Seem Childlike

Other indications of iodine shortage are childlike behavior, foolish and immature actions and notions. At other times, though less often, patients are violent, impossible to please, cruel, dangerous and unreasonable or jealous. Mind functions are not indicated by facial expressions; they impress others as harmless, jolly, innocent and agreeable. Eyes tend to roll and squint; speech may be garbled and unclear, as if the tongue were partially incapacitated. As a result of inability to self-direct mentally, the iodine-deficient patient does not have normal use of senses, eyes, fingers— causing objects to be dropped. He exhibits indifference, stupidity, dullness and lack of normal understanding, intellectual reasoning, consciousness and thought patterns. He appears to be in a daze even when awake, muttering to himself in a harmless manner. His actions are childlike, concentrating on trifles, obsessed with details of things most people would hardly notice. The brain is unable to function normally; it is degenerating, softening like a paste or becoming watery. The gait is awkward with difficulty controlling the feet, especially at the first steps; jumping is clumsy and so is running. An innocent, happy expression belies the true state of nervousness, restlessness and changeability.

Restlessness is Pronounced

When reclining or sitting, the patient is more perplexed and restless than when on his feet. A feeling of drowsiness is powerful, but sleep is not relaxed, may be frightening; sleep may be sound the first portion of the night and restless the remainder (after midnight). Interchanging waves of heat and cold wash over the body. Meeting strangers is difficult. The patient may shy away even from relatives and develop a hermit-like existence. On occasion, excitement is evident, with tendency to fidget or jump around from one place to another constantly; at these times, stillness is an impossibility. A rapid change to high elevation can cause heart palpitation and respiratory pressure.

Beginning Stages of Shortage Are Not Obvious

However, beginning stages of iodine shortage go unnoticed since they are undistinctive. The advanced stages are much more pronounced as the patient passes from anastasis to catastasis.

Iodine Deficiency Leads to Cell Destruction

As we have stated, iodine starvation results in pathology and retrogressive cell destruction, especially noted in the brain. Albuminous toxins are neutralized by iodine in many parts of the body. The skin alternates between dryness and stickiness. Warm, humid, sultry air makes breathing difficult. Wheezing, arm numbness, spitting of blood, rectal bleeding and bleeding gums and overly relaxed sensations in the body may manifest. When iodine reserves are exhausted, cells in the brain and other parts of the body destroy themselves. A patient may show evidence of poor comprehension in studies, enlarged lymph glands, myxomatous degeneration, stupidity, fatty degeneration. Lymph glands can become soft and movable or doughy. The blood is loaded with unneutralized toxins which are carried to the brain and other parts of the body. The brain is not oxygenated properly, resulting in anxiety state, inclination to mutter, slow comprehension, crying, false state of cheerfulness, swelling, eruption, primary anemia, scrofula, ulceration of arteries, headcolds with discharge, chronic catarrh, spinal meningocele, locomotive ataxia, insanity, arterial softening, spinal cord softening, degenerative bronchitis, scrotism, speech difficulty (especially pronunciation) and difficulty with phonics, cephalic coryza, idiocy and mental retardation. The expectant mother completely lacking iodine can bear a retarded child. Pleurisy, edema, strumitis, scrotal edema, sterility, miscarriage and spontaneous abortion, chronic glandular imbalance, corpulence, inner ear adhesions, scabby catarrh of the head and nose, bronchial pneumonia, pneumonia with cerebral complications, scrofula of larynx, trachea and adenoids, hydrocephalus are other disease conditions that may appear.

Cretinism Due to Iodine Starvation

It is interesting that congenital cretinism, degenerative cretinism and mental degeneracy—characterized by thick, bullish neck, stubby arms and legs, degenerate brain, shortness, flabby tissues, massive and flabby stomach, thick lips, protruding tongue and big, fleshy face and features, soft goiter, paste-like brain—are probably caused by iodine starvation. It is also known that an individual deprived of iodine before and at birth has difficulty utilizing iodine in its metabolism from that time on; the doctor and nutritionist should know both this and how to ensure assimilation and utilization of iodine in these cases. Mucus cells form in the brain and the body's connective tissues and thyroid gland can malfunction; pus forms in glands and brain; muttering deep in the throat as well as slow speech are often present. Additional symptoms of iodine depletion include thick, scaly, dry, occasionally pasty skin; vacant expression; protruding and fleshy stomach; mucus accumulation in entire body; myxedema; throat and thyroid gland swelling.

Brain May Soften

Manganese and magnesium assimilation is defective when iodine is missing. When iodine is completely absent in the thyroid secretion, the brain may become liquified, soft or doughy, leading to idiocy or toxicity; manic-depressive or other psychoses may result. Other dangers are crysepalatous eruptions, stinging neuralgia, swelling scalp, puffiness and swelling under eyes, perienteritis, distention of lower abdomen, mucus diarrhea, pyemia, mucus adenoma, sacculated gums, mucus inflammation of the bladder, fatty tumors, mucus neuroma, occasional inordinate appetite, neuralgia of uterus, atonicity of blood vessels, diaphragmatic neuralgia, glioma.

Heartbeat May Slow Down

Tachycardia may result from irritation of the medulla and inhibitory nerve of the heart; the heartbeat may become too slow. Nerves become very inflamed, notably the superficial cervical, opthalmic, splanchnic, sternal, lingual, perineal and superior laryngeal nerves, in addition to many of the plexuses, heart linings, uterine linings and other sensitive linings—evidenced more at the outset of the disorder; as the disorder progresses to chronicity these sensitive linings become numbed.

Throbbing Throat Indicates Deficiency

The patient may complain of throbbing in the throat or the thyroid gland and pulsation in the hepatic, gastric, splenic arteries, the temples and in most of the primary arteries. A throbbing throat is a definite sign of thyroid (iodine) deficiency.

Lymphatic System Needs Iodine

The lymph nodes can be sites of scrofula, under the armpits, in the groin, along the neck, on inner thighs or in the fatty part of the bowel. The lymphatic system functions in absorption and assimilating vital fluids of materials entering the circulatory system and in elimination of toxins. The lymph fluid penetrates areas too small for blood vessels and functions in the conversion of food to lymph fluid which enters the bloodstream. If the lymph system is malfunctioning, lymph, blood and chyle are not made of the best materials for nourishing the system.

Treatment Involves Diet, Medication, Climate

When iodine is unavailable, iron and calcium are improperly metabolized and oxygenation in brain and glands is decreased. When a child is born to parents with thyroid deficiency, he inherits a tendency toward pus formation in brain and glands and scrofulous cachexia. Nutrition will be poor whether the child is stout or lean. The only true remedy utilizes iodine food, thyroid-extract medication, high iron diet, cod liver oil, fresh air in hills and high altitude, dry climate, breezy weather.

Ailments Occur on Left Side of Body

Other indications of iodine deficiency are a small head or excessively large head and an underdeveloped body; frothy salivation; scars that break open; palpitation when climbing stairs or steep grade; brownish-red, violet, thick, acrid, scanty, yellowish-green, turbid or muddled urine giving off a strong odor; urine which is albuminous, bloody or contains a claylike sediment after standing; neuralgic pains in the diaphragm; sensations of pressure and fullness in the throat; alternating sweet and putrid saliva; many symptoms alternating; unilateral ailments, more often on the left side of the body; dull ache under the scapular bones; swelling of feet or toes; preference for standing and motion as opposed to sitting and lying; occasional extreme prostration; desire to wash the face, head and neck in ice water; tendency to grasp the throat; occasional sickness from odor of food; stinging eyes with poor vision; acuity of thought when working, walking or exercising but mental slowness when at ease; fear that a doctor will find incurable hereditary illness; fear that something dangerous is behind one; sense of compression in chest; exhausted feeling in lungs; left arm weakness; nerve tremors; tendency to yawn and feel sleepy day and night; awkward handwriting; painful shyness; alternating bluish, pale gray, pale amber, brown, red, claylike or earthy complexion; loss of hearing; fluttering in ears with feeling of warm waves washing through the ears; restless and rolling eyeballs along with pupillary dilation resulting in flickering light before the eyes, even occasional dimming of eyesight; tendency to push inward on eyelids to aid vision; muttering or even screaming while asleep; inability to control balance while moving; enlarged head; swelling, sunken, pulsating fontanelles (in children); squinting; water and pus in the brain causing excessive growth in brain; gnashing and gritting of teeth; dropping lower jaw or clinching jaws tightly occasionally; preference for milk because it furnishes calcium needed due to malfunction of thryoid metabolism; tender lower ribs. These symptoms are all attributed to iodine deficiency and call for a diet high in iodine, the "metabolizer" in the body.

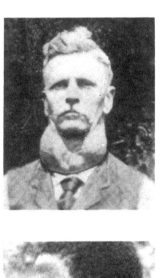

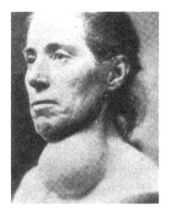

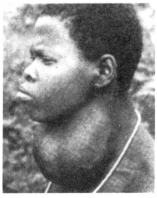

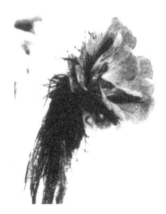

Goiters are caused as the thyroid attempts to compensate for iodine deficiency. The African woman had come to gather special plants such as the water hyacinth (shown) whose ashes prevent goiter.

201

═HIGHEST IODINE FOODS═

Kelp and dulse (Nova Scotia) head the list of iodine-rich foods. Others are listed below.

Agar	Mustard greens
Artichokes	Oats, steel cut
Asparagus	Okra
Bass	Onions, green & dried
Beans (butter, French, kidney, snap)	Oysters, raw
Blueberries	Peanuts
Brussels sprouts	Perch
Cardemom	Pike
Carrots	Potatoes, sweet, Irish
Chervil	Quail
Chives	Rutabaga
Coconut	Salsify
Cucumber	Seaweed
Eggplant	Silver salmon
Fish	Sole
Fish roe	Spinach, New Zealand
Garlic	Squash, summer
Goat cottage cheese	Strawberries
Goat milk, whey	Swiss chard
Green peppers	Tofu
Green turtle	Tomato, ripe
Haddock	Trout
Halibut	Tuna fish
Herring	Turnips
Kale	Turnip greens
Leaf lettuce	Watercress
Loganberries	Watermelon

IODINE MENUS

Salad made of salmon, raw asparagus tips, cabbage, avocado, leaf lettuce, green onions and sweet green peppers; whipped goat cottage cheese and pineapple dressing; glass of tomato juice and cod roe.

Steamed oats, fresh strawberries, blueberries, bananas topped with coconut cream, glass of goat milk and soft-boiled eggs.

Broiled haddock or sole, steamed green peas, steamed eggplant, tomatoes and green onions, concentrated fish broth with mushrooms, kelp and dulse seasoning.

Baked sweet or Irish potato, steamed brussels sprouts, steamed red beets; tossed salad made of anchovies, cucumber, summer squash, tomatoes, okra, leaf lettuce, watercress, parsley and green onions or chives.

Green turtle soup, wild rice (steamed), steamed okra, steamed Swiss chard or turnip greens, tossed green salad with mixed greens and leaf lettuce, tomato dressing.

SUMMARY OF IODINE

GENERAL CHARACTERISTICS

"Metabolizer" element

In thyroid gland secretions

Abundant in ocean water

No iodine type

IODINE IN THE HUMAN BODY

Aids assimilation of calcium, silicon, chlorine, fluorine

Vital to brain function

Prevents goiter

Affects teeth and bone metabolism

Essential for children

Found in spleen, blood, saliva, perspiration, tears

Vital for thyroid, spleen, liver

Neutralizes albumin toxins

Prevents sores, ulcers

SIGNS OF IODINE EXCESS (There is No Iodine Type)

Iodine excess rare

Nervousness, anxiousness

Protruding eyeballs

Acute sense of touch

Fear of future

Fear of sharp objects

Overly sensitive heart

Nerve tremor

203

SIGNS OF IODINE DEFICIENCY

Extreme nervousness   *Goiter*
Flabby, doughy skin   *Awkwardness*
Frothy salivation   *Childlike behavior*
Restlessness   *Much catarrh and phlegm*
Cretinism   *Mental degeneration*
Unreasonable fears   *Heart and lung problems*
Throbbing throat   *Gnashing of teeth*

HIGHEST IODINE FOODS

Kelp
Dulse
Sea plants and fish
Fish roe

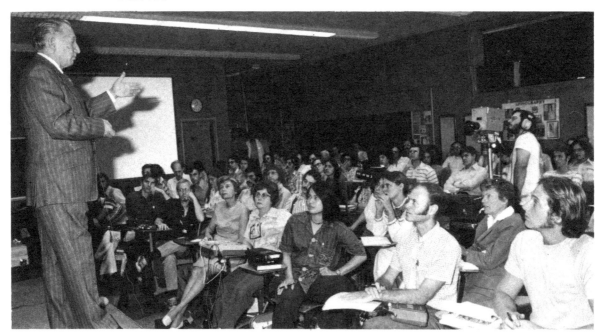

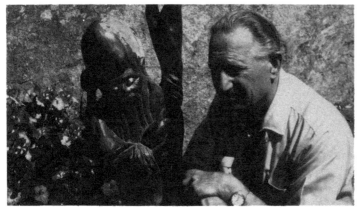 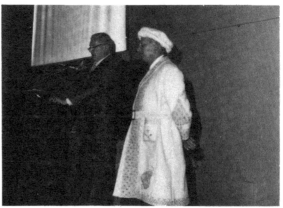

Who is going to teach people how to stay well? I have lectured before many audiences in many nations, but it will take many more years to get the idea across. The Chinese god of longevity symbolizes man's search for ways to stay healthy while growing older.

seven

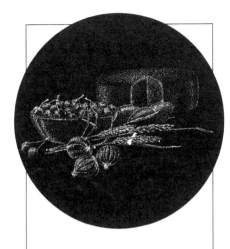

Iron, the "frisky horse"

A young lady once came to us from Canada with a severe anemic condition. A blood test showed she had a two million eight hundred thousand blood count, when the normal for a woman should be from 4.2 to 5.4 million. Serious consequences were developing in her body—menstrual disorders, lethargy, inability to walk properly, dizziness and upset equilibrium. One of the largest clinics in the United States told her that her blood count was so low that she needed blood transfusion. At 18, she was a third generation vegetarian. I respected her philosophy. She did not want meat or any of the high iron foods from the animal kingdom.

I went directly to iron from vegetarian foods. One of the best iron sources is liquid chlorophyll, and in four months, this young lady built her blood count to four million eight hundred thousand—a two million increase—by the use of liquid chlorophyll and high iron foods such as blackberries, black cherries and black cherry juice. We used an unusually large amount of liquid chlorophyll to bring the blood count up to normal.

Signs of Deficiency and Excess

In many patients we can observe anemia by looking at the inside of the lower eyelid where the blood is closest to the surface. If the inner surface is not red and the membrane is not criss-crossed by blood vessels, this condition suggests anemia and low blood count. Paleness generally indicates lack of iron and the presence of anemia.

In this context, Rocine frequently joked about how a person could make a "spook" out of himself by eating refined white flours or white "spook" bread. On the other hand, we can have the oxypheric condition, which represents an excess of iron and oxygen in the body. Such a person has a red, hot, burning face and needs to be cautious since this excess can lead to stroke due to the build-up of high blood pressure. Usually, however, we have iron and oxygen deficiency, rather than excess.

Low iron sometimes results from fasting and dieting without proper supervision. It can result from "calorie

Inorganic iron is valuable to industry but disastrous to the human body.

Iron deficiency lowers resistance to colds.

"Tobacco drieth the brain, dimmeth the sight, vitiateth the smell, hurteth the stomach, destroyeth the concoction, disturbeth the humors and spirits, corrupteth the breath, induceth a trembling of the limbs, exsiccateth the windpipe, lungs and liver, annoyeth the milt, scorcheth the heart and causeth the blood to be adjusted."
—Tobias Venner, 1620

Average smoker smokes 1-1/2 packs a day, says FTC.

Twenty-five percent of premenopausal American women are deficient in iron, and iron deficiency hinders lactic acid elimination, which results in fatigue. Chelated iron supplements should be taken with vitamin C if it is suspected that food sources of iron aren't providing enough.

counting" diets and from eating refined and processed foods. Or, it can result from poor assimilation due to a toxic bowel.

Oxygen Demands Iron

Iron is an important element because it is one of the great blood builders. Further signs of iron deficiency are blue lips, blue bags under the eyes or a bluish-whiteness of the eye. In these instances, due to insufficient iron in the blood, there is also insufficient oxygen. Oxygen is attracted from the air in the lungs when there is sufficient iron in the blood, so without iron reserves, no amount of breathing exercises will get more oxygen into the body. We can breathe until we are blue in the face, but if iron is deficient, we will not be able to hold the oxygen in the body.

As Rocine said, iron and oxygen are the two "frisky horse" elements. Additionally, oxygen is known as "the giver of life." Iron and oxygen demonstrate how chemical elements often work in company with each other; rarely does any one element function alone, but achieves its power through biochemical combination and relationship with other elements.

Iron is stored in every organ of the body, but particularly in the liver. Alcoholics are destroying their livers and making them hard. Now iron helps soften the liver so it can work properly, detoxifying the blood. One quarter of the blood of the body is in the liver at one time being purified; iron and oxygen work together to burn up waste material. We call the liver the "iron" organ, but it requires oxygen as well to burn up toxic wastes. Oxygen is additionally necessary in the body for providing the warmth to prepare foods for assimilation and elimination. Without oxygen, no burning or heating transpires—the life force is gone.

Bad Blood Chemistry

A United States government report has claimed that 92% of the people in this country are not healthy, and anyone who does not have a good blood chemistry, a high blood count, the proper nutrition and the proper biochemical balance is a member of this huge club of people. Above all, most people do not have the biochemical reserves needed for tissue repair, rejuvenation and rebuilding. If we are recovering from an illness, we need a high blood count, which is greatly aided in development through the proper amount of iron in the body.

My patients usually have what is called an "average blood count" by the standards of Western medicine. The average blood count for men is 4.7 to 6.1 million, while that of women is from 4.2 to 5.4 million. Most doctors say this amount is normal and acceptable. But if you are sick with an "average" blood count, you can't depend on it to get you well. It may, in fact, be low in terms of your own "normal" level. Get the blood count as high as possible. Indeed, iron is one of the first minerals I consider with patients, and much of my success is based on raising the blood count. A high blood count, in addition to iron, also requires manganese and copper in proper balance.

Sources of Iron

Pregnant women need extra iron. That person who is lethargic; who cannot keep up with the crowd; who cannot do daily work; who has menstrual disorders; or who does not produce healthy hemoglobin—needs iron supplements.

I can describe case after case of menstrual disturbances helped by iron and calcium. The more iron and oxygen we have in the body, the more heart trouble is reduced or prevented. Iron supplements and the increased oxygen supply they bring about, have helped many heart disturbances. All hearts are overworked when the blood lacks enough iron to bring in the oxygen needed by the body. Where do we get this extra iron?

First, we must not get it from an inorganic chemical or drug form. Iridology shows that these forms are quite constipating, settling in the intestinal tract and the bowel. Iron in chlorophyll, the link between man and the plant kingdom, is the greatest source.

We cannot live without greens. Through the process called photosynthesis, plant nutrients are developed through the combination of sunshine, water, earth and air, and greens must be considered one of the survival foods. Thus, greens and high iron fruits are two of the greatest of all sources of iron for building a good blood count and a good bloodstream. Further, we really should live surrounded by greenery because it helps keep the bloodstream healthy.

Additionally, black cherry juice, blackberry juice or liquid chlorophyll and green juices are excellent sources of iron. Cherry juice is especially good when iron is needed for the liver. In arthritic cases, cherry juice helps patients suffering from rheumatic and arthritic acids. Vegetarians, as a rule, get along well because they eat foods rich in iron, leading to a good blood count. However, I can't say that vegetarians are always balanced in the other elements, and this blood count strength may be misleading in terms of total health and expression. All of us, at any rate, should always make sure that plenty of iron is available to the body, in the biochemical or life-giving sources.

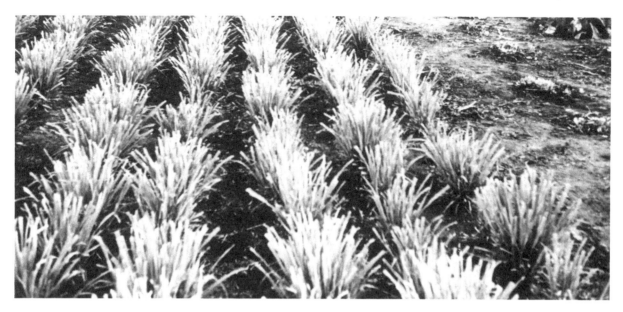

These are my gardens at the Ranch—lemongrass on the left; comfrey on the right. Chlorophyll-rich foods are usually high in iron and potassium, and help control calcium assimilation in the body. They assist in building up the blood and in cleansing it.

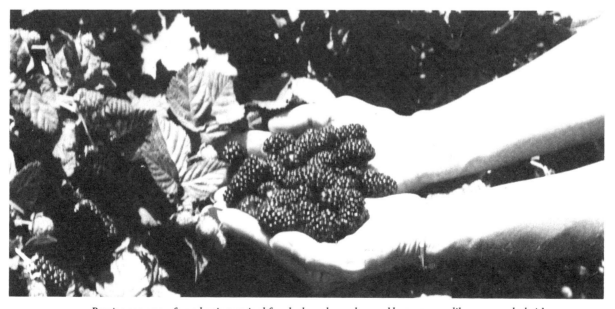

Berries are one of our basic survival foods, largely unchanged by man—unlike so many hybrid or genetically altered fruits and vegetables. Dark berries are good sources of iron. These are from my Ranch. We dried and froze them for winter use.

IRON
"The Frisky Horse Element"

GENERAL CHARACTERISTICS

Iron is a metallic element, gray in color and with a positive electrical charge. Its specific gravity is 7.80, its atomic weight 56. Inorganic iron is valuable to industry but disastrous to the human body. Rust is the product of oxygen and moisture attacking iron.

"Inorganic iron is valuable to industry but disastrous to the human body."

Iron Oxidizes Rapidly

Iron in biochemic form is susceptible to water and oxidizes rapidly when oxygen is present. Food should be steamed in very little water which should also be consumed in order to retain the benefit of food iron.

Iron Attracts Oxygen

Iron works hand-in-hand with oxygen. In fact, iron is responsible for attracting oxygen to the body and carrying oxygen to all systems, tissues and organs. Iron acts as an astringent upon tissues due to its contractive effects.

Iron Must be Eaten in Organic (Biochemic) Form

Inorganic iron is useless to man. It must evolve through plants which organize iron into biochemic form. Although overdoses of inorganic iron produce violent reactions in the body, there are rarely any complications from oversupply of food iron. Excess iron is stored in the liver, bone marrow and spleen where it is on constant stand-by duty for formation of hemoglobin. Its temporary sojourn in the bloodstream lifts vitality momentarily but is rapidly rejected and expelled by the body through the kidneys and bowel. This can be to the detriment of these organs.

"Inorganic iron is useless to man. It must evolve through plants which organize iron into biochemic form."

Chlorophyll Depends on Iron

Chlorophyll, the green color in plant life, depends greatly upon iron; chlorophyll is likened to the hemoglobin in red blood cells. In one experiment, the blood of rats was replaced with chlorophyll and they remained in good health. Chlorophyll is necessary for plants to manufacture food substances (carbohydrates or sugars) from

208

inorganic materials and minerals through photosynthesis in the presence of light.

IRON: ITS ROLE IN THE HUMAN BODY

Iron enters the human body to the extent of only about one-sixth ounce or 3.25 grams—enough to make a ten-penny nail.

Iron and Oxygen Inseparable in Bodily Functions

Iron and oxygen are the "frisky horses" in the body. Without an iron reserve, oxygen cannot be attracted to the body; the two are inseparable in their functions. The principal compound form of iron is iron phosphate.

Women Require More Iron

Newborn infants and animals have four times the supply of iron in the body that adults have. The mother supplies the offspring with enough iron, stored in the liver, for the entire first year of life. Because milk lacks iron, anemia develops in infants on prolonged milk diets. Women require more iron than do men due to their menstrual cycle and consequent loss of blood iron. Pregnant and lactating women should ensure a high iron content in their diets.

"Iron and oxygen are like the hand and the glove; one cannot be considered without the other."

Women More Often Deficient in Iron

The hemoglobin percentage in women is about 12.59 and in men 13.77. Yet women require more iron, especially during pregnancy, menstruation and lactation. It is found lacking in women much more often than in men.

Excretion of Iron

Worn-out iron is excreted through the serous and mucus surfaces, the bile, the urine, the bowel and even the skin.

An Iron Will and Vitality

Iron and oxygen are like the hand and the glove: one cannot be considered without the other. If they are present in normal quantities in the body, they ensure vitality, personal magnetism, charm, optimism, a sharp mind, a strong (*iron*) will, and courage—all of which add up to the power to accomplish. In addition, iron is the beauty element for rosy cheeks and lovely complexions, for feminity and masculinity. Together with oxygen, iron raises metabolism, promotes ambition and reasoning ability, moves one to sentiment and emotion, improves the appetite and the memory.

Iron Essential to Life

If iron were not present in the hemoglobin of the blood, man could not live long; like a fire without oxygen, he would suffocate and die. Metabolism would decrease and atrophy. Oxidation could not take place without iron (hematin) in the hemoglobin of the red blood cells. Oxygen is drawn to the body as if by a magnet when iron is supplied in the diet and well stocked in the body; this process contributes to magnetism, vitality, motivation and mobility. Oxygen burns waste materials to prevent them from overburdening and building in the body. Oxidation generates carbonic acid which must be eliminated by the teamwork of oxygen and sodium; together they also eliminate carbon dioxide through the lungs.

Iron Improves Circulation

Because iron entices oxygen to the organism and increases its free consumption, it intensifies motor force, mental vitality, liver, kidney and heart function, arterial elasticity. It raises blood pressure, improves circulation, digestion and elimination. In cooperation with potassium chloride, oxygen and sodium salts, iron augments tissue oxidation and muscular power.

Iron Lack Means Susceptibility to Colds

Patients short of oxygen and iron lack sufficient body heat and are therefore susceptible to colds, throat and chest troubles and catarrhal buildup. Muscles generate heat when oxygen and certain metallic oxides are at work in and with them. Persons who have much animal heat or magnetism have plentiful oxygen, iron and potassium chloride active in the body. These same individuals do not often suffer catarrhal ailments.

Iron-Oxygen Teamwork Enhances Love

Iron and oxygen are important in conception because they allow parents to pass on the highest genetic traits to the child. Oxygen invigorates each cell, motivates life force, nerve supply, sexual magnetism and reproductive power. Iron spurs the lover to romance; oxygen awakens sentiments, lends enthusiasm, emotions and literary or verbose qualities of love.

"The correct balance of iron and oxygen in the blood multiplies charm, comeliness, grace and personal magnetism."

Iron-Oxygen Balance Creates Alluring Women

The correct balance of iron and oxygen in the blood multiplies charm, comliness, grace and personal magnetism. A woman becomes animated, her personality bubbling, her complexion radiant and rosy. Her eyes have a hypnotic, alluring quality and her skin is crystal clear and blooming; her arteries are elastic and active and her blood is deep red and warm; the opposite sex finds her very alluring. Of course, sulphur is also vital in association with oxygen and iron for these qualities to manifest.

Oxygen and Iron Promote Youthfulness

The quest for youth is eternal in itself and is linked to the performance of oxygen and iron in the body. If oxygen and iron are lacking, men, women or children feel and look old when they are still young. Wounds, injuries, nicks, bruises, cuts, abrasions heal readily when these elements are present; the power of recovery lies in the blood.

Enthusiasm, Vitality Linked to Elements

Silicon affects the temperament in much the same way as do iron and oxygen. All three elements heighten optimism, ambition, vivacity, happiness,

vitality, liveliness. The joy of living, good health, animation and enthusiasm are dependent upon the proper balance of silicon, sulphur, oxygen and iron.

Iron-Hemoglobin Relationship

Biochemic (food) iron is evolved to be converted to hemoglobin in the bone marrow. Following this transformation, it is carried to the liver in preparation for oxidizing blood and tissues. At one time, red corpuscles in meat were believed to multiply red corpuscles, hemoglobin and the ferric element (hematin) in human blood, but this is not accurate; the human body must make its own hemoglobin, organize its own iron through biochemic iron as found in foods.

Iron More Easily Assimilated from Juices

The duodenum absorbs iron after the stomach has converted it to iron chloride through action of hydrochloric acid and digestive juices. Note that iron is more readily assimilated from fruit and vegetable juices than from solid food. Iron extracted from juices is held in the duodenum long enough to allow its absorption; much solid food passes through the duodenum with the iron still intact.

"The quest for youth is eternal in itself and is linked to the performance of oxygen and iron in the body."

Inorganic Iron Damages Kidneys

Inorganic iron taken into the body must be partly excreted by the kidneys, having a damaging effect on them. Drug injections of iron into the blood have similar effects, as well as a corrosive effect on the bowel. Metallic iron has a contractive effect on vessels, arteries and veins; it also affects the vibration of cells.

Inorganic Iron Causes Death of Mice

A Dr. Socin proved the detrimental effect of inorganic iron in laboratory mice. One group received an iron-free diet and drug iron (inorganic iron chloride). The other group was fed the same iron-free food, with the addition of raw egg yolk which contains a highly-evolved biochemic iron. In less than 33 days, the entire group receiving drug iron died; the other group remained healthy and gained weight.

Iron Found in Body Fluids

In addition to its predominance in the red corpuscles of the blood, iron is found in gastric juices, lymph fluid, bile, eye pigment, hair and skin. It functions in the body as ferric oxide along with the other organic colloids and compounds.

There is No Iron Type, *Per Se*

Oxygen is noted for its intense, even violent reactions in combination with other elements. The oxygen type possesses volatile, explosive, powerful characteristics and is known for a broad chest, deep booming voice and vice-like handshake. Iron is so closely related to oxygen in the human body that there is no pure iron or ferric type.

Iron in Food is in Compound Form

Iron is present in vegetable and animal food as a compound, not as pure iron or as a free organic salt. It is a vital part of the protein molecule. The color-producing (chromogenic) process in the hemoglobin or red corpuscles uses iron.

"Milk, as we have said, is a poor source of iron (goat milk is a better source)."

Iron Stored in the Body

Iron is utilized in the body many times before being excreted by the bowel and to a lesser extent by the kidneys and liver. It is placed in storage in the liver and spleen for when it is needed in the manufacture of red corpuscles.

Cow's Milk A Poor Source of Iron

Milk, as we have said, is a poor source of iron (goat milk is a getter source). Cow's milk contains only about three milligrams of iron in each thousand grams. The body's reserve supply of iron is rapidly precipitated through the high content of calcium, sodium, chlorine and potassium salts in milk, and this precipitation shows a deceptive temporary increase of hemoglobin. Continuation of a milk diet for months or years is therefore not advisable. The ultimate result would be total iron depletion and many attendant complications.

Food Iron Alleviates Ailments

Biochemic iron is beneficial for conditions of sexual debility, leucorrhea, spermatorrhea, anemia, nosebleeds and tendency to hemorrhages, erysipelas, chronic nephritis, amenorrhea, hematemesis, chlorosis, enterorrhagia, sterility (also needs vitamins). The idealistic, soulful, sentimental, emotional patient needs iron sulphide foods. The coarser, rougher, stronger patient can digest the rougher foods such as whole wheat bread, oatmeal, raw vegetables, tough vegetables and beans and utilize the iron in them. Not so the finer, weaker patient; he needs finer and more easily-digested foods.

SIGNS OF IRON EXCESS

The Brain Becomes Fogged

An excess of iron, whether in drug or biochemical (food) form, causes symptoms of hearing difficulty, absentmindedness, brain heaviness, dulled senses, heightened blood pressure, cranial pressure from within. When too much blood is channeled to the brain, mental hebetude, lethargic disposition, head pressure and tension, difficult concentration, inability to pay attention, faulty reasoning, disjointed thinking and incoherent ideas may manifest. Speech is impeded and mental faculties seem out of control; a fog seems to cover the brain. Thoughts and soul are in bondage; intellect is crippled; wits are lacking; manners are stifled and one is no longer himself; his head seems to weigh a ton.

Iron Excess Upsets Many Processes

Immoderate intake of iron agitates body functions; upsets digestive processes; changes blood chemistry; leads to anorexia, nauses, extreme thirst, fever, inner head pressure, dizziness, raised temperature. There may be face, back and chest acne and eruptions; plethoric ailments; vascular alterations; mucus surface hemorrhages.

Too Much Iron, Too Much Blood

An exaggerated iron supply in the blood, fluid and tissues can result in drowsiness, congestion, polyemia, moments of blindness, heavy breathing, vertigo, vomiting, general discomfort, internal overheating. Teeth, bones, kidneys, bowel, blood and digestive processes are adversely affected. If oversupplied, iron can enlarge blood corpuscles, increase fibrin, solids and albumin, and force the body to produce an overabundance of blood. Arteries may be in danger of rupturing due to high blood pressure, as may veins, vessels and blood pockets; blood becomes too thick; solids are excessive and the brain is under tremendous pressure.

Blood Vessel Congestion

Other indications of iron running riot are portal system congestion; lack of appetite; nosebleeds; swelling of medulla or cerebellum; inflammations; rushing, ringing, tingling in the ears; blood vessel dilation; headaches; heart palpitation; heart pressure; kidney malfunctions; depressed breathing; polyemia and plethoric symptoms such as dangerously high blood pressure; alteration in specific gravity of the blood; overconsumption of oxygen; bodily hebetude; venus congestion and bleeding.

Loss of Equilibrium from Iron Excess

Overuse of iron may manifest as constipation; discolored tongue; excessively dark feces; brain dullness; tooth discoloration; mottled tooth enamel; insatiable thirst; dazing headache; kidney, liver and spleen inflammation; toxic indications and symptoms; bulging eyes; enlarged veins and bloated flesh, especially in calves and thighs. Reeling of the head, loss of equilibrium or balance, incoordination, muscular control, especially in the fingers, all depict iron excess.

Excessive Iron May Damage Kidneys

As has been mentioned, the liver stores iron as does the spleen. If these organs become suddenly inundated with iron, whether by injection or food and drug consumption, they may swell and their functions become distorted. Sudden inundation of iron in the blood is felt acutely by the kidneys as they attempt to eliminate it. Even though they are not the major avenues of iron elimination, they may be considerably damaged.

Acne May Indicate Iron Imbalance

It is significant that acne (vulgaris) attacks the face, back, chest at the age of puberty, when iron consumption is highest and sexual prowess greatest, especially in strong types of people. Acne can indicate an excess of iron in the body and exaggerated vigor in the sexual mechanism. In this case, an iron diet is contraindicated.

Iron's Contracting Ability

As an astringent, iron binds, draws and contracts as if it were a sponge or a suction cup. It has this effect on the entire body. By contracting heart muscles, it causes the pulse rate to be quickened; blood pressure is increased by means of artery and vein contortions; by increasing muscle spasticity, it causes urine flow to increase and urination to become more frequent. Because the body retains more oxygen at high altitudes, ferric oxemia may be a problem.

SIGNS OF IRON DEFICIENCY

Lack of Iron Means Lack of Oxygen

Converse symptoms appear when iron is lacking. And when iron is absent, so is oxygen. Emotions, brain activity, sensations, habits, mental activity and personality are affected. Manifestations include poor recall, listlessness, depression, ill temper, ready annoyance, melancholy, lowered mental ability; nervous stress, agitation and excitement; delayed mental perception; laziness; difficulty with studies or mathematics; inability to formulate plans. Mental and emotional signs include crying, hysteria, complaints, actions or recreation without normal limits; insomnia and disturbing dreams; inordinate mental attitudes; hypersensitive nerves; short temper, subject to outbursts; laborious study and memory processes; sulking; worry about nonmaterializing problems; overpowering faintness at times; liveliness at night; greater turmoil in the morning; peevishness, nervousness, oversensitivity, and at times, even sadism.

Iron Lack Creates Hysterical Women

Females suffering from iron hunger are unnerved by expressions of displeasure from mother, father, siblings, friends or lovers. This may result in hysterical explosions. A woman may cry, wail, complain and seek sympathy in her self-pity; be afraid of crossing water; prefer forests and mountains; have an aversion to noise, bustle, hurrying, rattles, eccentric moods of others.

Iron Deficiency, Memory Deficiency

Memory courses may not be indicated so much as a diet rich in iron because it enhances nerve supply, brings more oxygen to the system, energizes the gray convolutions of the brain, enlivens speech, heightens passion and soul expression. Red blood rich in iron is necessary for a life of vitality and power.

Iron Depletion Brings Irrationality

Patients suffering from iron depletion are often hypochondriacs, antisocial and uncooperative. Their speech is in monotone. They blame others for their troubles and unhappiness; childish irrationality pervades.

"Converse symptoms appear when iron is lacking. And when iron is absent, so is oxygen."

Oxygen Lack Disturbs Respiration

When iron is in short supply, so is oxygen; and when oxygen-carrying capacity is cut down, oxygen hunger manifests, resulting in nausea, even actual illness; pulsating arteries; heart palpitation; quick breathing; faintness; an oppressive feeling; extreme muscular weakness; great sleepiness; throbbing head pain; giddiness; variable hunger. Oxygen shortage leads to disturbed pulmonary circulation; lungs feel uncomfortable and stiff; blood is channeled through lungs to left heart chamber with difficulty; there is lung pressure in vessels; blood is oversupplied to capillaries and alveolar cells and breathing is maladjusted for air requirements. There may be gulping or gasping for air.

Nervous System Suffers

The nervous system is disrupted; audio-chamber noises, head noises, dulled senses (namely sight and hearing) manifest; nervous bronchitis is probable. Patients exhibit a nervous cough and are out of breath as if from running up stairs. They desire alcohol and tonics. They experience nervous perspiration during the night which comes and leaves rapidly, and neurasthenia (fatigue, lack of energy, listlessness) due to poor nutrition and low vital force in brain and nervous system due to poor oxidation or lack of oxygen.

Menses Are Irregular

Female patients lacking iron and oxygen complain that their eyelids are weighty; lower backhead or cerebellum throbs painfully; head seems to be in a vice, as are the heart, waist, chest and other body areas; they get headaches from reading, writing or concentration. They may have falling hair, tender scalp, sore throat, dry mouth, blue lips, lackluster eyes, anxious face; foods taste acrid; appetite is not good; stomach feels swollen; heart flutters; muscles lack tone; menses are irregular; tongue and skin are colorless; conjunctiva lack color; eyelids swell; skin appears bloodless; pulse is slow and weak. Other signs include hot breath; taste of blood in mouth; fingers semitranslucent on edges; greenish-yellow or sallow complexion; burning urine; swelling in lower extremities; craving for fresh air, yet open air fails to invigorate because iron is lacking. The system becomes autointoxicated and carbon gases build up; knees feel weak; there is danger of falling down stairs; heart palpitates from exertion; carotids and jugular veins throb like the heart and beat faster under stringent activity. There may be a feeling of faintness; spastic muscles; neuralgic pains in chest, heart, nerves; cold extremities; thirst; chills; flesh flabby and loose; menses scanty and irregular; dry skin; scanty secretions; bushy or coarse hair. Bone marrow feels frozen; drowsiness overcomes during the day; restlessness comes after retiring at night; fear of pregnancy and therefore marriage is common. These symptoms may all indicate exhaustion of iron supply in the body.

Anemia A Classic Sign of Iron Loss

Classic signs of iron starvation are anemia, exhaustion, low energy, pale skin, lack of ambition, general debility, night sweats, low blood count, hemorrhages, dizziness, fainting, nosebleeds, acute infections, inflammatory diseases, obesity or emaciation according to individual tendencies. A patient has an aged look even when young.

Iron Depletion in Girls

If iron is depleted, young girls may suffer from chlorosis, pyorrhea, waterbrash, chin eruption, uterine pain, hoarseness and rash following strenuous exercise or work; sthenic fevers; certain manias; apyrexia; face acne; joint eruptions; uremic convulsions; falling hair; blood boils; chronic nephritis; mouth blisters; headaches with activity of tear ducts; narrowing of certain channels or ducts in the body, such as vesical, rectal, bilary, retrovesical and others.

Deficiency of Iron Aggravates Ailments

In cases of tuberculosis, anemia, neurosis, senility, chlorosis, dropsy in muscles, pain in small of back, asthma, bronchial and throat ailments, epilepsy, hemorrhoids, skin eruptions, nose troubles—iron salts are deficient. Throbbing in certain organs heralds an iron shortage, a sodium shortage or both. Pulsation in the throat, nervous goiter and a general debility in the nervous and sexual systems require a diet rich in iron and vitamins.

Extra Iron Helps Prevent Colds

Patients predisposed to colds should have extra iron in the diet because it improves oxidation and raises body heat. Cold extremities, catarrh, phlegm, mucus and moist skin need a high iron supply. In any case, where oxygen assimilation is not optimal, or in older patients or in cases of prostatic hypertrophy, deafness or frequent voiding of urine, iron is called for in abundance.

Spitting of Blood Indicates Iron Deficiency

Spleen problems, vertigo, insomnia, bladder disorders resulting from anemia of the medulla or insufficient oxidation—all indicate a need for more iron in the diet. When there is lung turgidity, spitting up of red, frothy blood or entero-colitis, iron is lacking; when there is itching, burning or tingling in some body areas, similar to symptoms of sodium hunger, iron is lacking as well.

More Signs of Iron Shortage

Patients may bleed easily because of low oxidation; they may exhibit chronic nephritis, adrenitis, acute arthritis, anasarca, copious menstruation, infectious rheumatism, chronic diarrhea, gurgling with palpitation, respiratory strain, tenesmus, glandular swelling, prolapsed female organs, vulvar pruritis, larynx phlegm, rectal and anal maladies, pharyngitis, urea complications, tendency toward albuminuria. Eventually these iron deficiency symptoms may progress to anemia, anemic corpulence or emaciation and dropsy.

Still More Signs

Still other suggestions of iron shortage include capillary congestion, leucorrhea, erysipelas, kidney inflammations, rachitis, amenorrhea, hysteria, chorea, hematemesis, enterorrhagia, larynx inflammation, consumption, glandular imbalances. Growth in children may be stunted (also when calcium is deficient or protein assimilation poor; in other instances, the cerebellum may have been afflicted by measles, whooping cough, scarlet fever or other infirmities resulting in corruption, toxicity or anemia). Nitrogen and phosphorus metabolism is undermined when iron and oxygen are not in liberal supply. This brings on feeblemindedness.

Iron Helps Slow Children

To help a slow-minded child evolve, feed him a diet rich in iron, nitrogen, sulphur, potassium, calcium and phosphorus. Include fresh air, physical exercise in the daytime and plenty of restful sleep at night. In cases of low vitality, iron may be lacking, as in instances of suppuration and necrotic diseases.

Mountains Are Beneficial

Not all patients can assimilate iron efficiently. In some cases, there is predisposition to bleeding or hemorrhage liathesis. A tonsillectomy may result in near-fatal bleeding; bruises heal slowly and with struggle. These types need a mountainous climate, moderate physical exercise and reinforced will to improve the uptake of iron by the bloodstream. People with undersized lung cavities and a deficient number of air cells do not attract oxygen in sufficient quantities, even when it is adequately supplied to the blood.

High Altitude Releases Iron Reserve

In cases of anemia or iron depletion, the hills or mountains are indicated because high altitude releases the reserve of iron in the liver and other storage organs, improving oxidation and iron assimilation, provided iron is supplied lavishly in the diet. Sea level builds a blood count of approximately five million red corpuscles per cubic centimeter; an elevation of 1500 feet increases the count to six and one-half million; 4000 feet and higher can produce a count of up to eight million. Altitude requirements vary for each individual, however, and there is an altitude limit for each person, evidenced by his inability to attract sufficient oxygen (and therefore iron) for metabolism when he is at or above that elevation.

Iron Needed for Red Blood Cells

Red blood cells decrease with advancing age; they become less active, efficient and animated. In progressed states of disease, the same is true. The system may fail to utilize the necessary biochemical elements even when they are available. Iron insurance must be provided via the diet from infancy to old age, as much as the other biochemical elements or salts. In case of depletion of any elements, the system may react violently if they are suddenly supplied in large quantities; but they must be supplied at any cost until the system accepts them and the reserve is reestablished.

"The average person's diet is deficient in iron."

Average Diet Deficient in Iron

The average person's diet is deficient in iron—especially the largely devitalized, demineralized, devitaminized, refined diet—because iron is not high in many foods. Foods normally containing a fair supply of iron may also be nearly devoid of the "frisky-horse" element if they are grown on iron-poor soils. A milk diet (especially cow's milk) is very poor in iron.

Doctors Recognize Symptoms of Iron Deficiency

Some of the dramatic symptoms of iron hunger that can be recognized by the doctor, nutritionist or dietitian are heart palpitation upon arising; one-sided facial sweat; complexion alternating between flushed and colorless, yellowish or ashen; depression, anxiety, irritability, cowardice, shrewishness, discouragement; swinging in disposition from confident to bashful; mountains made out of molehills; uncontrollable weeping; befuddled mental processes; vocabulary difficulties; fatigue from conversation or logical thinking. The mind is fuzzy and the patient may fear losing it.

Craving for Fresh Air and Hills

Pains may switch from spleen to kidneys; stimulants, coffee, tea, cloves, charcoal or other unorthodox foods are craved (sometimes called pica symptoms); there is a feeling of fullness in the throat region. Other deficiency signs are atonicity and displacement of stomach; heightened sexual desire with lowered physical desire; sneezing; dry, hacking cough; dry throat; heavy lower legs; trembling legs on occasion; cold hands and feet; catarrhal troubles; feeling of contortions in organs or of slackness; epigastric pulsations; throbbing in fingertips, pelvic organs, cerebellum, temples or other areas; annoying itches; flatulence; tightness in chest or head. Heart muscles contract; sight is dim, eyelids or eyes fatigued; a blur appears in front of the eyes; eyes are sore, caustic and tearful; sense of smell is impaired; nostrils are tender, voice husky, breath rasping; lung area is painful, as are shoulder joints; sleep is fitful; hills and fresh air are craved. Nerves are exhausted; tendons jerk spasmodically; head colds and coryza are common; arms feel better above the head; stretching appendages is helpful; morning is confused and slow, evening more lively; patient is oversensitive to criticism; fever in head occurs along with cold feet; sight is better in darkness. At times there may be a white-coated tongue, an unpleasant or bloody taste in mouth; extreme thirst alternates with lack of thirst, even when patient is feverish, dry or heated. In all such instances, iron is in demand.

Patients May Expect Sympathy

Still more indications of iron lack are offensive breath; weight in pit of stomach; dry throat and other organs; susceptibility to anemia; chlorosis, pneumonia, asthma; menstrual difficulties, hysteria, nervousness and exhaustion; feeling of suffocation; cramps in the spleen; incapacitated arms; stiff neck; ticklish throat and nose; nerve irritation; frothy saliva; oppression in chest; whitish tissues; white inside of lower eyelids; bloodless face. Sympathy is thought necessary. There may be pain over eyes, heavy head and brain tension, tender scalp; nerves are unsteady, liver often enlarged, spleen besieged; nerve plexuses are hot and dry; sexual organs are under stress; balance and coordination are poor due to cerebellum trouble; stiffness occurs in arms; underlip trembles, as do hands and voice; thrombin can form in arteries; ankles are weak; uterus may be dropped; muscles lose tone; bottoms of feet burn; a need is felt for something unknown or unidentifiable.

Symptoms Difficult to Diagnose

In times of iron starvation, urea decreases; so do calcium, potassium, nitrogen, magnesium, chlorides; water and fats increase. An aversion to the opposite sex develops; one becomes hypercritical of others. One may experience frequent micturition, greater at night; night sweats; heart murmur; food poorly and incompletely digested; rectal muscles lax; burning anus. Urine is red, stinging and torrid; symptoms of neuralgic pain develop; rest, solitude and relaxation are craved; bladder weakness may cause urinary inconsistency; tumors are likely in uterine tissues or other parts of organism; kidneys are lax and tubules narrowed; kidney cells may degenerate; blood is found in excretions; hearing is worse during mensus; stenosis of some body canals is possible. Others tend to believe patient's sickness is imaginary and doctors have difficulty diagnosing the symptoms.

Treatment of Iron Deficiency

Any and all of the above manifestations require a rich iron diet with deep breathing exercises before meals and at other times; hiking in the hills and forests; higher altitudes in general.

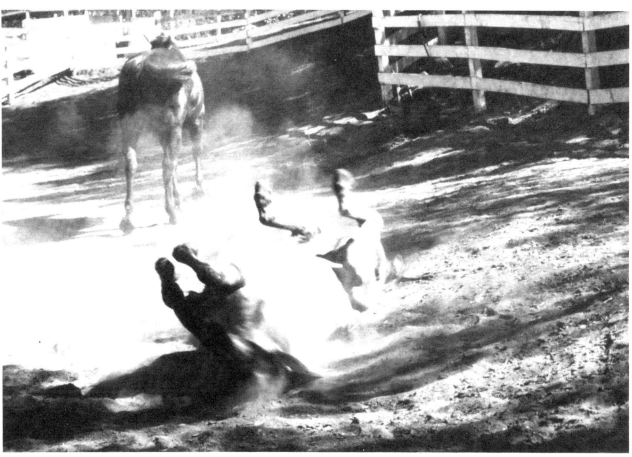

Iron is the "frisky horse" element we all need in order to have a high red blood count. Without sufficient iron, the blood can't pick up enough oxygen for the body to function with vitality and zest. And, by the way, this horse is getting a nice dust bath.

216

HIGHEST IRON FOODS

All foods are relatively poor sources of iron; even the highest iron-carrying foods have a low supply. Remember that boiling and soaking destroy iron, causing a loss of up to 46% unless the cooking water is also used as food. Iron foods should be cooked only lightly, preferably steamed; raw foods and juices are better. Only unsulphured dried fruits should be used.

Highest iron foods (*) include dulse, kelp, rice bran, greens such as spinach, dried fruits, black cherries and liquid chlorophyll. Iron-containing foods are listed below.

Agar
Almonds
Apricots
Bananas (red are best)
Beet greens
Blackberries
*Black cherries
Blackstrap molasses
Black walnuts
Butternuts
Cashew nuts
Dandelion greens
Dates
*Dried fruits
*Dulse
Eggs
English walnuts
Fennel
Figs
Goat milk
*Greens
Irish moss
Kale
*Kelp
Lentils, dried
Lima beans, dried

Millet
Mung beans, dried
Mustard greens
Parsley
Peaches, dried
Peas, dried
Pinto beans, dried
Prunes, dried
Pumpkin, squash seeds
Radishes
Raisins
Red beans, dried
Red peppers, hot
*Rice polishings and bran
Rye
Salsify
Sesame seeds, whole
Sorrel
Soybeans, dried
Spinach
Sprouted seeds, beans
Sunflower seeds
Swiss chard
Wheat bran and germ
White beans, dried

IRON TONICS

Black cherry juice with two egg yolks, beaten well.

Blackberry juice with two egg yolks, beaten well.

Strawberry juice with two egg yolks, beaten well.

Loganberry juice with two egg yolks, beaten well.

Celery, parsley, carrot juice and liquid chlorophyll.

Black salsify, spinach, sorrel, parsley simmered over low fire and seasoned with kelp, dulse or vegetable broth powder.

Black mission figs, goat milk, rice polishings, vanilla, beaten well.

Nut milk drink sweetened with raisins or dates.

Coconut milk, black cherry juice, egg yolk, beaten well.

IRON MENUS

Split pea soup; green salad made of spinach greens, leaf lettuce, parsley, sprouts, sunflower seeds, walnuts, broccoli, cauliflower, avocado, sundried black olives, leeks, cherry tomatoes; steamed Swiss chard, steamed corn on the cob; goat milk and carrot juice, half and half.

Clam chowder, spinach omelet, steamed okra, steamed Jerusalem artichokes, watercress salad with choice of raw vegetables, cole slaw, coconut milk dressing with nut butter, marjoram tea.

Lentil casserole with vegetables; green leafy salad with shredded beets and carrots, radishes, sprouts, bell pepper, green onions; avocado and caraway dressing; steamed collards or mustard greens, steamed beets, dandelion tea, prune whip.

Steamed rye cereal, poached eggs in spinach nests; four supplements: rice polishings, wheat germ, flaxseed meal and sunflower or sesame meal; peaches, pears, papayas and apricots topped with date coconut cream; goat milk.

Barley and green kale soup (with extra greens), roast leg of lamb; salad made of dwarf nettles, watercress, leaf lettuce, radishes, tomatoes, parsley, red peppers, sprouts, savoy cabbage, nut butter dressing; steamed onions, steamed dock or shallot, fennel and mint tea, rice pudding.

Dr. DeWitt Fox of the Neurological Center in Los Angeles, California, believes that the healthy nutrients in fruit and vegetable juices help "scrub away" sluggish waste accumulations in cells, blood vessels and organs.

218

SUMMARY OF IRON

GENERAL CHARACTERISTICS

"Frisky horse" element
Works in combination with oxygen
No iron type

IRON IN THE HUMAN BODY

Ensures (with oxygen) vitality, magnetism, optimism, will, courage

Converts to hematin to carry oxygen to cells

Attracts oxygen to the body
Promotes usefulness

Improves circulation, digestion, elimination, respiration

Augments tissue oxidation

Helps prevent colds

SIGNS OF IRON EXCESS (There is No Iron Type, Per Se)

Heaviness of senses, brain, blood and functions
Excessive blood and brain pressure, congestion

Lethargy, drowsiness

SIGNS OF IRON DEFICIENCY

Common, especially in women & elderly people
Depression, melancholy
Low oxygenation, oxidation
Low vital force in brain & nervous system
Susceptibility to colds
Spitting up of blood

Low blood pressure
Anemia
Slow speech
Poor memory
Poor respiration

HIGHEST IRON FOODS

Dulse, kelp, Irish moss
Dried fruits (unsulphured)
Black cherries

Greens
Liquid chlorophyll
Black berries

According to American Health magazine, hot foods like chili peppers, garlic and horseradish irritate the digestive tract, which stimulates an increase of secretions in the nasal passages and lungs, breaking up congestion due to sinusitis, colds or other respiratory problems.

---

eight

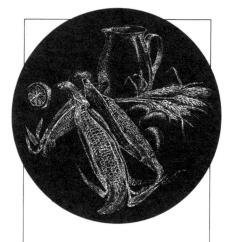

Magnesium, the "relaxer"

When we look at the rainbow of colors in nature's foods, we find that all laxative foods are yellow. Natural laxative foods include peaches, apricots, oranges, grapefruits, yellow summer and winter squashes, castor oil and senna. Above all, yellow cornmeal is a particularly good laxative food, even though it is a heavy starch, because it is high in magnesium.

Considered one of the strongest and healthiest of all peoples and said to be the only Indian tribe never conquered, the Yupi Indians of Mexico use cornmeal plentifully. In Guatemala and South America, too, we find people who use cornmeal as a staple and have no bowel trouble. If we go back in history to the Incas and Mayas of South and Central America, we find that in their statutes, inscriptions and codices, corn is held up as the staff of life.

Corn contributes greatly to the health of all peoples, especially when there is little or no meat in the diet. Yellow cornmeal is also 4% phosphorus as compared to only 2% in white cornmeal, and is high in vitamin E in the germ. Notice how corn oil is popular today in low cholesterol diets; indeed, yellow corn and cornmeal contain the natural magnesium that we all need.

Tension in Today's World

Tight, tense people are common today, and one out of every seven of the United States' populace is taking stress tablets or tranquilizers. People are so much on edge they need sleeping pills, something "to knock them out." Many mothers cannot go through delivery without a tranquilizer. In the past, we had much trouble with thalidomide, a sedative which caused severe deformations in unborn children. The search for relief from tension and stress through drugs has taken a terrible toll. In combating tensions of daily living, we develop constipation, colitis, ulcers and spastic conditions that will not allow the bowel to adequately eliminate toxic materials.

The Need for Magnesium

Most of my patients have constipation problems, I might add, and I feel that introducing yellow cornmeal

Magnesium is widely available in foods, but very little of it is absorbed. It is not what we eat that counts, but what we digest and assimilate.

Magnesium activates important enzymes, helps regulate body temperature and is needed for the synthesis of protein.

Weakness and mental depression may be signs of magnesium deficiency. Extreme lack results in tetany.

Chronic constipation is a sign of magnesium deficiency as are putrifaction in the bowel, indican and urates in the urine and sleeplessness.

Magnesium counteracts sulphur gases.

into their diet—one to two times weekly at the very least—has wonderfully improved bowel activity. What we should not be doing is reaching for a laxative drug that is not biochemical, not derived from food. Even worse is to reach for the cigarette or cup of coffee to help one relax. Magnesium, "the relaxer," is what is needed in the proper form. Children are especially in need of it for healthy bowel function.

Thus, we don't need to be spending millions of dollars a year on laxatives. All that people with bowel tension or colitis need to do is pay attention to magnesium, which is needed in the bowel wall. As the biochemical form of it becomes part of the bowel wall, regularity improves. We can feed magnesium properly, for example, by raw corn soup. To prepare this soup, use 1-1/2 cups corn-off-the-cob, 1-1/2 teaspoons vegetable broth seasoning, bay leaves (optional) and 1-1/2 cups raw milk or cream and milk (goat milk preferred) and blend until smooth. Strain to remove hulls, if desired, and enjoy cool or slightly warmed. Cornmeal, as one of the best sources of magnesium, should be prepared by slow cooking or steaming over low heat. Keep in mind that salads are also a good source of magnesium.

Many backaches that patients complain of disappear when magnesium is added to the diet. The colloids of magnesium silicate, magnesium carbonate and magnesium phosphate are effective in overcoming joint disturbances, especially in the back and lower spinal regions. Every chiropractor should be aware of the merits of magnesium as should any physiotherapist or mechano-therapist.

The best magnesium foods include savoy cabbage, dandelion, nettles, pomegranates, brown rice and rice bran, rye, barley, whole wheat, walnuts, beets, mustard greens, freshly-made bone gelatin, almonds, chestnuts and most other nuts.

Many patients complain that chiropractic adjustments of the spine do not hold because the vertebrae slip out of place again right away. Keep in mind that magnesium is found in the tendons and ligaments, and it is necessary to have a good reserve of it to make the vertebrae stay in their proper position. Moreover, when a person is relaxed mentally, we have fewer spinal problems and, of course, much less tension. The vertebrae will stay in place when the muscles are relaxed.

The Importance of Attitude

Along with including magnesium in our diets, we need to work on proper attitudes so as to reduce tension. We should keep in mind that troubles actually develop us and bring out the best in us. We need to be aware of the deeper spiritual dimensions of troubles, using our resolve to turn them into training. Magnesium, "the relaxer," will assist us in soothing the nerves for calm, but we can support it to this end with our minds.

The moment we take a natural food into the body, an infinitessimal amount of the elements needed are being picked up by the blood; but we must be patient because most foods will not cause visible improvement in less than a month. The moment you take oat straw tea, your hair is becoming better, but you won't recognize that for probably a month. The same for people who are high in sulphur and continually exploding with temper. Adding magnesium to the diet will help to gradually calm them, but the will and mind must assist. Li Ching Yun from Szechuan, China, a man said to have lived over 200 years, told us that he attributed his longevity to inward calm, suggesting that he not only had all the magnesium he needed but also the proper mental training.

The Natural Foods and Homeopathic Principles

I believe that the natural foods work similarly to homeopathic principles. The better mineral balance we have, the easier it is to attract more of the same into us. Like attracts like. We can attract certain kinds of chemical elements through living a life in accord with the laws of life. When we begin to relax in living, we will attract more magnesium to us.

Yogananda said that he could attract iron to his body through his mental concept about iron. Here is a very advanced idea. The nearer we are to the higher life of the soul, in other words, the more we have a balance in harmony with the finer forces of nature. There are those who can attract these finer forces when they merely pass by flowers. They can take in the odor and the color, and that color can be a food.

Again, as explained in earlier chapters, vibrations occur not only as specific frequency rates but in specific colors. We can put ourselves in a state of vibration that attracts to us what we need, or what we are short of. Every note in the scale vibrates to the seventh note below or the seventh note above. Wherever you are in the scale of life, it is possible to pick up what is higher or lower, according to your needs. We are speaking of a deep study which bears upon our potentials and our futures. Once again, we need to concentrate on how man is a unity of body, mind and spirit.

MAGNESIUM
"The Relaxer"

GENERAL CHARACTERISTICS

Magnesium, known as the "relaxer," is cathartic in nature, an alkaline metal which has alkaline reactions in the human body. Its atomic weight is 24.3; specific gravity is 1.75; the electrical charge is positive. The metallic form of magnesium is described as being grayish white, giving off a silver aura. Magnesium has a pungent taste, is light in weight, flexible and highly alkaline. It lends these properties to human and animal tissues making them limber, elastic, youthful and supple. Normal balance of magnesium in the body contributes to a love of motion, action and physical activity; if overbalanced, these qualities are intensified. There is not, however, a pure magnesium type. Magnesium takes the compound forms of magnesium carbonate, magnesium silicate, magnesium chloride, magnesium sulphate and magnesium phosphate.

Man Needs Organic (Food) Magnesium

Magnesia, an inorganic substance, is an earthy, white, insoluble, antacid, slightly cathartic, introceptive, tasteless powder, which is found in nature or manufactured synthetically and is actually a combination of oxygen and magnesium (magnesium oxide). Magnesium forms the metallic base of magnesia. Magnesia alba, a hydrated carbonate, is used extensively in allopathy. Inorganic magnesium is also employed in photographic processing. Man must have the biochemic (organic) form—food magnesium—rather than the inorganic form.

MAGNESIUM: ITS ROLE IN THE HUMAN BODY

Magnesium Counteracts Poisoning

Approximately one and one-half ounces of magnesium are found in the body tissues, and at times up to three ounces. Magnesium contributes to the alkalinity of the body and acts as a natural laxative for the bowel. In addition, it calms nerves, makes the body more flexible—especially in muscles, nerves, ligaments, tissues, joints and tendons. It influences glands of the body, mucus membranes, excretory nerves, secretory nerves, serous membranes and trophic membranes (pertaining to nutrition). The soothing properties of magnesium induce restful sleep, cool the body and purify or purge body tissues. Magnesium combats acids, toxins, gases and impurities. The nerves are cooled and intestines purified by its alkaline reactions; poisons are neutralized when magnesium is liberally available. In cases of poisoning due to albumin, lead, phosphorus, muriatic acid, antimony, chloride, ferrous sulphate or barium, magnesium foods in great supply are indicated; ptomaine poisoning also calls for magnesium. Magnesium prevents phosphates from depositing in joints and other dense body structures. If these deposits are allowed to go unchecked, arthritis, bone complications, gout may develop, especially when uric acid and urate are also found in fluids and tissues of the body, when eliminative avenues are partially blocked, hypoactive or when liver and kidneys are sluggish.

Magnesium is Soothing and Cooling

An active brain is indirectly benefitted by magnesium as it neutralizes phosphoric by-products of heavy brain usage or overconsumption of phosphorus foods. Magnesium soothes and cools the brain and nervous system in general. Sound sleep is encouraged when insomnia is due to harmful gases, toxins, acids or impurities. Congestion and hardening of tissues are prevented when magnesium is in good supply. Osmosis and infiltration are enhanced as are the eliminative processes.

Magnesium Has Sedative Properties

The patient who is highly nervous, excitable, overly emotional and erratic in actions needs magnesium as a sedative. Also for the individual who has a hyperactive nervous system, is hot tempered, overly active and agitated, magnesium is indicated.

"Magnesium contributes to the alkalinity of the body and acts as a natural laxative for the bowel."

Magnesium Compounds in the Body

Magnesium in the form of magnesium phosphate, present in nearly all tissues, fights acid buildup, neutralizes toxins, calms algesic activity and quiets nerves. Magnesium carbonate performs similar functions. Magnesium enters the construction of white fibers of nerves and muscles by utilizing albumin and water. In gastric hyperacidity, magnesium carbonate combines with stomach contents to produce gas and belching. But when the stomach is not overly acid, indigestible materials present due to improper diet are removed by that compound from the stomach and intestines.

Magnesia Versus Magnesium

It is important to make a distinction between the element magnesium and the compound magnesia. Magnesia, an earthy product, is an antacid which may form an earthy coating on the walls of the entire digestive tract; the walls may become gluey, which causes intestinal adhesion,

notably when there is a condition of nonacidity in the digestive tract. The laxative properties of magnesia react correctly only in the presence of much acidity in the stomach. Arsenic poisoning calls for magnesia (magnesium oxide). Magnesia outweighs the food element magnesium and is not readily joined as a hydrate.

Magnesium Sulphate Equals Epsom Salts

Magnesium sulphate, commonly known as epsom salts, combats autointoxication product buildup in the intestinal tract by drawing fluid from the intestinal structures and contents and eliminating them speedily through the feces. At certain times, a warm epsom salts enema is highly beneficial to the colon.

Magnesium Lowers Fever, Balances the Body

Fevers are lowered with magnesium, the liver is cooled, nerve ends and nerve nets are soothed; itching may be relieved, motor nerve contractions prevented, neurotic cramps ended, temper mellowed; pain in perineural, periosteal structures or linings with extremely sensitive minute nerves is stopped principally by magnesium's destroying acids, germs and bacterial life and quickly removing poisonous materials from the system. Extreme passions, hypnotism, strenuous healing work, overwork which dry brain and nerve oils and cause irritation, fever and dryness in those structures—all need a high-magnesium diet. If the mind does not concentrate well; when mental excesses are allowed; or when imagination runs rampant, magnesium is in order. Heavy brain activity or excessive consumption of phosphorus and sulphur foods must have magnesium for balance.

"Magnesium soothes and cools the brain and nervous system in general."

Magnesium Essential to Many Body Functions

The eliminative, neutralizing, laxative, sedative, calming, alkaline properties of magnesium are essential to the proper functioning of the body. Bones, brain, nerves, organ linings, membranes and tissues need magnesium for proper functioning. But this magnesium must be taken in biochemical, food form—not from drug compounds.

SIGNS OF MAGNESIUM EXCESS

Excess Intensifies Sedative Qualities

Excessive consumption of magnesium, whether in the form of food, drinks and tonics or drugs, produces symptoms of defective memory, drowsiness, sexual apathy, mediocre reasoning power and general sluggishness. Nerve matter is drugged and deadened, producing an inert nervous system and a feeling of lethargy. The brain is dulled, mind depressed, nerves hypoactive, perception slow and intelligence decreased. The calming, sedative qualities of magnesium are intensified.

Objective World Becomes Confusing

Sleepiness overcomes during working hours; algesic centers are hypoactive; sleep is unrefreshing; dreams of hazards, death, blackness, craggy roads, frightening scenes, funerals, corpses occur, due to centers of fear and perversion being adversely affected by overconsumption of magnesium. There is difficulty in recognizing people and identifying certain objects; objective world becomes confusing as to place, time, space, distance, size, shape, conformity.

Life Seems Uninteresting

Life may seem uninteresting, unimportant; there may be indifference toward any and all things except accidents, phobias, destiny, teasing. The patient walks as if sleepwalking, dazed, unworldly and not conscious of actions, conversation or others. He exhibits indolence, procrastination, languorous tendencies; low creativity; inertia; quick loss of interest; listless moods; expectation of an unhappy destiny; stubbornness; foul moods with occasionally jolly ones; over seriousness; sadness; laughter at ordinary things; preoccupation with dead animals, corpses, blood and surgery, both in waking and in sleeping states; extreme phobias in daytime, even visions. The nerves lining the digestive tract are adversely affected; caustic bowels cause some phobias; the patient has difficulty staying

awake at public functions; he goes to bed early; evening study is impossible for him. He feels a sensation of pressure; appetite is alternately poor and whimsical or ravenous; periods of gluttony alternate with abhorrence for food; feverish thirst cannot be satisfied; life is felt to be unsatisfactory in every way. He is apathetic toward all; depressed; irritable and quarrelsome at times; sleepy in afternoon, at sunset, in early morning and following heavy mental exertion. His brain is stupefied; mental concentration intensifies symptoms; there's mental unrest at night; frequent desire to urinate at night, but urination is difficult. All such conditions indicate the need for less magnesium in the diet.

The eliminative, neutralizing, laxative, sedative, calming, alkaline properties of magnesium are essential to the proper functioning of the body."

Brain Activity is Slow, Speech Incoherent

The student suffering from magnesium overbalance falls asleep in class; largely ignores interaction with students or teachers; cares little what people think of him; detests teasing by others. Brain activity is as if partially suspended or in slow motion. Sexual activity becomes passive, weakened; mucus membranes are irritated; generative organs are deranged as are regenerative processes; cerebral and white muscle fibers are weakened; nerve currents are short circuited in certain nerves; activities of brain, mind, nerves, membranes are disrupted. Nerves may be partially blocked; mental, sensory and motor directions are not transmitted properly by white nerve fibers. White matter is transformed to pulpy, mushy, putrid state, yet gray brain material is untouched; this contributes to lowered intelligence and paranoia. The brain may atrophy when magnesium is oversupplied, with rise of neuroglia and brain fluid quantity; white fibers are destroyed, accompanied by pulpy, mushy, gluey thickening of cerebral meninges resulting in poor perception, lack of reasoning power, loss of intellectual ability, lack of coherence, inability to control self, lack of emotional direction, incoherent speech. The ultimate result may be mental derangement.

Excessive Beer Drinking Overloads System with Magnesium

Veteran beer drinkers, those who drink excessive mineral waters high in magnesia and those who overconsume magnesium foods, often develop intestinal adhesions; their alimentary tracts become sticky; there is spontaneous gas generation from the bowel that rises to the throat in unpleasant belching; the digestive tract is in a state of irritation and atonicity which often causes abdominal protrusion or obese appearance. Lean patients become more there is fondness for acid food, drinks at this time. Spontaneous nausea is experienced at the dinner table; nerve networks smart after meals, as do linings studded with nerve fibers and teeth. Head is causing excessive consumption of liquids and forcing vital nutrients out of the system before they can be assimilated. Breathing becomes shallow when magnesium is too high; muscles are overrelaxed; brain cells are torpid; feelings are desensitized; sentiments are lacking; menstrual function is reduced; female organs are affected; romance is unimportant; there is a general state of paralysis, sedation, anesthesia, nausea, laxity, weakness. Excessive use of alcoholic beverages leads to alcoholic hypertrophy in addition to adhesions.

SIGNS OF MAGNESIUM DEFICIENCY

Nervous System Becomes Hyperactive

The nervous system is hyperactive if magnesium is short in the body. A patient suffering from magnesium deficiency is anxious, apprehensive, fidgety, overly concerned about work and industry, overly energetic and industrious about every venture. Eventually the patient is exhausted by intense mental and physical effort; his nervous system is hypertensive; cerebral neurasthenia and cerebellar fatigue are possible.

Symptoms of Magnesium Hunger

Specific symptoms relating to magnesium deficiency are vibratory tremors in the head, nerve endings and nerve networks; voice breaks and stammers; unclear conversation; quivering;

anticipations of doom; inclination to instruct, reprove, scold others and self; foreboding of danger and accidents; feeling of impending fate. Near evening nerve matter is dry from exertion of the day; there is fondness for acid food, drinks at this time; spontaneous nausea is experienced at the dinner table; nerve networks smart after meals, as do linings studded with nerve fibers and teeth; head is extremely heavy upon arising; top of head may be painful; there may be a crawling feeling in the scalp; sundown brings increased tiredness and drowsiness. Shoulder and neck muscles stiffen in the evening because muscles are congested with blood; nervous chills play along route of nervous system causing perspiration. All indicate magnesium hunger.

Neuralgia is Common

The patient is emotionally-charged, nerved and neuralgic. Neuralgic pains may be sharp, especially during night so that one has to get out of bed and walk or exercise for relief. Resonance of movement of trains, buses, cars, airplanes causes nerve pains, toothache, nerve quiver, neuralgia. Doctors diagnose such a patient as "nervous." Hermit-like behavior may develop; craving for sugar and sweet foods increases; walking produces pain and debility in back; sex brain is disrupted causing nervous agitation or even modified hysterical actions, weeping, spasmodic pains in women during monthly period. Jarring irritates nerve networks and nerves in viscera; so does reclining in curved position, stretching, bending to lift heavy objects. Symptoms are intensified when sitting but disappear when walking and moderately exercising; they reappear when sitting or reclining again.

Moods Swing Drastically

Prolonged magnesium poverty eventually inflames the nerves, destroys thoughts; ambition leaves; hopes change; desires are fitful; love is fickle. Direction is inconstant; habits sway; views change often. Personality is not centered or grounded; moods change drastically; wishes are inconsistent; tastes are whimsical; resolution is erratic; nerve messages travel spasmodically. Character changes often; conduct is inconsistent; attentions are fleeting.

Female Patient Has Unique Symptoms

The female magnesium patient is characterized by symptoms of ever-changing wants, whims, appetite, moods; psychotic signs, paranoia; fickleness; being upset by trifles; ticklishness; having many premonitions; fearing doom, accidents and disfiguration; wistfulness for something that cannot be identified. She may at times eat clay; her complaints are aggravated by worry, embarrassment, excitement and annoyance. She has an earthy or clay-like taste in her mouth; a craving for sweets and pastries; tingling, groping, stinging pains in pelvic organs with colic pains in transverse colon (abdominal) area. She persists in portending events; believes herself to be clairvoyant; is suddenly irascible but the mood disappears just as suddenly, followed by a short period of devotion, apology, gratitude, repentance or a pledge of undying love accompanied by a flood of tears. At times, food is detested and nausea washes over her. She stumbles over objects in her path because her mind is distracted and very troubled; she suffers nervous unrest and difficulty in relaxing.

She Expects Calamities

A woman patient suffering from magnesium hunger falls easily; this results in part from erratic impulses in motor nerves and resultant loss of brain control of movement. Left side of brain functions abnormally; left side of face and head are subject to stinging pains (even left ear, jaw and teeth). The worst is expected; she fears for herself, her family and friends; she has no concern for past or present, only for the future and its misfortunes; she feels that destiny is against her and those close to her; calamities are anticipated. He is suspicious of loved ones and hypersensitive to the point of tears if they try to help. There may be a craving for beer, tart liquids with a high magnesium content; liking for earthy substances such as minerals, metals, acrid mineral waters; desire for foods and drinks high in magnesium (considered "abnormal cravings"); indulgence in pastries and confectionaries. Severe pressure relieves pains in nerves by quieting algesic centers of brain.

Complications Are Varied

Symptoms and disease manifestations of magnesium hunger are both directly and indirectly related to the "relaxer" element. As a result of magnesium famine in the body, germ life multiplies; intestinal putrifaction products build up; urates and indican are found in the urine; dull headache in lower forehead where fresh air enters during walking or moderate exercise; dull aches and pains manifest throughout the body; bowel stasis results in poor digestion; feet burn and swell; bloatedness, constipation, influenza develop. Other indications are feverish brain; extreme emotions; congested and fevered liver; heated blood; pimples; nerve irritation; irritated linings of organs and membranes; dulled intellect; serious colic; spasms in pericranial, periostead centers; pericardial, perineurial, peritoneal symptoms; paranoid states; deranged brain; burning in urethral channels; extreme fever; fibroids; urine warm, cloudy, reddish, phosphorus laden; decreased generation of nerve force; neurotic spasms; psychological complications; occasional hysteria; grandiose fantasies; anal itch due to bacterial growth.

Disorders Caused by Short-Circuit in Brain

Schizophrenic tendencies; borderline insanity; behavioral inconsistency; neuroses; cataleptic afflictions; manic-depressive disturbance; claimed clairvoyant visions; hypnotic trance; abnormal moods, actions, fantasies—all are caused by breakdown or short circuit in communication in the brain's white fibers, as are choreic neurosis and many other mental symptoms and idiosyncracies. All mark magnesium impoverishment.

> "*As a result of magnesium famine in the body, germ life multiplies; intestinal putrification products build up; ...*"

Magnesium Lack and Hypnosis May Be Related

There are many other disorders which call for a diet rich in magnesium, the "relaxer." These include spasms due to presence of toxins and harmful germ life; peri-cardial complaints; ailments of the nervous system, some of which are caused by acids and toxins in the nerves; gout accompanied by nerve aches. Excessive participation in seances, overuse of hypnosis, overwork in healing practices and mesmerism brought on by strong individual's call for magnesium because nerve and brain matter are dried out, "burnt out," heated and inflamed.

Further Ailments Due to Magnesium Lack

Polyneuritis potatorum; alcoholic overindulgence; beri-beri; arthritis deformans; wandering neuritis fascians; muscular neuralgia; vasomotor neurosis; specific types of insanity; saturine epilepsy; infantile spasms—all can be benefitted by a diet emphasizing magnesium. Poor elimination; congestion affecting nerve ends and nets; itchy pimples; sexual system depletion; overexcitement; globus hysterious; whooping cough; annoying muscle twitches; hardened livery; nerve stress; hysterical outbursts due to pelvic region and sex brain nerve ends and nerve fiber irritation; headaches brought on by nervousness, nervous palpitation; urine retention; nerve-induced dysmenorrhea; ulcers as a result of acidity; acid bowel; extreme colitis; acute enteritis; acute diarrhea; edematous effusion; tetanic convulsions due to agitated nerves; anger; headache following emotional excess; lenticular cataract; eyes tearing excessively; nosebleeds; dim sight; swelling maler bone; motion-induced toothache; catarrh of the eye lens—all are disturbances related to magnesium hunger.

Magnesium Shortage Results in Digestive Problems

Fetid tubercles; stomach contractions; softening of splenic tissues; stammering; nervous blisters and eruptions; legs that feel like water; epileptic seizures related to nerves that are toxic, acid, impure, germ infested all call for magnesium. Nerve-irritated lumbo-inguinal pains; periosteal spasms; complexion eruptions; vomiting from motion; liver enlargement; cervical gland swelling; flatulent colic; belching; atonic bladder; orbital neuralgia; pelvic infiltration; chemosis due to conjunctiva nerve irritation. Contortions of diaphragm with pain; catarrh of digestive tract; periodic indigestion attacks; diarrhea in spring and fall; hematuria; menstrual dysfunction; fungus-related skin ailments; urethral atonicity; scrotal laxity; os uteri induration; prolapsed uterus; waterbrash; hemorrhage during menses; asthma related to nerve convulsions brought on by gases and acids; scalpular spasms; nerve spasms during

sleep; stenosis; alternating ravenous appetite and disgust for food; prostration without warning; laryngeal epilepsy; lung hemorrhage; stumbling epileptiform cramps; emotional upset with related dyspepsia—all are likewise complaints of the magnesium patient. Though they are not entirely attributable to magnesium starvation, magnesium has a bearing on such complaints and is one of the remedies.

Complaints Include Head, Sinus, Eye Pain

Further complaints include bloody diarrhea; painful, swollen hemorrhoids; swelling of labia majora; metritis; tympanitis; heart pains; lochial suppression; partial paralysis of lower legs; mulberry rash; axillary gland swelling; thumb cramps; unrelenting headache; headache which intensifies after menses; numbed body surfaces and other areas similar to partial paralysis and due to nerve debility; sensation of pulling in head; nearsightedness; painful eyes; freckles; sinusitis; nerve structure ruptures; oppression from summer heat; seborrhea; inclination toward infection and germ invasion; overconsumption of phosphorus and sulphur, resulting in fermentation; mucus accumulation in nasal passages or at the base of the brain; wax buildup in ears. The above are complaints and complications related to magnesium poverty.

Children Conceived When Magnesium Lacks in Parent May be Hard to Control

If a child is conceived at a time when magnesium is lacking in a parent, when the parent's brain is fevered and nerves inflamed, depleted or irritated, the child is likely to be hot tempered and difficult to control—even vindictive and sporadic in disposition. Magnesium is needed for such a child.

Cigarette Smoke Annoys the Patient

Tobacco smoke is extremely annoying and frightening to the magnesium-deficient patient, especially the feminine or child patient. The senses of smell, taste, hearing are distorted; there are phobias about cleanliness and aversions to dirt; memory is defective; sense of balance is deceptive; patients are highly reactive to drugs, anesthetics; mental instability is likely and even insanity is possible in advanced cases. There may be atrophy of brain faculties; cells vibrating excessively in brain and nerves; head pulling backward due to cerebral anemia and nerve tension; cerebral fatigue; hypersensitivity to sound, temperature, color, magnetic, electrical, atmospheric, metallic, psychic vibrations; respiration occasionally labored; aversion to heavy clothing, especially wool fabrics; unnerving by trivial things; echokinesis; crying spells; manic tendencies; epholia and additional hysterical mimicry—all signal the need for magnesium in the diet. Children of spirited temperaments, particularly girls, may exhibit fits of rage with spasms. Highly emotional women may act hysterical, neurotic, psychotic at times. Both lack magnesium or need an ample supply in the diet to offset emotions and nerve stress. Magnesium is necessary to calm nerves; quiet algesic centers in the brain; neutralize phosphorus by-products; disarm toxins, germs, acids, gases; promote good elimination and keep the digestive tract clean and sanitary.

Signs which alert the doctor, nutritionist, dietician and nurse to the fact that magnesium is wanting include poor nutrition without a definite cause; nasal, bronchial, secretory, eliminative membranes laden with catarrh; putrid discharges; acidity throughout the body; feces backed up in the bowel."

Overheating, Insomnia Symptomatic

Signs which alert the doctor, nutritionist, dietician and nurse to the fact that magnesium is wanting include poor nutrition without a definite cause; nasal, bronchial, secretory, eliminative membranes laden with catarrh; putrid discharges; acidity throughout the body; feces backed up in the bowel; catarrh not readily eliminated; sour small of feces; emaciation; acid blood; pale, sickly, mottled complexion. Ambitious mental workers may be weakened by jaundice; children may suffer during teething due to extra activity of teeth breaking through gum tissues. Gas pockets may be formed by phosphorus products; insomnia develops due to

bacterial toxins in the bowel; headache, nerve troubles and syncope symptoms appear in young girls; anemia of medulla (chest brain) causes circulation to suffer, possibly resulting in catalepsy; emotional women faint in cars, planes, trains, buses or other public places; chorea is apparent in active, growing boys; dysentery occurs during hot summer months; brain and nerve matter are plagued by excessive heat; overheating of blood inflames myolin cells, sometimes partially melting them; toxic substances cause sunstroke or heatstroke. For any of these conditions, magnesium is imperative.

Increased Magnesium Beneficial in Many Conditions

At still other times, magnesium is invaluable: in cases of peritonitis, bloating, fevers, cholera; at any time when nerves or nerve networks and endings are painful and irritated. Magnesium is not the only answer, but in conjunction with other remedies and treatments, it can be very benficial. Extra magnesium is in demand when the nerves are under stress or depleted; when one is an extremely intellectual thinker; during times of intense study because the brain disintegrates much phosphorus and this breaks down the supply of magnesium in the body.

Negative Emotions Destroy Magnesium Reserve

Negative passions such as hatred, temper outbursts, jealousy, quarrels, resentment, bitterness, hostility, selfishness, greed need magnesium; so do fears, dreads, worry, panic, paranoia, nerve shocks, overwork or over study, loss of a loved one. Such emotions break down phosphorus extensively and the nerves and brain become overheated; then magnesium is essential. The more phosphorus used by the brain, the more phosphates must be eliminated by the body, and this process calls for magnesium. If magnesium is not available, the liver is overstrained, the bowels cannot eliminate properly, more gases are generated than can be easily eliminated, acids infiltrate the body and toxins enter the brain and nervous system to a great extent. At such times, the patient is in dire need of magnesium, nerve oils, nerve salts, liver salts, blood salts, sulphur, sodium, iodine, phosphorus, iron, fresh air, sunshine, exercise, rest and sleep. Negative emotions are disastrous to health even under the best of care.

Further Complaints of Magnesium-Short Patients

Other complaints registered by magnesium-deficient patients are pains in alternating teeth; spasms in children; neuroses; fondness for earthy and metallic substances; metallic taste in throat originating in stomach; inclination to overwork because of hyperactive nerves; stiffness in neck and shoulders; tendency to overlook need for rest, sleep and relaxation; poor memory for details; yellow expectoration; catamenial flow lightest in afternoons, heavier when reclining or first arising; tardy and scant menses with headaches, chills, backache, sore throat, loss of energy; bloody, knotty expectoration in adults; yellow white of eye; susceptibility to infections; sensitivity to electrical appliances and motors or electrical vibrations in the atmosphere; whirling sensation in the head; grippe symptoms likened to flu; sore calves and legs; face and neck evidencing oily perspiration; moods swinging from elation to depression; visions just before falling asleep; inability to withstand pressure from clothing; restless desire for motion; great oppression from normal summer heat; craving for negative foods and cool clay pack on body; restless fingers and eyes; headache from tobacco smoke; legs fatigued when walking; heated feeling from nerve endings at skin; skin extremely sensitive to external preparations.

"Negative passions such as hatred, temper outbursts, jealousy, quarrels, resentment, bitterness, hostility, selfishness, greed need magnesium."

The Beat Goes On

Patients may complain of heat in head, hands, feet, face, liver, nerves, with skin color alternating between red and pale and earthy; pressure on bladder felt upon getting out of bed or rising from sitting position; skin of face feeling too tight; toothache from walking; motion sickness; nausea at mealtime; oily, acrid perspiration which stains light-colored clothing; sensitivity to strong light; brain seeming partially paralyzed; symptoms more pronounced during night; difficulty maintaining balance when standing for lengthy periods; chills after getting into warm bed; nerve shocks to body during sleep; rheumatic pains that leave with action; pain and other sensations rising in intensity, climaxing about every six weeks; feeling tired when sitting; heart palpitation after sitting for lengthy periods; burning of vesicles in mouth; inclination for tart fruits, prunes, pomegranates, endive, celery, raisins, figs, nuts, grapefruit and other citrus fruits and other preparations high in magnesium; sensitivity to vinegar, pickles, tomatoes. Activity makes the patient feel better; atmospheric pressure and humidity cause itching; eyes burn in warm room; neck and jaw muscles twitch; fear of operations is pronounced; headache is joined by feeling of depression and hunger; flatus occurs at night; there is a feeling that the head is in a vice or is under extreme pressure, resulting in vertigo when head is too warm or wrapped. There may be predisposition to neuralgia; coughing and simultaneous chest contractions occur if patient bathes in water high in magnesium; babies may clench fists, scream and push fists forward and up, even stuff the fist in the mouth (as when suffering from colic). Music has an immediate soothing effect but later causes headache and heightened cell and nerve activity; strong coffee, motion, enjoyable tasks, fresh breeze, pressure, cold compresses, exercise, immersing head in cold water, clay packs on head and other areas, violent thunderstorms, running water, babies crying, white cloth, colorful surroundings, pastel fabrics, magnetic massage—all have a soothing, calming, restful, peaceful effect in cases of magnesium hunger.

Secondary Signs of Deficiency

Other symptoms offer indirect evidence that magnesium could be helpful. Scalp and hair follicles are tender; fatigue and prostration result from work. Glasses do not solve vision problems. Feces of children may be green and bloody; tongue may feel parched and burned; strength vanishes rapidly when massaging others; heat causes itching; sleepy feeling vanishes after walking outdoors; bowel movements are difficult. There is a craving for activity and excitement; batteries have an adverse effect; a ball seems to rise from stomach when belching, with sulphur odor and taste resulting; nervous tumors may form beneath teeth; sheer fabrics, fresh, breezy areas and brisk walks are favored; eyes and head have pulling sensations from reading or musical strain. Other secondary indications include itchy

229

rash on abdomen; nervous stomach; longing for hills; frequent urination; burning sensation after urination; light yellow-colored urine; indican in urine; fluttering in ears; soreness, tenderness, itch in lower back region; tingling ache which travels toward fingers; fainting following meal due to gas pressure buildup prior to eating; blue aura seen surrounding artificial lights; stomach discomfort; sleeping with eyes half open; spasms of muscles and nerves; blood veins pulsating in neck (symptom indicative of other elements also lacking); stuttering and stammering speech; weakness or paralysis of thumbs; cramps in motor nerves; crying in sleep; mouth and chin developing blemishes; irritable disposition; painful fears; dull headaches starting in tentorium cerebelli and traveling to forehead, often in afternoon, accompanied by nausea and dull pain over eyes.

"Remember magnesium when a natural antispasmodic is necessary."

Magnesium Antispasmodic

Women who suffer from magnesium destitution often have a light complexion. The nervi-motive type is most vulnerable to magnesium depletion. Men suffer magnesium insufficiency much less often than do women. Coffee, alcohol and tobacco, as well as refined sweets, have a disastrous impact on magnesium metabolism. Remember magnesium when a natural antispasmodic is necessary.

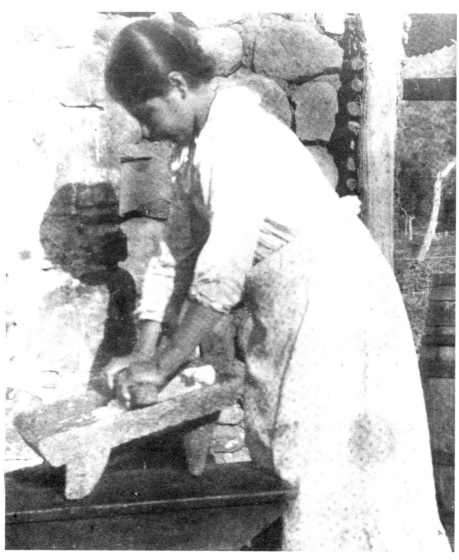

The yellow corn used by American Indians of the Southwest is high in magnesium, the "relaxer."

HIGHEST MAGNESIUM FOODS

Magnesium is highest in certain nuts and whole grains. Unpolished rice has eleven times the magnesium content of polished rice; rice polishings are an even more concentrated source. Wheat germ is another high-magnesium food. Other food sources of magnesium are listed below. Always include yellow cornmeal.

Apples, fresh & dried
Apricots, dried
Avocados
Bananas, dried
Beans, dried white, fresh lima, garbanzo, snap
Beet tops, greens
Black walnuts
Brazil nuts
Cabbage
Cashews
Coconuts
Comfrey leaves
Corn, yellow sweet
Cornmeal, yellow
Dates
Dulse
Endive
Figs, dried
Filberts
Fish
Gelatin
Grapes
Green pepper
Goat milk
Hickory nuts
Honey
Lentils
Mint
New Zealand spinach

Nuts
Oats
Okra
Onion tops
Parsley
Peas, dried
Peaches, white fleshed & dried
Peanuts
Pears, dried
Pecans
Pistachio nuts
Prunes
Rice, wild or brown
Rye (whole)
Sorrel
Soybeans, dried
Soy milk
Spinach
Sunflower seeds
Swiss chard
Turbot
Tofu
Turnip greens
Veal joint broth
Walnut, English
Watercress
Whiting
Whole Wheat

MAGNESIUM MENUS

Steamed yellow cornmeal topped with sunflower seed meal, flaxseed meal, rice polishings, wheat germ, sesame seed meal; grape juice, black raspberries, black cherries, loganberries.

Cashew loaf, steamed parsnips, steamed beet greens; leafy green salad with shredded beets, shredded turnips, sprouts, shredded carrots, endive, parsley, green onions, comfrey tea.

Veal joint broth, steamed brown rice, steamed brussels sprouts, steamed kohlrabi, leafy green salad, avocado dressing, alfalfa mint tea.

Barley and green kale soup, steamed broccoli, steamed New Zealand spinach, baked potato with skin (or sweet potato); green salad with romaine, spinach, mint leaves, sprouts, cauliflower, sweet green pepper, tomatoes, summer squash, garlic and oil dressing, glass of soy milk.

Broiled whiting, cole slaw, steamed beets, steamed beet greens, sliced eggplant topped with nut butter, celery stuffed with nut or seed butter, carrot juice and goat milk (half and half); gelatin mold of sliced bananas, peaches, cherries and walnuts.

SUMMARY OF MAGNESIUM

GENERAL CHARACTERISTICS

"Relaxer" element
No magnesium type

MAGNESIUM IN THE HUMAN BODY

Vital for solid teeth and bones

Fosters cell growth

Increases tissue elasticity

Calms nerves

Counteracts acid poisoning

Necessary for lungs, brain functions

Promotes excretory processes

Adds alkalinity to fluids

Promotes sleep

Lowers fever, cools and soothes

SIGNS OF MAGNESIUM EXCESS (There is No Magnesium Type)

Defective memory

Deadened nerves

Slowed perceptions

Incoherent speech

Sleepiness, sluggishness, apathy

Dulled brain, intellect

Indolence, inertia

Anesthesia, numbness

232

SIGNS OF MAGNESIUM DEFICIENCY

Hyperactive nervous system   *Aches and headache*
Sleeplessness   *Nerve pain and congestion*
Fainting   *Stiff muscles*
Neuralgia   *Drastic mood shifts*
Great forgetfulness   *Overheated blood*
Sensitivity to cigarette smoke *Hot temper*

HIGHEST MAGNESIUM FOODS

Nuts
Wheat germ
Whole grains
Greens
Berries
Yellow cornmeal

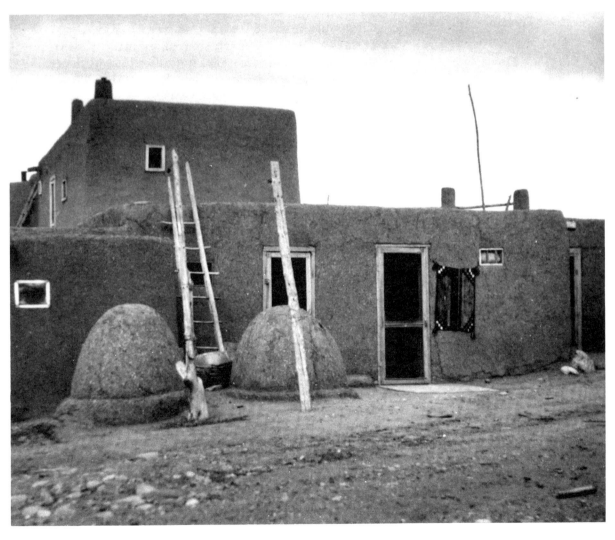

Cornmeal, nuts and seeds—high magnesium foods—were staples of the Hopi Indians.

nine

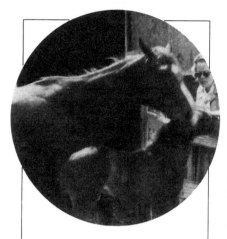

Manganese is the "mother love" element. Animals deficient in it show no concern for their offspring.

Chemical manganese poisoning, after long-term exposure, results in weakness, staggering, trembling and brain disturbance.

Bone metabolism and many enzyme reactions require manganese.

Manganese is lacking when ailments become worse at night or when sitting still; when we have angry silent moods, shriveled skin, a greasy taste in the mouth.

Manganese, the "love" element

I have tried to impress upon people, as Dr. Rocine did, that whenever we have a disease, we have a shortage of one or more of the chemical elements. More subtly, we are talking about imbalance. Suppose, for example, we have an excess of calcium in the form of calcium deposits, perhaps in the joints. Are we going to cut out the calcium in the body? No. The calcium is out of solution, out of balance. In fact, all arthritic people **need** calcium but in a different balance. Thus, we look at arthritis, not as an excess of calcium and not simply as a shortage of sodium, but as a need for the balancing of these two elements.

The same is true of the need for potassium as a heart element. If we have too much sodium, a doctor is likely to put us on a sodium-free diet. But it is, possibly, better to add potassium for balance rather than cut the sodium. If you cut the sodium too much, you see, you will have a good heart but end up with arthritis. Balance is what we must strive for, because without it, we become out of harmony and suffer dis-ease.

Manganese has a definite impact on a person's mental activities, and if the mental faculties are to remain well-balanced and under control rather than unruly and chaotic, manganese must be balanced and supplied in proper quantities. Because it occurs in very small proportions in foods, it is difficult to determine how much manganese, as well as lecithin, and it is generally deficient in the population. As with other elements, it must be supplied by foods that have evolved this substance biochemically from the dust of the earth.

The Function of Manganese

Manganese is a brain and nerve food element often found stored in combination with lecithin. Lecithin is a brain and nerve fat. Manganese acts upon the linings of the brain and cranium, upon nerve conduction and the tubular walls of nerves, the ganglia, nerve plexuses and nerve trunks. It gives us strong nerves, coordinates our thoughts and produces elasticity with quick recuperative ability. We also find it in the lining of the heart.

234

Manganese is found in the bloodstream, and its metabolism is similar to that of iron. Like iron, it helps carry oxygen from the lungs to the cells; however, it is different in molecular and atomic structure, and is not hematinic. Further, manganese has a beneficial effect on the general glandular system by acting upon the visceral lining, the biliary passage, laryngeal lining, excretory duct of the liver and gallbladder, the ovaries, the linings of the generative organs and upon the periosteal structures.

Poor memory may indicate a shortage of manganese, because with nerve depletion goes memory. Memory is not stored in any one area of the brain but functions more like a computer drawing on a vast "bank" of related information. Manganese is part of the entire brain computer system and is used whenever any of our over 100 different mental faculties is utilized. It is also important for mental activities requiring commanding, supervising and organizing.

The Impact of Deficiency on Attitudes

Manganese is called the "love" element, because signs of manganese deficiency are vindictiveness, meanness, irascibility and sadism. When manganese is taken away from an animal, it will not nurse its young. It loses ability to associate and to become fraternal or maternal. Anyone who lives in a prison, any criminal is likely to be a good candidate for manganese shortages.

An incident occurring at the Ranch perhaps illustrates what I am saying. One night three of our helpers were robbed by two men. They were going to take a guitar from one of our boys, but he pleaded with the robbers. "I implore you to leave that guitar with me. It is my only way of making money!" When the robbers conceded to leave the guitar, a conversation ensued and the two thieves explained that they had returned from Vietnam and for three years had been unable to find jobs. They did not feel welcome

anywhere and had turned against society. A few days later they were apprehended.

It seems to me that these two typify problems of manganese deficiency. Good, no doubt, lay buried in them, but due to many factors, including poor environment, they had turned destructive. Where would they get the manganese they needed? Three sources are greens, nuts and particularly Missouri black walnuts. I'm sure they had never heard of a Missouri black walnut. More likely, they had been living on hotdogs, soft drinks and white bread sandwiches, consuming devitalized foods. No doubt they were unfit to handle a job requiring balanced thinking. They were victims of imbalance.

Finding Manganese

Manganese is another food that a person clearly has to seek out. It is only found in the most natural of foods and in foods not commonly eaten by most people. Raw nuts, such as English walnuts, almonds, pecans, hickory nuts, butternuts, pignolias; in foods such as pineppples, blueberries, carob, steel-cut oats; and in many of the raw greens. Baking or refining tends to remove traces of manganese from foods.

Other signs of deficiency are sensitivity to the slightest wind touching the skin; piercing, spike-like feelings going to parts of the head; and offensive bowel gas. Excess may be indicated by clothing irritating the oversensitive skin and by gritting the teeth.

Deficiency is, usually, the problem, so attention to proper sources is needed. Dr. Rocine greatly favored the Missouri black walnut because it is also rich in lecithin. Vegetarians, although familiar with the importance of the nuts I have mentioned, sometimes lack manganese because they eat preshelled nuts wherein the oil is dried out. Always seek out nuts in their shells so as to be sure the oils have not disintegrated or oxidized.

Manganese is used in the buildup and breakdown cycles of protein and nucleic acids, according to Dr. Carl C. Pfeiffer, and is needed in the formation of thyroxin, produced by the thyroid gland. Manganese chloride has been successfully used in the treatment of schizophrenia.

MANGANESE
"The Love Element"

GENERAL CHARACTERISTICS

Manganese has many properties similar to those of iron, but it is not a hematinic. The "love" element is a grayish-white or silvery-white metal; its electrical charge is positive; specific gravity 8.0; atomic weight 54.93. Manganese occurs principally in oxide form. Oxidation takes place rapidly when it meets air, and water decomposes it which results in liberation of hydrogen. Manganese may be termed wiry, elastic, tractable; these properties lend it to the manufacture of metals, metallic goods and articles. In combination with iron, manganese possesses great strength, resiliency, rigidity, elasticity which are beneficial in forging and tempering iron, steel and metal products. Manganese reduces the tendency to corrosion in some metals. Manganese ore, or peroxide, is integral in production of chlorine for bleach manufacture.

MANGANESE: ITS ROLE IN THE HUMAN BODY

The human body contains only a trace of manganese, about half an ounce. Traces enter red blood cells, specific solid tissue and other areas. Its major influence is upon heart linings, bone linings, cranium linings, visceral membranes, abdominal cavity membranes, joint capsules and all joint structures. Bones and other hard tissues are strengthened and elasticized. Manganese also influences the intestinal tract lining, biliary lining, laryngeal passages, excretory duct of the liver and gall bladder (ductus choledochus communis). Manganese is best known for its control of nerves, resistance fortification, thought and action coordination, memory improvement. It is closely related to bile activity as well. The term "love" element is derived from the fact that parents deprived of manganese turn hostile or in test mice, canabalistic toward their young.

"...parents deprived of manganese turn hostile, or in test mice, canabalistic toward their young...."

No Manganese Type as Such

Noticeable improvement is evident in bones, linings, tubular walls, motor nerves, organ linings and membranes when extra food manganese is added to the diet. As was described under properties of the metal manganese, it adds rigidity—in the body, to tubes, linings, membranes, periosteal structures, bones and fibers. The linings of the sexual organs are strengthened and catarrh eliminated when manganese, silicon and fluorine are provided in liberal quantities. These three chemical elements enhance physical qualities of power, stamina, elasticity, toughness, wiriness and heat endurance. However, there is no manganese type as such.

"In general, manganese deals with the following functions in the human body: helps brain fibers make connection, encouraging coordination of thought and purpose; improves eyesight, benefit small-print and distance viewing."

Manganese Similar to Iron

In general, manganese deals with the following functions in the human body: helps brain fibers make connection, encouraging coordination of thought and purpose; improves eyesight, benefitting both small-print and distance viewing. Nerve problems call for manganese; so do stuttering, chaotic judgment, fretting, mental depression. Manganese is found in the red blood cells, enabling more oxygen from the lungs to reach the cells. The glandular network—notably the kidneys, spleen, liver, pancreas, heart and brain—depends upon manganese because of its great influence on secretions. Memory is heightened by manganese through brain and muscle coordination; concentration becomes easier and nerve circuits are electrified, guarding against nerve depletion and worry. It is important to remember that manganese influences the body in much the same way as does iron, performing similar functions; therefore, iron-rich foods are also good sources of manganese. A diet which includes plenty of iron, phosphorus and vitamins also ensures adequate intake of manganese.

Manganese Influences Recuperation

The "love" element combats certain metabolic acids and by-products, helping to neutralize their power in solid structures. To a slight degree, manganese counteracts damage of certain veneral diseases; it reinforces recuperative ability of the body; acids, toxins and germ life are attacked;

septic, gouty and rheumatic complaints are battled by manganese. It is a preventive measure against malignant growths in linings, membranes and organs. Metabolism is balanced in the membranes of joints. Bone anabolism and catabolism are favorably influenced by manganese; so are building of joint, tendon and ligament substance, as well as bone ablution, cell affinitization (attraction) in bone tissue, sterilization of bone and ligamentous structures. Resiliency of nerves, nerve conductivity and transfer of nerve messages increase with manganese. The intercommunication network of the brain is more efficient when manganese is supplied in ample quantities.

Manganese Affects Oxidation

Oxidation of plant life is affected by manganese; in humans, the oxidation in skeletal and ligamentous cells is affected.

"...iron-rich foods are also good sources of manganese...."

Some Uses of Manganese

Medical and pharmaceutical preparations utilize manganese in the form of oxides, sulphates and iodides. It is effective both as a food supplement and as a medicinal ingredient. Manganese oxide is a constituent in chlorine gas manufacture; manganese sulphate is a passable emetic and cholagogue for jaundice and biliary duct catarrh symptoms. Manganese is used at times in treating chlorosis and anemia, even though it is not a hematinic. It operates as an emmenagogue (to bring on menstruation), acting on the uterine lining when administered a few days prior to the catamenial period. Manganese is to be considered when a tonic or favorable effect is desired on linings, membranes, joints, ligaments, galatinous and tubular structures.

Manganese Small But Vital

Manganese, along with several other elements, is found in minute amounts in the human body. The others are sulphur, fluorine, potassium, sodium, magnesium, iodine, silicon, iron, with the smallest traces being of iodine and manganese. Without exception, if any one of these elements is missing, good health is impossible until it is replaced. In every instance, these elements must be supplied in the food form alone; drug forms are not organized nor evolved for compatibility with the human organism.

SIGNS OF MANGANESE EXCESS

Excess Extremely Rare

Due to the relatively minute quantities of manganese found in food, it is nearly inconceivable that any man, woman or child suffers from its excess. Even the best source of manganese, the Missouri black walnut, contains only a paltry amount of the element. The majority of foods, especially manufactured and processed foods, contain only infinitesimal percentages of manganese if any at all.

Reasons for Excess

In rare cases, as a result of body chemistry, temperament or diet, manganese may be excessive in the body; these persons have overindulged in greens, nuts, seeds, tonics or mineral water rich in manganese.

"Manganese is to be considered when a tonic or favorable effect is desired on linings, membranes, joints, ligaments, gelatinous and tubular structures."

Symptoms of Excess are Varied and Pronounced

Symptoms of manganese excess, determined by observation of persons on a high-manganese diet, are varied, pronounced and chaotic. On occasion, patients are puzzled, embarrassed, unable to focus on where they are; walk is unsteady; direction and regulation of mind, muscles and nervous system are nil; intellectual ideas are abundant; trivial matters and details worry them unnecessarily. There may be exaggerated laughter, crying, worry and sorrow; extremes of optimism alternating with pessimism; joyful surprise which is upsetting; occasional fear of death along with simultaneous cold shivers and feverish sensations. Deep, spontaneous emotions cause weakness; cravings, aversions, joy, sorrow, grief, vexation, wonder, hopelessness and other emotional manifestations are exaggerated. Movement, activity, exertion, passion invigorate physical functions, particularly the sexual. Excitement brings on chest heaving; underlip is quivery; nerves of extremities tremble. Feelings become hypersensitive, disposition cantankerous; moods swing from hysterical, apprehensive, timid, afraid to ecstatic, laughing, happy; laughter resembles girlish giggling; animosity intensifies. Eyesight improves to ability to read fine print; objects at a distance become easier to detect. Faculties of perceiving and observing are intensified; intellect becomes sharper. Almost imperceptible changes in location, motion and position are noticed.

"The five senses—taste, touch, sight, hearing, smell—become more intense when there is manganese excess."

Further Symptoms of Manganese Excess

The five senses—taste, touch, sight, hearing, smell—become more intense when there is manganese excess. Pulse is seemingly audible in the ears when out of doors, though not in darkness; there is greater awareness of internal body processes; senses are energized. Movements are hyperactive; the slightest noise awakens one at night; touch by others is like an electric shock; the brain is super charged with tension; teeth nerves are more sensitive; the entire nerve network is more keen and tense, responding to emotions and stimuli acutely. Pains plague the nerves; spinal perspiration appears from physical exertion; darkness brings stiffness and chill; the chest heaves more noticeably in normal respiration; repeated swallowing efforts are noted in the open air, as if something is caught in the throat; vocal chords feel as though they are enlarged; throat walls seem puffed out, but not at night. The appetite may become more ravenous; meals are eaten in haste; sweating is accompanied by thirst; icy drinks or food produce nerve spasms and aching tooth nerves; cold food or liquids intensity the current mental state—an ecstatic person becomes more ecstatic and a depressed and morose person sinks into deeper depression; aversions are magnified. Sexual activity may be increased and the skin becomes greatly heated and dry during sexual play.

Excess Symptoms in the Female

Other manganese excess symptoms may be frequent and copious urination; mental confusion; watery diarrhea; hiccough; warm, whitish leucorrhea. Female patients complain of discharges coexistent with vulvular pruritis; the lower abdominal area becomes painful as though nerves are aggravated. Intense study of difficult subjects brings on headache on one side (hemialgia), as if the head were being pierced by a spike, which may persist for a day or longer; headaches are accompanied by reddened eyes and pupils that contract and dilate excessively. Both internal and external stimuli have extreme impacts; abdominal colic, offensive flatus may manifest. Loose clothing and thin fabrics are preferred to heavy, tailored clothing, as pressure from clothing is offensive. Nerves of teeth ache until cavities are suspected; morning produces hoarseness; larynx may be feverish, arid, raw or even wheezy; chest oppression is experienced in the morning; a hacking, dry cough may plague her.

Excess Symptoms in the Male

Masculine patients may complain of many of the same symptoms, such as crural neuralgia; sciatic nerve pressure accompanied by pain; black-out spells; perspiration beads on spine during physical labor; nocturnal shivers, twitching pains, warm water waves over and through spinal area, along with dry heat production. Nearly imperceptible air movement is felt by the skin; rash is concurrent with adverse moods and actions; cowardice is experienced at times; moderate signs of stroke occur when gnashing of teeth, extreme excitement, head rolling, near paralysis in one arm, and feeling of losing balance beset him. Blood seems to gurgle; head feels heavy at times; ears crackle; ear noise seems to stem from the center of the head; senses are sharp and responsive to emotions; nausea washes over at times; teeth nerves are hypersensitive to pain; full sensation in throat cannot be shaken; stubborn nosebleeds recur frequently.

SIGNS OF MANGANESE DEFICIENCY

Manganese deficiency produces varied and peculiar symptoms and complaints. As stated earlier, manganese is almost never in excess; rather, it is lacking in many cases because it is found in only minute traces in some foods and is totally absent in many. In times of manganese poverty, the patient may suffer memory defect and mental confusion. Teamwork of mental faculties is disturbed; muscular coordination becomes difficult; handwriting is chaotic; sentence structure becomes garbled; memory is faulty; ability to order, supervise, instruct, direct is impaired; the subject may seem disjointed. The patient is susceptible to absentmindedness; grammatical errors in speaking; loss of subject recall and tendency to omit clauses, phrases, words and verbs in verbal and written communication; written messages may be unfinished and incoherent because details of accuracy, organization, regularity are ignored. Business management often suffers, due to incompetency and oversight in commands and directions, verbal or written; details necessary to a specific subject are not understood; chain of thoughts is not cohesive; mind strays easily and is perplexed.

"Manganese deficiency produces varied and peculiar symptoms and complaints. As stated earlier, manganese is almost never in excess; rather it is lacking in many cases because it is found in only minute traces in some foods, and is totally absent in many."

The Manganese-Deprived Patient Detests Work

Any job is detested, especially mental work; effort is deplored; will power is unstable; nerve impulses are spasmodic; mind is incapable of making decisions. The manganese-deficient patient is easily riled, impatient, quarrelsome, moody; he fires employees with the speed of lightening; office

239

managers throw the office into chaos. Judgment wavers; speech is disjointed, halting; accent is unsure; pronounciation is stammering; doubtful feelings hang on; incentive and direction are indecisive; problems are anticipated; the future appears gloomy; anxiety, uncertainty concerning health, diseases, job and position are a burden. The objective world appears sinister. There is considerable preoccupation with self, likes and especially aversions. Doubt, confusion, indecision, bewilderment overcome the patient; his information is faulty; mistakes are numerous, but he or she is not aware of them.

He Craves A Calm Environment

Chills wash in waves over and through the body; energy comes in spurts; din, clanging, fuss, high winds, dissonance, disagreements, dissension, one's own voice and the mingling of many voices simultaneously are distressing. Parents are disconcerted by sibling noisiness; nerves are on edge; depression lingers; dread feelings are bothersome. Anxiety is constant; a calm environment, relaxation, rest, contentment and kind treatment are craved.

Dizziness and Nausea Are Problematic

Dizziness comes from bending over, dancing, leaping, turning, jumping quickly from bed, facilitating suspicions that the brain's gray matter has shrunk, producing a vacuum next to the outer cranium. The patient may assert that his brain is loose, rolling from side to side or front to back when he leans over. Indeed, the cerebellum is adversely affected by leaning over; bending causes objects to swim or dance before the eyes; turning over in bed or pivoting on the feet produces a revolving sensation of objects; dancing or whirling causes such adverse sensations that it is nearly impossible. Vomiting may result. Motion of a boat, car, train or airplane is nauseating and fosters dizziness. Fresh air and exercise is pleasant; sunshine and quiet are preferred. Features may become puffy, feverish, reddened and swollen as if the cerebellum is inundated with too much blood (hyperemia of the cerebellum); the scalp crawls and itches; the lower backhead is heated and feverish.

Physical Senses Are Altered

Physical senses of the manganese-impoverished patient are dulled and blunted; eyes feel pressured from within, causing the patient to close them often for relief; myopia may manifest; optical illusions are evident, possibly due to pressure and adhesive friction in the optic nerve; spots appear before the eyes; eyes may itch and burn. Ears detect feeble, far-away noise that interferes with normal hearing and may create mental derangement. Cerebro-spinal fluid is not secreted amply or is possibly dried up, resulting in shrinkage of the brain's gray matter and dryness which disturbs cerebral intercommunication and deters intellectual activity. Taste buds are erratic, ranging from an overly-sweet taste to metallic, oily, putrid, rotten, offensive, tastes; seemingly without reason, food tastes rancid, oily, fatty, disgusting. All such symptoms indicate manganese shortage.

Stomach and Appetite Suffer

Appetite for food is reduced greatly; coffee may be the dietary staple, along with occasional sweets or acid drinks. When hunger is pronounced, even a small meal disagrees; the stomach may bloat from a glass of milk alone; it feels shrunken as if there is no room for food. Thirst is absent; inner stomach fever demands cooling liquids; drinking irritates symptoms. The throat feels full and raw and the voice seems distorted; the tonsils feel swollen and the esophagus parched.

Tenderness, Rashes and Swellings

Tenderness is felt in lower back, hip region, thighs and sexual organs; these also develop grasping and pulling pains; arms and legs feel immobile; heart nerves convulse, with resulting weeping, light flashes before the eyes, momentary insomnia, sweating, trembling, falling, breathing oppression, fainting and epileptic sensations. Chest becomes covered with a rash, as may the back and face; hands are unsteady glands swell; bones crackle, evidently from lack of lubricating oil (synovia). Organs are sluggish and cramped, due to specific gases generated in the digestive tract; yawning during the day and evening is common, especially when reclining. Other manifestations of manganese hunger are daytime sleepiness between noon and three p.m.; restlessness between midnight and three a.m.

Characteristics of the Female Patient

The female manganese-deficient patient is impetuous, impatient, easily affronted and difficult to please; insignificant matters upset her world. Evil is imagined influencing happenings around her; surprises startle and disorient her; her nerve power is constantly depleted; disagreements and altercations are easily provoked with repentence afterward; emotions are unrestrained. Female manifestations differ from those of males in that the woman cries while the man curses prolifically.

Signs of Manganese Deficiency

Such a patient is likely to moan, whine, grunt and groan when exercising, working or exerting himself in some way; moods are silent; temperament is reserved; a heaviness and clumsy feeling is noted. The brain is obstructed; nerves are blunt; eyes are cloudy and heavy; dreams are vivid; heat waves wash over the body, usually commencing in the central brain area and moving downward to the feet; cerebrospinal fluid secretion is adversely affected; taste and appetite are distorted. Other areas unfavorably affected are stomach, sexual organs, nerves of arms and lower legs, heart nerves, circulation, skin activity (elimination), several glands, synovial membranes, emotional stability, stamina, the five senses, recti-muscles, brain circulation, relaxation and regeneration of the nervous system, heat perception, the cerebellum, objective impressions, judgment of gravity and balance, thirst signals. Bone ablution is damaged; tissue and ligamentous matter suffers; oxidation is crippled; recuperative ability, magnetism and resilency are reduced.

Gout Fostered by Manganese Lack

Manganese symptoms are difficult to fathom but realistic in severity. Absence of manganese facilitates disease manifestations in bones, joints, tubular tissues and membranes followed by bone sores, tumors, throat ailments, periosteal complications and pericranium problems which are not easily remedied. Periostitis, stiff tendons and joints, laryngitis, painful motor nerves, gouty joints, throat and larynx consumption, tender bones are other results. Periosteal aches are distinctive, more pronounced in nocturnal hours when quiet, immobile and asleep; normal balance of manganese encourages restful sleep in dark hours. Light, movement, air invigorate manganese, while darkness and tranquil states affect it adversely. Without manganese, bones are susceptible to gout; bones and joints become painful. An idiosyncrasy of gout is that it is more volatile in night hours when the patient is reclining; a diet high in manganese helps nullify gout symptoms at night.

Further Signs of Manganese Deficiency

Other related manganese poverty indications are burning rheumatic pains and swellings; leaping gouty aches; rheumatic pains in shoulder joints springing to tips of fingers by way of nerve impulses; gouty pains in finger joints, ankles, hips, knees, wrists, spinal vertebrae, maxilla (upper jaw), which invariably criss-cross and proceed downward, never up; tremors and palpitation; poor equilibrium and unsteady walk; tense and stiff tendons; feverish sensations in lung tissue; premature menstruation with stinging waves of pain; late menses, excessive or skipped entirely; stinging, sharp pains in scrotum accompanying urination; frequent urination, even copious or difficult, with urine assuming a purple cast or earthy color; blood sputa, catarrh and mucus; coughing causing pain in the cranial bones; colitis symptoms along with bowel tension and tightness in the rectum and anus making evacuation difficult; inflamed stomach with heat production necessitating cold acid liquids; atonicity of abdominal canal; throat congested with dry phlegm; stomach, pylorus and colon catarrh and mucus; toothaches characterized by sharp pains routed toward the auditory nerves and membranes of the ears; puffy eyelids; defective hearing; congestive headaches; cerebral tension and mild cerebral congestion; tender, sore and bulging piles (hemorrhoids); tongue inflammation (glossitis); convulsions of cardiac muscles; pseudoangina; pain sensations beneath skin; pylorus distension; night sweats due to cardiac complications; aching and cramped heels; anal tenesmus; watery, blood or cloudy leucorrhea; menstrual cramps before period; cramps in periosteal matter with convulsions and tension; predisposition to chlorosia rubra, notably in young females. Instead of being normally alkaline, bowel waste is acid, sour, offensive.

Emeregence of Gout Symptoms

Women patients, particularly gout patients, deprived of manganese foods for a considerable length of time, may develop symptoms similar to those experienced when sodium is deficient. Other complications are erratic pulse; painful chest; constricted throat and stomach; hoarse voice in the morning; heart tremor; chilled sensations; body temperature alternating between fever and chill; heat waves infiltrating spine and face. Sultry weather oppresses greatly; ears feel as if water is swirling through them; breath is hot; cough is dry; skin and palms of hands may itch and burn. Lower legs are senstive and tender; nose and throat are congested with dry catarrh; stomach feels heated and arid; drowsiness manifests after noon; bones crackle in joints; hip bones are painful as if pain is in nerves (actually pain is in sensitive joint matter). Numerous gout symptoms emerge.

Extreme Irritation Causes Anger, Depression, Pain

Prolonged manganese starvation results in complaints of cold ankles or a cold area on the crown of the head, in the left arm, in various bones or other areas. Pupils dilate; eyeballs are painful; brain membranes are bothersome; blood gurgles; hearing is reduced; blood causes arteries to expand; pains are fleeting and chaotic; joints and ankles are feeble; bones become sore; tendons lose tractability; cranium muscles enlarge; other bony structures ache; periosteum is damaged; legs become stiff; thigh muscles contract; fingers become arthritic (gouty); elbow tendons are painful; sciatic nerves, from hips down through legs, are painful; even big toe or other toes are painful. Irritation and dry inflammation is noted in heart linings, cranium linings, brain and spinal cord coverings, periosteum and other extremely sensitive structures; this irritation explains why manganese patients display fits of anger, irascibility, depression, fear, anxiety, indignation and hypersensitivity; it is also responsible for boring, burning, stinging, constricting, yawning, stretching, fleeting, alternating, pressing, itching, trembling, grinding, stitching, stabbing pains. The digestive center located in the spinal cord and other brain faculties are disrupted. Gouty arthritic pains are attributed to the sensitive bone linings.

Manganese Deficiency Ailments

It is worth noting that patients in whom bony structures are active and bone-building elements in great demand manifest gouty ailments when manganese, silicon, fluorine and sodium are delinquent. Exceedingly active bone metabolism gives rise to by-products of a toxic and acid nature. If the bones are unable to eliminate these harmful agents, they settle in and adversely affect bones, nerves, joints, blood, linings, membranes, nerves and nerve linings. Blood corpuscles need minute amounts of manganese, which enters the manufacture of blood corpuscles in bone marrow and affects cementation, resiliency, tractability and cleansing of bone cells. Without manganese, the brain shrinks, as do bones, marrow, linings; synovial fluid in the joints dries up; bones and joints crack and creak.

Treatment of Manganese Deficiency

The described symptoms can be removed when the diet is abundant in manganese, silicon, fluorine, sodium and also potassium, magnesium, vitamins. It is also necessary that the patient be moved to a dry climate at a high altitude and that acid-forming foods are avoided or minimized. The time required to completely remove the symptoms ranges from one to seven years.

Symptoms of Manganese Hunger

Manganese hunger symptoms that can be observed by the doctor, nutritionist or patient are itching during and after sweating; gouty, arthritic and rheumatic afflictions; extremely cold hands and feet; tense and itchy hollows of knees; aversion to touch; downward shooting pains; copious perspiration; pain due to hot, humid weather. Cold food and liquids aggravate symptoms or cause toothache; movements make a rushing nose in ears; periosteal and bone pains are coupled with swelling and shiny joint surfaces and skin; body feels as if it is on fire; hot, humid, foggy weather intensifies symptoms and complaints; senses are duller in fresh air; joints are weak; leaning head backward causes neck muscle stiffness; rawness between fingers or toes is accompanied by increased gouty pains from touch or movement. Motor nerves are keyed up; knees feel like buckling, leg tendons draw and twist; joints of fingers become swollen and ache; nerve pains shoot from shoulders to ends of fingers or from hip down to toes; spinal nerves are afflicted with drilling, constant pain; pulse is feeble and light; heart or other areas exhibit shaking, bobbling, rushing sensations; chest throbs. Discharges contain blood. Dancing, laughing, conversation, walking, breathing cause headache; throat is scratchy and ticklish in the morning or when in sunlight; the scrotal area itches; spermatic cord pulls and burns.

Further Signs of Manganese Shortage

More manganese shortage indications are difficult bowel movements and frequent urination; urine takes on clay-like cast with violet sediment after standing; stool is yellowish; anus is contorted; bowels are loose; stomach is gassy; maxillary joints are painful; rectum is crampy and painful after meals. Stomach cramps and distress follow meals. Patient is only thirsty if throat and stomach are parched. Appetite is poor or absent; pressure and heaviness in stomach follow meals, along with splenic symptoms with contortions of stomach, bowel and other organs or swelling of one side of the groin; the liver swells; undigested food is expelled through the colon due to the generation of specific acids and/or toxins capable of hindering normal digestive function.

Sensitivity to Temperature Changes

Additional manganese-deficiency symptoms include a stinging itch with stabbing sensations in the ears; nodes of the periosteum or of tendons are indurated, even at base of tongue, on hands or tendons of fingers; mouth has greasy taste; scalp is greasy. Perspiration is rancid; stool is rank. Drafts cause sudden sensitivity; chilly night breezes are unpleasant; cold, damp rooms are offensive; sudden change from cool air to heated rooms causes one to catch cold. Face appears gaunt, shrunken, colorless; tip of nose is sore; bones of face are neuralgic; eyesight is defective in daytime; eyeballs are sore; eyes tire easily; objective world is fuzzy and seems to move slightly; fluorescent light for reading causes eyeballs to ache.

Disposition Becomes Irritable

Further symptoms include angry, silent moods; aversion to society, work and business; irascible disposition. Objects appear outlined by a light purple border; eyelids are feeble; patient falls asleep during the day or fights drowsiness. There may be sneezing spells; enlargement of ovaries with painful urination; nipples sore or tender at time of period; thighs cramping and contracting during menses; griping and colic in lower abdomen during menstruation, along with heardening of breasts. All are signs indicative of the demand for manganese.

Cracking Joints and Bad Dreams

Ankles may be cold; shoulder joints bruise easily; finger joints and others crackle; gait is unsteady; tremorous spells manifest on occasion; nerves are unsteady and weak; dry, open air is craved, along with sunlight. There is aversion to moisture, either chilly or hot and humid; sensations of warm water wash through the body. Dizziness comes from leaning over; gums are sore and tender; nose discharges watery, stinging mucus; nerves of teeth are easily aggravated; vesicles develop at root of tongue and swallowing becomes stressful. Skin becomes dry even when perspiration is excessive, notably at night; menstrual cycle may be premature; distress develops over heart symptoms. One may experience shaky hands; nightmares concerning peril, snakes, frogs, heavy equipment, dogs, homicide, funerals, blackness, ghosts, gales and combat (which are produced by autointoxication in bones and ligaments); apprehension and superstitiousness as a result of bad dreams; faulty bone and joint metabolism due to toxic settlements which interfere with cellular chemistry and bone and ligament catabolism. In these conditions, manganese foods in liberal quantities are crucial.

A University of Rhode Island study of 94 adults following a macrobiotic diet showed that iron and vitamin B-2 levels were low in many. No deficiencies were found of vitamins A, B-12, C or folic acid. The wise vegetarian can avoid deficiencies, but must know which foods have the nutrients he or she needs.

HIGHEST MANGANESE FOODS

The Missouri black walnut is the highest source of manganese. Other fair sources are almost any nuts and seeds and the foods listed below.

Acorns
Almonds
Apples
Apricots
Beans, young green & French
Blackberries
Blackeyed peas
Blueberries
Breadfruit
Butternuts
Cardamom
Celery
Chestnuts
Egg yolks, raw

English walnuts
Leaf lettuce
Marjoram
Mint
Oats, steel cut
Olives, sundried
Parsley
Pignolia nuts
Pineapple
Rye meal
Walnuts
Watercress
Wintergreen

MANGANESE MENUS

Tossed green salad made with assorted leaf lettuce, parsley, celery, sprouted alfalfa seeds and lentils, olives; celery stuffed with Missouri black walnut butter; blackeyed peas; steamed greens; marjoram tea; apple betty (apple crisp); nut butter dressing.

Steamed rye cereal; apricots, pineapple, apples and peaches; nut butter made from walnuts, almonds, pignolia nuts and rice polishings; apple juice.

Tossed green salad made with watercress, sprouts, cooked green beans, endive, nasturtium leaves, topped with chopped assorted nuts and seeds, nut butter dressing; mint tea; broiled halibut; French beans; gelatin made with black cherry juice, pineapple, walnuts, apples, celery.

Chop suey made with almonds, chestnuts and chicken; leafy green salad; steamed greens; green beans; cardamom tea.

A person so tired that they cannot stand up straight is lacking calcium and manganese.

SUMMARY OF MANGANESE

GENERAL CHARACTERISTICS

"Love" element
Wiry, elastic, tractable

Strong, resilient
No manganese type

MANGANESE IN THE HUMAN BODY

Controls nerves
Increases resistance
Coordinates thought and action
Increases ability to see clearly
Enhances recuperative ability

Improves memory
Acts upon body linings
Related to bile activity
Increases tension
Enhances intellectual power

SIGNS OF MANGANESE EXCESS (There is No Manganese Type)

Intensified sensation
Exaggerated emotion

Excess extremely rare
Improved eyesight

SIGNS OF MANGANESE DEFICIENCY

Ailments worse at night
Profuse, burning perspiration
Mental confusion
Quarrelsomeness
Headache from any motion
Senses dulled, blunted, erratic
Swollen glands
Anger, depression

Aversion to being touched
Aversion to work, effort
Impatience, anxiety
Craving for calm environment
Nightmares
Reduced appetite, thirst
Cracking joints
Gout symptoms

HIGHEST MANGANESE FOODS

Missouri black walnuts
Nuts and seeds

ten

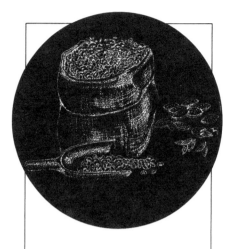

Nitrogen, the "restrainer"

1. Nitrogen, as found in food or in air, is a restraining element, the opposite of oxygen. Oxygen is like fire; nitrogen is stillness itself. Either one separately would kill us. Oxygen without nitrogen would burn us up and life would cease. All protein foods contain a high percentage of organic nitrogen.

2. Our main supply of nitrogen is obtained from the proteins. Nitrogen acts as a vitalizer and tissue builder.

3. An excess of nitrogen in the body results in diseases of many kinds including goiter, enlargement of the heart, neuritis, autointoxication, swelling, sciatica, bronchitis, neuralgia, liver and kidney disease, epilepsy. Many diseases may also result from nitrogen shortage. They include paralysis, feeble health, muscular exhaustion, abstractmindedness.

4. Nitrogen may be needed when we feel confused or when the brain is under high pressure; when the heart flutters and the pulse is changeable; or when there is no desire to work.

5. An excess of nitrogen may result in autointoxication, kidney and liver disease, insanity, decay of brain, mania, crime, wild deeds, etc.

6. Plants fix nitrogen from the air and store it in the leaves and roots. Legumes are particularly abundant storehouses of nitrogen, taking it from the air and storing it in nodules on the roots. If the roots are allowed to remain in the soil and decompose, the nitrogen is released as nitrates and greatly enriches the soil, adding to its vitality. The process called "green manuring" refers to plowing green plants back into the soil rather than harvesting them, to allow the nitrogen and other manufactured plant foods to enrich the soil.

7. Composting is the primary method of creating nitrogen-rich organic fertilizer. The greater the variety of materials that go into the compost heap, the better the quality of the resulting fertilizer. Animal and plant wastes are mixed and something like calcium carbonate may be added to counteract excess acidity. The compost heap is kept moist, and the decomposing wastes heat up sufficiently to kill most harmful microorganisms as nitrogen is fixed. The process must take place by fermentation, not putrifaction, or the fertilizer value is largely lost.

246

NITROGEN
"The Restrainer"

GENERAL CHARACTERISTICS

Nitrogen Restrains Oxygen

Nitrogen is the restraining element that balances the radical, explosive qualities of oxygen. Oxygen is active, while nitrogen is largely inert. Nitrogen is a colorless, odorless, gaseous element; it is nonmetallic, incombustible, slightly water soluble. It makes up four-fifths of the atmosphere we breathe. If nitrogen replaced the oxygen in the air, respiration would be cut off and dealth would ensue; on the other hand, if nitrogen were removed from the air, oxygen would disintegrate or burn all forms of life out of existence in an instant. Each element balances the properties of the other, and together, they ensure the continuation of life. Without either element, life could not exist.

"By itself, oxygen is too volatile, whereas nitrogen is overly lethargic and sluggish. Oxygen has a positive charge and nitrogen a negative; positive charges tend toward action, while negative charges are passive and receptive...."

By itself, oxygen is too volatile, whereas nitrogen is overly lethargic and sluggish. Oxygen has a positive charge and nitrogen a negative; positive charges tend toward action while negative charges are passive and receptive—as with oxygen and nitrogen. When combined with oxygen, nitrogen is more active; combined with some other elements, it is less active; with the majority of elements, it is inert. Nitrogen may be described as preservative, protective, conservative, suppressive. Its atomic weight is 14.0067.

NITROGEN: ITS ROLE IN THE HUMAN BODY

One-Fifth of Human Flesh is Nitrogen

About 3.8 pounds of organic nitrogen may be found in the body of a 160-pound man. Its chief function in the body is as a vitalizer and tissue constructor. Free nitrogen is absorbed by the skin and some is utilized in the liver, but in general, it is eliminated retaining its free form. The inert quality of nitrogen prevents it from uniting with any elements, even in the presence of heat. Although nitrogen is present with oxygen during combustion, it is unscathed and escapes in its original form. One-fifth of our flesh is made up of this element, obtained from lean meat, fish, fowl and vegetables. Plants, animals and man must take up nitrogen as it is combined in chemical form. Decomposition following death is largely attributed to nitrogen's instability in combination.

The Nitropheric Type Described

Although nitrogen is itself colorless, individuals retaining much nitrogen in their bodies (Nitropheric) have a dark complexion; this is due to the ability of nitrogen to magnify the solvent power in the body so that more plant pigments are extracted. The longer nitrogen is held in the body, the more pigment is absorbed. These pigments are absorbed by the skin, secretions, tissue and body fluids; a more swarthy complexion is the outer manifestation. Individuals who have a light complexion do not retain nitrogen in the body for long; it cannot therefore influence their physical and mental characteristics to any great degree. Free nitrogen remains longer in the bodies of brunettes, melanic, dark people and olive-skinned individuals. A study of human characteristics—mental, spiritual and physical—discloses that the blond differs markedly from the brunette; the body magnetism and electricity of each is unique.

Racial Differences

A comparison of races reveals the basic differences. Countries whose natives are darker skinned tend, in general, to be less advanced technologically. Sanguine and blond-peopled nations are more progressive and civilized. For example, the Spaniards, Chinese, Japanese, Muscovites and Semites are more conservative, reserved, less advanced and deeper in soul qualities. They are slower to develop their capabilities, as compared to their fairer counterparts. Their qualities resemble those of nitrogen: repressive, concealed, conservative.

Characteristics of the Nitrogen Type (Nitropheric)

Generally speaking, the nitrogen type (Nitropheric) is a "late bloomer." His talents are slow in developing, unlike the oxygen type (Oxypheric) who blossoms in glory and self confidence or the sulphur type (Exesthesic) who is outgoing and proud. Free nitrogen escapes continually through the pores of the skin, but it escapes more rapidly from the blond than from the brunette; the latter has the ability to retain nitrogen to a greater extent, even if his body absorbs less nitrogen than does that of his blond counterpart.

The genuine nitrogen type possesses a less efficient motor network; weaker tendons; undersized joints and bones; thinner, more delicate muscles; less powerful ligaments and heart muscles; feebler muscles covering the entire involuntary system; diminished working capacity in physical functions. Strenuous physical labor and protracted work is impossible for the weak musculature of the Nitropheric type. Protein metabolism is less efficient in the nitrogen individual.

Nitrogen-Containing Substances

Albumins, proteins, alkaloid agents, ammonia and its products are rich in nitrogen. Secondary nitrogen-containing substances include gelatin, casein of milk, chrondrin. The complex molecule of protein is especially saturated with nitrogen. Proteins are notably plentiful in solid and elastic tissues; approximately thirty percent of tissue is made up of histons, the form of protein in spermotozoa and hemoglobin. The serum-albumin form of protein is present in the tissues of the chyme, lymph, blood and other body fluids; lact-albumin is present in milk; myo-albumin is found in muscle plasma; serum-globulin is the other protein found in blood serum and lymph tissue; para-myosinogen is a protein constituent of muscle plasma, as is myosinogen. Crystallin is found in the crystalline lens. Chrondrigen is the organic foundation of cartilage. Ossein enters the fibrous connective tissue and bones. Elastic is resident in the yellow elastic connective tissue. Fibrin belongs to the blood. A protein agent possessing phosphorus, a nucleo-protein, is found in tissue cells. The epithelial cells of mucus membranes and related glands contain mucin, a protein constituent. Myohematin is a protein found in muscles which, according to spectroscopic analysis, is implicated in blood oxidation in muscular tissue. Vitellin, another protein, is the life principle found in egg yolk and related to sulphur. Still another protein, keratin, resides in the nails, skin, hair, as well as in scales, horns and other horny tissue; it is distinctive in that it contains a high percentage of sulphur.

Nitrogen Essential to Metabolism

The main protein found in milk is caseinogen; calcium phosphate is also a constituent of milk and is essential for coagulation. Nitrogen is part of each protein to a greater or lesser degree, whether in plants, animals or man. Nitrogen, in conjunction with the other three vital elements—hydrogen, carbon, oxygen—is important for power and vigor of all organisms. For instance, myosin, the principal protein of muscle, is made up of about seventeen percent nitrogen. Almost sixteen percent nitrogen is found in casein and serum-albumin; fifteen percent in egg albumin. Nitrogen has a vital role in life; in order for metabolism to be complete, nitrogen is essential.

SIGNS OF NITROGEN EXCESS

The Nitropheric Female

The Nitropheric female possesses distinctive characteristics. Her skin is sensitive and tissues tender; aversion to drugs is inborn; her character is receptive, negative; her personality is passive (true of men, as well). She is characterized by an aristocratic selectiveness, haughty pride, remote and conservative bearing, slowness; she prefers sitting occupations; she is described as obtuse, unenergetic, apathetic, strengthless, sorrowful. Melancholy moods accompany rainy, cloudy weather; stuffy or crowded rooms and sultry temperatures cause her to pale and weaken; as evening progresses, she loses energy. Her skin is clammy, cold; she abhors excessive physical effort and finds arguments and jostling intolerable; she sleeps a great deal. Her skin is cold because nitrogen influences it powerfully (conversely, the skin of the Oxypheric type is ruddy and feverish). Nitrogen types are fleshy, especially with advancing years. More weight is carried below the waist (in hips and thighs).

Appetites of the Nitrogen Female

Generalizations about the Nitropheric type do not include all dark-complexioned individuals; dark complexion alone is too general a criterion. Some brunettes possess flexible, velvety-smooth, spongy tissues or steel-spun muscles. Only the fleshy, swarthy-skinned brunettes with qualities of nitrogen are referred to as the Nitropheric type. This female builds her diet around starches, pigment foods, acid vegetables. Her system assimilates these foods readily: tapioca, corn, rice, rye, barley, spaghetti, macaroni, buckwheat, white bread, condiments, pastries, spices, chestnuts, horseradish, mustard—all nitrogen-dominant foods.

The Nitropheric Woman is an Enigma

The Nitropheric woman is an enigma, deep and unfathomable, mysterious, passive, romantic, dreamy, contemplative, meditative; strong and selective in associations, undemonstrative in love by speech or action; slow to fall in love, she keeps her lover or husband mystified; she demands great adoration from him but does not outwardly return it. Neglect alienates her and drives her away; she grows more appreciative when apart from her loved one; her mind entertains many romantic fantasies: her mate must be as strong as the rock of Gibraltar, an accomplished lover, warrior, businessman, etc.

The Nitrogen Woman Needs to be Humored

A Nitropheric wife distrusts her husband, believing he is not truthful; she uses many ploys to test his love. If he speaks complimentarily of another woman the wife becomes distraught and does not forget the incident. She needs to be humored, fawned over, romanced. Not expressive of love and feelings in words or letters, she becomes attached to people nearby and ignores others; she maintains a close-knit circle of family, loved ones and friends. She loves nightfall, as its qualities are similar to those of nitrogen; evening is a romantic interlude; she is emotional, deep, reserved, romantic, fond of starry nights and moonlight; she often retreats into her personal dream world.

The Nitropheric Female Craves Power

The Nitropheric woman is capable of learning the deepest secrets of others, but she does not reciprocate. She slows a more energetic husband down; she disdains others with icy rebuttal. She is serene, while the oxygen woman is a tempest of feelings. The nitrogen woman makes decisions based on her feelings but is practical where the necessities of life are concerned. She is reverent, full of awe, thankful, admiring, tender. Even though she is easy-going, slow, cautious; she hungers for power, prestige, fine clothes and sumptuous living. She abhors grime, physical labor and miserly men. Men of power, position and fame attract her as do mansions, expensive clothes and jewelry, opulence, aristocratic associates, elaborate decorations and furnishings, expensive cars, abundance. She is inclined to be remote, isolated, serene, gentle, cautious in speech and action, reticent, undemonstrative, slow to develop.

She Holds onto the Past

Other qualities of this type are procrastination, prevention, regulation, restriction, avoidance, sound judgment, determination, respect for rules, stalling, prudence, caution, cunning, inclination to follow in one direction, abhorrence for change and revolution, love for establishment and tradition, enjoyment of horrible scenes. She may plan a trip and back out at the last minute; moving, change and newness are frightening to her. She is sober and believes the world is strange; serious consequences are funny to her and trivialities are depressing. Although she is remote, she likes activity within her view. She is slow in all actions; finds decisions, plans, direct questions unsettling; prefers the past to the future; is silent in large crowds but perceptive, able to recall details of the event but troubled by generalities. She holds onto past memories, good or bad; apprehensions and beliefs stay in her mind; deaths or mishaps remain in her memory indefinitely. Poisonous snakes and other reptiles terrorize her. She loves the hills unless she fears they harbor rattlesnakes.

Characteristics of Nitrogen Men and Women

The nitrogen brunette is conservative, deliberate, selective, a creature of habit, slow in study and movement, adverse to change, slow to fulfill duties and obligations. Any quest for attainments, aggressiveness, temper, bravery, verbosity, impulsiveness are lacking. This individual is habitual, dreamy, persistent, aloof, selective, sentimental, almost inert, hesitant to mix with strangers, not strongly attracted to people in general, inclined to long illnesses and accompanying tissue disintegration, soft-spoken, neutral in intellect, sulky at times, passive, not passionate, modest, serene, suspicious, distrustful, curious; has a cold sense of humor; prefers sedentary activities.

Weak Spots in the Nitropheric Body

Weak spots in the Nitropheric body include cardiac centers, involuntary muscles, motor equipment, vocal structures, vision, coordination and equilibrium centers in the brain. Vocal cords may be damaged by extensive and stressful use of the voice; the voice is usually good but the individual is probably better at playing an instrument than at singing; laryngitis may appear at times. Nerve nets of physical senses, sensory nerves and sense perception are acutely sensitive; thus physical control is lacking, sudden falls are likely and are potentially injurious to fragile bones and joints. Muscle impulses are feeble and muscular structure sensitive and fragile, accounting for aversion to physical labor. The effort of exercise for muscle strengthening and building is not considered worth the energy expended.

Keen Senses of the Nitrogen Type (Nitropheric)

During infirmity, this patient's emotional feelings are aggravating; anesthetics and drugs have a disastrous impact upon the delicate nervous system and brain faculties; diseases and disorders are difficult to correct; sometimes a change of scene is the best medicine. The patient's physician will discover that pills, food additives and preservatives, sweeteners, acids and aromas are always detected, no matter how cleverly disguised. The nitrogen brunette has a lively imagination which insists that offensive odors are everywhere; an exceptional sense of smell which never misses gases, taints in the air, house, clothes, water, basement or backyard. The olfactory faculty is keener than psychic and occult senses; the sensation of heat, cold and moisture is also acute.

Treatment of the Nitrogen-Excess Patient

The patient's heart is unfavorably affected by deep emotions; the liver is poisoned by negative passions and pessimism; in the presence of sorrow, quarreling, noise and stress, improvement is prevented. He or she must experience quiet, serenity, freedom, a clear blue sky, arid air, lovely scenery, sunny weather and an altitude of about 2000 feet, in order for recovery to take place.

The Obese Nitrogen Patient (Nitropheric)

If this patient becomes obese, he usually shuts out others, becoming secluded at home, immovable, antisocial, neutral, more passive and negative. Even the establishments, government, regulations, laws, politics, religion hold no interest for him or her.

Physical Problems of the Nitrogen Type

In persons retaining larger quantities of free nitrogen in the body, certain characteristics predominate. Heat generation is low; tissues are tender; complexion is olive or somewhat swarthy; makeup is phlegmatic; oxidation is faulty; there is a predisposition to specific, chronic, atonic, cataleptic, pathetic, nervous or brain infirmities. There is delicacy in the heart system, in the motor, cerebellar, visual and voice areas, in the equilibrium and auditory centers. Vitality and normal functions are often hindered; blood is short of fibrin and specific alkaline elements; calcium and silicon are deficient in some solid tissues; protein is in short supply in muscles; involuntary muscles are feeble; rejuvenation ability of the body is inefficient; tissues are frail, sensitive and may develop internal growths.

Manifestations of Pain and Weakness

Other nitrogen-excess manifestations include lethargy, death-like sleep; maladies of parotid glands, cervical glands or groin glands; loose teeth; quivering spells; waterbrash; bowel convulsions and constrictions; groin swelling; dyspnea; catarrh which is difficult to remedy; acute neuritis appearing and disappearing spontaneously; rheumatic pains soothed by cold water and vinegar compresses; hand and foot swelling; feebleness of arms; weakness in knees, fingers, back, ankles; sensations of numbness; a phlegmatic type of consumption; a rolling inner motion caused by specific body gases; abscesses and/or respiratory complications.

Healing is Slow

Fractures, wounds, cuts, abrasions, burns, scalds, boils, sores fail to heal well. Throat troubles develop, as do sciatic pains, rheumatic heart valve and intestinal disintegration of food, which causes nausea and bile-related headaches. There may be chilled feet; menstrual hemorrhages; congestive and defective, oxygen-based pneumonia; nervous debility; paralysis or numbness of part of the motor neurons of the cerebral cortex nerve departments; enteralgia; tetanus of flexors; phlebitis; venous throbbing; contusions; effusion into synovial sacs of joints; eye and vision complications; unexplainable exhaustion; hernia; phlebismus; obesity of phlegmatic origin; swollen glands; blood fermentation; ruptures. All of the above infirmities indicate excessive nitrogen consumption.

Ailments of the Nitrogen-Excess Patient

The ailments of the nitrogen type are opposite those of the oxygen individual; nitrogen is cold and oxygen on fire, so to speak. In the nitrogen type, liver, kidneys and intestines are overworked and are usually massive. Bones and joints are highly susceptible to injury. Eustacian tubes are often blocked, causing hearing difficulties. The eliminative channels as a whole are overtaxed, so diseases are readily contracted. The entire body runs at a subnormal rate; blood pressure is low. Symptoms include states of unconsciousness, mental melancholy, fears and anxieties; swooning after extreme mental effort; severe absentmindedness; headaches on one side; sleepiness; sneezing coryza; feebleness; dropsical puffiness; necrosis in times of disease; heart dilation; nausea spells; suffocation sensations and wheezing asthma during sleep in the lower side of the body. There are also likely to be acute fevers, bronchitis, typhoid-pneumonia, rheumatic pleuritis, humid asthma, perspiration of palms of hands, lethargy, glandular dysfunctions, nephralgia, mental confusion, uncontrollable discharges, metritis; anoxemia in high or low altitudes, due to superfluous generation of carbonic acid in the body, or when carbonic acid is found in the air or when free nitrogen is retained excessively in the body.

Vital Immunity is Deficient

The nitrogen-excess patient contracts typhoid readily; his vital immunity is deficient; involuntary muscles are feeble; infections develop easily, as do cramps and neuralgic symptoms; neuralgia is commonplace in the nitrogen type. There may be infrequent intestinal stasis or stasis of heart, lungs, liver or muscles, or other signs of sluggishness in the body; anemia heart failure due to medulla anemia and cardiac contractions; epileptic vertigo; uterine or intestinal hemorrhages which develop spontaneously.

The Nitrogen Type Generates A Harmful Acid

The nitrogen type generates a certain acid that attacks the ligaments, capsules, bone linings, certain sensory and motor nerves and some muscles, notably the trapezius, deltoid and some neck muscles. Ligaments exhibit pain and tension, usually in the plantar cunecuboid, in long plantar or in tarsus ligaments. This acid is also at the basis of neuritis, sciatica, rheumatic aches, neuralgia, headache, heart failure, cataleptic stages, sleepiness, memory failure, sluggishness, paralysis and numbness and other nitrogen-type afflictions. A general soreness in muscular tissue is due to acid production; this soreness may result in trembling, feebleness or swooning spells.

Symptoms of Nitrogen Excess

The Nitropheric type is subject to being affected by the rolling, swaying, swimming movement of boats, ships, swings, trains, airplanes. Further symptoms resulting from excessive nitrogen retention in the tissues include thrombosis, aching pubic bones, morning diarrhea, catarrh of membranes, psychical moods, phobias, fantasies— due to the inherent sentimental qualities and imagination of the nitrogen type. Prolonged imprisonment of free nitrogen makes such a patient very susceptible to the influence of drugs, anesthetics, disease fumes, metallic acids, malarial taints, food preservatives and additives, offensive odors from septic tanks, wells or garbage collection areas. Powerful drugs disturb the sensitive nervous system and lead to later serious diseases. The female Nitropheric type particularly should avoid drugs and surgery, which may result in massive hemorrhaging, blood poisoning, infection, gangrene, nerve shock and ultimately death.

Phobias and Weaknesses

There may be nerve shock from apprehension, sorrow, failures, grotesque sights, hideous reptiles, savage animals, bloody operations or accidents or any experience that shocks their high-strung nerves and emotional soul characteristics. Extreme phobias may lead to a form of epilepsy. There is a possibility of nerve center paralysis, cerebro-emotive center paralysis, as the sensory-motive system dominates the motor system. The Nitropheric woman's reproductive system is weak and miscarriages are possible. If nitrogen is inadvertently held for lengthy periods, the imaginative, emotive, intellectual centers of the brain may become distorted, with abstraction being the result.

Individual patients may differ in manifested symptoms, but the basic causes and disease inclinations are similar.

SIGNS OF NITROGEN DEFICIENCY

Reasons for Nitrogen Deficiency

Nitrogen deficiency may originate from two sources, either from organic causes or due to lack of free nitrogen retention. A certain type of individual is unable to retain free nitrogen for any length of time in the body. When free nitrogen is short in the air or fails to remain in the body, the effects upon the patient are evident in mind, passions, inclinations, enterprises, thoughts and goals.

Oxygen-Nitrogen Relationship

Patients who consume excessive oxygen, do not retain sufficient nitrogen in their bodies; oxygen has control of the body and functions much like a prairie fire out of control. Such an idividual, then, does not have control of his emotions, thoughts, inclinations; he is observed to be fiery, energetic, vivacious and passionate. His speech is too fast; he rushes through life with no concern for the results of his actions, thoughts, passions, emotions. He is incapable of staying with any one thing for long; he is restless, tempestuous, volatile, explosive, chaotic and undependable.

Nitrogen-Deprived Patient A Hypochondriac

The patient suffering from nitrogen hunger is a hypochondriac: every little ache is exaggerated and observers would assume him or her to be dying. Tendencies are extreme and hyperbolic: either worthy of heaven or deserving of hell; black or white, with nothing in the middle. The patient is subject to extreme variations in mind, nerves, body functions, causing excitement, overindulgence and superfluous rush of blood to those brain faculties which are active; such an excessive flood of blood to any area of the body or brain produces hyperemia and causes the current thoughts, activities, feelings, emotions, goals, mental state, romantic inclinations to become overpronounced. The mind is changeable. On occasion, an individual may become so agitated that intracranial pressure is produced with such intensity that a momentary mental breakdown or temporary insanity is the result.

Characteristics of Nitrogen-Deficient Patient

This patient's career is chaotic, his actions unpredictable; he is occasionally subject to drinking spells; he overreacts to love, disappointments, unhappiness, anger, animosity, investments, interpretations, comments. His optimism is rapturous and his depression destructive; he is funny when happy, enthusiastic when enthralled, overzealous if activity is pleasurable. His body is under the influence of exaggerated alterations: he dives into business; he invests intemperately; he views work as play and vice-versa; he may also confuse success with failure. An elopement with quick regrets would be typical.

Passion and Temper Manifest

When nitrogen is lacking, oxygen characteristics are pronounced. Hence, the patient may disregard conventionality and social etiquette in favor of rash behavior, familiarity, impatient and impulsive actions. His attention is secured quickly but just as quickly vanishes; temper outbursts follow in rapid succession; moods are fickle; passions are intense, ardent. He is tactless in speech, animated in gesture, restless in mind. He is inattentive, irrational, incongruous, unsettled, verbose, explosive, inclined to travel; overly strict or overly flexible, he is unable to achieve balance. He has little or no patience; impulses rule him because the repressive, restraining nitrogen is absent; inner fantasies, inclinations, aversions, preferences, moods overwhelm him. His personality, thoughts, emotions, impulses, goals change incessantly; he tends to speak excessively or remain excessively silent.

Physical Results of Nitrogen Deficiency

When nitrogen agents are insufficient in the tissues, albumin-uria manifests; tissues refuse to accept albumin and it cannot be utilized; tissues become protein deficient. Though the causes may be numerous, the principal cause is inability of tissues to assimilate and metabolize nitrogen substances. Purpura, scurvy, sepsis, pyrexia, anemia, phlegmosis, toxic-laden blood, lead accumulation, epilepsy, dyspepsia, extreme mental and physical strain, pregnancy when the woman is in weakened condition—all may result in albumin-uria due to systematic weakness and inability of tissues to utilize nitrogen. Sexual functions are also disrupted when

there is lack of nitrogen; leucorrhea, spermatorrhea, sterility and impotence are possible indications.

Paralysis and Blood Clots A Danger

Inability of tissues to utilize nitrogen may result in prostration (exhausted muscular force). If prostration is not corrected, the outcome may be paresis, which may terminate in paralysis. Symptoms of encroaching paralysis include weakness in the muscular system, paralytic numbness, fatigue, sore muscles, paresthesia, gastric sourness, peritoneal tenderness, acid production, analgesia, stumbling and writer's cramp. When cerebellar force is deficient, nitrogen cannot be metabolized; body heat is not balanced; blood clots (thrombi) may develop, causing complications in the spinal cord, brain, blood pockets and motor and mental activities with resultant suffering, insanity and ultimate death. Any agent disruptive to nitrogen metabolism may culminate in albuminuria, insanity and paralysis.

"The body mechanics are chiefly motor, muscular and cerebellar. When nitrogen metabolism is optimum, vitality is great; if the reverse is true, the brain is likely to manifest a weakness."

Muscles, Membranes and Tissue Metabolism Affected

Many agents are destructive to nitrogen metabolism, including: drugs such as arsenic; syphilus and gonorrhea (which also destroy cerebellar energy and specific tissue salts); insanity and mental disorders such as periodic, impulsive, confusional, hereditary, paralytic, hysteric, epileptic, volitional. A patient displaying inherent weakness in nitrogen metabolism may suffer from prostration, muscular tremor, paresis, albuminuria, sexual neuresthenia, myodemia, feeblemindedness, muscular tremors, muscle softening, paralysis, neuralgic rheumatism, myonosus, compensatory hypertrophy, myopia, pericarditis, insanity, myalgia, hernia, muscular induration, palsy, myosis, connective tissue inflammation, muscular tension, stricture, contraction of specific canals, tetanus, contraction of reflexes or of motor nerves or of the cerebellum itself, tonic muscle spasms, membrane inflammation and many other maladies.

Nitrogen Affects Vitality

The body mechanics are chiefly motor, muscular and cerebellar. When nitrogen metabolism is optimum, vitality is great; if the reverse is true, the brain is likely to manifest a weakness; also noted may be asthenia in nerves, sluggish intellect, muscular default, weak will, lack of ambition, feeble body, atonic sinews, blood clots, weak sexuality, dull mind, coarse thoughts, lack of ambition and effort, ill-advised judgment, idle comments. If nitrogen metabolism is optimal, the individual is alert and intelligent; when the reverse is true, the person is dull, apathetic, slow, absent-minded or contemplative.

Nitrogen Balances and Soothes

Without nitrogen, protein could not exist. Nitrogen adds regulation, strength and vitality to life. Without it, oxygen would rage through the universe, burning up all in its path. Nitrogen balances the explosive qualities of life. In times when sedatives, tranquilizers, suppressants are common, a diet rich in nitrogen is indicated, as it is a natural tranquilizer and sedative, calming and soothing nerves and inducing restful sleep; its effects reach tissues, blood, brain and organic functions. Nitrogen is dominant in a serene disposition, in an individual with quiet nerves, a still mind, a reserved manner, an olive complexion, organized thoughts and powerful protein metabolism. Nitrogen is lacking in cases of tense nerves, excessive fever, muscular weakness, mental turmoil, high brain pressure, chaotic functions, erratic pulse rate, heart palpitation, reckless tendencies, temper and cases of anemia in some parts of the body and hyperemia in others; a diet high in nitrogen is clearly indicated, as is a climate facilitating greater nitrogen influence on blood and body activities.

Symptoms of Nitrogen Lack

In cases in which men are inclined toward turbulent actions, drinking excesses, ecstasy one moment and depression the next; overcheerfulness followed by deep melancholy; overly influential ideas, urges, emotions, inclinations; being ruled by impulses, business, romance, quarrels rather than by sound judgment, reason, common sense, the wisdom of others' experience or the examples of balanced persons; fads and fantasies; temper; contempt for tradition and the establishment; instability; idealism; dizziness; extremes in actions and notions, in sorrow, illness, fever, discontent, failure; imbalance—all are indications that nitrogen foods are in demand, as is a climate with a nitropheric atmosphere: a low altitude with nitrate-rich earth, warm temperature; a climate conducive to healthy nerves, sweating, evaporation, elimination and increased nitrogen assimilation in skin and tissues; a climate which encourages nitrogen to remain longer in the body for its restraining, repressive, tranquilizing, calming qualities; a place where more urea is expelled and urine's specific gravity is stable.

Loss of Free Movement and Energy

The holding power for free nitrogen is diminished when albumin is found in the urine, indicating that tissues are rejecting the albumin. Symptoms include urea registering excessively high or low (briefly); specific gravity of the urine being overly high or low; dropsy symptoms; feebleness of some sexual system activities; numbness, exhaustion, prostration, paralysis; a certain form of autointoxication; muscular quivering; hysterical inclinations; sensations of prickling in the skin and tissues. Thin persons lose weight and become sicker; tumors develop; muscle tissues disintegrate. Chiropractic adjustments and deep massage are helpful, if not essential, in treating loss of free movement, poor muscle tone, tension, contraction, pain and soreness, heat, fever and inflammation. Blood clots develop in vessels, endangering brain, spinal cord and vital functions. There is lassitude in motor nerves, lack of energy and vitality, feebleness in the brain, dull intellectual processes, absentmindedness due to low nerve force and vital energy, buzzing in the ears, coldness or fever in the limbs, aching eyes, paralyzed or numb tongue, stiff eyelids, aches in joints or tendons, colic and convulsive pains in the stomach, difficult urination, exhaustion of nerves, superfluous or nonexistent action in some organ or body function. A nitrogen diet is imperative because nitrogen metabolism is deficient.

Complications from Poor Nitrogen Metabolism

The doctor must be cognizant of the fact that when free nitrogen remains too briefly in the body, brain, muscles, nerves, blood, tissues throughout the body become overheated, fevered, agitated and excessive in activities which precipitate sodium salts at an alarming rate or they are removed from the body by excessive water consumption; dyspepsia and gas formation in the digestive tract result. If nitrogen metabolism is deficient in the tissues for a prolonged period of time without correction, the results are albuminuria, suppuration, exhaustion, insanity, dropsy, paralysis, paresis, impotence; death may ensue in spite of medical and surgical efforts; nor will osteopathy or chiropractic manipulation rescue the patient. Unless the right scientific diet is utilized, along with a good climate, enjoyable and manageable work and the services of a good nutritionist or doctor, the patient is unlikely to recover.

Treatment of Nitrogen Deficiency

Diet alone will not remedy the condition; and drugs only mask symptoms temporarily. Free nitrogen is essential, but inorganic nitrogen is not advisable. A warm, balmy climate is beneficial, as in parts of California, Egypt, the Mediterranean coast, regions of Italy, Algieria, parts of Florida. Such locations with low altitude and lush vegetation encourage improved nitrogen metabolism and longer nitrogen retention in the body.

HIGHEST NITROGEN FOODS

Foods high in nitrogen are high-protein foods. They include:

Almonds	Peas, dried
Beans (dried lima, French kidney, garbanzo, horse, navy, pinto, soy)	Pignolia nuts
Blackeyed peas	Quail
Bluefish	Red snapper
Butternuts	Salmon
Caviar	Sardines
Cheeses (cheddar, cottage, cream, goat, limburger, roquefort, skimmed milk, Swiss)	Sea bass
Chicken (tough meat)	Tunafish
Codfish and cod roe	Turbot
Gelatin	Turkey
Haddock	Veal, lean
Halibut	Veal Joint jelly
Herring	Walnuts
Lamb and mutton	Whitefish
Lentils	Whiting

NITROGEN MENUS

Broiled bass, tomato juice and cod roe, green salad with assorted sprouted seeds and beans, roquefort dressing, celery stuffed with almond butter, steamed broccoli, fish bone broth; gelatin mold with walnuts, apples and pineapple.

Veal joint broth, lentil casserole, green salad with assorted sprouts, chilled three-bean salad, steamed asparagus, steamed eggplant and tomatoes, cottage cheese dressing, cheese sauce.

Leg of lamb, chicken bone broth, green salad with sprouts, julienne Swiss and jack cheeses, steamed green kale, steamed beets, celery stuffed with walnut butter, nut butter and caraway dressing.

Goat cottage cheese, goat cheese, Swiss cheese, cheddar cheese, mixed nuts or nut butter, sesame seed crackers, almond nut milk drink, persimmons, apricots and papaya slices.

SUMMARY OF NITROGEN

GENERAL CHARACTERISTICS

"Restrainer" element	*Makes up 4/5 of atmosphere*
Largely inert	*Nitrogen type = Nitropheric type*

NITROGEN IN THE HUMAN BODY

Vitalizes, builds tissues	*Found in body fluids, elastic and connective tissue, hair, nails, skin, lens of eye*
Essential for complete metabolism	

SIGNS OF NITROGEN EXCESS (Characteristics of Nitropheric Type)

Fleshiness	*Fondness for evening, nighttime, the past*
Romanticism	*Mysteriousness*
Susceptibility to disease	*Drowsiness, forgetfulness*
Sensitive, fragile bones, joints	*Keen olfactory sense*
Lively imagination	*Low heat generation*
Slow healing	*Deficient vital immunity*
Passivity	*Dreaminess*

SIGNS OF NITROGEN DEFICIENCY

*Feebleness, numbness, muscular
exhaustion, fatigue*
Absentmindedness
Sexual weakness
Hypochondria
Lack of desire to work

Danger of blood clots

Cramps in tendons
Unpredictability, passion, temper
Brain weakness, dullness

HIGHEST NITROGEN FOODS

High protein foods   *Nuts*
Spices   *Pasta*
Fish   *Cheeses*
Condiments   *Pastries*

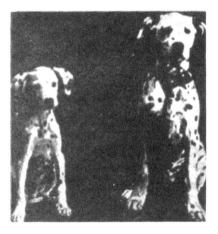

Same-age puppies; larger one had an abundance of milk and sunshine; smaller one had plenty of foods other than milk and no sunshine.

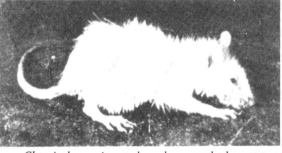

Chemical experiments have been worked on rats as shown. Compare the animal which has been fed improperly with the larger healthy one which was fed on a chemically well-balanced diet.

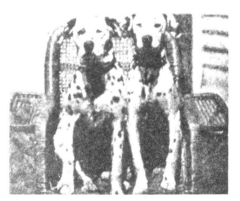

Same puppies four months later after both had been well supplied with milk and sunshine. The one at the right was formerly stunted.

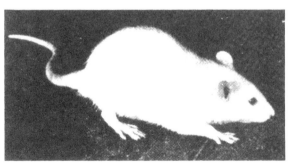

Rats have been experimented with for many years and every disease has been produced in them that man is heir to. The sad mistake is that these same experiments are going on with human beings daily.

eleven

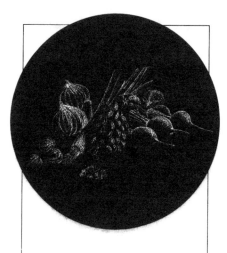

Oxygen, the "giver of life"

When I considered purchasing the Health Ranch in the hills outside of Escondido, the oxygen available at that altitude strongly influenced me to settle there. I needed that oxygen and pure air in my lungs more than anything else, because the lung area is my weakness.

Afterwards, people arriving at the Ranch for some sanitarium work would always remark on how wonderful the air was, and within two or three days they would be saying to me, "I feel better, doctor. I don't know why."

Whenever we have a lot of oxygen in the body, all faculties are improved and no doubt it was the air and the exercises we were doing that greatly contributed to my patients feeling better. Their nerves, emotions and activities were becoming more stable.

Oxygen is the "life giver." Life demands heat and we cannot have heat without oxygen. Every faculty of the body must have oxygen, particularly the brain—the most active part of the body vibratorily. The brain requires more than four times as much oxygen as the rest of the body to repair and rebuild tissues. Additionally, it takes four times as long to break that oxygen down, but it is also one of the great oxygen-holding organs in the body. The oxygen, of course, is coming through the lung structure, requiring us to have good lungs. We must also have a good brain to have good lungs; they work hand in hand.

How Oxygen Works

I always insist that patients in need of extra oxygen must have enough iodine for good metabolism and sufficient iron to attract the needed oxygen. Many people need more oxygen, particularly those living in smog-ridden cities.

Oxygen builds the efficiency of the medulla oblongata, the chest brain, to improve respiration. The medulla is a phosphorus/sulphur organ, also needing plenty of iodine. (Generally, sulphur, phosphorus and manganese are the brain elements along with oxygen.)

The body requires sufficient heat for various reasons. It is necessary to burn off waste material and eliminate toxic conditions, a process impossible without oxygen.

A slow-burning process called metabolism is ongoing in the body. Anabolism (building) and catabolism

Oxygen has more life than food.

Persons in polluted areas such as Los Angeles have only one thousandth as much air to breathe as they would under normal conditions, a leading American environmenmtalist has said.

Residents of Fairbanks, Alaska, produce 10 to 100 times as much carbon monoxide pollution per capita, as residents of Los Angeles, says a University of Alaska scientist.

"Air, or rather oxygen, it can rightly be maintained, is a part of food...it has peculiar importance in assisting at so many vital processes of movement and energy that it has to be constantly added to the blood by the special lung apparatus."
—G. T. Wrench, MD

(destroying) are combined to make up metabolism. Anabolism breaks down food so that it may be assimilated for tissue building, repair and fuel for running the human machine. Catabolism follows, breaking down the toxic waste material and worn out waste material to prepare it for excretion. As tissue and cells disintegrate, they are broken down into various acids and by-products carried off by the body elimination channels.

Our bodies are constantly on fire, so to speak, at a temperature of 98.6 degrees Farenheit, whether we are at the Equator or the North Pole. Regulated a good deal by oxygen intake, the temperature should remain uniform. Additionally, oxygen is vitally important to hematin and hemoglobin, constituents of the blood.

Oxygen for Rebuilding

We need to think of oxygen when the heart is going poorly or the lung structure needs improvement. In replacement therapy, where we are replacing old tissues with new tissues, always think of oxygen. Whenever we have to get rid of wastes, fresh oxygen must replace the morbid gases, which are produced when tissues break down. Our goal is good oxygenation.

Often yawning is a sign that the brain needs more oxygen. It may be a sign that a person is lacking calcium and potassium and cannot breathe deeply. Yawning may also be a sign that the medulla oblongata is broken down. The medulla can break down from a shortage of nerve supply as well as a lack of phosphorus and vitalin (a part of lecithin). If we are inherently weak in any of the mental centers or have broken them down by studying too much, for example, we need oxygen to rebuild us. In fact, pure oxygen therapy, under the supervision of

medical personnel, has been highly successful in a number of cases, even when persons have been thought to be on their death beds.

Excess and Deficiency

The oxygen type of person—or "oxypheric"—is an active, optimistic person, usually insistent on doing what he wants to do. He's likely to be living on stimulating foods, steaks and spices. He burns up oxygen fast and needs to replace it. Whatever he does, he does intensely. If he chases a woman, he chases her diligently. We can all use some of these characteristics to some degree, but, as Rocine indicates, the oxypheric person tends to go too far.

On the other hand, with insufficient oxygen, we tend to have difficulty accomplishing tasks; we lack enthusiasm. Sociability requires a good oxygen supply, for when you're oxygenated, you're vivacious. A person lacking oxygen carries grudges and tends to hold on to feelings for weeks.

The Importance of Climate

There are people who feel "stifled for air" or short of breath, suggesting that iodine is needed to help bring in more oxygen by raising the metabolism of the body. Going to a higher altitude also helps quicken the breathing, which in turn draws more oxygen to the body than does living at sea level. Indeed, anyone who has tissue toxicity or wants to get rid of catarrh should go where it is dry and oxygen is abundant. A humid climate does not work in our favor when we need oxygen for the tissues. Climate is an important consideration in the healing process as it influences our chemical balance.

A U.S. Department of Agriculture survey has shown that 20% of the population in the U.S. is deficient in iron. Of 12,000 children surveyed, 30% had iron deficiency anemia. Foods rich in iron include spinach, walnuts, prunes, raisins, eggs, lima beans, liver, wheat germ, blackstrap molasses, dandelion greens, organ meats, peas and mustard greens.

I consider iron and oxygen the two "frisky horses" in our body chemistry. Iron picks up oxygen from the atmosphere. With these two elements, our bodies can be clean, active and vital. These elements help prepare nutrients for the cells and energy for release in activity.

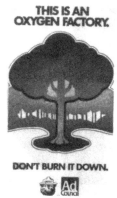

The U.S. Forest Service has produced ads like this to help Americans understand how important trees are.

OXYGEN
"The Giver of Life"

GENERAL CHARACTERISTICS

Oxygen Misnamed

Oxygen, the life-giving element, is actually inappropriately named. "Oxygen" is a Greek word meaning acid producer, which property the element simply does not possess; hydrogen is the acid producer. Yet, even after chemistry discovered its error, the name oxygen remained.

Oxygen Combines with Almost Everything

Oxygen is the "giver of life" in the body. Colorless, odorless and tasteless, it combines with all elements except fluorine, the "resistant" element. Oxygen is absorbed rapidly by positive elements and slowly by negative ones. Oxygen is explosive, spontaneous, volative and unstable. It is never stationary, immobile, fixed or motionless but craves activity, motion and work. It is always hasty, never deliberate. It penetrates everything, no matter how solid or where located.

Oxygen Important in the "Wheel of Health"

We speak of the "wheel of health," meaning that all must return to nature for recycling; the cycle of disintegration is only complete with regeneration. Disintegration is one of oxygen's major functions.

Rubble, garbage, junk, refuse, debris are destroyed by oxygen. Only the resistive qualities of fluorine can resist for a time the ravages of oxygen.

Oxidation is the merging of oxygen with other elements. Part of the process of oxidation includes heat generation and decomposition. Bacteria and germ life need oxidation for propagation.

"Oxygen is the 'giver of life' in the body."

The Oxygen Cycle

Oxygen is manufactured by plants through the decomposition of carbon dioxide and water; it is essential for all forms of life on earth although it comprises only one fifth of the total atmosphere. Carbon dioxide and carbonic acid are the by-products of oxygen utilization in animals and humans. If it were not for plant life, no other life forms could exist, because plants consume carbon dioxide and carbonic acid and manufacture or recycle oxygen for the rest of life. The cycle has no beginning and no ending.

Massive quantities of oxygen are imprisoned in plants, food, seas, lakes and other bodies of water. The surfaces are much more oxygen charged than are the depths or ocean beds.

Ozone (O3) Versus Oxygen (O2)

Ozone, a normal constituent of air, is a form of oxygen; ozone's molecular structure has three atoms as opposed to oxygen's two; the volume of oxygen is reduced by one third when converted to ozone. Electrical action, pure dry oxygen and moderate temperature favor formation of ozone, so forest, mountain and seashore atmospheres contain more ozone. Ozone contributes to greater oxidation in the human body and functions as an antiseptic and tonic for the body.

Oxygen Similar in Function to Heat

Terms descriptive of the activity of oxygen in nature and in the human organism are these: constructive, destructive, fiery, corrosive, degenerative, regenerative, revolutionary, life sustaining, spasmodic, climactic, extreme, fleet and excitable. Oxygen is similar to heat in that it disintegrates, regenerates and purifies. Nature could not function without this powerful agent of change.

OXYGEN: ITS ROLE IN THE HUMAN BODY

A man weighing 150 pounds has some 90 pounds of oxygen in his body. Oxygen lends its properties to the temperament and physical characteristics of man according to its consumption relative to that of the other 15 elements.

Oxygen Enhances Life

Through combustion, heat is produced from oxygen, as are physical and mental energy. The medulla oblongata is affected strongly and circulation is raised; the muscular system is stimulated through the brain centers; metabolism and regenerative functions are strengthened by oxygen. The mind is inspired to greater activity; oratory, zeal, laughter and speaking ability are promoted. Physical functions, blood count and outlook on life are all elevated. There is an optimism for living and a zealous pursuit of pleasure when oxygen is in good supply.

Oxygen Infiltrates Every Cell

Because oxygen generates heat, liberal oxygen available to the body improves oxidation, growth

> *"Because oxygen generates heat, liberal oxygen available to the body improves oxidation, growth and catabolism."*

and catabolism. Manufacture of red blood corpuscles in the blood is increased by the presence of much oxygen. Oxygen infiltrates each individual cell in the body, influencing building and demolishing processes. Oxygen's mission in the body is dual: both organic and functional. In combination, oxygen enters catabolic and eliminative processes.

Oxygen Affects Each Individual Differently

A concept important to understand is that oxygen's effect on each individual differs according to the leading chemical elements in that person's makeup. If carbon is predominant, for example, additional oxygen is required for good health; if a patient lives on excessive carbohydrate foods, fats and proteins, oxygen is often deficient because it is required in mammoth quantities. Those who are overweight are not inclined to deep-breathing exercises, physical exertion and other methods for improving oxidation, and they may be lethargic or lazy; consequently, overweight people lack sufficient oxygen. Nitrogen and hydrogen diminish the power of oxygen if supplied in larger than normal amounts. Potassium and iron are necessary in blood and muscular tissue to attract oxygen; if they are deficient, oxygen is also deficient and carbonic acid generation is increased in the body, with its attendant ailments.

Oxygen Vital for Youth and Health

An ample oxygen supply in the lungs, blood and tissues fosters radiant health: the arteries are elastic, eyes glow with magnetism, heart is active and agile, pulse is strong, skin is rosy, mind is positive, gait is springy, emotions are uplifted and temperament is enthusiastic. Assimilation and utilization of nutrients are improved by oxygen. Quality of life is improved, notably in areas of sexuality, anabolism and manufacture of red blood corpuscles. Life can be sustained only seconds if oxygen is withheld. The fountain of youth is likened to oxygen, Nature's beautician. Youth and health demand oxygen.

Oxygen in Respiration and Circulation

Hemoglobin and hematin, the iron constituent of hemoglobin, are inundated with oxygen drawn into the lungs. From the lungs they are transported to all parts of the body through the blood. Carbonic acid and carbon dioxide are the waste products produced through tissue oxidation; the blood must then carry this waste back to the lungs where it is replaced with oxygen. The lungs thus serve a double purpose: inhalation of oxygen and exhalation of carbonic acid and carbon dioxide. (Urea produced by nitrogen must be eliminated by the kidneys.)

Hematin, as has been mentioned, retains oxygen in the blood's hemoglobin. Air pressure has much influence on this process: pressure of a minimum 30 to 50 mm/hg promotes oxygen's merger with the blood. Heat and chemical affinity bring about hemoglobin's conversion to oxyhemoglobin. These forces counterbalance one another; heat hampers hemoglobin's oxygen saturation while chemical attraction facilitates transformation of hemoglobin into oxyhemoglobin.

"An ample oxygen supply in the lungs, blood and tissues fosters radiant health."

Individual Oxygen Requirements Vary

Oxygen requirements vary according to many factors, internal and external—such as body temperature, age, emotional makeup, amount of food consumed, type of work, climate. An estimation of the oxygen required by a man resting is 575 liters (a liter is 1.056 liquid quarts) in a 24-hour period. During activity, the requirement rises to 700 liters per 24 hours. Iron content of an individual's hemoglobin determines its capability for absorbing oxygen. The health and vigor of the red blood cells and the man himself are also influential. The greater the percentage of carbonic acid in the blood, the lesser the ability of the hemoglobin to absorb oxygen. At times when the sexual system is depleted or enervated, hemoglobin is weakened and oxygen is

deficient, even when iron is present in normal quantities.

Air Pressure Must be Within Certain Limits

Oxygen pressure in the atmosphere must be within a certain range. A pressure three times normal atmospheric density is detrimental to any form of life; five to fifteen times normal is fatal to animal, vegetative and microscopic life forms. When placed under high stress, oxygen becomes noxious, damaging and destructive. If air pressure is quickly intensified, blood vessels show signs of anemia and conjunctivae grow pale. A slight increase in oxygen pressure lowers the function ability of plant and animal life. Reduced air pressure has a similarly disastrous effect on all life forms. Atmospheric air pressure half as great as normal causes birds to become agitated; one third normal pressure causes staggering, vomiting and prostration in animals. Normal atmospheric pressure is well-suited for all life forms.

Sunlight Enables the Body to Absorb Oxygen

Certain light vibrations magnify oxygen motion, as typified in the utilization of carbonic acid by plant cells. During this process, free oxygen is extricated. The sunlight spectrum has great influence on plant life. Blue, violet and ultra-violet rays are most refractable and are termed chemical (biochemical) rays. At the opposite end of the spectrum, red and ultra-red are least refractable. Chlorophyll processes in plant life utilize intermediate yellow rays extensively in splitting carbonic acid for use in plant cells, resulting in liberation of free oxygen. When plants are placed under red light, growth is improved; under blue light, growth is stunted. When exposed to sunlight, plants grow better and animals take up more oxygen as does man. Humans placed in darkness soon suffer oxygen shortage. Animals starve under violet light much sooner than under red light if food is withheld, because the red light stimulates absorption of oxygen. Dark clothing inhibits oxygen ingestion, as does closing the eyes. Powerful rays of sunlight destroy certain bacterial species. Blue, violet and ultra-violet rays act as an antiseptic and germicide on the skin and penetrate to tissues; red-yellow rays penetrate twenty times more than blue-violet; ultra-red penetrate twenty-eight times more than blue-violet rays.

Direct Sunlight Vital to Health

From the foregoing, we conclude that direct sunlight is vital to the health of man; his eyes should receive these life-giving rays. Nude sunbathing is to be desired and light clothing is advisable whenever possible; both improve the uptake of oxygen, providing the necessary iron and potassium are present in the blood. However, individuals differ and climate, altitude and weather conditions are also influential in oxygen induction. If air is too rare or too dense, oxygen admission is curtailed.

Ozone Helps Remove Wastes

Every person's organs imbibe oxygen and eliminate carbonic acid, to be expelled as carbon dioxide (carbonic acid gas) by the lungs. Muscles require more oxygen than do other structures. Bones demand less oxygen and therefore excrete the least carbonic acid. Ozone helps remove waste material and impurities from the body as well as from the air. Providing the ozone quantity in the air is not too high, it has a tonic effect on lungs, nerves and bloodstream.

"Muscles require more oxygen than do other structures."

Summary

In summary, to ensure the proper functioning of oxygen in the human framework, sunlight on the body and optic nerves, deep breathing and foods rich in oxygen, iron, potassium, sulphur and phosphorus are to be emphasized.

SIGNS OF OXYGEN EXCESS

The Oxypheric Type

Persons possessing large quantities of oxygen in their system are sanguine, buoyant, active; skin is radiant, chest expansion great and skin warm. Much heat is generated within the body; passions are intense; lungs are well developed with large lobes and active air cells. A man's associations with women are uninhibited; he often works with animals and in the outdoors; red meat is a staple in his diet as are stimulating tonics, both of which increase free oxygen importation. The oxygen man is active, impulsive and hot blooded; he is an extremist—emotions soar and plummet alternately. Optimism, enthusiasm, spontaneity, recklessness are his characteristics. He has more than the average amount of oxygen and other elements in his system. We call him the Oxypheric type.

Oxygen Lends Passion, Intensity, Vigor

When free oxygen is performing powerfully in blood and tissues and throughout the body, all processes are escalated. Ambition is raised; sympathy promoted; intellect stimulated; sense of freedom sharpened; passions fired; emotion compounded; pulse quickened; joy enlivened; despair intensified; awe inspired. Fever is incremented; love enlivened; lust excited; heart activated; wonder excited. Oratory becomes ardent, nerves high pitched. Brain sharpens; anger boils; desire deepens. Both positive and negative qualities are invigorated and magnified.

Oxypheric Type is Optimistic, Expansive

The oxygen personality is optimistic, spontaneous, jolly or angry with great force, constructive and creative, violently impulsive, intensely passionate. He believes in freedom. His temper is revolutionary; aversion spontaneous; manner excited; mind responsive; senses finely tuned; moods fluctual; appetite hearty; speech fluent. Grudges are rarely held long; mind is commercial; emotions are fickle; ideas are promotional; attention is wandering; voice is booming; poise is unsteady; relationships are familiar. An oxygen man is impatient, generous, good-hearted, hospitable and freedom-loving. He rapidly negates jealousy and envy. His mental state constantly fluctuates; mentality is climactic; fortunes are made and lost by cycles. He joshes, jests, ridicules, criticizes, jeers at public functions in a sporting manner; he provokes friends by joking in an innocent way, but no harm is intended.

Oxygen types work excessively, play hard, become intoxicated with life; they adore pleasure, sociability, liberty, romance, festivity, happy companions. Interest in and enthusiasm for any one thing soon disappear; waiting is unbearable; progression and promotion are foremost. Extemporaneous speech is easy; imagination is vivid; knowledge of life is instinctive; manner is blustering but generally harmless. Value and quality of anyone or anything are well-judged. Generative, cardiac, brain systems are active. Heat is dissipated rapidly but replaced quickly. They are communicative, honest, opinionated, expressive. Stride is lengthy; gestures are expansive and manner imitating or mocking. The mind has many rooms.

Oxypheric Type Experiences Extremes

The oxygen man climbs to great heights, then plunges to the depths. Business reaches a climax and bankruptcy may follow. Undaunted, he begins again to amass as much or more; the cycle is repeated over and over. He experiences culmination in all facets of his life, whether personal or business. Sickness tends to be intense—high fevers, excruciating pains, extreme illness—but recovery is phenomenal. His health breaks after a life climax but he quickly recovers. Depths of despondency make him a worrier and a complainer, insisting that he is about to die, that all is lost and hopeless; he threatens suicide and insists that he be waited on hand and foot. He calls in several doctors and nurses; enlists aid of as many wise people as he can find; but recovery is miraculous and speedy. Life, energy, vitality, strength are regenerated rapidly. This pattern is repeated many times. The unstable, unpredictable quality of oxygen is responsible for such pendulum swings. When the oxygen man is ailing, the symptoms are intense, gaining momentum until the bursting point or crisis. Then he becomes well again, and his health is equally intense.

Sociability of Oxygen Type (Oxypheric)

Voluminous oxygen intake inclines a patient toward sociability and public interaction. Associates come from every walk of life; acquaintances are beneficial personally and industrially or financially. Interests are varied and numerous; partnerships are entered in many areas; ownership may stretch around the globe; businesses are created and left to the management of others. Brain faculties dealing with love and sex are active when oxygen is prevalent in the system. There is a tendency toward polygamy and many sexual encounters; romantic and platonic love is not strong but passion is forceful, rising and abating fast. In youth, the oxygen man gravitates to parties, dances,

clubs and other social functions where the opposite sex is found.

Typical Characteristics of the Oxygen Woman

The oxygen woman is flirtatious. If her emotions incline toward love, faithfulness and honor, she can be a worthy mate. On the other hand, she may be free in love and disinclined toward marriage.

Typical Characteristics of the Oxygen Man

An oxygen man is often remorseful, self-punishing, self-condemning, conscience-stricken for no apparent reason. Out of the blue, he may return money he has had for years, saying that it is bothering his conscience.

Emotions Rule Oxygen Type (Oxypheric)

Oxypherous types are ruled by their feelings, their heartfelt impressions, reproductive instincts, pleasure senses, food and drink appetites, self-preservation motivation. In some cases, however, these tendencies are controlled or transmuted by culture, diet, religion, self-restraint or self-discipline.

Career May Be Impressive But Brief

The revolutionary quality of oxygen lends itself to invention, genius, great accomplishment, fiery passions, expansive ideas. An oxygen person's career may take on great fame, inspire wonder in others, but it is brief and transient. At times oxypheric characteristics can be potentially harmful to their possessor as well as to others.

Changes, Cycles, Extremes

Oxygen contributes a spirit of diligence, disquiet, motion and vigor to the individual endowed with a high supply of it. It moves in periodic cycles in work, pleasure, health, activity. Energy is channeled into accumulation and accomplishment until the climax is reached. A man having much oxygen is rarely lazy, though at times he may take a rest from the world of action; he then emerges from seclusion and tackles life with characteristic gusto. Again we see changes and extremes. At times, the mind can run rampant, temperament ramble and personality exhibit inconsistency and transiency.

Pure Vegetable Diet is Overstimulating

High-oxygen foods stimulate the brain. A strict vegetarian diet (only vegetables) is high in oxygen, but it also contains oxalate of lime and oxalic acid. Its early effect is one of intellectual stimulation, increased energy, emotions and passions; but gout, urinary complications and other ailments develop later. Initially these foods elate, exhilarate, stimulate mentally, emotionally and sexually to a point where control is difficult; the result is positive overstimulated brain, compensated for by later weakness. A vegetable diet stimulates the brain, spinal cord and heart and adversely affects the voice and vocal cords.

Excess Oxygen May Cause Disturbances

If excessive amounts of oxy-acid and calcium oxalate are found in the body from too many vegetables in the diet, gout may result. Symptoms of overconsumption of oxygen in free form and in foods simulate to a lesser degree those of oxalic acid poisoning: there are heat flushes even when immobile; face reddens near evening; neck and small of back are chilly, numb; back feels too weak to hold up the body. Deltoid muscles feel effects first; aches manifest beneath scapula traveling toward loins through nerves. Wheezing asthma or hoarse, whistling breathing is noted. Sexual drive is heightened to point of incorporating vulgar language and lewd preoccupations. Stomach troubles bother when one is reclining; glucose-containing foods cause colic; bloating occurs at work but not when relaxing; symptoms vary between work and relaxation; headache occurs the day after wine drinking; face is feverish and hot; one feels heat inside and chill outside; thirst is accompanied by depression or weakness; weak sensation vanishes after reclining or sitting momentarily; head swims occasionally when rising suddenly, as though the world were spinning. Executive propensity is pronounced, as are intellect, reasoning ability. Perception is keen.

Vegetable Diet May Cause Hardening Symptoms

The individual who consumes too much oxygen enjoys onions, tomatoes, radishes and other high oxygen-carrying foods; indulgence in these foods burdens the system with oxy-acid, oxalate of lime and oxygen, both organically and functionally. Deep breathing is practiced, which adds to symptoms. At times there is a sense of a boring behind the ears in bones or periosteum. A vegetable diet contributes to formation of gravel, ossification, hardening of the arteries and varied mental and brain symptoms resembling oxalic acid poisoning. (It is noteworthy that horses eating principally hay and green grass develop kidney and urinary troubles or symptoms of excessive oxalate of lime in the system.)

Treatment of Oxygen Excess

The oxygen-excess patient should minimize foods high in oxalic acid, oxygen, oxy-acid, oxalate of lime and depend instead on salty foods, milk products, raw egg yolks, a combination of distilled and lime water. At the outset, milk is disagreeable but nonetheless must be persistently taken.

Arid climates cause the oxygen patient to generate more heat than can be given off from the body unless great quantities of liquid are consumed to induce perspiration and lower body temperature; if breathing and evaporation are active, heat is exuded easily from the body. At these times, milk beverages, mulberry juice and distilled water are beneficial for bringing on perspiration and heat evaporation. Warm baths open skin pores and invigorate skin. Balmy, moist climates favor the oxygen patient. Lower altitudes are beneficial; high altitudes, cold, dry climates and humidity are not indicated. Cold water, in moderation, is good; overuse of cold water in drinking or bathing adds to body weight, favors animal heat generation within the body and increases the consumption of oxygen.

Sickness Results from Intemperance

The oxygen type is healthy because he has perfect oxidation, hematin (iron) is abundant, heat is amply generated and red corpuscles are vigorous. Yet the very nature of oxygen predisposes this type to unjudicious eating, drinking and other habits that are destructive. Sickness is self imposed through intemperance. For example, the diet may consist of highly-seasoned and spiced foods, oily and fatty foods, sweets, seafood, steaks, potatoes, rich gravies and sauces, cabbage, cakes, biscuits, cucumbers, dumplings, grapes, candy, cream, ice cream, syrup, molasses, pepper, condiments, canned and processed meats and fish, doughnuts, fried eggs, fried food, pork, ham, bacon, sausage, butter, chocolate, alcohol, coffee and sweetened tea—foods which cause the brain, liver, bowel, kidneys, nerves, blood to be besieged, overheated and aggravated. Blood pressure may soar; plethora may appear; specific gravity of blood is upset. Excessive heat is produced; the body is an inferno. Fevers rage and the battle between health and disease intensifies; infirmity attacks without warning and is vanquished just as suddenly. The climactic cycle is violent and extreme.

Oxygen Patient Unreasonable, Irrational

Immoderate oxygen intake accelerates functions. Sex drive is heightened; brain activity is escalated; brain is intoxicated; blood pressure rises; arteries become stressed; heartbeat and pulse quicken; bowel develops adhesions; base of brain becomes congested. Insomnia bothers occasionally; cranium is feverish; actions become violent and hopeless; mental faculties fail suddenly. Anger, unreasonableness and irrationality manifest. As a result of heat creation, the bowel, rectal muscles, cardiac muscles, kidney and liver become inflamed, atonic and sticky; this weakens the bowel, contributing to adhesions, intestinal stasis and fever and eruptive diseases caused by vegetable poisons. One consolation is that the patient will never develop tuberculosis!

Excess Oxygen Disturbs Vital Functions

At times when the atmosphere is oversaturated with oxygen or the air is more compressed, hunger is amplified and digestion enhanced in patients lacking oxygen. But excess oxygen disturbs the vital functions. Urine is copious; stimulants and spices are craved; sexual system may be overstimulated leading to congestive or hyperemic conditions. Other possible complications are psychotic and frenzied behavior; nosebleeds; membrane congestion; agitated brain functions; cardiac disturbances; rectal weakness and bleeding; tinnitus aurium; vascular fatigue; cardiac auxesis; flatulence; plethora; rupture of certain blood vessels, hyperemia at the base of the brain; emotional agitation; spontaneous pain in hands and arms with partial paralysis; sexual overindulgence and resultant venereal disease; extreme nerve stress; intense unrest; skin ailments; overheated body;

superfluous perspiration; enlargement of liver, kidneys or heart; suicidal considerations; plethoric hemorrhages; congestion of meninges (cranial membranes); convulsions and coughing. The oxygen-excess patient cannot hide from his ailments; each is forced to the surface for open battle with his vital forces. Oxygen stirs up the patient, his brain and nervous system, blood, toxins, germs, acids. Health generally wins out because of his innate vigor and strength. After a crisis, health generally returns rapidly.

SIGNS OF OXYGEN DEFICIENCY

Nervousness Increases

Nervous irritability intensifies when oxygen is lacking because oxidation is diminished. Other indications of oxygen hunger are sleeplessness, frightening dreams and phobias, discomforts, emotional instability and agitation, and inability to perform mental tasks.

Senses Are Dulled

When air is rarified or oxygen lacking, a man is erratic and easily angered and his appetite is extreme. He complains of noises in the ears and of dizziness. His senses are dulled; sight, touch and hearing are below par. Intellect is crippled; mental grasp is slow. Planning is perplexing; calculations are a struggle; trivial matters are upsetting. He has a greater-than-normal need for sleep. Senses are rattled; muscular coordination is difficult; laziness overcomes. There is an aversion to conversation and lack of social inclinations. Prolonged oxygen poverty in bones, tissue and brain manifests symptoms similar to calcium shortage because calcium metabolism is also disturbed and bone oxidation impaired. When calcium, potassium or iron are in short supply or even sodium and chlorides, oxygen is also lacking. Then carbonic gas and certain acids and ferments tend to develop. Symptoms seem to merge together, producing modified deoxidation signs or carbonic acid-poisoning indices.

Energy Decreases

Carbon dioxide trapped in the body makes a patient susceptible to climatic changes, storms, humidity, rain, wind and electrical tension in the atmosphere. Symptoms include a heavy feeling, tiredness, depression without explanation. Sunrise intensifies depression, but improvement is noted toward noon because the vegetative kingdom is absorbing carbon dioxide and producing more oxygen at that time. Sunshine draws carbonic acid from the body and improves nerve functions. As the sun sets, carbon dioxide increases and so does depression; nervousness, anxiety, unrest and irritability increase toward nightfall. A patient exhibiting a high percentage of carbonic acid and reduced oxygen dreads nightfall because oxygen is lowered in the air at night, aggravating symptoms and causing more congestion, heavier depression, lowered energy, depressed breathing. In these cases, sunny climates, much sunshine, arid weather, high altitude, coolness, energizing atmosphere and dry oxygen are all indicated.

"Oxygen shortage harms general nutrition in body and mind."

Patient Becomes Stubborn, Hypersensitive

Oxygen shortage harms general nutrition in body and mind. Moderate delirium is symptomatic of both oxygen hunger and excess. Oxygen deficiency heralds lowered vitality, dulled senses, weakness in respiratory center of spinal cord and reduced oxygen in tissues and blood. As oxygen starvation advances, nerve supply and vital energy drop; mental depression sets in; fainting spells may come on; confused states manifest; stupor overcomes at times; collapse is possible; speech is difficult, as is swallowing, due to swelling of the esophagus. Expression is irritable; solitude is preferred to social interaction; little regard is held for others; studies are preferred to people. The patient disdains others when they talk, frowning and believing they are unknowledgeable; he has spells of forgetfulness; he maintains secretiveness about his plans, studies, life, habits; he appears odd to other people. The oxygen patient is hypersensitive to scrutiny, churlish when criticized, cantankerous and waspish in disposition if watched closely; opposition draws bitterness, resentment, acerbity, pugnacity, shrewishness. He takes displeasure in everything; is ill-tempered and moody; is cross with doctors,

nurses and others. Women cry easily; men explode angrily. Notions become stubborn; motion, change, din are disturbing; interruption is disliked; irate moods hang on; forgiveness and forgetfulness come with great difficulty; conversation offends; diligence is applied to work. Some patients are listless, apathetic, bored, impatient, indignant, nervous, pouting, patronizing. Slow detail work is favored; painstaking research or investigation of scientific nature is indicated; sedentary jobs are preferred. Mind, work, ideas, aptitudes are creative. In such work, patience is exercised. A patient develops many reservations, coldness and remote, stilted, disinterested tendencies.

Digestion is Poor

When oxygen is insufficient, digestion is poor and food is not assimilated properly; this encourages overeating because nourishment is needed. Hunger is monstrous; appetite for unusual items such as clay or chalk may develop. Chlorine and sodium foods are desired so foods are oversalted. Craving for stimulants, salt, tonics, spices and alcohol increases. increases.

Memory Declines

Recall faculties are weakened; memory for names, dates, places, words is faulty; memorization is difficult; learning must come through understanding. Laws of nature, men, governments are understood, but expression of ideas is arduous. All such symptoms are oxygen hunger signs.

Emotions are Unrealistic

In addition, emotions are unrealistic, imagination lofty; regard is for future rather than present; great things are anticipated in the future; one clings wildly to life; trivial matters spark cynicism; optimism and positive attitude are held about future; complications of the future are expected but not accepted as reality.

Breathing is Adversely Affected

Disease manifestations of oxygen hunger are varied and generally are in direct opposition to oxygen-excess maladies. They include weakened sexuality; reduced personal magnetism; predisposition to consumption; tubercular tendencies resulting from faulty tissue oxidation, absence of sufficient free oxygen in lungs, blood, tissues and shortage of biochemical elements. Pulmonary, respiratory and breathing apparatuses are disadvantaged. High percentage of calcium and phosphorus encourages low oxidation; free oxygen needed by lungs, tissues and blood is deficient; germ life flourishes; pus increases; tuberculosis-related troubles appear. Consumptive germ life assaults tissues, bones, lungs, bowel, kidneys, glands, with tuberculosis as the ultimate result if oxygen and other therapies are not provided.

Germ Life Multiplies

Oxygen poverty causes memory defects; nutritive weakness and irregularity; brain dullness; vertigo; night sweats; ear noises; bluish or pale complexion; lack of appetite; depression with nightfall; craving for hills, mountains, forests; craving for seclusion from friends, loved ones, family; aversion to people; anemia; catarrh; colds; blueness of white of eyes; weak eyesight; indigestion; reduced power or sway over public; cold and moist skin; emaciation; heavy head; tickling irritation in throat and nose; mental confusion; sedentary preference; muscular laxity; sleepiness; face wrinkles; aged look; feeble and short pulse; loss of ambition and animation. Low oxidation opens the door to germ life and carbonic acid so tissues become inundated; secretions become acrid.

Patient Predisposed to Congestion

Reduced oxygen quantity predisposes a patient to head, chest, spleen, portal and capillary congestion; stinging sensations in many parts of the body; burning pain with weight in the spleen; frequent sneezing and overall discomfort. Spine is cold, tender, tense, notably in respiratory, interscapular and upper dorsal regions; throat tickles; hot weather is malevolent; cold, humid, dank weather intensifies condition; specific glands may solidify. Morning brings turbulent coughing.

Urine Changes When Oxygen is Lacking

Sometimes a gelatinous substance becomes visible in the urethra, causing difficult urination. Urine may be pale, sometimes reddish or bloody, at other times pale amber or milky. It may even assume a sweet odor on occasion. Acetic acid may be found in urine, detected by vinegar smell. Diacetic acid or hippuric acid may also manifest.

Likelihood of Bleeding Increases

Oxygen deficiency sufferers experience inflation pressure in chest and abdomen, to the point where stomach feels it will explode, especially after eating starchy, fatty, sweet foods or drinking coffee, because these foods are highly acidic and result in acerbity and bitter belching. Lungs, spleen, liver, spinal cord and other organs may succumb to gas pressure symptoms. Heart trouble may be wrongly suspected. Following meals and between two and five a.m. the patient has his worst gas pressure symptoms. Increased likelihood of bleeding, typhus, pythisis, diabetes, dropsy, throat ailments, abscesses, aches in spine, feebleness in lower legs, hyperactivity of sensory nerves and sensoria of brain, hemorrhages of bowel, nose, rectum, stomach, uterus, spleen—all signify low oxidation. Respiration is depressed and patient claims he does not breathe well. Venous system is mildly stagnated; pulse is feeble, short and shallow.

"When oxygen is insufficient, digestion is poor and food is not assimilated properly; this encourages overeating because nourishment is needed."

Sitting Comfortably Becomes Difficult

Preliminary signs of oxygen starvation include cold knees, perhaps even numbness; extremities go to sleep easily; legs are numb from knees down. There may be a feeling of partial paralysis in extremities; crampy calves; fingertips or palms damp, dotted with white spots; elbow joints sensitive to touch; aching shoulder joints; small of back, scapula or sacral region sore, making it eventually almost impossible to sit comfortably; cramped, tight neck muscles and bones; shooting pains in lungs, ribs, spleen, chest or small intestines. Alimentary tract is sluggish and inactive, resulting in bowel torpidity even without constipation. Morning diarrhea may manifest in some cases.

Skin Affected by Oxygen Deprivation

The countenance turns hot and rosy when congestion is present, then muddy, waxy, purplish or earthy and claylike, changing with mental and physical symptoms. Skin may flake and scale at times. Tiny bluish skin tumors may develop on various parts of the body. Lips may take on a bluish-red cast.

Symptoms of Oxygen Deficiency Vary

Many oxygen patients complain of bleeding gums so tender, soft and touchy that chewing is painful. The tongue may be paralyzed or weighty, which makes speaking difficult; silence is preferred. At times, tongue is dark and speckled with fleshy pustules; throat is sore; mouth becomes dry as oxygen starvation increases. One may gnash teeth at night; jawbone joints throb; ears feel congested; hearing is defective or lost; hearing faculties develop fuzziness; pressure in temples and pulling sensation occur along with tender scalp; hair often falls out; whites of eyes dull; pupils fail to respond properly to light, causing patient to stare dumbly; dark spots appear to drift in the air; warm room makes sinuses active; nasal membranes become inflamed; pounding in head results from inhalation; brain spins because blood is rushed there; sight is blurry and deceptive; eyes feel pressure.

Patients Avoid Helpful Activities

Ironically patients subject to oxygen deficiency breathe only shallowly, neglect tissue salts capable of attracting more oxygen, take insufficient exercise outdoors, sit in closed offices with artificial air circulation, disdain trips to the hills or residence in higher elevations or ozone belts—in short, they avoid all considerations which are vital to good oxidation. Sedentary jobs and heavy mental work make such a patient his or her "own worst enemy," so to speak.

At High Altitudes Oxygen is Less Plentiful

In instances of oxygen scarcity in the air, digestion is upset; constipation may persist; nausea, heart palpitation, dizziness, collapse, muscular weakness, drowsiness, pounding arteries, headaches, depressed functions, faintness, fast breathing may manifest. These indications may materialize in high elevations—especially over 15,000 feet—or in patients suffering oxygen hunger at lower altitudes. However, high altitudes affect various people differently; each person has a specific altitude limit, evident by his inability to attract sufficient oxygen for metabolism at or above that elevation.

High Altitudes Induce Breathing Difficulties

When an individual over reaches the limit of his normal oxidation range, lungs become torpid and stiff; blood is funneled through the lungs to the left heart chamber with difficulty; pulmonary artery oppression increases; capillary congestion of alveoli contributes to lung swelling. Adjustment of lung respiration to air needs is difficult in rarified air; congestive stiffness institutes inhalatory and expiratory dyspnea because lungs cannot expand and contract properly. In times of emergency, artificial oxygen may be crucial.

High Altitude May be Beneficial or Detrimental

High altitudes can also act beneficially, as a tonic and stimulant to the metabolism. Cold, dry air stimulates external and internal parts of the body—especially mucus membranes of lungs and bronchial tubes. But if the altitude is too high, rarified air or diminished oxygen affect circulation unfavorably and promote cracking and bleeding of skin. Skin becomes dry and parched and moisture is evaporated. Cracked skin causes nosebleeds, bleeding of lips, eyes, fingertips and other areas. Arteries, venules, veins, capillaries become engorged due to oxygen hunger.

Tubercular Patients Need High Altitude

A consumptive patient convalesces at a higher altitude, as it fills his normal needs. Where soil is sandy or rocky, air dry, sunlight brighter, ozone content higher, air cleaner and cooler, metabolism is increased, lung exercise improved, urea reduced; less carbonic acid is produced and circulation is improved.

Oxygen Starvation Undermines Sexuality

Excessively high altitude is unfavorable to the sexual function, as is rarified air, altered air pressure, extreme cold, powerful wind or intense dryness of the air. Oxygen starvation undermines sexuality and the sex brain is enervated, causing sexual excitement with impotency.

Certain Activities Increase Demand for Oxygen

Physical activity raises oxygen consumption and the production of carbonic acid. During relaxation, less oxygen is required and less carbonic acid created; work demands more oxygen and more carbonic acid results. Digestion entails more oxygen, and more carbon dioxide must be eliminated as a waste product. Rise in temperature reduces need for oxygen but dropping mercury means more oxygen is in demand. (Cold blooded animals are oppositely affected.) Youth requires more oxygen because cells are more active, eliminating more carbon dioxide. Fevers and inflammations heighten respiration by heating medulla (chest brain) and respiratory centers. High fevers cripple the hemoglobin's ability to hold oxygen. Fevers also harm respiration and lower general oxygen supply in the body; thermopolypnea (fever breathing) may ensue. Labored breathing (dyspnea) is the result of excessive muscular activity in patients who are not in good condition. Emotional states induce the need for more oxygen. A highly-sexed individual has an increased oxidation rate; sterility lowers oxidation and the oxygen supply in the body. Mental depression reduces oxygen attraction and augments production and elimination of carbon dioxide. If oxygen is depreciated in blood and tissues and carbon dioxide increased, the patient exhibits signs of oxygen hunger (dyspnea).

Lack of Iron or Hemoglobin Means Lack of Oxygen

Inhalation is more pronounced or exaggerated when oxygen is short, and exhalation is more pronounced because carbon dioxide is excessive. Exhalation centers of the medulla are agitated when carbon dioxide is overbalanced, as are spinal cord centers. The entire body is oxygen-starved if hemoglobin is lacking or iron is deficient. Nervous asthma, nervous catarrh, watery coryza (head cold) are possible outcomes. Eventually, if oxygen starvation continues, the blood constituency changes and diseases appear.

Asphyxiation is Oxygen Starvation

Asphyxiation is merely oxygen starvation with excessive carbon dioxide. The word asphyxia means "no pulse;" when carbon dioxide is excessive, respiratory centers are paralyzed and pulse is suspended. Skin turns blue (cyanosis) and white of eye becomes bluish. Spontaneous oxygen removal and oversupply of carbon dioxide bring on contortions, collapse, loss of consciousness, failure of reflexes, muscle relaxation, retarded heart action, cessation of pulse, respiration stoppage, cyanosis and, ultimately, death. Pale skin and bluish whites of eye are direct evidence of oxygen hunger, even if the patient denies it. Oxygen starvation progresses in many stages; consumption, colds, catarrh, mucus, phlegm, asthma, anemia, dyspnea and other afflictions are due to oxygen shortage, along with other pathologic, nutritional, climatic, hereditary causes. In cases of asphyxiation, oxygen supply is voided and the respiratory system paralyzed.

Mental Depression Depletes Oxygen Supply

Unfavorable oxidation effects arise from mental depression, excessive masturbation or hypochondriasis. Mental depression robs oxygen from the body, dissipates tissue salts and disrupts oxidation. Calcium oxalate may form and appear in the urine.

Oxygen Shortage Has Definite Symptoms

The list of oxygen-deficiency maladies and symptoms is definite: Pott's disease; dyspnea; catarrh; phlegm and mucus; tuberculosis of the larynx; throat consumption; short, shallow and difficult inhalation; sighing; vertigo when walking with eyes shut; staggering when walking in darkness; foreboding of something dreadful; pressure within the head; clammy perspiration at night; buzzing in ears; sensitivity to temperature and climate changes; coryza; blood or salty taste in mouth; tissue tenderness; flatulence; asthmatic respiration; coughing; heart palpitation; lower legs numb and chilled; dull head with dizziness and mental confusion; exaggerated reserve, anxiety and indifference; raw, sore throat; respiratory attacks; gasping for air from exercise, work, climbing stairs, yawning; coldness; reduced body temperature; faulty oxidation; ashen-blue or bloodless skin; irritation from cold; susceptibility to pulmonary oppression; suffocating night coughing spells; heightened arterial stress; heat flushes; foamy, thread-like expectorations; faintness; muscular debility; high pulse; fast breathing; inclination to hemorrhages; pulsation of arteries; drowsiness; headaches, dulled perception; sluggish senses; constrictive lung pains. In all such cases, intake of oxygen must be increased and facilitated.

HIGHEST OXYGEN FOODS

Organic oxygen is found in all foods, but free oxygen is attracted to the blood by iron. Therefore, iron foods are of prime importance in attracting oxygen to the body. Foods containing liberal quantities of calcium, potassium, iodine, fluorine would also be used. Red, juicy meats are high in oxygen; so are iron tonics, nuts and seeds, liquid chlorophyll. Vegetables and fruits in general, and especially their raw juices, are high-oxygen foods.

Fresh mountain air, clean air, higher altitudes are the best oxygen "foods" for the respiratory system. A diet high in protein, carbohydrates, starches, sugars, fats, sulphur and heavy meals in general lowers oxidation in the body and should be used only in moderation if additional oxygen is needed by the body.

Oxygen-carrying foods include:

Beets	Nuts and seeds
Blueberries	Dried olives
Bone broth	Onions
Carrots (red)	Parsnips
Figs	Raisins
Fish	Sea vegetation
Goat milk products (raw)	Sorrell
Grapes	Spinach
Green peppers	Tomatoes and juice
Horseradish	Turtle
Leeks	Wild cherry juice
Mustard greens	

OXYGEN MENUS

Chef's salad including sprouts, raw goat cheese, avocado; carrot juice and goat milk (half and half); celery stuffed with nut butter; sundried olives.

Assorted fruits, cheese sticks, nuts and fruit juice, figs stuffed with nut or seed butter, raisins.

Turtle soup, rare beef, large green salad, steamed beets, steamed sorrel, comfrey tea, tomato dressing.

Bone broth, broiled whitefish, steamed parsnips, steamed spinach, leafy green salad with sliced tomatoes and olives, green vegetable juice (with liquid chlorophyll).

Breathing the oxygen in air has a deeper dietetic meaning than even food, but the oxygen should be vitalized by sunshine, by the motion of air and by the life given off by plants, trees and flowers.

SUMMARY OF OXYGEN

GENERAL CHARACTERISTICS

"Giver of life" element
Active, volatile, unstable
Combines with almost everything

Powerful agent of change
Oxygen type = Oxypheric type

OXYGEN IN THE HUMAN BODY

Strengthens metabolism
Elevates mental activity
Enhances cell regeneration
Infiltrates every cell

Fosters radiant health
Improves assimilation of nutrients
Promotes enthusiasm, youthfulness
Ozone helps remove wastes

SIGNS OF OXYGEN EXCESS (Characteristics of Oxypheric Type)

Optimism, expansiveness, heartiness
Cycles, extremes, pendulum swings
Disquiet, motion, vigor
Hardening, weakening, flushing symptoms

Spontaneity, "joie de vivre"
Ruled by feelings, instincts
Brain overstimulated
Tendency toward intemperance

SIGNS OF OXYGEN DEFICIENCY

Nervous irritabililty
Susceptibility to climatic changes
Stubbornness, hypersensitivity
Increased germ life
Changes in skin
Asphyxiation

Dulled senses
Dulled brain, forgetfulness
Poor digestion, respiration
Congestion and bleeding
Weakened sexuality

HIGHEST OXYGEN FOODS

Iron foods and tonics
Red meats
Greens

Nuts and seeds
Watery vegetables and fruits

Oxygen is the principle element of sanitation. It purifies the blood, strengthens the lungs and improves the chest brain.

---

twelve

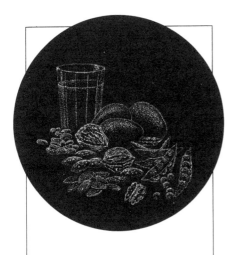

When you are angry, drink a quart of mulberry juice and it will help you lose the anger. During anger, the blood secretions and urine become acid. Mulberry juice helps neutralize the acid.

Phosphorus hunger symptoms include nervous prostration, lack of vitality and sexual interest, general debility, nervousness and dizziness.

Excessive use of the brain weakens the general physical strength. The brain uses much blood when very active. When you use the brain vigorously, from 10 to 20 times as much blood as normal goes to the brain. If you become very excited, the blood flows to the brain tremendously, and the red corpuscles are worn out in great numbers. At last, the brain becomes hyperemic, over-charged with blood. This affects the health.

Lecithin, a phospholipid rich in choline, helps feed the nerves and builds the important neurotransmitter acetylcholine. Researchers have reported that lecithin added to the diet helps keep blood cholesterol down.

Phosphorus, the "light bearer"

Today is a day of phosphorus hunger. Our abundant financial, marital and social problems create tensions which severely tax our phosphorus reserves. Fears, drudgery, monotony, study—all heavy mental activity burn up this element to create phosphorus hunger. Of course, we must think and concentrate in this world today, but it is **how** we think that matters mostly. We can be overly intense; we can be excessively driven—to make money, to prove ourselves, to advance and succeed—and find that we are depleting the brain and nervous system.

Intense brain and nervous system activity utilizes nutrients that maintain nerve cell function so fast that the supply of needed chemical substance for this process must be kept up. It must be replaced quickly. If the brain and nervous system are not working well, all physical activities are threatened. Diabetes, digestive disorders, ulcers and anything from sciatica to shortness of breath can be traced to inadequacies in the brain and nervous system. Of course, phosphorus is not the only chemical element we need here; it must be balanced with calcium, iodine and magnesium. But brain cells predominantly need phosphorus.

Two Kinds of Phosphorus

There are two kinds of phosphorus, a brain and nerve phosphorus and a phosphorus for the bones. What we need for the bones comes from vegetables, but the brain and nervous system require phosphorus from animal products—dairy, eggs, meat, fish and fowl. From the animal proteins we derive much of our lecithin, a nerve fat carrying phosphorus and other brain elements. We should notice that brain and nerve phosphorus and lecithin are not found in liberal quantities in a vegetarian diet. Thus some animal products—goat milk and egg yolks—should be included by the vegetarian. Bone-building phosphorus alone cannot supply all the body's needs. The highly-evolved phosphorus needed for the nerve and brain functions must come from animal protein.

We must keep in mind that the brain is always at work, and, therefore, needs its food twenty-four hours a day. Moreover, it works on a high vibrational level, at a fast rate of speed. Phosphorus is called the "light bearer,"

273

aiding us as we search for light or enlightenment. Enlightenment, joy, happiness, peace and harmony are all forms of vibration working in various brain faculties, and each brain faculty must have the proper amount of phosphorus to work efficiently.

Ways to Deplete Phosphorus

I am very familiar with the excessive use of phosphorus because as a student with Dr. Rocine, and later counseling, lecturing and analyzing patients, I was burning it out too fast. Dr. Rocine explained that when the inner part of the ear constantly flaked a powdery-white substance, and scabs formed on the ear itself, a phosphorus deficiency was indicated. All conditions of neuralgia, neuritis, neurosis, neurasthenia and other nervous problems show a need for brain-building phosphorus.

Different temperaments offer us clues to phosphorus deficiency. One like myself, who perhaps drives too hard, who thinks that eating and going to bed are a waste of time, who doesn't like exercise, and who lives primarily in the mind—such a person may not be taking care of his or her mind. A sign that a person lacks the nerve force to build a good nervous system is found in the digestive pole in the temple area of the head, when it is sunken or indented. A weak digestive pole suggests lack of nerve force. A narrow chin is likely to indicate one mentally inclined and headstrong in many faculties, with a tendency to rapidly break down the brain and nervous system.

Additionally, there are people who become neurodemic or "brain children"; they may be geniuses as they are constantly using their minds. They may also forget their bodies and lose their health. In contrast to the phosphorus-using temperaments, there are people who never move fast enough to burn out any of the brain and nerve elements. They tend to be quiet, serene, humble and easy-going. They do not need to worry much about lecithin depletion. However, the person on a spiritual quest may not belong in this category; sufficient intensity even here can cause the brain to go hungry.

Fatigue and the need for a great deal of rest are also indications of phosphorus depletion. Moreover, optimism and idealism can dwindle or vanish. There is difficulty in responding to stimuli. We need to be particularly careful with fevers, because phosphorus has a low melting point, between 108 and 111 degrees. A continuously high fever, therefore, can burn out the phosphorus, potentially causing brain damage. The same thing can happen due to the excessive heat in a sunstroke, with the phosphorus literally melted away.

With any mental disturbances, we need to look at the body's supply of phosphorus. The brain works with our awareness, thinking, intuition, projection, recognition, visualization, etc., and moves as fast as the speed of light. It is light in the brain that determines how alert we are and how high in mental energies; thus, we must care for that element which bears light to us.

Remedies

Additional to animal protein, phosphorus is abundant in fish eggs, especially cod roe. Throughout Europe, caviar, sturgeon's eggs, is considered one of the finest brain and nerve foods available, but it is usually very expensive. Next to the sturgeon is the "poor man's" fish egg product—cod roe. We have used this food for many patients in order to repair, rehabilitate and rejuvenate with the phosphorus, lecithin and nerve fats it supplies. To prepare, place one tablespoon of pressed cod roe in a blender and blend with one glass of vegetable juice, tomato juice or vegetable broth, taking one cup two or three times weekly.

We must also pay attention to joy and other positive mental qualities. When we are working joyfully, we don't produce the acids that come from working under stress in a job we detest. Joy, happiness and cheerfulness do not wear out the mental faculties as fast as activity done under friction. To help us along in today's stressful world, we need relaxation, good company, hobbies or physical activities and what pleases the mind. Sometimes we need to let go and wear this world like a loose coat.

After the age of 45, we need less fats and sugars and more chelated mineral salts.

274

PHOSPHORUS
"The Light Bearer"

GENERAL CHARACTERISTICS

Originally called *Lucifer*, a Latin term signifying "carrier of light," the element phosphorus now bears the Greek word for "light bearer." Phosphorescent qualities are inherent in many life forms, such as the glow worm or the firefly; scores of polyzea and microscopic organisms residing in oceans, marshes and streams contain enough phosphorus to appear to be illuminated or flaming. Phosphorus is the lamplight of fish, animals and mineral forms. It is symbolic of man's intellectual faculties.

Phosphorus Has to do with Intelligence

Phosphorus is synonymous with intelligence—the medium for coupling the soul with matter. It combines with sulphur in food form and with specific nerve and brain fats within the body. It is chiefly assimilated in the form of lecithin.

"Phosphorus is synonymous with intelligence."

Phosphorus Glows in the Dark

The "light bearer" is a highly toxic, nonmetallic, yellowish-white, waxy element. Its atomic weight is 31. It burns with a white flame; combustion takes place in air in average temperatures. Phosphorus appears luminous in the dark. It is insoluble in water and does not conduct electricity. Its melting point is between 108 and 111 degrees.

Phosphorus Compounds Essential to Life

Phosphorus unites with several other elements—as phosphates of iron, potassium, sodium, magnesium and calcium, the most important being calcium, sodium and magnesium phosphates. These compounds are essential to plant and animal life. Phosphatic manures (consisting of bone phosphates and other phosphates) revitalize depleted soils. Phosphate of lime is an effective fertilizer. Phosphoric acid is found in soil, mainly in unity with lime (calcium) as phosphate of lime. Plant life takes up phosphorus from the soil; a substantial phosphate supply improves nitrogen assimilation in plants.

PHOSPHORUS: ITS ROLE IN THE HUMAN BODY

About two pounds of phosphorus—enough poison to kill everyone in a small city—are found in a man weighing 150 pounds. Phosphorus is found in the nucleus of each cell, in body fluids and in solid tissue as potassium phosphate; as calcium phosphate it enters the bony structure. Bones are made more dense and nutrition of nervous system

275

tissues is improved by phosphorus. Sensory seats in the brain, nerve networks, sympathetic (autonomic) nervous system, nerves, ganglia in general (especially those connected with the heart) and sensory nerves are under the influence of phosphorus. The reproductive organs and bone-producing functions are favorably affected when phosphorus is supplied in proper quantities. The higher intellectual capacity depends on phosphorus—psychic perceptions, idealistic tendencies, humanitarianism, philanthropy, the subjective functions of the brain, physical brain sensations (especially taste and touch). The organic (food) form of phosphorus, sulphur and nerve fats vitalizes and regenerates brain and nerves. Phosphorus is a nerve and brain tonic. In cooperation with more powerful food elements, it is capable of strengthening tissue integrity and tissue function or metabolism. Because it combines into five phosphates, it is plentiful as a general tonic.

"The higher intellectual capacity depends on phosphorus— psychic perceptions, idealistic tendencies, humanitarianism, philanthropy, the subjective functions of the brain, physical brain sensations (especially taste and touch)."

Thinking Consumes Phosphorus

The "light bearer" becomes the medium of the soul's expression through the brain faculties. But to get to the evolved form necessary for the brain to assimilate, phosphorus must undergo transformations beginning in the mineral kingdom, moving from there to the soil by decay, then into seeds and grains, into animals, fish and birds, and ultimately into the human brain. Without phosphorus, we could not study, memorize, read, reason, create, visualize, comprehend. With each thought, phosphorus is used up; each activity of every brain and nerve cell requires phosphorus. The mental worker particularly needs phosphorus, as do writers, students and expectant mothers. The

correct balance of phosphorus ensures the proper acid/alkaline ratio in the blood and digestive juices and instigates proper liquid distribution in the tissues. Cells divide normally due to the presence of phosphorus. Thinking consumes phosphorus. The broken-down phosphate waste material from brain and bone catabolism must be eliminated by the liver. Tests have proven that after extreme mental exertion, there are greater quantities of phosphorus in the urine. This is a dramatic argument in favor of adequate phosphorus in the diet.

Brain Phosphorus and Bone Phosphorus Differ

There is a distinction between the phosphorus needed for bones and that needed by the brain; they are vibrationally different, in that brain phosphorus is more highly evolved. Brain phosphorus comes from the animal kingdom (meat, fish, eggs and dairy products), and bone phosphorus is derived from the vegetable kingdom. Phosphorus is integral to bone formation and repair, and it also nourishes the brain and nerves. It increases the number of red blood corpuscles. It improves tissue nutrition in general. But its greatest function is in the brain and nervous system.

Lack of Phosphorus Causes Serious Problems

Without phosphorus, bone tissue becomes soft. Rickets may develop, indicating that phosphorus, phosphoric acid and calcium, as well as other vital elements, are in demand. Mucus membranes are adversely affected. Sterility is possible. The brain softens and decays. Pus is generated. Neuralgia develops. Intellect atrophies and vanishes. Children or anyone studying hard in school must have brain phosphorus in the daily diet.

Phosphorus Needed for Lecithin Production in the Body

Lecithin, which in its Greek form means egg yolk, is a complex fatty compound necessary in the human body. It is present chiefly in semen, bile, milk, nerve tissue, brain, white and red blood corpuscles, lymph and serous fluids, blood and pus. Its primary constituents are carbon, hydrogen and nitrogen, but it also contains oxygen, phosphorus, fluorine, iron, calcium, sulphur and certain nerve fats, chlorine and glyco-phosphoric acid (stearic). If the diet is deficient in vitamins, nerve fats, phosphorus, oxygen, sulphur and specific nerve salts, lecithin cannot be manufactured within the body; if this is the case, impotence, neuratrophia, brain decomposition, feeblemindedness, physical debility, suppuration and low nerve vitality are among the manifestations. If phosphorus is deficient, lecithin cannot be formed properly in the body.

"Without phosphorus we could not study, memorize, read, reason, create, visualize, comprehend. With each thought, phosphorus is used up; each activity of every brain and nerve cell requires phosphorus."

Phosphorus Vital for Brain and Nerves

The nervous system that pervades the entire body is extremely important. If nutrition is poor, the blood cannot nourish the brain and nerves. When phosphorus is deficient in the diet and sufficient lecithin is not manufactured, the brain and nerves atrophy, the brain decays and phthisis and neurasthenia appear.

Phosphorus' Role in Reproduction

The egg yolk contains vitelline which is the creative principle. Vitelline is a nucleo-protein containing a good deal of phosphorus. Phosphorus is thus necessary for reproduction in man and animals and for their proper growth.

Blood Needs Phosphorus

White blood corpuscles are composed of about ninety percent water, proteins rich in nucleo-albumin and cell globulin which consists of much phosphorus (up to ten percent). Additionally, white cells contain lecithin, glycogen, fat, earthy and alkaline phosphates. Phosphorus is as important here as anywhere in the body; absence of phosphorus causes lowering of metabolism and depleted general health.

Phosphorescence

The fluorescent quality of phosphorus is vital to life forms. Phosphorescent fish generate greater electricity; more animal heat is manufactured in phosphoric animals, and greater tissue activity and muscular heat are generated. In man, the luminosity of phosphorus serves the above purposes in addition to heightening his mental activity (This is where he differs from animals.). The phosphorescent characteristics act differently in various individuals—in some, the action is more in the brain and nervous system and in others it is more in the tissues. It may be said that phosphorus holds the soul in the physical body, imprisons that life spark sometimes referred to as spirit. Phosphorescence is believed by some to be the "astral body" or the "aura."

Phosphorus and ESP

The properties of phosphorus implicate it in telephathy, ESP (extrasensory perception), dreams, wireless etheric communications, suggestive treatments, mediumship, psychogenesis, physical sense perception, sensory impulsion, obsession, delusion, hallucination, hypnotism, psychometry and other purported "strange phenomena."

Calcium Phosphate Essential to the Body

Calcium phosphate is essential to the body for favorable osteosis, bone metabolism, bone building and repair; it prevents excessive generation of pus and brain disintegration. Phosphorus is imperative for the brain, for all thought processes, emotions, organogenesis (along with sulphur) and optimal internal pressure.

SIGNS OF PHOSPHORUS EXCESS

Optimism and Autosuggestion

Excessive phosphorus, whether entering the body in food or drug form, is disastrous to the body's economy, emotions, personality. The individual suffering from phosphorus excess spends money prodigally. Idealistic emotions rather than sound judgment and practical action direct his life. His philosophy is that "thoughts are things." Autosuggestion, mental healing and Christian Science healing are attractive to him. The power of suggestion has great influence on his illnesses, as well as on his health. Platitudes such as, "Believe in disease and it shall come to pass," and, "As you think, so you are," are expounded often. His optimism follows certain directions, such as those of speculative and idealistic philosophy. Speculation is constant; his imagination is prolific. His faith is in the future, in mental conditioning; he has less faith in work, diligence, diet and material concerns. He can read volumes of idealistic philosophy, but goals and optimism outweigh his power to accomplish. The deluge of blood in the brain overstimulates the higher mental visualization centers. Optical illusions and visions are possible. Novels are of interest to him, as are fantastic tales of adventure, mystery, psychic phenomena, travel. His faith is in the infeasible and he dislikes everyday reality.

"Phosphorus overconsumption affects the brain, personality and actions."

Emotions are Volatile

Phosphorus overconsumption affects the brain, personality and actions. Such an individual finds it easier to study at night between ten and three than during the day. He may be a sleepwalker—subjective mind alert while objective brain faculties are in slumber. Internal manifestations of phosphorus excess are many: brain and nerves may be feverish; the patient may feel a craving to know what the future holds, frequenting palm readers and psychics; he may entertain superiority feelings regarding his abilities, positions, genius; he may insist that he is influenced by invisible forces, receiving cosmic revelations—information from angels, space beings, saints and discarnate spirits—relevant to the code of ethics of the universe and the laws that govern the destiny of men. The manner is haughty and proud; emotions are volatile; thoughts and visualizations are vivid. Excitement causes faintness or weakness. Joy is ecstatic; laughter, excessive. The mind overworks, while will power, decision-making ability, practical judgement and concentration ability are feeble and faulty. Vigorous thoughts and emotions result in excessive heat production in the brain revealed by a feverish forehead, chilled feet and hands, and inflamed

nerves. Mental orientations are chaotic, instantaneous, immoderate and intermittent. Merriment, optimism, speculation, hope and confidence are exaggerated. Stimulants are desired.

The Self-Proclaimed Prophet

The patient suffering from immoderate consumption of phosphorus often considers the knowledge of others almost nil and belittles them. He is under the delusion that he is highly intelligent and more wise than anyone. This delusion encourages feelings of false pride, insolence, tyranny, especially with respect to doctrines, theology, canons, philosophies, miracles, psychic phenomena. Such a patient believes he is a chosen one to preach to others and manipulate ecclesiastical activity. He is of the opinion that he is qualified to run the lives of others, dictating their activities and beliefs. He is arrogant, vain, bombastic, autocratic mentally, ethically, theologically, philosophically.

"The patient suffering from immoderate consumption of phosphorus often considers the knowledge of others almost nil and belittles them."

Phosphorus-excess patients are under the delusion that they are more knowledgeable than in actuality they are. They particularly overrate their theological knowledge. Some may dream about the universal plan, utopia, the great unknown, magnetic qualities, essence of spirit and detest practical activity and everyday reality, money, matter, work and manual endeavor. Heat is produced in the brain as a result of sorrow, passion, rage, excitement and hyperemia in the sexual glands and genitals. The outer world may be regarded as deceptive, unimportant, deficient—especially mentally. These patients are animated, energetic, nervous and restless, but are incapable of self-sufficiency, concentrated work, executive command or business judiciousness. Extreme effort and lengthy labor are impossible for them; their dexterity is with the mind, with thinking, psychic endeavors and creeds.

278

The Neurogenic Type

Excess phosphorus facilitates brain and nerve metabolism and hampers osteosis. Consequently, the phosphorus type—the neurogenic—is small-boned, mentally precocious, with overactive nerves and brain. The movements of phosphorus-excess patients are quick and agile. They are animated, swift, spirited, keen, quick of reflex, alert, quick to grasp and memorize new ideas but equally quick to forget. They have restless and mobile hands, feet, tongues, senses, arms, legs. They are unable at times to direct energies productively; their energy soars for a time, then vanishes and ambition leaves. Hard work is not possible on a continuing basis. The realms of theology, philosophy, psychic phenomena attract them as do human magnetism, energy healing, psychotherapy, electrotherapy, magnetic and polarity treatments, Christian Science healing. Magnetization can relieve their pains, as can psychotherapy, electrical therapy, animal magnetism, hypnosis, mental suggestion. The world of reality is often more than they can cope with and they long for "never-never land" and the etheric plane or heaven and its peaceful valleys. Their actions are speedy and slight. Dirt, work, disease instill fears in them. They can create castles with thoughts but cannot build a house with bricks or stones. Study is excessive to the detriment of health, sleep, physical exercise, nutrition, dietetics until exhaustion overcomes them. Some are impractical. Some gesticulate wildly when speaking. Phosphorus-excess children shoot up rapidly but are as lean as fence posts. They crave sensationalism, even if it is violent.

> ## "Excess phosphorus facilitates brain and nerve metabolism and hampers osteosis."

Phosphorus Excess Means Total Mental Orientation

Phosphorus predomination precludes earthiness and practicality. The patient tends toward occult subjects, spiritual and mystical activities and philosophies, and the world of the mind and the etheric plane. The atmosphere, space, ether, light are of interest. Riding on a magic carpet, sailing on clouds are preferable to three-dimensional reality.

Upper story dwellings are favored. Harsh treatment and heavy blows are intolerable. Injury comes easily and there is great sensitivity to pain and internal injuries. Elite businessmen are despised for their wealth. Work is considered debasing. The phosphorus-excess patient favors and dignifies oratory, occult occupations and psychic performances, doctrine making and psychic research. The likes and dislikes of others are often ignored. His mental orientation is extreme.

> ## "The phosphorus-excess patient favors and dignifies oratory, occult occupations and psychic performances, doctrine making and research."

Periodically he may cry, laugh or leap for pleasure. He experiences phobias, extreme superstitions, excitable moods, sexual passion, sensation and sentimental moods by turn. His nature is sensual, yet physical prowess is lacking. Feebleness and worthless feelings predominate. Spiritualistic and occult circles are preferred to the family circle. This patient takes avid interest in aviation, marine-related subjects, space, astronomy, high-speed travel, inventions, revelations, electricity and magnetism, idealistic enlightenment. He lives within his mind and an inner reality rather than with the outer world of physical labor. Reasoning power is devoted to mental and spiritual endeavors rather than earthly matters. He has trust in mental healing and faith healing rather than physical effort. He believes that he can "think and grow rich." His confidence is in the mind and thoughts rather than in science, labor, business, actions or exertion. He lives in an imaginary land of his dreams, in the ethers, until it is the only reality he accepts. The ultimate results may be neurasthenia and extreme phobias.

Practicality Requires Other Elements

When phosphorus joins forces with silicon, calcium and other strong elements, genius is

> ## "The movements of phosphorus-excess patients are quick and agile."

279

probable—a practical genius. But if the phosphorus is preponderant, intense concentration is not feasible. Genius comes when phosphorus binds strongly with calcium, silicon and fibrin. For example, Thomas Edison, the inventor, exhibited a good physique, superior bone development (signifying plenty of calcium), intense mental concentration and had excellent use of his brain, nerves and senses. Surplus phosphorus encourages impracticality, loathing for work and extremely arduous concentration, inability to utilize mental and physical powers, less-than-successful breadwinning. Money is squandered foolishly.

"When phosphorus joins forces with silicon, calcium and other strong elements, genius is probable—a practical genius."

Characteristics of Female Phosphorus-Excess Patients

Female patients displaying phosphorus excess may be painfully selfconscious, hypersensitive to criticism of appearance, full of false pride, deficient in muscle and bone development, will power, mental concentration, attentiveness, independence, selfsustenance and business management talent. The occult world is more real to them than outer reality. Love is craved but returned negatively. Nothing short of expensive dress, furnishings, jewelry or autos will suffice; but these do not satisfy. Change is a recurring fancy. Anything pleasing is received with ecstasy. Solid food has little appeal, but frothy drinks do. Candy, confections, dainties, fruits and novels are longed for. Late hours are kept. Nervousness and weakness mount, promoting the use of coffee, tea, stimulants, magnetic and polarizing treatments, health spas or Christian Science healing. But sleep, relaxation, deep breathing, proper nutrition and adequate exercise are neglected. There is an unfounded restlessness and sentimentality. Excitement, plays, travel, entertainment, change and profuse spending are preferred. The phosphorus-excess female seeks society life, champagne suppers, moonlight strolls, expensive vacations, extravagant home and clothing, glittering jewelry, patronizing doctors, poetry and a life of leisure rather than labor. Imaginary romances are dwelled upon. Airplanes are appealing. Rocking chairs are comforting. Money is spent lavishly and foolishly.

Characteristics of Male Patients

The male patient suffering phosphorus indiscrimination may be sensitive and frail. His mental powers are excitable, but he is physically weak. Prophetic inspirations come to him. He becomes obsessed by ideas. His conversation is disjointed, sentences unfinished. His arguments lack foundation. Graphic descriptions of nertain diseases produce the symptoms personally. He operates on sheer nerve energy, and his imagination and visualization are prolific. Skin pigment may be ash-gray; heat in upper forehead and central tophead is intensified; thyroid gland pressure causes eye pressure; eyes and nose water excessively; lower jaw falls out of place easily when tired; facial muscles are taut, causing expression to twist; ear wax stiffens.

Prophecy and Imagination in Neurogenic

A phosphorus-excess patient is likely to predict the future of others—prophesy about the future of his associates, family, city, nation, world and the universe. His imagination becomes dominant over three-dimensional reality. The mind is clouded, wandering, meditative, mediumistic, subject to self-hypnosis, mysterious and mystical. Moods vary from verbosity to silence and sullen periods. Strength alternates with debility and helplessness.

Physical Signs of Phosphorus Oversupply

If phosphorus is oversupplied, the secretion may take on a luminous aura. Urine develops whitish, foamy bubbles. Pulse becomes weak. Urine is scarce and may include phosphorus, bile casts, ammonia or its smell, sugar, albumin, sarcolactic acid, leucine, tyrosine or even oxalic acid. Breath may be foul and similar to rotting vegetables.

"If phosphorus is overconsumed for a prolonged period of time, the lungs and kidneys are damaged and their efficiency reduced."

Possible Damage to Lungs and Kidneys

The lungs and kidneys expel the greatest percentage of worn-out phosphorus. If phosphorus is overconsumed for a prolonged period of time, the lungs and kidneys are damaged and their efficiency reduced. Neurogenic (phosphorus) types are notably weak in the kidney and lung structures, often inherently. Oxidation in tissues and blood is injured by an excess of phosphorus by-products in the body; in this case, neurasthenia, neuralgia and hepatic complications are likely.

Fresh Air Important to Recovery

It is important to recognize that recuperation from phosphorus deficiency or excess is lengthy and arduous due to emaciation, low oxidation, malnutrition and partial tissue disintegration. High altitude, breeziness, cool air, fresh and outdoor air, proper exercise, abundant ozone and oxygen are important to the recovery.

Jawbone May be Afflicted

In the event that phosphorus is overconsumed or excessive from birth or before birth, there is a tendency to become a neurogenic type—the cerebral or phosphorus type. Overconsumption of phosphorus is unlikely in types other than the neurogenic, but it does occur. Characteristics of phosphorus overusage are distinctive. They may include fatty degeneration of the liver; fatty degeneration of muscles, kidneys, heart, intestines, glands of the stomach; progressive weight loss; deterioration of connective tissues. Predisposition to afflictions involving the maxillary bone are common when phosphorus is oversupplied to brain and nerves.

Youthful Signs of Phosphorus Excess

In youth, the bones of the neurogenic type may not develop properly due to poor assimilation of bone elements (salts). He may be delicate and thin. His body is small, mind precocious, brain large and vigorous, skin pale and gray. Nerves are edgy and restless. Physical labor is declined. Sexual appetite may be excitable in adolescent years but unmatched by physical stamina in the sexual function.

Complaints of Women with Overabundant Phosphorus

The female patient suffering from overutilization of phosphorus demonstrates many peculiarities. She may complain of stiff knees, foot pains that move up toward the hips, cramps in finger tendons along with numbness, arm weakness, stinging with pain in restricted areas of the small of the back (usually relieved by gentle massage, mental suggestion or Christian Science techniques). Spinal bones are sensitive or sore. Physical effort is very difficult. She is plagued by indecision. Bone metabolism is unfavorably changed. Her brain generates excessive heat and there is a battle for enough oxygen. (Men who have phosphorus excess carry hats rather than wearing them.) The patient holds hands to head as if there were trouble there. Spinal ganglia express tension. Heat sensation is felt in upper spine or lower back of head along with heat and stiffness in the brain. The phosphorus-excess female also drops her lower jaw when tired or overworked. Her head is feverish and body cold, attended by flushed face; or her face may be colorless, and neck and face beaded by perspiration with alternating heat waves. Nights may be sleepless due to undue heat production in the brain, restless nerves, motor nerve neuralgia, hunger pangs. Temper fits are frequent.

> ## "The female patient suffering from overutilization of phosphorus demonstrates many peculiarities."

Sleepwalking and Peculiar Sleep Habits

She is very gifted psychically, and she impresses people. The phosphorus-excess female may demonstrate somnambulism, but during sound sleep she resembles a corpse; low oxidation develops. Color returns in daytime when she is active and outdoors, but some paleness remains. Her stomach is under attack of smarting pains and cramps following physical exertion, along with constant soreness in peritoneum and whole abdominal area. The stomach is frequently acid. There is a predisposition to vomiting after meals. She experiences infrequent fainting but is energetic otherwise. The medulla is weakened and the circulatory system suffers. The blood lacks fibrin and organic salts. The lips may become indigo or bluish white and shrivelled. Shooting pains move through teeth. The throat may be arid and weak. The esophagus burns. Feet tingle. Tendons convulse in spasms. There may be a painful spot in the temple region or lateral area of forehead and frequent rolling motion in the ears coexisting with chilly feelings in the body and a feverish forehead. When slumbering, the feet are drawn up toward chin and straightening legs out causes pain. The day brings yawning, notably near nightfall because strength is flagging and more carbonic acid is present in the atmosphere. Thighs are sore and organs feel enlarged, atonic and malpositioned. There is an inclination to sweating when excess carbonic acid is in the body. The sexual system is weakened; the nervous system is agitated; carnal thoughts are entertained; nasal bones are tender; arterial walls are weak; catarrh settles in the walls of the digestive tract.

"There is an inclination to sweating when excess carbonic acid is in the body."

Pains and Shortwindedness

Other general symptoms of phosphorus-excess women are diminished urine flow; disrupted liver function; acidity of digestive tract; complexion turning yellow or milky yellow; restlessness in dead of night promoting tiredness in the morning, greater fatigue upon rising than when retiring at night; flushing and crawling waves moving toward the head; bronchitis with foamy and slightly bloody discharge; shortwindedness; rapid walk; chaotic breathing, episodes of suffocation. Lungs do not oxygenate blood properly. Digestion is poor. Stomach is heated and large amounts of water are consumed after meals and during the night. Stomach has gnawing, grinding sensation. Patient experiences bowel cramps. Epigastrium is atonic and tender. Throat is raw. Tonsils are swollen. Muscles are painful. Salivation increases. Nerves are razor-edged because acid is formed which attacks nerve tissue. Phosphorus-excess women may present neuralgic pains in cheek bones, ear noises, eye weakness of optic nerves, blood rushing to brain. Ears experience abnormal sounds because

acids and toxins are disrupting cells in the basal membranes.

She May Become A Religious "Fanatic"

If objects are scrutinized for any length of time, they appear to alter in color. High altitudes are preferred where air is cool, fresh and arid; the ozone she needs is found in mountain regions. Her hair may turn gray prematurely and she may appear aged. Her moods are variable, her strength absent. Suicide is contemplated because she finds no reason for life. The brain is never still. This patient is energized easily, readily irascible, cantankerous and difficult to please. Physical work is detested; brain work is acceptable but sometimes difficult. She may become a religious fanatic; she may engage in deep study of metaphysical and occult subjects. Heavy brain use results in harmful aftereffects. Electrical changes in the atmosphere cause her to respond. The phosphorus-excess female may demonstrate optical illusion, poor bone metabolism, craving for stimulants, propensity for Oriental beliefs, love of mystery and suspense. She is susceptible to quackery, idealistic doctrines, speculation, superstition, exaggerated imagination, visions, insomnia. She has a craze for talking. Metaphysical subjects are her chosen avenues of preaching, teaching, writing, lecturing.

Phosphorus-Related Physical Ailments

Disorders directly or indirectly related to phosphorus intemperance include hematuria, stomach pains, diarrhea, cystitis, phosphaturia, pyelitis, exaggerated brain activity and nervous ebullience, brain fatigue, atrophy of muscular tissue, atonicity, chest pain, leucocythemia, dense urine, asthmatic complications, vomiting, bloody discharge, hemorrhage of mucus membranes, albuminuria due to destruction of kidney cells, thirst, restlessness, painful liver enlargement, cramps in finger tendons, nervous unrest, volatile temper outbursts, somnambulism, hypochondria, flatus, eructation, shaking, jerking in tendons, raw throat, sagging spine, night sweating, atonicity and softening of arterial walls, jaundice, aching teeth, bleeding canker sores, itching (especially on knees or elbows or both), extreme nervousness, spitting of blood, weak lung activity, complications of trachea, double pulse, rush of blood to brain and lungs, poor calculation of distance so falling is likely, drugged stupor, painful and feeble muscles, tonsillar swelling, paratrophy, heart disorders, left shoulder pain, swelling of auxillary glands, trembling of hands, unsteadiness of lower legs, near exhaustion in the morning, episodes of suffocation, chronic salivation, inflammatory neuralgia, bronchitis, below-par digestion and nutrition, neuritis (especially due to drafts), toothaches caused by moisture or cold. Phosphorus may be found in the urine as may ammonia or its smell; bubbles form in urine. Unrestrainable delirium may manifest occasionally. Other manifestations in phosphorus-excess women include convulsions, hemorrhagic complications, sexual system hyperesthesia, religious fanatacism, weakened pulmonary and circulatory activity, phosphaturia (phosphorescent urine). The religious, spiritual, metaphysical brain faculties are affected. Bone nutrition is sabotaged; liver and kidneys are damaged; sexual system is atrophied; brain and nerve nutrition is abnormal.

SIGNS OF PHOSPHORUS DEFICIENCY

Weakness is Nearly Constant

The patient suffering from phosphorus shortage has a ravenous appetite but is not hungry at the table. Tissue oxygenation is low; assimilation capacity is below the needs of the body. In bed the patient is hungry, but not at the breakfast table. Faintness is constant. Lack of appetite alternates with extreme hunger. Sexual system is weak. Desire for cold drinks or food is strong. Nerve pain intensifies with position changes. Reasoning seems extremely difficult and often causes headache. Study or ebullience cause anxiety and nervous sensations in the epigastric plexus; unfavorable information is exhausting; entire nervous system is weak; power of self direction is lacking. The patient does not command power or exhibit executive activity. Nervous collapse succeeds excitable periods. His sickness is all-important, leaving no room for consideration of others; he constantly talks about himself. Mental states fluctuate from apprehension to gaiety and laughter, from uncommunicativeness to verbosity, from optimism to extreme depression. Dangers are imagined above, around, near or beneath him. Crying periods may manifest and then change to hysteria and laughter. Brain weakness exists continually; stimulants are desired; helplessness and weakness are almost constant.

> "The patient suffering from phosphorus shortage has a ravenous appetite, but is not hungry at the table."

Personality Characteristics of Patients Deficient in Phosphorus

The personality, nerves, heart and brain cells are under siege when lightning and thunderstorms take place. Women, especially, feel like hiding at these times; the heart beats rapidly from fear. Courage, will power, decision-making ability, activity, ambition are lacking. The brain does not serve well; ideas do not come easily; mental confusion takes over. Loss of intellectual ability is dreaded. Fine lines appear all over the face giving an aged appearance. The phosphorus-deficient patient is sleepy, dull during the day. Night brings fear, shyness, depression about one's condition. The patient is very sensitive to criticism. Unfounded and unidentifiable foreboding hangs over him. Noise is extremely irritating; trains, planes, cars, buses, ships, machinery, children's noise, city bustle are intolerable. Peace and serenity are desired. Will power is absent. He becomes disgusted with the world status and his own. He may harbor an extreme desire for shunning society, for life as a hermit in the hills or forest. He ignores his own good qualities but finds imaginary shortcomings distressing.

Females Evidence Lack of Phosphorus

The female phosphorus-deficient patient may be painfully sensitive to flaws in her appearance and, at times, refuse to be seen in public. In public, she imagines all eyes are scrutinizing her; she feels self-conscious, hypersensitive, nervous. Her mind is weak, nerves starved, brain tissue toxic and nerves acid. Nerves crawl when under criticism, accused of something, reprimanded; these experiences further deplete the nerves. Her imagination is morbid; people are frightening; self is punished. She feels apprehensions without cause, aversion to noise, qualms about accusations, gruesome fear of disease, worry. Phosphorus-deficient patients may detest foods they once liked and have a craving for coffee, tea or other stimulants. They take pleasure in sensationalism. They exhibit fatigue, self-judgment, hopelessness, self-pity, weeping, misgivings, proud self-consciousness, mental inability, exhausted nerves, uneasiness, indecision. Crying comes easily.

Weakness Overcomes Patients

Patients who lack phosphorus think they are weaker than anyone, too weak to put effort into obtaining luxuries, food, drink and shelter. They experience daytime sleepiness but cannot sleep well at night. Parts of their bodies have sensations of semiparalysis, especially the tongue. Infections overcome them easily. All things black, worrisome, noisy or unfavorable have a harmful effect on mind and nerves. Arms and legs tremble and shiver. There is possible extreme heat production in the brain, attended by much nerve weakness. Phosphorus-deficient patients may exhibit numbness of hands, ankles, feet; swollen ankles; taut skin of feet and ankles; taut but shriveled face skin. They are keenly responsive to drafts but like cool mountain air. They experience congestion of chest from strong emotions. Involuntary activities may refuse to obey the will because of incapacitation. Senses are not properly oriented and mind concentrates with difficulty.

Patients Create Their Own Diseases

Many phosphorus-impoverished patients cannot stand to hear or read about graphic disease symptoms; they find a morbid reality in them too painful to withstand. They prefer treatments such as mental healing and Christian Science. They are intensely sensitive to what is heard; distasteful conversations have a deep impression. Diseases have a great influence on them, resulting in hypochondria. The mind stands in morbid vigilance due to acidity in the nerves, autointoxication of the brain or tissues; the autotoxins create the sense of morbidity and abandonment characteristic of the phosphorus-depleted patient. Poisoning himself with his own waste material he often believes others are trying to poison him.

Females May be Afraid of Males

Female phosphorus-deficient patients describe their afflictions and symptoms dramatically. Such symptoms may include phobia of men, matrimony and married life. They exhibit lack of energy in the morning, sneezing and coryza, chest oppression in the morning, bluish cast to skin, shaky hands, drowsiness toward evening, temple pain brought on by bright light, depressed breathing and chest activity due to unfavorable atmospheric alterations. The skin pales occasionally. Moisture is chilling. Chills are accompanied by face flush, stinging palms, burning soles of feet upon staying for long in a warm room. Temperature changes affect throat. Head and neck perspire mainly at night. There may be excruciating neuralgic pain coupled with heart palpitation. Pains jump from place to place, but centralize in the head, face and teeth. In the early morning thinking is intolerable.

"The phosphorus-lacking patient hankers for love, affection, sympathy and gratitude."

A Woman Describes Her Symptoms

Another patient might describe her symptoms as follows: decisions are impossible; weakness confines her to bed nearly all day; her tongue seems half paralyzed; spinal bones feel disjointed and displaced; sensitivity is severe; mental activity is aggravated; circulation is extremely poor; hearing is distorted; brain is cloudy; mind is confused and breathing difficult; insomnia is produced by overactive mental faculties at night. Other symptoms may be weakness in bones, nerves, brain and muscles; shirveled or dry and feverish skin; shallow wrinkles forming a net over face, on hands, neck, nose, forehead and ears to give an aged appearance; transparent skin showing blue-vein network below; swollen roots of nails; worried, dispirited and listless eyes. Head is overheated and the body chilled. Mind is morbid, depressed and hypersensitive to all said or done. Trivial matters are upsetting. Work is detested. Nerves manifest terrific pains. The phosphorus-deficient female suffers from delusions, quarrelsomeness, irascibility, restlessness and nervousness, inability to concentrate, inattention, worry, pessimism, sadness, loneliness, dejection, gruesome and morbid emotions. Nothing seems to bring her relief.

Patients Lack Confidence

The phosphorus-lacking patient hankers for love, affection, sympathy and gratitude; misery and self-depreciation set in. Age brings a hollow chest due to drooping of shoulders. Morbid fears develop. Sleep seems drugged. The patient runs on nervous energy. His eyes are listless, cheeks hollow, appetite poor, fingers sometimes blistered, face furrowed, eyes contracted. His nerves are under attack by sharp, stabbing pains. Bronchial tubes are rough and throat raw. A tickling cough teases him; the nerves of the throat sting and pulsate. There are stitching indications in facial nerves. He is clumsy, making false judgments of distance and stumbling. He is sluggish and indifferent, pessimistic in attitude, but optimistic in religion and conversation. His desire to recline or sit is strong. Disappointment alternates with optimism and irritability. Bones of lower spine are tender and sore. Such a patient often seeks comfort in religion for melancholy souls. Confidence is lacking. Malevolent suggestions are frightening. There is great demand for positive thinking, optimistic doctrines, merry friends and uplifting sermons. Self-confidence founded upon a diet rich in phosphorus is needed.

Fears and Dread of Future

There is a feeling among phosphorus-deficient patients that others have no faith in them. Nutrition is crucial, but food is not digested properly. If the proper help is not obtained, the patient may grow discouraged with life to the point of suicide. The body feels almost dismembered. There is love of water because it is symbolic of reaching another plane of existence. Solitude breeds depression and develops fears. Association is exclusive. Congenial friends are almost impossible to find. Dread clouds the brain, but there is an irrepressible curiosity about one's future destiny. Horrible, unidentifiable happenings are expected. A fatality looms ahead. The patient is a coward; he appears deficient in his own eyes; misfortunes are viewed with dread, but when they actually arrive, he is less concerned. A tiny mouse may drive a woman patient to distraction. There is a constant foreboding of something fatal, ghastly, paranormal. The patient can sit for great lengths of time without taking action or making a decision.

A Male Describes His Symptoms

A male phosphorus-starved patient might describe his symptoms in this way: he feels constant depression; everything appears impossible; he fears for the salvation of his soul; he imagines poisoning; he feels he is being chased by evil forces, hostile enemies; he is suspicious of others. He feels worthless in his own estimation, but is too cowardly to commit suicide. Engagements have been broken because he cannot face the marital responsibilities. His mind is unable to concentrate on studies, problems and labor; scrutinizing objects for some time causes mental confusion. His neck is always sore. He puffs when exhaling and during sleep. He collapses from utter weakness. Bright sunshine produces headache and neuralgia. He is tired of living, filled with apprehensions, jealous, argumentative, hypersensitive, bombastic, enterprising yet feels worthless. He is overwatchful and painfully self-conscious. His temper flares explosively. He mumbles to himself. He feels irrational fear of ghosts, evil, old houses, dark alleys. Study of disease, anxiety, passion, anger, excitement, affect him unfavorably; nerve tension or strong emotions exhaust him for hours.

Some Individuals More Prone to Phosphorus Deficiency

Inherent qualities, brain development, personality incline some individuals to phosphorus deficiency more than others; in their bodies phosphorus is precipitated rapidly by the brain, nerves and tissues. There is a stronger propensity for certain maladies and complications in some people as a result. Phosphorus-deficient individuals suffer from neuralgia (sciatic, crural, intercostal, cervico-occipital, tri-facial, cervicofacial, lumbo-abdominal), nervous diseases and disorders, enteralgia, odontalgia, coccygodynia, visceral neuralgia, leucorrhea, rickets, hemicrania, ganglioma, ganglitis, softening of bones or brain and nerves, neuriasis, neuroglioma, mucus membrane disorders, impotence, brain decay, stupor, spermatorrhea, abdominal spasms, spinal irritation during menses, poor blood due to deficient oxygenation and lack of red blood cells. Other common symptoms are sleeplessness, lassitude, neuromyelitis, debility of various body functions, eventual nervous exhaustion, paralytic muscle twitch, angina pectoris, neurotabes, incapacity for prolonged mental concentration, extreme shyness or aversion to society, fear of possession or hypnotic control. Locomotor ataxia is prevented if the supply of phosphorus is adequate.

Blisters, Poor Circulation & Respiration

The phosphorus-deficient patient may manifest migraine, photesthesia, photalgia, lung hemorrhages, neuratrophia, frontal headache, severe ache in temples, hay fever or asthma, various pains (extremities, stomach, sides, heart), erysipelas, corneal ulcers, predisposition to ague, teeth disorders, typhus, mouth blisters, salivation and throat ailments, faintness, throat ulcers, hoarseness, floating or wandering liver with chance of liver abscesses, lumbar hernia, distension and debility, rectitis, renal problems, edematous ailments, purplish blisters, bleeding wounds, cerebral exhaustion, pericardial pains, spleen complications, metrorrhagia and other metropathic ailments, aphonia and throat spasms, heart rheumatism, chills, nightly sweating, intermittent fever, inflammation of cellular tissue. There is also greater inclination toward epilepsy though it is not directly attributed to phosphorus shortage. There is danger of gangrene when operations are performed on diseased tissue. The skin may be nearly blue (cyanosis) indicating that oxygen is deficient in blood and tissues. The left lung may be easily implicated leading to respiratory troubles. Excessive drinking is a danger because the liver is diseased and the mind warped.

Digestive and Heart Problems

Other symptoms of phosphorus deficiency include inflammation of the psoas muscle (psoitis), bone decay, foot and toe disorders, intestinal problems, ovaritis with severe uterine pains. Headache and profound neuralgia of the face and teeth may together overcome the patient if phosphorus and other tissue salts are wanting. Loss of speaking ability, weak thighs, uremia, premature gray hair, temporary blindness, aching eyeballs, alternating dry and liquid coryza, polypi of the ears, glaucoma, mental confusion, chest cramps, extreme groin pain, nervous convulsions, susceptibility to scarlet fever, nasal polypi, nasal membrane inflammation, earache, bone function disruption with bone enlargement, hydromania, joint enlargement, hip bone diseases with watery pus and dark edges, lower jaw complication, peromelia, muscular angina, stricture of esophagus may be presenting symptoms. Phosphorus-deficient patients may also demonstrate gastro-adenitis, tympanitis in the colon, colon enteritis, greenish bloody discharge from bowel, nausea, polydipsia, cardiatrophia, softening of heart structures, hydromyelia, chronic diarrhea, bleeding piles, rectal ulcers, pyloritis, hydrocele, phlebitis, pyemia, hydremia, involuntary stools, faulty bone metabolism, improper tissue nutrition, gurgling in the stomach.

Treatment Includes Exercise, Diet and High Altitude

Young people deficient in phosphorus (both girls and boys) may develop glycosuria which requires living in the mountains, proper diet and the correct exercise program. Other phosphorus-deficiency patients experience venous stagnation, heart dilation, disturbance of the right heart artery. Swelling of joints may occur due to faulty bone metabolism. Joints are easily dislocated. Glands are enlarged. Ankles show evidence of edema. Cranial abnormalities may appear. Sores, boils, pimples may manifest. Injuries leave ugly scars when phosphorus and other tissue salts are in deficit. Prolonged phosphorus starvation results in afflictions that often cannot be cured unless the patient is relatively young. In any case, recuperation takes a great deal of time and effort including proper diet, appropriate altitude, pleasant environment.

Deficiency Symptoms May Be Chaotic

The symptoms of the phosphorus impoverished patient are chaotic. Psoriasis may appear on knees, ankles, elbows, hips. Blood disorders of a nervous or bacterial origin are likely.

Symptoms in Children

A certain type of child suffers from malnutrition causing pus generation similar to tuberculosis and often mistaken for same; but it is really phthisis—pus formation due to lack of oxygen, phosphorus and specific vegetable salts. This child is characterized by stagnant and inactive bowels, scrofulous tendencies, emaciated arms and legs, purulent glands, swollen joints and poor blood. Neurogenic children are precocious and are excellent pupils in school. They resemble alabaster or fine porcelain in appearance and seem old beyond their years. Nightmares trouble them. They may present problems with adenoids, adenosis, faulty teeth, small bones, weak legs. Their intellect is advanced, but they tend to die young because vital force is lacking; exhaustion often overtakes them.

Bones and teeth give them trouble. They are afflicted with headaches, hydric tendencies, pain in long bones (mistakenly termed growing pains), fainting caused by brain anemia, lack of nerve and brain energy, chronic eczema between fingers and toes. Some grow rapidly in height, but do not develop properly outwardly. Their chests are small and sunken; shoulders are square and often sloped; hips and waists are small; face is elongated—sometimes pear shaped but long. Eyes are set low on the face; cheeks are hollow, chin small, ears thin, skin soft and milky white or pale gray, voice high-pitched, hair fine, features shapely and sculptured, feet long and slender, nature idealistic, lips thin, disposition exclusive, movements smooth and easy, eyes large, movements speedy, expression intelligent. Their walk lacks power and force. Their appetite is minimal and subdued with ease. They are considered "frail" or "delilcate" children. They are considered tubercular; but, in actuality, they have pus formation due to low oxygenation, poor blood, deficiency of phosphorus, lack of blood and necessary tissue salts. They are ruled by the brain; it robs the rest of the body of vital elements. Education is their only interest, yet it is their undoing. They often die young after graduating from college and failing to make use of their education due to debility. It is a mistake to send neurogenic children to college with poorly developed bodies and poor bloodstreams; their vitality should be built up first.

Hereditary Weaknesses Intensify Problems of Phosphorus Shortage

Each emotion and thought disintegrates phosphorus in the brain. In the event phosphorus is expended to excess, phosphorus by-products are released in such massive quantities that, if the eliminative organs are not active and efficient, metabolism is disturbed. Neurogenic patients are identified by a slender waist and, consequently, a diminutive liver; small liver and small kidneys are a disadvantage in correlation with a large, prolific brain because excessive cerebral waste products are released hourly. If phosphorus by-products are imprisoned in the body, the mind is darkened, nerves weakened and bone metabolism undermined. Digestion, nutrition, circulation and oxygenation of blood and tissue are adversely affected. The result is weakness, nervousness, depression and excessively meticulous (compulsive) habits.

Breathing Problems

Oxygenation is slow in any phosphorus-deficient patient. The condition calls for fresh air, windy climate, enjoyable exercise, sandy soil, a home in the mountains, pleasant environment, frequent physical activity, considerable sleep and a phosphorus-rich diet (also rich in blood and tissue salts). The neurogenic type abhors exercise and dislikes deep breathing which he needs to overcome his weakness; it is essential to place him in an environment where nature helps do the work of rehabilitation.

Symptoms More Subjective Than Objective

Phosphorus poverty symptoms are decidedly subjective rather than objective; a number of them are recognizable to the doctor, nutritionist, nurse, parent. Included are neuralgia, brain softening, debility, impotence, pale and bloodless complexion, aversion to exertion, listlessness, sleeplessness part of the night (tossing in bed for hours with sleep coming near morning). Action is possible only under stimulating or exciting circumstances; collapse follows the excitement. The patient may experience gloomy moods and a gnawing sensation in his digestive tract. He has a false appearance of health, but feels as if death is approaching. It is incorrectly assumed by physicians that the patient is a victim of his own imagination. The future is dreaded; ailments hold great concern. The patient may report throbbing in head or chest; prostration during menstruation; distorted sensations of touch and motion; numbness in specific skin areas of finger, toe, leg or arm; acute sensitivity to pain, cold or heat; loss of finger control or of normal use of hand, arm or tendon; momentary paralysis of a part of the body; twitching muscles, notably the eyelid muscles with resultant involuntary winking. The patient exhibits painful shyness; intermittent symptoms; neurasthenia; constant scrofula; pain in small of back, sides, hips or stomach; hardening of ear wax; milky-blue or milky-gray skin tone; sores with dark-blue or dark-green edges; gnawing in stomach; sensitivity to pressure; a heavy feeling; disdain for executive work; weakness; emaciation; aversion to society, especially the opposite sex; brain exhaustion; excessive growth in height yet underweight; general weakness of constitution; a fine porcelain or alabaster appearance in youth;

287

faulty bone metabolism; degenerative alterations in joints; extreme emaciation of arms and legs. Total mental and physical disintegration is possible.

Children Are Mentally Precocious But Physically Weak

Phosphorus-deficient children are slow in learning to walk but precocious mentally. They may awaken at night with screams of agony. Joints may swell; upper vertebral bones may be sore, painful, stiff, swollen, weak. Neurogenic children suffer malnutrition. They have finicky appetites with preference for candy, sweets, apples, orange juice, stimulants. Their faces may be puffed but bodies emaciated. Body temperature varies; blood is feverish because it is not oxygenated. These children may present a deep cough, pea-like knots in glands of neck, fleeting pains, insufficient oxygenation of blood and tissue. They are often kept home from school because of weakness. Teeth are poor and bones small. The child's head jerks when he is sitting still; head draws backward. Excitement produces heat in the head and a flushed face. Pushing tongue out of mouth is difficult; tongue trembles when this action is attempted. Teeth decay. Forehead is unusually feverish. Tip of tongue develops blisters. Saliva is foamy, profuse, tenacious. Bones are curved. Reclining causes heart discomfort. Toes tingle.

Further Symptoms of Phosphorus Shortage

Other phosphorus starvation indications are fainting episodes; numbness; scalp contraction; agitation in spring and summer heat; lung congestion from strong emotions; stooped, bent chest; morbid imagination; piles that bleed easily; frothy, soap-like bubbles in urine; shiny, greenish or phosphorescent stools; hair graying prematurely; insufficient oxygen level in blood and tissues exemplified by pale or milky skin tone (bloodlessness); bluish skin cast; sweating of head, neck, face (more at night); craving for massive amounts of water. Other indirect symptoms of phosphorus deficiency include a deflated feeling, meandering aches and pains, fatigue, tender and sore spine, shooting pains in abdomen and chest, spinal irritation during menstruation, itching, constant neuralgic pains, aspasmodic dyspepsia, limb convulsions. Often the complexion is waxen or clay-like, dirty or greasy; skin tone may be pale, bloodless.

Indirect Symptoms are Many

There may be loud, humming, whirring noises in the ears. Appearance may be deceptively healthy, hale, rosy and phosphorus still lacking. Other patients may demonstrate debility, weakness, small frame, neuralgic tendencies, minor illnesses, lack of appetite, weakness in lower back, invalidism, debilitating headache, prickling feelings, pains appearing and disappearing without reason, formation of nerve tumors causing excruciating pain, angina pectoris caused by pressure from an enlarged blood vessel (aneurysm). All are indirect evidence of phosphorus hunger. Other symptoms are hearing difficulty, stomach acidity indicating lack of oxygen, cyanotic skin, oily pimples on face.

Male and Female Coimplaints Differ

Male patients lacking phosphorus have neuralgic pains in hips, stomach, sides, small of back. Women complain of neuralgia in face, teeth, lower back of head, ears, temples and pubic region. However, it is important to remember that phosphorus is not the sole cause of neuralgia. Other contributing factors may be lead poisoning, hereditary syphilis, toxic metabolic products of excess brain activity, drug poisoning, malaria, autointoxication waste, metabolic toxins and gases, latent gonorrhea, among other causes.

Further Signs in Children

All precocious, predominantly intellectual, nervous, thin and slender children lack phosphorus. They suffer also from poor blood, low oxygenation, malnutrition, susceptibility to colds, foot trouble, glandular tubercles, earache, catarrh, tonsillitis, ill effects of cold air and moisture, fever accompanied by cold feet. They are irritable and difficult to please. Weaknesses exist in respiratory system, digestive system, heart, lungs, kidneys, liver, circulatory and sexual systems. The body is thin, lean and sore; joints swell often. Bowel is sluggish. Nails grow long and curve outward. Forehead is large; temples are indented; head is large. Brain is energetic, but body suffers from emaciation. They may be diagnosed as tubercular, but blood tests are negative. Saliva is profuse; roof of mouth is tender and sore; fauces are purple. Perspiration is clammy, throat tender, arms weak, bladder painful. Such children complain of gnawing in stomach. Appetite is slight and they feel worse after eating.

288

The Symptoms Continue

Phosphorus-deficient patients may present still other symptoms: feet swelling; hip tendons contracting with pain; thighs contracting painfully when walking, exercising, working or otherwise exerting; weakness on left side with pain running throughout the body; extreme weakness, fainting or prostration in spring or during heat waves are all direct or indirect symptoms of phosphorus deficiency. Brain complications, brain shrinkage causing peculiar symptoms when the patient moves (turns, jumps, leans, stoops or is jarred), hypersensitivity to noises, facial cramps, neck cramps with tension in neck and shoulders, abdominal pains, numb joints, intolerable neuralgic pains, ear congestion attended by pain, nasal membrane inflammation, neck and throat weaknesses, nervous deafness, weakness in sexual system, utter disgust for sexual activity, intense nevousness, inability to think, feverish forehead, mild fever running throughout the system, low energy, various neurasthenic symptoms—all are

"Individuals differ in their phosphorus demands; some need more than others."

direct and/or indirect indications of phosphorus lack.

Types of People Prone to Phosphorus Deficiency

Individuals differ in their phosphorus demands; some need more phosphorus than others. Frequently deficient in phosphorus are cerebral types, neurogenic types, emotional types, atrophic types, highly intellectual and extremely precocious children, those who do intense brain work, students, lawyers, doctors, teachers, musicians and other individuals engaged in nerve/stress occupations. These individuals must have a diet rich in phosphorus.

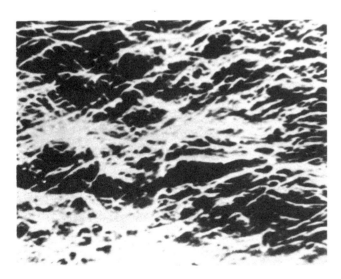 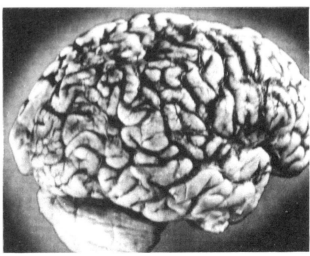

Phosphorus is a critical element to the brain and nerves, and they cannot function effectively without it. Some neurotransmitters need phosphorus, which is found in eggs, milk and all lecithin foods. Over 30 neurotransmitter chemicals have been found in the brain.

HIGHEST PHOSPHORUS FOODS

We must differentiate between a "brain" phosphorus and a "bone" phosphorus; the latter can be obtained from the vegetable kingdom, but brain phosphorus must be derived from animal products. The sources of brain phosphorus are meat, egg yolk, fish, fish roe, dairy products. High phosphorus foods of the vegetable kingdom are almonds, rice bran, rice polishings, wheat bran, wheat germ, pumpkin and squash seeds, sunflower seeds, lentils, dried soybeans. Phosphorus-containing foods are listed below.

Almonds
Barley
Bass
Beans (broad, lima, red, white, mung)
Black fish
Bone broth
Bone marrow
Cabbage (common, Savoy)
Cardamom
Carrots
Cashew nuts
Cheeses (roquefort, Swiss)
Cod roe
Corn
Dairy products
Dulse
Egg yolk
Eggshell broth
Fish
Fish broth
Fish roe
Goat butter, butter-mild, cheese, clabbered milk
Haddock
Halibut

Herring
Kelp
Lentils, dried
Milk (raw cow or goat)
Millet
Oats
Oily fish
Olives, ripe
Pecans
Pumpkin seeds
Rice, unpolished
Rice bran
Rye
Sardines
Sesame seeds
Shad roe
Sole
Trout
Turbot
Veal joint broth
Vegetable marrow
Walnuts (English, black)
Whiting

PHOSPHORUS MENUS

Tomato juice and cod roe; celery stuffed with almond butter; leafy green salad with shredded carrots, cauliflower, green peas, sprouted lentils, black olives and chickpeas; egg yolk dressing; fish broth; broiled haddock.

Poached eggs; steamed rye cereal topped with rice polishings, wheat germ, sunflower and sesame seed meal; goat butter; goat buttermilk; revived raisins; revived peaches.

Chef's salad made of greens, sprouts, onions, sardines, julienne Swiss cheese, goat cheese, jack cheese, shredded carrots, ripe black olives, savoy cabbage; nut butter and egg yolk dressing; goat milk and carrot juice (half and half); veal joint broth.

SUMMARY OF PHOSPHORUS

GENERAL CHARACTERISTICS

"Light bearer" element   *Responsible for phosphorescence*
Symbol of intelligence   *Phosphorus type = Neurogenic type*

PHOSPHORUS IN THE HUMAN BODY

Stimulates intellect, thinking   *Improves nerve nutrition*
Acts on bone and brain   *Stimulates sexual functions*
Affects muscle tissue   *Necessary for reproduction*
Agent for growth and life   *Vegetable phosphorus feeds bones; animal phosphorus feeds brain*

Present in white blood cells

SIGNS OF PHOSPHORUS EXCESS *(Characteristics of Neurogenic Type)*

Tissue degeneration   *Optimism, idealism*
Progressive emaciation   *Suggestibililty*
Volatile emotions   *Exaggerated confidence*
Overly-mental orientation   *Vivid imagination*
Somnambulism   *Religious fantacism*

SIGNS OF PHOSPHORUS DEFICIENCY

Constant weakness   Neuralgia
Brain softening, fatigue   Fearfulness, gloom, dread of future
Sensitivity to noise, criticism   Numbness
Morbidity   Lack of confidence
Slow oxygenation   Subjective symptoms

HIGHEST PHOSPHORUS FOODS

Brain Phosphorus: *Meat, egg yolk, fish, fish roe, dairy products.*
Bone Phosphorus: *Almonds, rice bran and polishings, wheat bran and germ, pumpkin and squash seeds, lentils, soybeans, sunflower seeds.*

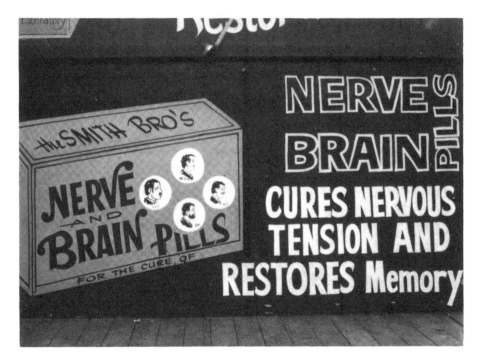

There are many dietitians with many diet theories around these days. My approach is comparatively impersonal, based on chemically balancing the body through proper foods.

People are still trying to "cure their nerves" through drug remedies, not realizing that nutrients—not drugs—are needed. The nerves need phosphorus as found in lecithin-rich foods, of which eggs are the best. The first step is to stop breaking down as a result of mental strain and stress. The next step is to revitalize the nerves with the right nutrients.

One of seven people in the U.S. is taking tranquilizers. If only they understood how to take care of the chemical needs of the nervous system, they wouldn't need drugs. Yet, life in the U.S. is fast-paced, high-tension, hard on the nerves. Stress from the marriage, finances and job can be a factor in nervous breakdowns.

The chemical story is needed to teach people how to get well and keep well. Everyone should have an education in right living, including chemical balancing, to keep body and mind at the peak of health.

thirteen

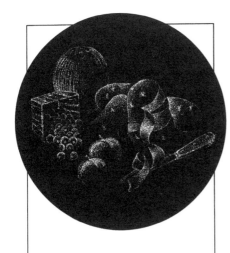

Watercress is one of the highest foods in potassium.

The most popular source of potassium is bananas, and one of the highest sources is olives.

Potassium and sodium work together in every cell of the body. In nerve cells, they shift onto opposite sides of the cell membrane to polarize the membrane and let the nerve impulse through.

Potassium is necessary to take care of internal fevers, muscular atrophy and fallen abdominal organs.

An estimated thousand to two thousand tons of potassium per million persons in the U.S. and Europe is annually poured into the rivers, lakes, underground water and sea.
—G. T. Wrench, MD, in
The Wheel of Life

Potassium, the "great alkalizer"

Nearly all my patients are in need of potassium, the "great alkalizer" for the body. Americans, however, have gone wild over alkalinizing foods and drugs as everyone tries to make the bloodstream alkaline instead of acid. But some people have gone so far that the urine becomes alkaline, a diseased, abnormal condition requiring correction. The urine should be acid in pH balance. Nevertheless, potassium's importance needs to be stressed, along with keeping one's system in a proper balance of foods and habits.

Generally, potassium assists the recuperative powers, helping to restore the rich alkaline salts to the blood. Potassium and sodium work together in all cells of the body, including at the nerve synapses, to maintain or restore membrane potentials and to assist in metabolic processes. Injuries, cuts, and bruises heal faster when potassium is in balance, and the enthusiasm and vitality are stimulated. Stored in the muscles, potassium assists in neutralizing muscle acids. Throughout the body, it is useful in preventing the spread of disease, constipation and the formation of uric acid and urates. It aids hair growth and tone and contributes to our sense of well-being.

For more serious problems, it is needed by people who have lost their equilibrium and cannot walk a straight line or who lack muscle coordination. Case after case of rheumatic or arthritic conditions have changed remarkably in a week or two, as acids leave the joints and stiffness eases as a result of consuming potato peeling broth. Potassium is beneficial in breaking up lymph gland congestion due to overconsumption of sodium foods and not enough potassium foods. Here it is not necessary to cut out sodium foods (table salt intake should be cut out) if potassium is added to balance the sodium levels.

While we do not treat cancer in our practice, I would note that Dr. Gerson suggested in his therapy that a person with degenerative diseases should use more potassium in the diet, while sodium should be cut down. Potassium helps to carry off some of the fluids due to lymphatic gland congestions often found in the average American diet, which is heavy in table salt and sodium foods. Sodium holds water in the body, impeding cleansing. But to turn to diuretics for this problem is not the answer, because forcing the kidneys to work also forces the potassium out of the body. Instead include potassium, which stimulates the kidneys and thus assists in carrying off fluids.

Potassium for Heart Problems

The heart is a potassium organ. Experimenters have taken a heart and have circulated sodium salts through it, to find it beats for only fifteen minutes. Then they ran potassium salts through the same heart to find it beats for three hours and fifteen minutes. Now sodium, as indicated above, holds excess water in the body, leading to disturbances of the muscles and the heart. Even the strongest heart can be weakened by too much sodium. Of course, we must be careful of the sodium-free diet, when sodium **food** (not table salt) is restricted. Here we run the danger of imbalance with calcium.

As long ago as 1967, Dr. Demetrio Sodi-Pallares, noted Mexican heart specialist, challenged the use of drugs for treatment of heart conditions, saying that the cure is achieved more effectively by a low salt and high potassium diet. He was particularly critical of using diuretics due to loss of potassium, essential to normal heart function. He recommended a diet with an abundance of fresh citrus fruit, bananas, figs, potatoes, tomatoes and other high potassium foods, with sodium foods restricted (and anything with the preservative sodium benzoate cut out). He pointed out that his theories were widely accepted in Europe and South America, but not in the United States. Even today, American medicine continues with drug therapy for heart problems.

Potassium Foods

A primary reason most people are lacking potassium is that it is found in bitter foods, especially greens. Who wants bitter foods? Even though potassium is one of those "spicy" elements people want little of, we need the variety for the "spice of life." I advise most people to include six vegetables, with two greens in their daily food routine. We find potassium in the tops of vegetables and watercress. Dr. Jarvis, in his book *Folk Medicine*, recommends apple cider vinegar—another high potassium food.

One of the best sources of potassium is in sundried black olives. You can make a tea by taking 10-12 olives and steeping them in a cup of water for 10 minutes. Remove the oil that collects on top and drink the remaining tea daily (as directed) for building the heart structure or getting additional potassium.

Perhaps the finest alkaline producer in the potassium realm is potato peeling broth, which we have used in sanitarium work with great success. I recommend one cup a day for one month. In severe cases, I suggest two cups a day over a period of a month.

Potato peeling broth has been a champion remedy in times of fever and in helping patients successfully through healing crises. At these times, such a broth and other light foods or drinks are most helpful. Curiously, most people eat the inside of the potato, discarding the skin section where potassium is stored. Once again we see how, through imbalanced food habits, we deny ourselves proper nutrition and bring on illness. The potato peeling broth will help to provide us with the potassium we have left behind through our daily living habits.

Potato Peeling Broth

Use 3 large potatoes. Cut peeling one-quarter-inch thick. Throw the center of the potato away; this is the acid part of the potato. Use four carrots, eight sticks of celery and a handful of parsley. Put all of this in about a quart and a half of water. Simmer for 20 minutes. Strain off and drink about one pint of this liquid daily for 30 days.

The Indian is known for a high-potassium build relating to keen eyesight and physical agility. Potassium types make excellent athletes due to their speed, balance and muscular control.

294

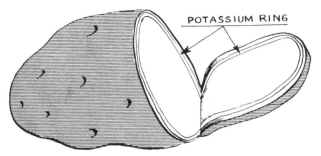

POTASSIUM RING

Sixty percent of the potassium in a potato is directly beneath the surface. When potatoes are peeled, the potassium is largely lost. This potassium ring is the reason we use potato peeling broth so much. It is the highest potassium broth you can get.

POTASSIUM
"The Great Alkalizer"

GENERAL CHARACTERISTICS

Potassium, or kalium (K), is a bluish-white, metallic element, silver in color and light in weight, having an atomic weight of only 39.1. The "great alkalizer" is known for highly alkaline properties, as an excellent neutralizing agent, a preservative and a cooling and antiseptic product. Due to high explosive properties, it is valuable in the manufacture of gunpowder.

Potassium Combines with Phosphorus, Sulphur, Chlorine

Potassium occurs commonly in compounds with phosphorus, sulphur or chlorine. When in combination with chlorine, potassium is a glandular element; with sulphur, it is more for oxygen transfer in cells; and with phosphorus, it is a main constituent of the gray nerve fibers. When potassium is lacking, sodium and chlorine are also easily exhausted or precipitated.

Potassium Increases Physical Activity

Since early recorded history man has used the olive (black, dried) to enhance cunning; olives are one of the highest potassium sources. Persons having an abundance of potassium in their makeup display physical activity, stamina and love of motion; they may exhibit cunning, as well. The Indian is known for a high-potassium build relating to keen eyesight and physical agility. Goats and leopards are potassium animals. Potassium types make excellent athletes due to their speed, balance and muscular control.

Potassium Promotes Growth, Protects Against Disease

Potash, potassium carbonate, is abundant in the soil and extremely important to healthy plant life. Without it, crops are scant and fruit does not mature properly. Potassium promotes the proper growth of stems, flowers and fruit and the general maturing of the plant. In addition, it protects the plant against diseases and germ life much as it does the human body. Sour, anemic-looking soils are deficient in potassium and thus the plants grown in it and the animals that graze it also lack potassium. It is known that potash is vital to formation of carbohydratets (sugars and starches) in plants.

POTASSIUM: ITS ROLE IN THE HUMAN BODY

Potassium Enhances Health

Only about three to four ounces of potassium are found in the human body at any one time, but a tremendous amount is utilized during a lifetime. Individuals who attract more potassium to their bodies are likely to have a greater supply of oxygen, a more alkaline system, higher blood alkalinity, a stronger general system, and a muscular system especially efficient and well developed. There is a vim and vigor inherent in such individuals and they recuperate readily. Brain and muscle tone is excellent, giving them power to carry things out in the world. Health in general, mental and physical, is accentuated by potassium. Potassium improves the assimilation of albumin, casein and fibrin. When potassium and other alkaline salts are high in the blood, injuries heal quickly and recovery is rapid due to an abundance of fibrinogen and serum-albumin in the blood and oxygen in the tissues. Albumin is principally a carbon material but is also high in oxygen and nitrogen and contains hydrogen and sulphur to a lesser degree; the albuminous substance is generously present in those with much potassium in their systems—potassium types or Myogenics.

"Potash, potassium carbonate, is abundant in the soil and extremely important to healthy plant life."

Activity, Efficiency of Body Processes Increased by Potassium

Elimination, respiration, arterial and venous circulation, recuperative ability, sexual system functions, muscular efficiency, hematogenesis, heart function, blood oxidation, internal oxidation, rest process of the nervous system, secretions, brain performance, cell life and function, balance of body heat, blood alkalization, nerve conduction, hair growth and abundance, skin activity, fibrin production, albuminogenesis, muscle coordination, internal oxidation, thermogenesis, distribution, memorization, equilibration, electrovital phenomena, neuricity, evaporation, capillarity and any other physical, biochemical, mental or vegetative processes are highly active and efficient when potassium is liberally available in the body.

Healthy Hair in Potassium Type (Myogenic)

Men and women with much potassium in the body never go bald but generally have excellent hair growth and a full head of hair. Hair color is usually good, roots strong and strands thick. Women of the potassium type often grow very long hair.

296

"Only about three to four ounces of potassium are found in the human body at any one time, but a tremendous amount is utilized during a lifetime."

Muscles, Nerves Are Healthy

Muscular men have a high percentage of potassium in the body. Abundant muscular energy, love of athletics, fire industries, heat vocations, explosives, ballistics, aeronautics, physics, forestry, action, dancing, fencing, martial arts, skating, hockey and other strenuous sports appeal to the potassium temperament and physique. These people study life in the arena of life itself, not in books; nature is their best-loved professor. The vegetative (autonomic) nervous system and counterparts in motor nerves and brain are well-formed in those with potassium strongly active in the body. Because it has an affinity for oxygen, potassium increases tissue oxidation, vitality and the desire to climb, hurl or move is intensified. Such a person is mobile, enthusiastic, impatient and impulsive in action. He does not like to be still and seeks change and excitement constantly. A violent temper may be evident, along with stubbornness to opposition. He may be a difficult patient when ailing. His actions may be monkey-like. He enjoys hobbies, freedom and action of all kinds. A dangerous vocation is in line.

"Muscular men have a high percentage of potassium in the body."

Potassium Vital to Elimination of Wastes

Potassium is excreted mainly through the kidneys but is also found in fecal matter, perspiration, milk, tears, gastric secretions and in many body acids, even in muscles. It is also eliminated to a lesser degree through other channels. Saponification (transformation of fat into soap) in the body depends upon potassium. If secretions lack potassium and sodium chloride, the intestinal waste product ferments and putrifies in the presence of body heat, producing gases, toxins, acids that are reabsorbed by the bloodstream and carried to the weakest organs of the body. If not for the presence of potassium and other elements which improve bowel elimination, the body is subject to autointoxication and self-poisoning.

"He does not like to be still and seeks change and excitement constantly."

Potassium Increases Alkalinity, Reduces Acidity

Potassium chloride and sodium chloride work together in nearly all departments of the body. They are vital to the neutralization of acids and toxins. Potassium chloride is found largely in the muscular tissues, nerve tissues and red blood cells. Potassium reduces gastric acidity, intestinal acidity and promotes good peristalsis of the stomach and intestines; potassium phosphate performs a similar function in the body fluids and solids. Alkalinity of blood and lymph is increased and every cell saturated by these and other biochemic salts. Heart action is supported, arterial pressure stabilized and circulation promoted by potassium.

"Potassium chloride and sodium chloride work together in nearly all departments of the body."

Muscles Need Potassium for Energy

Waste products produced in the muscle structure are monopotassium phosphate, paralactic acid, carbon dioxide. If these are not removed effectively, the muscles cannot function optimally. The principal source of muscular energy is tissue oxidation produced by conversion of glycogen. Potassium salts are a major ingredient of the tissue oxidation process; if potassium salts are missing from the tissues, oxidation is impaired, sufficient heat is not generated, glycogen consumption is cut

down, muscle activity is lowered and some tissue salts are precipitated. If potassium is lacking, starches and sugars are not assimilated properly and may be rejected by the system. Diabetes, dropsy and countless other complications may arise.

Potassium Helps Kidneys, Bowel

The "great alkalizer" has a diuretic effect on the body to favor good kidney action. Other functions include calming heart and nerves, reducing pain, preventing constipation and dehydration, improving the performance of adrenal and pituitary glands, and increasing bile production for good bowel action. It acts upon serous cavities and mucus surfaces, strengthens the heart muscle, unites with albumin to form gray matter of the brain. Potassium compounds are important to all elimination channels.

"The 'great alkalizer' has a diuretic effect on the body to favor good kidney action."

Potassium is Analgesic

Potassium is a natural pain desensitizer in the body for controlling convulsions, headaches, neuralgia, strictures, migraine, trifacial neuralgia, cerebral congestion and uterine pains. It is also beneficial to sound sleep, sensory neurons, sensoria in the brain, sensory and motor nerves, all algesic functions. Stress, worry, fear, anxiety, depression, excitement, grief, disappointment, hysteria, pain symptoms are reduced by potassium. Acidity is neuralized by potassium in all parts of the body. Extreme passions are mellowed by potassium; sexual excitement is reduced. When it is necessary to reduce sexual excitement, potassium and magnesium are both helpful. Nymphomania, hysterical convulsions, satyriasis, priapism, leukorrhea, uterine convulsions, spermatorrhea and menstrual pains are diminished by potassium. Catamenial complications are averted by puberty if potassium is in ample supply.

Potassium Prevents Ailments

Other benefits of normal potassium balance are prevention of the following: ulceration, holding of excess water in tissues, gangrene, cutaneous skin ailments, ingrown toenails, death from poisonous snake bites.

SIGNS OF POTASSIUM EXCESS

Slight Excess is Not Detrimental

A diet slightly higher than normal in potassium is not detrimental. Potassium acts powerfully on the muscular system, the mind, mental capability, talents, aspirations, personality and temperament. It gives physical energy, strength and inclination for sports, heat industries, explosives, aeronautics, physics, thermics, ballistics, forestry, dancing and active sports. Action can be explosive and erratic at times. Potassium helps eyesight, as mentioned in regard to the American Indian.

Excess Potassium Weakens Nerves

When there is too much potassium in the system, the effect is weakening, depressive, even paralytic to the autonomic nervous system, the motor and sensory nerves and specific brain faculties. If an overamount of potassium is assimilated and accumulated, sodium and chlorine are precipitated or exhausted. Preserved meats and potassium drugs, such as potassium bromide, potassium phosphate, potassium carbonate, potassium sulphate, can be given in excessive amounts; even a diet too high in potassium foods can overload the body with potassium.

"Potassium is a natural pain desensitizer in the body for controlling convulsions, headaches, neuralgia, strictures, migraine, trifacial neuralgia, cerebral congestion and uterine pains."

Brain Becomes Dulled

Results of potassium excess are thought confusion, muddled reasoning and ideas; reflex activity may be reduced; sensitivity becomes deadened; cortical nerve cells of the gray convolutions may degenerate, notably the sensory and emotional areas and motor brain areas. The brain can become mystified, senses dulled, imagination and creativity dulled, memory defective; drowsiness plagues, touch sensibility is reduced and the brain is overburdened with blood to certain areas, causing wild or violent impulses. The cerebellum is partially incapacitated affecting the gait and balance, even finger coordination. Faintness may manifest, as may anxiety, abhorrence for work, daydreaming, forgetfulness, sleepiness. Such a patient may be unaware of his actions, what he says, where he is, how to take care of himself in the face of danger or how to handle special situations. The normal perception of gravity is distorted.

"Potassium acts powerfully on the muscular system, the mind, mental capability, talents, aspirations, personality and temperament."

Bloating, Perspiration and Weakness

More specific tendencies and disease symptoms relevant to excess potassium include increase in pulse rate and arterial pressure. The bladder is overstimulated; so is kidney activity. Sudden flatulence is a result of potassium excess, which in turn, depletes sodium and chlorine; hot, salty water relieves that flatulence. Perspiration and muscular weakness are noted, as animals grazing on grass rich in potassium often bloat, become weak and perspire heavily.

Excess Potassium Means Overalkalinity

Too much potassium attacks hemoglobin, causes extreme thirst, vomiting, stomach pains and cramps, eventual heart failure, coma, jaundice, convulsions, uremia, depressed respiration, diarrhea. It is often responsible for the appearance of albumin in the urine. Nervous system, spinal cord, brain, medulla and some sensory, motor and psychological centers of the brain are affected. Skin ulcers, stringy secretions, ulcerous and false membranes, papules of the skin, excess alkalinity (in tissues, secretions or fluids), tissue dryness, fibrous tissue irritation and skin pustules are other indications.

Digestion May Be Disturbed

Other complications are neutralization of stomach secretions (acids), increase in waste products, weakened metabolism, burning sensation of mucus surfaces throughout the digestive tract to the anus. Sodium secretion is increased to the point of depletion and digestive disturbance is the outcome. The esophagus is constricted. If a patient tends toward obesity, he gains weight; if toward emaciation, he becomes more emaciated. Ear tumors may appear. Complaints include constant thirst with chills and heat without thirst. A heavy meal causes perspiration on the upper part of the body. Drowsiness bothers in day and early evening, but insomnia is experienced the rest of the night. Body temperature is lowerd and appendages feel cold and weakened. Joints itch and ache; fingers are numb in the morning and the spine feels broken or tender as if bruised. Valvular pathology may result from shrinkage. Heart rhythm becomes irregular—sometimes strong, at other times weak. The neck feels puffy and the entire body is so tender that the touch of persons or things is unpleasant. The chest is the site of watery phlegm causing lung and heart pressure. There may be rectal weakness; kidney pain; gas in stomach; stitching and pressure pains in abdomen; acrid taste in mouth; navel pulsation; fondness for acid and bitter foods; emotional faintness; loose teeth; tooth nerves inflamed and bothersome; toothaches; congested nose; nostrils crusty and bloody; frequent coryza; vision obstructed; sensitivity to drafts. All are indications of potassium overbalance.

Excess Potassium Bromide Complications

Potassium bromide taken as a remedy may lead to bromism characterized by anemia, acne, partial paralysis, burning stomach, gastric upsets, bloody stools, stricture of esophagus, stomach ulcers, collapse of muscles, stomach contraction, dyspepsia, bad breath, depression of brain functions (sensory, motor and psychological), paralysis or weakness of eyelids (levator palebrae) causing ptosis.

Treatment: Intake of Potassium Must Be Reduced

Potassium excess adversely affects fibrous tissue in joints. It causes diarrhea, vision loss and loss of muscle coordination. Urine becomes too alkaline. Blood fibrin increases abnormally. Intestines become inflamed. Nervous system is depressed. Urinary function is hyperactive. Lungs, stomach and mucus membranes are inflamed. Salivation becomes chronic. Cardiac nerves and heart muscles malfunction. Eventually muscular prostration, collapse, oliguria, gastro-enteritis, gastric ulceration, intestinal malfunction or kidney problems may result. All require reduction of intake of potassium whether in food or drug form. All drug forms are contraindicated.

"Extreme fears, especially fears of being alone and fantasies that death is near, plague the potassium-deficient patient."

SIGNS OF POTASSIUM DEFICIENCY

Deficiency Fosters Fears

Extreme fears, especially fears of being alone and fantasies that death is near, plague the potassium-deficient patient. He is easily startled by noises and other surprises. He may insist that supernatural beings or the police are pursuing him. His imagination runs to beasts, enemies, thieves, detectives or ghosts plotting the destruction of his business, health and reputation. He has an extreme fear of poverty and insanity. The female patient is inclined to weeping, staggering, despondency and depression, isolation and even fears of going to work alone. Pride and interest in dress are lost; she may feel there is no purpose in her living, to the point of wishing for death to end it all. Emotional stress makes her want to scream. A wife lacking potassium may hire private detectives to report on her husband.

Patient is Nervous and Afraid

The polygamous instinct may surface as potassium hunger becomes more pronounced; and the mind may turn to espionage, treachery, deception, sensational scandals, mutiny, poisoning and similar fantasies. The more chronic state of potassium deficiency increases fear of poverty, fondness of acid foods and desire for narcotics. The mind may succumb to anthropophobia. The potassium-deficient patient is distressed by the most minor annoyances. His hands are restless, nerves agitated and mind distrustful. Evil forces are thought to be closing in on him. His ability to recognize and place things in proper perspective may be lost. There is the impression of nervous delirium.

Moods are Changeable but Mostly Negative

Moods fluctuate during chronic potassium hunger, running from enthusiasm to cynicism; from trustfulness and stubborn carelessness to lonely and sad withdrawal; from friendliness and affection to yielding to hostility, irritability, ugliness, coldness. But depression, fears, suicidal impulses pervade. The patient may sleep for many days, then be unable to sleep for some time. Talkative spells alternate with silent periods, mirth with depression, superstition with religious rapture. He may decide to starve himself and believe it is healthy for others to do likewise.

Violence May Increase

Complete potassium depletion can foster an insane longing for hiding; arsonist impulses against residences or haystacks; desire to commit violent crimes against property, animals or people—even killing. The potassium-depleted patient may take pleasure in the suffering of others and want to throw bombs or other explosives to destroy the government or a fictitious "enemy." Life in every aspect appears dark and depressive. The nerves and mind become inflamed and he only sees the negative, dark side of life, blaming a wrathful god. Optimism increases with moonlight.

Chronic Potassium Starvation May Bring Mental Illness

As the potassium reserve is increasingly precipitated, symptoms become more dramatic. In early stages, depression, brooding moods, staggering, weeping, fears, eccentric hobbies are noted. When chronic proportions approach, suicide is contemplated or attempted, violent crimes acted out, alcoholism developed. Insanity may necessitate commitment to mental institution. Diabetes and premature death may occur. Mental institutions are the home for many victims of potassium starvation.

Patients are Suspicious, Unpredictable

Mental symptoms indicating potassium deficiency are dramatic. The mind becomes chaotic, unpredictable, highly imaginative and unorthodox. States of mind alternate between joy and melancholy or even excitability. At one time, the patient may be verbose and at another, taciturn and uncommunicative. He may mock people in jest or become agitated and irritable to the point of quarreling. He is highly suspicious of the motives of others. Family affairs are difficult to cope with. Trivial occurrences are upsetting and disturbing. Spirits droop and indifference appears. Sensitivity is intensified. He tends to scold, becomes absentminded and perplexed as if intoxicated; is childish; craves sympathy and is almost impossible to please.

Signs of Potassium Lack

The head may feel enlarged and contractions in the head or the cranial membranes may be felt. The patient may claim that his head has caved in or is under hydraulic pressure from the sides. The skin seems to crawl and sting from underneath. Mind and nerves function erratically and do not have control over muscular movement. Shivers and chills pass through the nervous system. Climbing fatigues one rapidly. The script is scrawly; handwriting is nervous and fingers do not respond well to the mind; spelling becomes difficult. The brain functions poorly during the day and better at night; the potassium-depleted patient is sour in the morning and more alive at night. Sleep is troubled and restless; dreams are vivid; habits alternate. Explosive sounds are imagined in the ears; the patient perceives sounds others cannot hear. The body is so tender that to be touched is painful. The mind is vindictive and nerves revolutionary.

Ambition and Drive are Absent

Extreme hunger is experienced, but the odor of food destroys the appetite. There is extreme thirst which is not satisfied by water. Ambition is lost because the person is no longer himself. Work becomes deplorable and the open air inviting. Tasks easy in the past become hard. The patient insists that his power, ambition, courage, memory, speech, vocabulary and drive have fled. His answers are often foolish, and his perception seems distorted and dull. Noise interferes with speech, thought processes and study. Dictation and mental concentration in a noisy office would be nearly impossible to bear.

Patient is Sensitive to Weather Change

Weather changes are irritating to the potassium-deficient patient, and sudden changes in barometric pressure are unbearable. Approach of a storm produces depression, desperation and even suicidal action; but violent storms produce wonderment and pleasure when they arrive.

Characteristic Moods of Potassium-Deficient Patient

Moods of stubbornness, sensationalism, unfounded fears, irrational temper and self-torture mark the potassium-deficiency case. Depression can become so intense that the patient will take poison or turn on the gas and await the end with a liquor bottle and Bible. He flirts with death by taking many dangerous changes. He may experience intense jealousy, deep despair, violent temper fits, intense hatred, storm-tossed passions or overpowering emotions. The body chemistry is adversely affected by the mental imbalance, increasing acid formation and taste for alcohol, narcotics and other destructive habits. Physical symptoms are irritated by the mind. Intense tension aggravates nerves to the point of desperate actions. Passion further aggravates the state, as do deep emotions and physical stress. Men feel like cursing; women feel like screaming.

Potassium Starvation Produces Exclusiveness and Cynicism

Other forms potassium hunger takes include disgust with life, cynicism, hermit-like behavior, unsociability and loneliness. The patient may be contemptuous, defiant, warlike, explosive in temperament. His speech is scorching and often shameless and abusive. A wrong deed may inspire great wrath. Fascination with witnessing and commiting horrible acts increase because he has an aversion to almost everything. He expounds against evil with great exaggeration. Religion may appear to him to be a childish deception; politics may also be viewed as manipulation and trickery. People are considered "no good," the government a farce; the spy, laborer and anarchist may be considered respectable, but no othes. The educational system, religion or government are worrisome. A minority movement may be a focal point of feverish devotion.

Severe Potassium Depletion Causes Severe Reactions

As has been noted, the more severe the potassium depletion, the more pronounced the symptoms. Loss of intelligence, muttering to self or raving may be observed. A type of anmesia may result in separation from self or friends and family. The potassium-deficient patient may suddenly commit suicide because of inner turmoil that others cannot fathom. He may fancy possession or a hypnotic spell or believe he is Christ, Buddha, Moses or another famous figure or feel that a spirit guide is near. Seances and mediums become fascinating and necessary to him. Imaginary evils are a constant plague.

Potassium Lack Causes Oxygen Lack

Because potassium is vital for attracting oxygen to the tissues, lack of it reduces tissue oxygenation, produces lax muscles, causes vital organs to sag and the heart to weaken. Digestion and assimilation of albumin, fibrin, gelatinous substances and sugar are impaired. The patient may have distress in the epigastrium, saying that he feels better in fresh air. There may be throbbing pain above the eyes, tendency to fall and fleeting pains. Headaches come at intervals. Eyes are sunken, dull, heated, reddened; the patient rubs them often, feeling as if sand is in them. There may be dropsy in ankles; sweating; skin dryness; green-tinged mucus discharge and sputum; numbness accompanying tingling neuritis; muscular atrophy; nerve sensitivity; tenderness and weakness in tendons and muscles; pain in lower back of head; poor bowel activity; intestinal stasis; internal fever; crawling sensation in feet, beneath skin or at roots of teeth; skin itch; ataxia; rosy patches on skin; many or burning scabs; intense itching around former injuries and scars; skin inflammation; blisters; painful pustules; fiery red ulcers; moist eczema on legs. All are indications that potassium is needed. Lack of potassium opens the door to germ life in the body.

Feet are Painful, Walking is Difficult

Nocturnal restlessness (tossing, turning, throwing arms and legs about) characterizes the potassium-hungry patient. Dizziness is produced by getting up quickly from a reclining position, turning, stooping and raising the head quickly. Bottoms of feet are often red, burning, tender or swollen. Corns and callouses are tender. Feet seem weak and unable to provide good support. Running downstairs is difficult. Walking causes weakness. Immediately after returning home from an excursion, there is an urge to disrobe (especially to remove tight-fitting garments and shoes). Organs feel prolapsed, and heart is cramped and painful. The throat and stomach feel dry and parched. There may be side pain and urethral contractions; rectal muscles tingle and burn; stomach is swollen; excitement, worry or heavy emotions produce nausea; the stomach is inflamed, burning, parched. Sour food and cold drinks or water are craved; the taste runs to acid drinks, pickles, lemonade, beer. Vesicles, tongue and teeth throb; smell is poor; the nose is filled with a fetid odor; the nose bleeds easily. One ear is hot, the other chilled; one ear is pale, the other reddened. There is an acid taste in the mouth. One cheek is cold, the other feverish. Eyes puff or bag underneath. Motor nerves and muscles are spasmodic. There is a feeling of paralysis in the appendages. The face changes from flushed to gray. Walk is unsteady. Distance perception with feet is unsure. Abdominal muscles are convulsive. Achilles tendons become sore after standing a long time, and legs feel as if lead weights are on them.

Nose and Throat Suffer

The patient may feel that food sticks in his throat. Pains and aches run in cycles in the stomach. The bladder burns and aches, as may the urethra or another body part. Fleeting, rapid pains and aches cause torment. Nose is ticklish; pains shoot in the jaws; parotids are swollen and fevered; arteries are weak; tongue is covered with yellow coating; saliva is foamy, salty, acrid.

Varied Signs of Potassium Lack

Earaches are common in the potassium-starved patient. Also common are miscarriages, fainting, typhoid fever and fevers due to bacterial toxins, dysentery or intestinal inflammation. Susceptibility to infantile pneumonia is noted. Vesicles form in the

302

heart and mitral valves suffer. Limb movement is spasmodic, tissues edemic. Nerves burn and twitch; teeth gnash; dreams are unpleasant. Body heat is low, with accompanying internal fever and outward chill. Veins lack tone. Erysipelas from incubation of streptococci is likely. Pyorrhea may develop. Muscles reject sugar which is expelled through urine; phosphate and albumin may appear in urine. Spinal meninges are congested. Nerves are high strung. There may be vertigo, sclerosis, conjunctivitis, indigestion, eye problems, swelling, angina pectoris, axaluria, croup or sepsis. Sleepiness may occur in early stages, insomnia later. There may be paroxysm; shaking limbs; sore knees, ankles, muscles; iritis; blindness; atonicity of muscles; poor and shallow breathing; inclination for alcohol consumption; periodic debility; inflammatory catarrh; underactive secretion. Scarlet fever is a possibility when potassium is in demand. Frontal sinuses are irritated; rami of lower jaw are painful. There may be dizziness; gastritis; peritonitis; backache; itching sensations in hair roots; fibrous tumors; rheumatic aches in tendons; rheumatic acids caused by germ life and cold extremities with flashes of heat and sweating. All require potassium in food form.

"Lack of potassium increases skin eruptions because tissue metabolism is disturbed."

Further Symptoms of Depletion

Lack of potassium increases skin eruptions because tissue metabolism is disturbed. Other symptoms may be mental dysfunction, cyclic neuralgia, eneuresis, sores and rash in mouth, throat ailments, tympanitis, arm paralysis, liver malfunction, edema of eyelids, measles, whooping cough, burning coryza, bloody or mucusy vomitus, parotitis, sores, wheezing, mumps, bronchial congestion, muscular anemia, suppuration of tonsils, hallucinations, stammering, brain congestion, pityriasis, lack of muscle coordination, tenesmus, pruritis, stuttering, numb tongue and mouth, summer ailments, prostration, poor tissue oxygenation, head jerking, arm muscles pulling, tumefaction, otitis, lassitude, bleeding and cracked lips, mental disturbance, colic of uterus, aphonia and general debility. Other indications include spasmodic choking, lung inflammation, lumbago, systolic heart murmur, pulmonary stagnation, multiocular pleurisy, aphonia, odorous foot sweat, temple headache, phlebitis, migraine, specific forms of lupus, sudden collapse, myasthenia, febrile excitement, mental disorders (especially thanatomania, mania feriosa, nymphomania, suicidal and homicidal tendencies, athymia, pyromania and abnormally strong sexual impulse before puberty). Other potassium hunger manifestations are painful hemorrhoids, paragraphia, myitis, abnormal sleep patterns similar to narcosis and integumentary swelling and tension. Female patients may exhibit membranous dysmenorrhea, myectopy, emotional hyperactivity, maramenia, uterine inflammation, chondritis, rash, chorditis and even tumors or sarcoma in cartilage tissue.

Complications Due to Loss of Other Elements

As stated above, lack of potassium in the diet or its excessive elimination also precipates sodium, chlorine and nitrogen. As a consequence, paralysis may develop, as may painful erections due to inflammation of cerebellum or genitals. Chorea, paralysis agitans, idiopathic atrophy of muscles, athetosis, inflammation of crura cerebelli leading to loss of equilibrium, cystitis or strangury are possible end results.

Atmospheric Electricity Affects Nerves

If potassium reserves are exhausted, it is likely that albumin, sugar, gelatinous substances, sodium and chlorine are also in short supply or not fully assimilated. Weather changes are painful to this patient because respiration and oxygenation are reduced. Electrical ferments and impurities and germ growth are generated during these changes which affect tissues, body heat, fluids, blood, metabolism, nerve impulses and their conduction, mental areas of the brain, nerve cells and especially the cerebellum. For this reason potassium-deficient patients experience increased problems during storms and weather changes.

Low Potassium Affects Many Body Processes

"Goose pimples" (cutis ansera) are a result of the erector pili muscles and hair follicles becoming irritated and inflamed when potassium is deficient. Consumption of fatty foods by individuals low in potassium produces heartburn, scorbutic cancers, leukemia, congestion of cerebral meninges resulting in psychosis and uterine subinvolution. If potassium is short, certain acids, toxins, gases, odors, metallic fumes are detrimental to health. Extensor muscles become weak when potassium is needed. There is greater danger of acidosis and autointoxication, diphtheria, bile dysfunction, catarrh of the duodenum, dysuria, Bright's disease, striditis, cramps, laryngismus, morning sickness, sea sickness, air sickness, bunions, phimosis, uterine and menstrual difficulties, gangrene, ingrown toenails, bromidrosis and putrid ulcers.

Nerves and Muscles Need Potassium and Oxygen

Nerve force is dependent upon oxygen. Because potassium foods attract oxygen to the body, potassium indirectly generates stronger nerve force. Power, vigor, vitality, enthusiasm and optimism come from oxygen. A form of neurasthenia is facilitated by low levels of potassium although phosphorus and iron shortages also produce this condition. Remember that potassium is active in the autonomic nervous system, in skeletal and involuntary muscles and sugar metabolism and apply food chemistry accordingly.

Potassium and Chlorine Reduce Water Retention

Water is drawn from the system by potassium, a process which is especially necessary in cases of edematous obesity. Chlorine also removes water. Water-carrying types need potassium and chlorine foods, dry food and climates and stony soil to reduce water retention in the body.

Syphilitics Need High-Potassium Diet

Syphilis germs generate poisons in the system which destroy potassium, fluorine and other biochemic salts. This infectious disease, which can be contracted or inherited, calls for a high-potassium diet.

Diabetics Need High-Potassium Diet

Diabetes, which involves reduced tolerance to sugar, indicates a lack of potassium. Tissue waste products, tissue water, acid and glucose stress the kidneys. In time, the sugar that is refused by the body passes through the kidneys and is often diagnosed as kidney disease when potassium hunger is the actual cause.

***

"Lack of potassium encourages gas generation, intestinal fermentation, flatus, germ propagation and organic dysfunction."

***

Potassium Lack Allows Acid Formation

Acid formation is minimized when there is plenty of potassium in reserve in the body. More potassium also assures more oxygen (as does adequate iron), thus ensuring disease resistance. Lack of potassium encourages gas generation, intestinal fermentation, flatus, germ propagation and organic dysfunction.

Potassium and Iron Needed for Energy

If the body has lost the power to utilize potassium properly, the oxygen supply is also diminished. This adversely affects the nervous system as explained above. Oxygen is the catalyst for mental and physical vitality and for nerve functions. If vital energy has been curtailed and biochemic salts (or elements) have been broken down or not supplied in the diet, or if organs fail to function in assimilation of certain elements, the level of necessary elements in the body will be lowered because greater muscular and mental energy is essential for assimilation, utilization and storage of reserves in blood and tissues. For example, there may be abnormally low levels of such chemical elements as potassium, iron, silicon and calcium. During such times, potassium and iron are of supreme importance in the diet. Massage, osteopathy, chiropractic, electrical treatments, homeopathic remedies, allopathic drugs alone are not sufficient methods; proper diet must be followed, as well.

Conditions Demand Potassium

Potassium-deficient patients may complain of objects reeling, indifference to and loss of interest in people and life, terrific pains, bluish skin tone, cold, hunger which disappears when they get to the table, pain deep in the eyes and eyeballs, tired eye muscles, taste of metal or putrid taste in mouth, intestinal

pain searing or ripping through the body, heart flutter, jumping and fleeting pains, weary thighs, chronic tiredness, excessive passions, inability of lower limbs to support the body, bluish calves, bruised calves, tissue anemia with a good blood count, sudden prostration, cold feet, pleurisy pains, stools slimy or knotty, burning urine, stringy discharges. In these instances, potassium is in immediate great demand.

Further Manifestations of Potassium Deficiency

When glycosuria manifests, self-preoccupation is noted. Other signs of potassium deficiency are ataxia; weak ligaments; subnormal protein metabolism; difficult bowel elimination; urine foamy, milky, sweet-smelling, red, slimy, hot, greenish, albuminous, dark in alternation; vaginal canal sore or constricted causing difficult urination; irritated erectile muscles and extreme amatory impulses; menses accompanied by cramps and pains; sore gluteal muscles (nates); lack of air in lungs; spasmodic coughing and throat tickling; difficult expectoration; dry cough without mucus discharge; ticklish sensation in uterus, vulva, spermatic cord, anus, skin, tongue, nose with simultaneous stinging sensation; lung weakness predisposing one to pneumonia, pleurisy, throat ailments; rushing, gurgling sounds in the heart indicative of heart muscle weakness and lack of tissue salts (elements); muscle throbbing; pains migrating from head to arms and down to finger joints and tips; purplish-rosy fingertips; skin moon-pale; amorous dreams; somnambular sleep patterns; neurotic reflexes; bluish-red cast to scars; pustular complexion. All such symptoms implore a potassium diet.

Easily-Recognizable Symptoms

Other indications that the doctor, nurse, dietitian, nutritionist should learn to recognize are oppressive breathing, poor finger usage, systolic heart beat, nervous script, tearful lachrymal glands, stiffened integument, tympanic and crampy abdomen, pruritic vulva, prolapsed uterus, swollen glands, spasmodic and cramped wrists, worry regarding work; dancing which lacks grace; heavy eyes.

304

Occupations Requiring Potassium

If the vocation induces cramps—such as in occupations of driver, writer, typist, stenographer, violinist, treadler, milker, weaver, glassblower, telephone operator, computer programmer, switchboard operator, tailor, of similar sedentary jobs—a diet high in potassium is necessary. Palsy and neurosis also require much potassium.

Potassium Must be Supplied in Food Form

Potassium, the "great alkalizer," is important to every man, woman and child, so long as it is supplied in biochemic (food) or supplement form. Following is a list of foods highest in potassium, which should be included in the diet without fail. Know when they are in greatest demand and where to get them when potassium reserves need to be rebuilt.

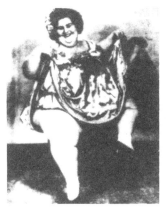 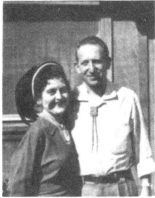

The two pictures above show a little lady who reduced from over 500 lb to 118 lb. When excess sodium favors water retention in the tissues, potassium helps drive the water out. Right: The potassium and sodium foods neutralize acids in the body.

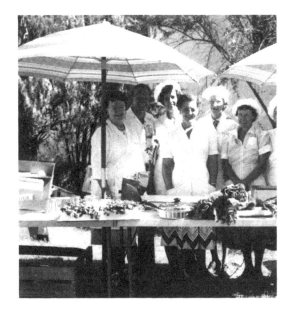

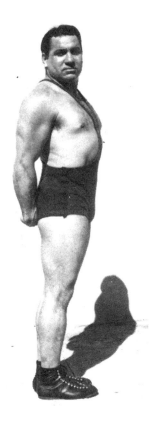

Left: Muscular men have a large amount of potassium in their bodies. Joe Tonti, the strongest upside-down man in the world in his time, walked on his hands up every flight of stairs to the top of the Woolworth building in Chicago. Right: Many of the fruits and vegetables we grew and served at the Ranch were high in potassium.

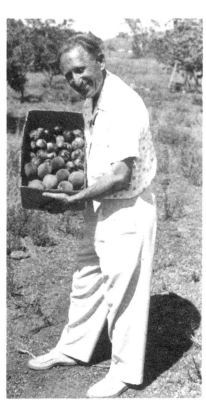

305

HIGHEST POTASSIUM FOODS

Sun-dried black olives and potato peeling broth are two of the best sources of potassium. Dulse, kelp and Irish moss are also high. Other good potassium foods are listed below. Remember that excessive heat destroys potassium, as does food processing.

Almonds	Kale
Anise seeds	Kelp
Apples	Leaf lettuce
Apple cider vinegar	Lentile
Apple peelings	Lima beans, dried
Apricots, dried	Olives
Bananas	Parsley
Beans (dried red, pinto, white, mung, string)	Parsnips
Beets (red, yellow)	Peaches, bitter
Beet greens	Pears, dried
Black cherries	Pecans
Blueberries	Potato peelings
Broccoli	Raisins
Brussels sprouts	Rice bran
Carrots	Rice polishings
Cashews	Sage tea
Cheese, brown	Sesame seeds, whole
Cucumbers	Soy milk
Currants	Soybeans, dried
Dates	Spinach
Dulse	Sunflower seeds
Egg white, beaten	Swiss chard
Escarole	Tomatoes (red, yellow)
Figs, dried	Turnips
Fish	Walnuts
Goat milk	Watercress
Grapes	Wheat bran
Green turtle	Wheat germ
Jerusalem artichoke	

POTASSIUM MENUS

Steamed green kale; salad made of red and white cabbage, sunflower seeds, cashews, green peppers, yellow tomatoes, pineapple; mayonnaise dressing; steamed beets and baked potato with skin; sage tea.

Spinach loaf; steamed carrots; steamed broccoli; salad made of mixed greens, cucumbers, sun-dried black olives, cauliflower, alfalfa sprouts, bamboo shoots, radishes, tomatoes; glass of goat milk and carrot juice (half and half).

Green turtle soup; grated carrots, red beets and parsnips on leaf lettuce; celery stuffed with nut butter (almond, cashew, sunflower, etc.); steamed Jerusalem artichoke, steamed asparagus tips; tomato-style lentils or soybeans; hops tea.

Steamed rye or millet cereal topped with sesame and sunflower meal, rice polishings, wheat germ and flaxseed meal; revived raisins and apricots; fresh blueberries; coconut milk.

Broiled white fish; vegetable casserole; steamed brussels sprouts; waldorf salad; fruit gelatin made of bananas, cherries, strawberries and pineapple; glass of grape juice.

SUMMARY OF POTASSIUM

GENERAL CHARACTERISTICS

"Great alkalizer" element
Potassium carbonate (potash) vital to plant life and soil

Potassium type = Myogenic type

POTASSIUM IN THE HUMAN BODY

Supports muscular system
Enhances recuperative power
Increases efficiency of functions
Aids in waste elimination
Reduces pain

Increases blood and tissue alkalinity
Promotes vigor and health
Supplies healthy hair, nerves
Reduces acidity
Prevents ailments

SIGNS OF POTASSIUM EXCESS (Characteristics of Myogenic Type)

Weakened nerves
Bloating, flatulence
Disturbed digestion
Precipitation of sodium, chlorine
Strong, healthy hair

Dulled brain
Overalkalinity
Loss of equilibrium
Exhaustion
Love of motion, athletics

SIGNS OF POTASSIUM DEFICIENCY

Fearfulness

Fantasy

Tendency toward violence

Suspiciousness

Loss of ambition, drive

Reduced oxygenation

Acidity

Restlessness, nervousness

Negativity, cynicism

Mental illness

Oversensitivity to touch

Exclusiveness, isolation

Pains and aches

Low energy

HIGHEST POTASSIUM FOODS

Sun-dried black olives

Dulse, kelp, Irish moss

Potato peeling broth

Bitter greens

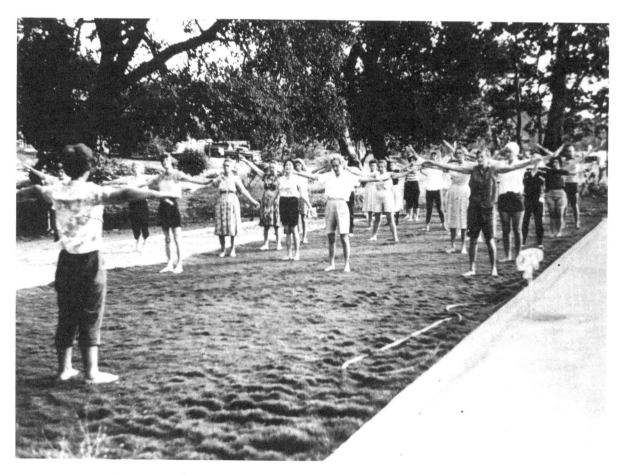

Potassium is the great neutralizer of muscle acids and is needed to get the most good out of exercise. Potassium is called "the alkalizer." All greens and tops of vegetables are high in potassium, which builds grace in the muscle structure. Potassium is the bitter element in foods. (Sodium is the sweet element.)

fourteen

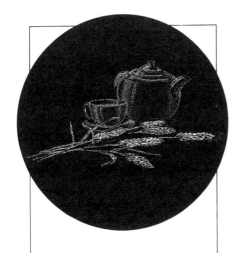

Nerve transmission would be impossible without silicon, which carries the electrical nerve impulses.

Nails, hair and skin derive their sheen, resilience and smoothness from silicon. If silicon is observed to be lacking in any of these, it is deficient throughout the body. Silicon is also found in traces in the bones and teeth.

Silicon acts as a link between blood and nerves.

The earth's crust is about 25% silicon. It is second only to oxygen as a constituent of our planet's surface.

Sprouts and rice bran are among the highest sources of biochemical silicon.

Silicon, the "magnetic" element

A lady patient once complained to me that her fingernails were three-fourths black and that she was not well. She asked when she would be well again. I told her that when her fingernails came in all pink she could expect to be well. You cannot be well without the correct silicon balance and proper silicon reserves, which are stored highest in the hair, skin, fingernails and toenails. When the patient's fingernails came in all pink, she was on top of the world! Silicon is one of the biochemical elements that I have used for the past 50 years with the most dramatic results.

I find very few people who do not need silicon, the "magnetic" element, which is reflected in the charming, magnetic personality and in beauty of movement, as in dancing. Animals, too, need silicon and show its presence with a glossy coat, indicating good health and spirit. A goat with a shiny coat gives good milk, and when I go to buy one, I feel the hair. Silicon is a protector to the skin and body, as well as an insulating agent.

It gives firmness to stalks of grains and produces a polished, hard outside surface to oats, barley, rice, corn, and other cereals. It also gives hardness, firmness, elasticity and polish to bone, teeth and tendons in animals and human beings. Thus, just as silicon supports the outer linings of many foods in the plant kingdom, similarly it protects the outside linings of animals and humans.

Silicon Deficiencies

Silicon, as part of the nervous system, helps the nerve messages or impulses of the brain to reach the various organs they are intended for. If this process slows down, silicon reserves are depleted. Additionally, varicose veins call for silicon, as do catarrhal conditions, constant colds, flu, nervousness, confusion, frustration, lack of concentration and problems with the skin, nails and hair.

When the proper biochemical elements are added and the major symptoms have been cared for, the minor symptoms disappear. We can notice symptoms of silicon deficiency in children, which include gritting the teeth during sleep, scratching the rectum, biting the fingernails and picking the nose. Interestingly, the "cribber"—a horse that chews the wooden corral fence—is in need of silicon.

Iridology shows the presence of nerve rings in the iris, an indication of much nervous tension. Nerve rings call for silicon to feed and restore the nervous system to good working order. Proteins feed the nervous system in general, but silicon is always additionally needed. It is also beneficial for impotence and sexual weakness by increasing working energy and sexual power, endurance and vigor. Overall, it makes flesh firmer, joints more elastic and veins stronger.

An Important Distinction

In the future, we are going to discover that vitamins are not as necessary in the body as minerals. Minerals control or hold the vitamins in the body and build the "temple beautiful," the gem of the earth that is the human body. Vitamins help run the temple. Like gasoline in an automobile, vitamins act as catalysts and provide fuel. Gasoline runs the automobile but does not build it. Silicon, in contrast, controls calcium to a certain extent (as does iodine) and assists in its evolution to a higher vibratory state.

Additionally, we can demystify the ingredients and supplements we are using for nutrition by realizing that what we need is always available biochemically from "the dust of the earth." Dr. Rocine helped me to this realization in the very beginning of my studies with him. At the time, I was using an extract of Avena sativa, which I was unfamiliar with, except that it was a homeopathic remedy. Dr. Rocine informed me that Avena sativa was an extract of oat straw tea. I wondered why I needed to be paying so much for this extract. Then he showed me how I could get silicon from oat straw tea, several cups a day of which would build up sufficient silicon reserves. Since that time, I have greatly appreciated being able to derive the same results from foods as from the homeopathic cell salts, potentized by nature to restore the right balance in the body.

Silicon Sources

Over a period of years, we have found that silicon is found in the outside of seeds, nuts, grains and the outer peelings of fruits and vegetables. It is highest in rice polishings. We have used rice polishings a great deal, feeling that it is one of the supplements which makes up

for what people have omitted from their diets. Almost everybody has used devitalized and refined or polished foods which lack silicon. Additionally, the other three supplements we recommend are wheat germ, flaxseed meal and sunflower or sesame seed meal—one tablespoon each on cereal in the morning.

Invariably, the comment I hear from my patients after they have been under my care for three to six months is that their nails do not peel or break as easily as they did in the past. They also say that their skin has changed, being not as dry as it was before, and that their hair has attained a new resiliency without troublesome split ends.

I have depended on rice bran syrup and rice polishings because they are the highest sources of silicon and several B vitamins (thiamin, riboflavin and niacin). In the experiments in which the B vitamins were discovered, polished rice, lacking silicon and the B vitamins, was fed to pigeons. Within a four-day period, they would flap backward and die. But if given the rice polishings—the part of the rice the miller throws away—before they were too far gone, they would recover. Chickens fed polished white rice developed "droop wing," but this condition also cleared up with the rice polishings. Once again we see the health penalty paid due to the refining process.

Oat straw tea is another of the champion silicon sources, as before mentioned, assisting even my varicose vein cases through the use of cloth packs soaked in oat straw tea and applied externally. Shavegrass tea not only supplies silicon but acts as a diuretic. I have had many doctors say, "I use nearly the same program as you but I don't always get the same results." My secret is that when I give something as a remedy it often serves at least two purposes, as indicated here with shavegrass tea. Alfalfa tablets are a high source of silicon, too, building a glossy coat for a horse and bringing in a full head of hair (or preventing it from falling out) for a person.

A Classic Silicon Case

To conclude, we are reproducing a classic silicon case from issue 3 of the *Iridologists International Instructor's Manual for Research and Development*, including photos to illustrate the dramatic changes that took place in one of my cases as a result of a high silicon diet and silicon supplements such as rice bran syrup.

A Classic Silicon Case—Mr. RP: His Own Story

Mr. RP, age 64, came to us with a severe skin condition; he was allergic to many things. The iris disclosed extreme acidity and catarrh and the skin elimination was poor. Also, both kidneys were underactive, especially the left kidney. The patient had many enemas, heavy supplements for the kidneys, many protomorphogens. The pancreas was performing poorly, preventing proper digestion of starches and proteins, possibly contributing to, if not causing, the allergic reactions.

Other iris manifestations were an acid stomach, acidity throughout the entire body, bronchial catarrh, poor leg circulation, inherent weakness in bowel and bronchial tubes, sluggish liver, lymph gland congestion, nerve rings, pancreas weakness, scurf rim, back weakness (lack of calcium). The large colon was pocketed (diverticula). The only operation had been for a hernia. Blood pressure was normal.

RP had exhausted his body's reserve of the "magnetic element," silicon, through extreme use of the nervous system, unsuitable occupations, resentment and resistance possibly, mental strain. As we have said, silicon is stored in the skin, hair and nails mostly. If they are in poor condition, the nervous system is likely encumbered or even incapacitated. A sick person lacks silicon for the nervous system.

In reference to the article "The Executive Dilemma," *Instructor's Manual,* Issue 2, RP is analytical, critical, serious—faculties which use the nervous system harshly. His nervous system was not depleted to the point of producing physical pain, but the skin area was adversely affected first as seen in photos. Skin improvement was noted as healing signs appeared in the rest of the body (and iris). Following the progress through iris analysis, healing signs appeared in proportion to skin improvement; skin texture was transformed.

We explained to the patient that the nervous system requires quadruple time to repair as compared to other parts of the body.

Each organ demands silicon to transmit and receive nerve impulses. If communication between the brain and organs is weakened or destroyed, many organic conditions can result.

RP sought aid earlier from a dermatologist without success. He states it as follows: "He told me to put some ointment, that I purchased at the drugstore, on the psoriasis. It would quiet it down for a few hours, but then it would come right back again."

RP describes the skin manifestation: "These spots were on top of the head, and they went to the back of the head and then appeared on the elbows. These spots were there for years and I'd keep putting salve on them occasionally when they bothered me. Then I would forget about them for awhile. A doctor prescribed a salve—some tar product—and it would loosen it and relieve the itching. A few times I thought I had it under control and I'd forget about using the salve. However, it kept growing and finally I began to notice a difference in the appearance; it was spreading and increasing in severity. It had a secretion underneath that would burn out and then reappear in another area. I didn't know what it was until last year when we were on vacation. I'd get up from watching television and could hardly move around. My knees bothered me—like arthritis and stiffness was in them. I thought rheumatism was coming on."

The iris mirrored extreme acidity in the body, denoting that rheumatic condition. It was an extreme acid, a catarrhal condition invading the joints. More than the element silicon was deficient—sodium had been precipitated from the joints in an attempt to neutralize some of the acids producing the arthritic or rheumatic condition.

A doctor back in 1951 had advised an extreme diet, cutting out eggs, meat and fish, limiting the patient largely to vegetables and green salads. He had recognized that the acids in the body were at a danger level then. We believe this was too extreme a diet, however, the doctor gave further advice:

"He said for me to find a chiropractor to relieve my stiff and painful back. He advised me not to return to any chiropractor who didn't give me relief by the time I got off his adjustment table."

During this interval, the skin condition was worsening rapidly. It was spreading to the rest of the body. RP describes the sensations thus:

"It all started spreading from the back of the head, like sutures or something. All at once the skin dried up and began forming scabs and scaling. Then it spread to the abdomen and the whole body. It broke out all of a sudden after I had started using a shampoo for controlling psoriasis.

"I first noticed it a year ago last June (first visit was July), especially up in high elevations. A couple of years ago, we crossed Colorado by bus and I could hardly breathe all night."

The patient explained that he had no evidence of particular food allergies at that time. "I thought I had heart trouble most of that night. One doctor told me it was my liver. He gave me bile mints and it straightened out immediately."

But this was only the beginning of his troubles: "Then it came down both legs and there didn't seem to be anything to stop it. It left my skin awfully rough, scaly and coarse. It still itches in places yet. But it is getting better now, in spite of lots of ups and downs (healing crises). I forgot to take some of my protomorphogens last Sunday and it got pretty bad."

The protomorphogen is designed for the brain and nervous system. Again, we are feeding the nervous system.

"The legs are much better these days. I use a steel rasp to file the rough, scaly dead skin off. We used to have to trim horses' hooves with this rasp so they could walk straight. It helps when my skin bothers me severely: I could pinch the rough dead scales and not even feel it. The skin feels different now. It's more alive. The wrists and ankles are still the main problems. There isn't the oozing that started out with the condition, but sometimes when I knock the scales off, it is kind of wet underneath."

RP originally looked extremely pale, white and anemic with the adverse condition at its height; he was very weak. He sustained many extreme crises and harsh elimination processes. He describes some of the symptoms he had to endure:

"A sticky, smelly kind of bloody mucus dropped into the throat often. It felt like congestive spots all over.

"I had trouble taking baths for a long time. The skin dried up and tightened, then began to itch. I don't use water on my hands even now, rather glycerine and rose water instead.

"I had to wear rubber gloves for a long time my hands were so bad. The fingernails have given me a lot of trouble. Under the nails it gets black and dark.

"The bowels are good these days—loose, in fact—and the kidneys are quite active." (The bowels were not moving properly when he first came to us.)

"Urination is about every hour. I noticed more frequent urination when the skin trouble was most severe."

When the skin is not working well, the kidneys must overwork.

"My appetite was kind of poor for a time, but generally it has always been good. Since I went on juice fasts and lost all that weight (18 pounds), my appetite picked up and I wasn't able to fill up for a long time. Now I seem to be filling up and satisfied after a meal."

We estimate that the elimination and reversal process (according to Hering's law of cure) is about 75% completed. The patient admitted that even his mental attitude and philosophy have greatly improved. He is confident that he will be completely well very soon. RP has progressed and matured in his outlook tremendously through this extreme experience. He has decided to work for himself in the future. He has acquired a spiritual contentment that everyone should seek.

Program

The program was set up for RP nine months before "after" photos. Dr. Jensen's Regular Diet: No citrus fruit, no head lettuce, no bread, no wheat or oatmeal, 50-60% raw food daily, 80% alkaline foods (fruits and vegetables) and 20% acid foods (proteins and starches); the proportion was 6 vegetables daily, 2 fruits, 1 starch and a protein. He was advised to add sprouts to the daily diet and to use only one of four special starches daily: rye, brown rice, yellow cornmeal, millet—steamed as a cereal not in baked goods.

The major supplements were silica, rice bran syrup (silicon and vitamin B), protomorphogens for the brain and nervous system, a starch and protein digestant, diuretics (kidney and bladder herbs and protomorphogens), vitamin A, vitamins C and E, bone marrow and a protomorphogen to drain extremely congested lymph glands.

RP was counseled to use a natural bristle brush over the whole body for the skin condition and to exercise on the slant board. Also, he used a modified fast of vegetable juices, flaxseed enemas frequently. Potato peeling broth was for the extreme acidity and was taken daily.

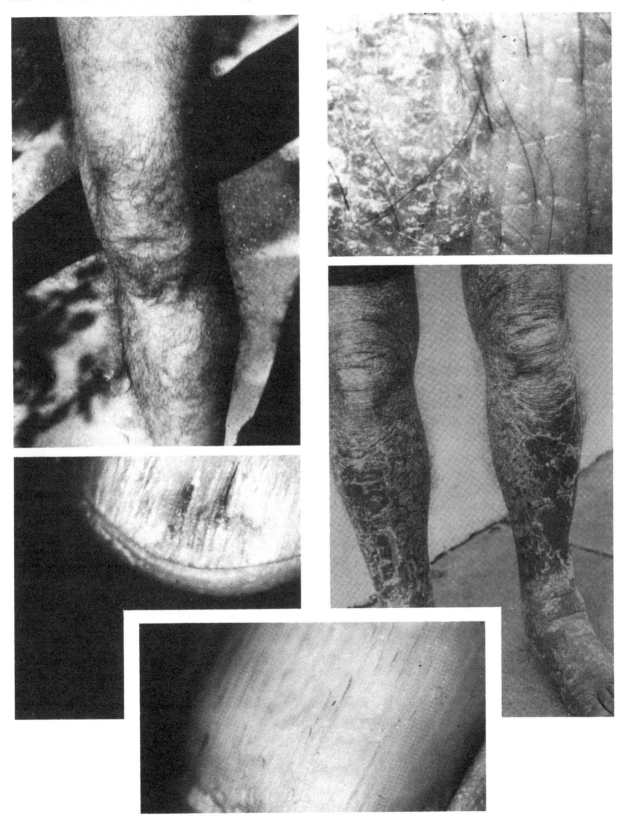

This is a classic case of silicon deficiency, before and after treatment. Nature heals, but sometimes she needs a helping hand.

SILICON
"The Magnetic Element"

Silicon, bearing the symbol Si, is a light-brown, nearly colorless element with a powerful electrical charge or "magnetism." Its atomic weight is 28.3; specific gravity, 2.49. It is almost odorless and tasteless. Acids join easily with silicon and are neutralized by this "magnetic" element. Thus soil is formed and broken down when silicon and water are at work together. Grain stalks are given rigidity by silicon; such grains as corn, rice, oats and barley owe their highly-polished, tough outer covering to silicon. Animals and humans receive firmness, elasticity, toughness from silicon; bones, teeth and tendons all need the "magnetic" element.

Silica is a Silicon Compound

Silica, as it occurs in the earth, is a compound of silicon and oxygen found in nearly all earthy minerals. It enters into such precious stones as jasper, onyx, opal and amethyst, among others. Next to oxygen, silicon is the most abundant element in the earth's strata, forming (as silica) almost one-fourth of the earth's crust. Silica acts as a plant support in the soil and is found in many mineral waters which are known to benefit health. Grains such as oats and barley are high in silicon and require a sandy soil. Oats contain about 39.2 percent silicon in their total ash content of 3.02 percent, higher than any other grain.

Oats a Favorite Source of Silicon

Oats also contain alkaline phosphates, starch, gluten, diastase, phosphorus and traces of sulphur, chlorine, iron, magnesium, calcium, sodium and a large amount of potassium (17.9 percent of the total ash content). Avenin, an agent which has powerful influence on the sexual system and is an aid in times of sexual neurasthenia, brain weakness, nervousness and breaking smoking or drug habits, is also present in oats. Oat straw tea is an excellent source of the properties needed in the above-mentioned conditions.

Historical Notes

Why do we call silicon the "magnetic" element? Tracing back to the origin of the word "magnetic," we find it springs from the name of the city Magnesia in Thessaly; words such as magnet, magnesia and magnetism have the same root. Magnesia and other similar words can be traced even farther back to magus, magh, and especially the Sanskrit word *mahaji*, meaning great, learned, wise. From the same etymon are derived our words magi, magic, magician and others of Latin descent. Most European languages, and many others, had their beginnings in ancient Sanskrit.

Ancient priests, magis or the "greats," used magnesian stones in curing people and in magnetizing wedding bands. These stones were found in the city of Magnesia, which was named in honor of these priests, the magi; the stones were called magnesian, Herculean or Heraclean by the plebian or peasant class.

SILICON: ITS ROLE IN THE HUMAN BODY

The body of a 150-pound man contains approximately one-and-one-quarter ounces of silicon; free silicon is used liberally in the body before being excreted. Silicon is found in all animal and vegetable tissues, especially in resistive tissue such as the skin, tendons, dura mater, fascia, hair, nails and birds' feathers. Silicon is responsible for making muscles firmer, blood warmer, hair more luxuriant and shiny. It reinforces all membranes, ligamentous tissue, arterial walls, throat walls, inner and outer organ linings, uterine lining, walls of the digestive tract, spinal and cerebral dura mater, nails and skin. It has a vital influence on the nervous system, the brain and the sexual system. In short, the whole body is invigorated and energized by silicon.

"Silica, as it occurs in the earth is a compound of silicon and oxygen found in nearly all earthy minerals."

Silicon Affects Tissues, Bones, Nerves

Much silicon in the body makes tissues very alkaline; the brain and nervous system are greatly influenced; the pulse becomes more rhythmic; bones are more efficient; the entire body is more alkaline. Nerve impulses are more efficiently transferred when silicon is in reserve in the body. There is a general disease resistance, as well, because silicon lends antiseptic protection.

Silicon Vital for Healthy Hair

United with sulphur, silicon works effectively in hair and nails. Growing children must have these elements well supplied for shiny, healthy, strong hair. Such animal kingdom representatives of the silicon type as sheep, foxes, bears, bison must have silicon and sulphur for glossy and healthy coats; their lives depend upon warm, protective coverings.

Silicon Combats Sexual Disorders

A diet rich in silicon is effective against impotence or sexual feebleness. The patient who suffers from ovarian, hysterical and menstrual complications needs silicon. Nicotine or drug habits are more easily overcome when silicon is well supplied. Neurasthenia and nervous prostration due to excessive work or passion are benefitted by silicon. The mental worker needs silicon in the diet to accomplish more with less tiredness. Nervofibrosis tendencies call for silicon. General appetite and feelings of well-being are enhanced by silicon.

"Silicon is found in all animal and vegetable tissues, especially in resistive tissue such as the skin, tendons, dura mater, fascia, hair, nails and birds' feathers."

"Old-Age" Complaints Lessened with Silicon

Silicon benefits elderly persons crippled by "old-age" complaints and weather conditions. Joints are made more elastic, eyesight is improved, varicose veins are reduced, polypi decrease, complexion improves, flesh is made firmer, scabs vanish; hair becomes more abundant and shiny when silicon is in proper balance in the body. Circulation is also improved.

Diseases Prevented by Silicon

Nations with the lowest cancer rates are known for diets high in silicon and formic acid. Malaria is also combatted by silicon foods. Catarrh, tuberculosis, tumors call for silicon; so do apoplexy, bruises, rheumatism and throat consumption. Autointoxication is prevented or reduced by silicon. Foot perspiration is counteracted by silicon and formic acid; animals developing foot rot need silicon also. Pus generation and suppuration due to infected wounds or sores need silicon, as do reactions from vaccination serums. Syphilis and gonorrhea are benefitted to some extent by silicon; they also require fluorine, sulphur, potassium chloride and other tissue salts destroyed by germ life in times of venereal disease.

Silicon Fights Numerous Ailments

In cooperation with other foods rich in potassium chloride, silicon ensures against paralysis. Nervous prostration demands liberal silicon. Circulation, arterial walls, testicles, ovaries, inguinal glands, the cerebellum and the epidermis need silicon. Pyorrhea, measles, many swellings, suppuration, self-poisoning are all benefitted by a rich silicon diet.

"Nicotine or drug habits are more easily overcome when silicon is well supplied."

SIGNS OF SILICON EXCESS

The Sillevitic Type

A person with great quantities of silicon in his body is quick, agile, lean, nimble and very active. His body molds to an abundance of silicon so the body is generally alkaline; sodium, potassium and magnesium are alkaline elements which are very active in the body in conjunction with silicon. A Sillevitic, or silicon type is light and optimistic; the Latin word "levis" means light and easy, both Sillevitic characteristics. The person having much silicon in the body is light-hearted, gullible, happy, fun-loving, funny, boisterous, carefree, unworried and inattentive. No circumstance, no matter how disastrous, wilts his spirits; poverty, misfortune, illness and disregard foster few or no complaints. The Sillevitic type is quick-acting, hearty, but fickle in affection; the personality changes constantly; the imagination is colorful. This type has a big heart; he is sociable and friendly; his ready smile can melt icebergs. Life is exciting and challenging to the Sillevitic type; he is kind, even-tempered, happy, cordial, agreeable, playful, teasing, quick to laugh; he likes to sing; social and business affairs are of great interest to him. In fact, he is an irresistible charmer.

316

Animal Silicon Types

A person who has silicon dominant in his system may be likened to some of his silicon counterparts in the animal kingdom—the gazelle, chamois, addax, mountain goat, eland, steinbok, elk, gnu, antelope, mountain deer—which are known for grace, speed and fleet-footedness.

"Silicon benefits elderly persons crippled by 'old age' complaints and weather conditions."

The Sillevitic Salesman

Silicon may not produce genius, but this type is well-qualified in business, even as a highly-paid executive capable of making dividends and sales soar. Salesmanship is the forte of the Sillevitic type, due to his friendly personality and persuasive manner and speech. He can make the most shy person feel at home; he makes an optimistic writer or a positive doctor or lawyer.

Happy, Breezy Sillevitics

A silicon man or woman favors happy, bright colors and lightweight, free-feeling clothing. Less sensitive to cold weather, these people prefer light clothing to heavy woolens, no matter the time of year.

The Unpredictable Silicon Type (Sillevitic)

Love is a passing fancy for the silicon type; changing affections leave broken hearts behind. A female silicon type is not a home-loving wife; she prefers changes and travel to housework and cooking. As an employee, she is unpredictable and may quit on the spur of the moment because she needs a change. She cultivates friends easily and the friends value her joking, lighthearted personality.

Silicon Oversupply is Uncommon

In rare cases, silicon may be so oversupplied that many symptoms develop, but this is not at all a common occurrence. When it does happen, the face may become flushed; fingers and feet are unable to stay still. The patient feels as if he is walking on pillows or riding a kangaroo. He is perpetually hungry, preferring bread and cereals rich in silicon, but he remains very slender.

Characteristics of the Silicon-Excess Type

Decisions are easy and spontaneous for the silicon-excess patient; he was born ready for anything. His speech flows as easily as if a phonograph needle served as a tongue. He takes in all details quickly; few things take him by surprise. Skates, skateboards and machines are easy conquests for this type. He or she is successful in occupations which capitalize on finger dexterity, such as typing, stenography, piano playing and other musical pursuits.

Mental Processes are Quick

Excess intake of silicon causes an overactive intellect, but the reasoning is nevertheless excellent. The emotions are subordinated to the mind. The person dwells briefly on one subject, then springs to a new one; his speaking is rushed; his observations and ractions are keen and quick; his mental processes are characteristically rapid.

"Nations with the lowest cancer rates are known for diets high in silicon and formic acid."

Overconfidence of the Silicon Patient

An overabundance of silicon produces a false sense of worth and potential; the individual believes he is a wise sage or a daring entrepreneur who can overcome the greatest adversity. He is sociable and detests solitude. He is apt to take very liberal views and throw away money freely. Mirth, powerful optimism, daring speculation, keen sense perception, a jovial and teasing manner, expansive gestures, verbosity, fickle affections, changing ideas and temperament, obsession with fantasies or excitement are qualities of the silicon-excess patient.

Sillevitic Innocence

The silicon type or silicon-excess patient may be a chatterbox, scatterbrained, flighty, disorganized, a braggart, an extreme idealist, prone to unconscious exaggeration and inconsistent reasoning. Yet there is an innocent quality, a childish idealism and a highly imaginative faculty about this patient. He often becomes conceited about his alleged accomplishments, blowing them out of proportion in a pompous way; exaggeration of anything that strikes his fancy is likely to go to extremes. But his tales of fantasy are true in his own eyes; there is no malicious intent in any of his talk. It is simply that his imagination is so vibrant and prolific that he is able to believe his own stories.

"A person with great quantities of silicon in his body is quick, agile, lean, nimble and very active.

Restlessness of Silicon Type (Sillevitic)

A patient suffering from excessive silicon consumption is unable to be calm and still, even at home in the evenings; his mind races like a playful squirrel, inventing games and tales and merriment; it seems his mind never sleeps. His moods are jovial and he finds humor in all things; he is a natural comic; whistling, dancing, leaping around are all common actions for him. His mind is an unlimited storehouse of ideas and he is incessantly jubilant; he often sings to himself at the slightest provocation and even sings in his sleep. Sleep is little needed by this patient; he retires in the early hours of the morning and arises early. He is a "workaholic," an indefatiguable student who has some peculiar habits.

Hyperactivity Causes Complications

Excessive heat is generated in various parts of the body when silicon is overconsumed. The mental faculties become hyperactive, resulting in mental stress and overfunction of the motor areas; locomotor parts are hyperactive, the cerebellum painful, the blood overly alkaline, secretions overalkaline, lower part of backhead fevered and inflamed, work desire abnormal; desire for activity is abnormally great, leading to paresis, neurasthenia and fever in solid body structures.

Craving for Sunshine and Hills

Silicon-excess sufferers crave sunshine constantly; they also long for hills and mountains. Salivation develops chronic symptoms; various solid structures harden and develop fibroids. There is an abnormal craving for cold water, ice cream and frozen foods. The blood darkens; excessive heat is generated in the body; fevers and alkalinuria manifest. Overwork and hyperactivity and poor assimilation of tissue salts result in emaciation. The ears may have a humming sound; there may be herpetic eruptions, optical illusions, malnutrition of tissues, total fatigue from overwork and hyperactivity, swelling of lymphatic glands; eventually psychentonia appears. An acid develops which, attacking the bones and fibrous tissue, may cause necrosis. The glands undergo dangerous catabolic alterations; mucus surfaces disintegrate; fibrous tissues are destroyed; pus is generated in bones.

"A silicon man or woman favors happy, bright colors and lightweight free-feeling clothing."

SIGNS OF SILICON DEFICIENCY

Psychological Signs of Silicon Lack

Psychological symptoms of silicon shortage are pronounced. The patient becomes overly anxious about his health and welfare; he feels he is facing death. Morning brings more optimism and depression appears toward evening; crying spells come on without provocation; he may feel like screaming or become hysterical; his disposition alternates between submission and stubbornness or willful behavior; at one time he is cowardly and weak-willed and at another, may be irascible, uncontrollable, irrational, angry.

Sensitive Nervous System

Motion, bright lights, noise, bustle, loud conversations are intolerable to this patient. His

318

nervous system is sensitive to the slightest noise or commotion; his ears may be acutely sensitive to the smallest sounds; his body is chilly because heat production is reduced, causing him to bundle up in blankets or warm clothes and huddle in a warm, dry, quiet room.

"Decisions are easy and spontaneous for the silicon-excess patient; he was born ready for anything."

Brooding and Feelings of Hopelessness

Life may seem hopeless and worthless to the silicon-deficient patient. Excruciating headaches cause him to fear losing control of his mind and reasoning ability. He constantly broods over ethics and principles which are trivial to others; he becomes agitated, menacing over insignificant happenings, argumentative and ungratified, uncommunicative and hostile, overconcerned, shy and withdrawing; his speech is evasive, his sense perception chaotic, his temper uneven, his spirit bashful, his feelings hypersensitive, his wants unsatisifed, his thoughts taxing, his memory cloudy, his nerves on edge; he finds conversation, reading or writing fatiguing; he gets drowsy from riding in automobiles.

Physical Indications of Silicon Lack

Bones and membranes undergo destructive changes; connective tissues may swell and joints crack. The diaphragm becomes enfeebled and some weakened parts of it may cause respiratory disturbances; the pleura may generate catarrh; some membranes or coatings may produce pus, as may walls of the digestive tract; other body canals may be plagued by catarrhal coatings. The head may become inflamed; the bottoms of the feet may sting and smart. The patient becomes adverse to being touched or coming into close contact with others. Weeping spells may be prolonged. When the silicon reserve in the body is depleted and silicon foods not provided, brain damage of a permanent nature is possible.

Abscesses, Suppuration and Scabs on the Skin

In addition to the above, the lips become dry and may develop scabs; skin is dry, scabby or scaly; ringworm may develop; dry scales and dandruff are found on the scalp. As silicon poverty advances, disorders of the ear membranes develop and scabs develop behind the ears. Carotid arteries swell and caries or pus appear in the mastoid process. Tiny, annoying, stinging scabs form high in the nose canal; the tip of the nose may itch and sting. Roots of teeth may abscess; small sores or ulcers form on the gums. Eyelids may be troublesome; yellow patches may be found on the skin—on arms, the outside of the hand, the forehead, the neck or in other locations. The anterior chamber of the eye may become suppurated. Fistula develop on various parts of the body. Eyes may discharge hot tears; membranes may become suppurated with granulation tissue (proud flesh); indurations, abscesses, blisters and inflamed areas may develop on the skin, along with fleshy warts and stinging, painful skin eruptions; all are silicon-shortage disorders. Suppuration may result from the most minor wounds or injuries; lymphatic glands become pus-laden and catarrhal. Patients may complain of a bloated feeling; sensitive, painful skin; soreness between toes.

"An overabundance of silicon produces a false sense of worth and potential; the individual believes he is a wise sage or a daring entrepreneur who can overcome the greatest adversity."

Children Susceptible to Scrofula

Children lacking silicon are susceptible to scrofula (tuberculosis of lymph glands of the neck), because silicon poverty contributes to skin disorders, bone pathology and chronic symptoms in membranes and canal walls.

Silicon Deficiency Contributes to Many Maladies

Activities of cartilage are abnormal. The rectum becomes atonic and inflexible so that waste matter is not properly expelled; at other times, the rectal pouch is unable to hold fecal matter. Frequent urination is a result of loss of tone or contractive ability of the bladder; enuresis, involuntary urination may also develop. It must be understood that silicon deficiency is not the sole cause of these and other disorders and diseases, but it often contributes to such complications and maladies.

"Silicon-excess sufferers crave sunshine constantly; they also long for hills and mountains."

Violent Pain is Symptomatic

Catarrh, phlegm and mucus may almost fill the bronchial tubes when silicon is deficient in the body. There may be fetid discharges from various parts of the body; bleeding of stomach, bowel, lungs or other organs is another indication of silicon insufficiency; violent or chronic headache is a further symptom. Pain is intensified by motion, sudden jarring or vibration; pain may be severe, pressurizing, ripping.

Lower Spine is Tender

Tendons become tender; motor nerves contract; nails become brittle and break easily; forearms jerk convulsively; nerves of arms are feeble; blood and muscles have gurgling, pulsating sensations; pain in lower abdomen stretches to lower back; tenderness or soreness in lower spine facilitates pain from sitting, horseback riding or reclining on the sore spot. There is a tendency toward spinal curvature and afflictions of the spinal membrane.

Sense of Taste May be Lost

Tumors may develop in cartilage; abscesses may form in loins; parotid or cervical glands may swell; the tip of the tongue may have a tickling, creeping, stinging feeling; some cells of the tongue may harden—for example, taste bud cells, causing loss of the sense of taste. Deep breathing is difficult; the voice is husky or hoarse in the morning. Parts of the body may develop lumps, notably in the tendons, membranes and gristle.

319

Silicon Shortage Intensifies Gout Symptoms

Germ life is allowed to flourish when silicon is exhausted; tumors in the dural sinuses are likely; lack of cerebral, spinal or sexual fluids may become a problem, contributing to rheumatism of the occipito-frontalis muscles, brain tumors, meningitis, brain inflammation, mental weakness, foot perspiration, cerebral fatigue, violent headache, cranial growths, brain softening, cephalomata, chills that last and last, scabs, integumentory tumefaction, sweating of head and face, cerebropathy, cephalemia, weighty feeling in limbs, gouty headache, dangerous ulceration, poor eyesight, chronic headache accompanied by intolerance for light and noise (cephalea), nausea, glandular swellings, carbuncles, corneal ulceration, ozena. Gout is intensified by silicon shortage; proper body temperature is not maintained, so the patient is perpetually chilled; colds are easily contracted.

"When the silicon reserve in the body is depleted and silicon foods not provided, brain damage of a permanent nature is possible."

Ailments Due to Silicon Deficiency

Ligaments are weakened and unable to support the body properly; bone nutrition is faulty. Other signs of silicon deficiency include dental caries; defective eyesight; symptoms of stenosis; mental disorders; bone problems; inability to think clearly; hemeralopia; neurasthenic psychosis; gruesome fear of cold (psychrophobia); pyelitis; suppuration; blockage of eustachian tubes; crusty scabs; pycnosis of tendons, membranes or linings; swelling of lachrymal sacs; stye formation; intolerance or dread of noise; faulty or hyperactive generation of nerve impulse, facilitating spasms or jerky movements; cataracts; induration of cellular tissue; anal itch; lip sores or gum boils.

Further Signs of Silicon Deficiency

Still other complaints or manifestations of silicon poverty include voracious appetite, eructation, liver abscess, flatus, lumpy feces, fissured colon, urinary troubles, pyloritis. Lack of

tone in testicles and other testicle problems such as inflammation, tumors, atrophy are additional silicon-shortage monitors in males. Amenorrhea, prolapsus due to myelitis, cysts in the vagina, hardening of, or pus generation in mammary glands, nipple ulceration and formation of lumps are indications of silicon depletion in females.

Lack of Silicon Reserve

When silicon reserves have been precipitated from the body, possible manifestations include hydrocele, scrotal hernia, dandruff, scirrhus, thyroiditis, pleural inflammation, varicella, sacral disability, spina bifida, contractions of flexor muscles, ingrown toenails and other nail abnormalities, cramps and tension in ovaries, echondroma.

Vaccinations are Dangerous

Body activities become spasmodic and chaotic when silicon is in great demand. Vaccination serums are exceedingly harmful to the silicon-deficient patient (and are detrimental to the average person, as well); injections are harmful to this patient, as are pus germs and suppuration. Snoring may come as a result of throat scrofula. There may be inflammation of fibrous constituents; growing pains in children; boils, rhagades, defective metabolism; soreness between vertebrae; increased predisposition to variola, boils, various types of zona, intestinal gas generation and gas pressure (flatus).

Symptoms of Low Silicon in the Body

A number of symptoms should be easily recognized by the trained doctor, nurse or nutritionist. These include buzzing in the ears; touchiness and agitation from sound, noise or commotion; declining eyesight; flying specks before the eyes; tingling in various parts of the body; neuralgic aches; numbness of various body parts; morbid vigilance; neurasthenic symptoms of almost every description; oppression; emotional and intellectual gullibility and impressionability; sleepiness alternating with insomnia; mental confusion; lethargy; aversion to work, motion and exertion; hysterical schizophrenic, neurotic and psychotic inclinations—all alert the doctor or professional to possible silicon deficiency.

The Silicon-Deprived Patient is Susceptible to Many Ailments

The silicon patient finds conversation extremely tiring; insignificant things worry him; he imagines he has contracted some dreadful disease. General health declines; vitality is being destroyed—but a doctor finds no indications of pathology and is inclined to believe the patient has psychosomatic or psychoneurotic problems. The spine is tender and pains dart through the chest and abdomen; arms and legs have muscle spasms; head or chest may have pulsating pains; there is insomnia and tossing at night, nervous indigestion, self-destructive tendencies which are latent or active and due to depletion of nerve force; numbness in body parts or skin for hours or days at a time; extreme awareness of temperature alterations in joints of arms or legs; loss of finger control; twitching in left eyelid or uncontrollable winking. Head and face sweat but body temperature is low and cold; drafts are very uncomfortable, especially on the left side of the body. Extreme mental exertion, catamenial symptoms that differ markedly from those in times of health, severe mental depression, listlessness with exhaustion, peculiar bashfulness, shyness, lack of self-confidence, sexual system weakness causing hermit-like preference, melancholic behavior, feebleness of body functions, back weakness, transient pains, nauseating headache, susceptibility to cholea, hysteria and schizophrenic behavior—all demand a diet high in silicon.

The Head is Painful and Eyesight Deteriorates

Motion which causes vibration of the brain and nerves is intolerable to the silicon-deficient patient; he longs for hot compresses on his head. Fatigue is precipitated by excitement or emotional stress. As the reserve of silicon in the body is exhausted, symptoms become more serious. The obese individual gains more weight; while appearing ruddy and healthy he is actually ill and constantly complaining. Massage produces temporary relief, but it lasts only a few hours and symptoms reappear soon. Classic signs of silicon deficiency are dim eyesight, feeble ankles, painful thighs, nearly incessant odorless flatus and crippled sensations in the sacrum.

Urine is a Barometer of Silicon in the Body

The urine of the silicon patient may be similar in hue to cider vinegar, or it may be pale amber, dark amber or pale yellow; red, sandy or milky sediments may be found in it. The urine is acidic; urates may appear after it stands, or a white sediment may manifest. Indican or phosphates may be excreted through the kidneys. Frequent, involuntary, painful urination is due to sphincter muscle contraction.

Strengthlessness and Drowsiness

Shortage of silicon results in almost strengthless arms and legs; small, hard, rapid pulse alternating with slow; perspiration and stinging of fingertips; itching feet; uncomfortable feelings in epigastric plexus (pit of stomach or solar plexus); inclination to snoring; transient and variable symptoms, covering several phases in a single day; cracking of gristle in knees or other joints; afternoon drowsiness; fleeting pains in genital organs.

Patients Vary Greatly

Symptoms vary vastly from patient to patient. One may exhibit rheumatic and neurasthenic symptoms; another may manifest gout and profuse perspiration. Urates may appear in the urine and its specific gravity may rise to 1028 or above; lithemic diathesis may cause excretion of excessive phosphates through the kidneys. The sexual system and nervous system are undermined when silicon reserves are exhausted.

Further Symptoms of Silicon Depletion

There may be complications with the catamenial periods; inclination toward tobacco and drug habits or dependence upon them; propensity to development of sores, scaly skin, blood poisoning, boils, vaccinosis, herpes facialis. Suppuration from toxic bites or stings may leave disfiguring scars. This patient is likely to perspire merely from descending a staircase because his ligaments are so feeble. His shoulder joints may gurgle, as may the spleen, lower legs or blood vessels. There may be heart pressure, kidney pain, stiff neck and occasional staggering to the right when walking; loss of hair or premature graying; extreme excitement with globus hystericus in high-strung patients.

Sleep is Preferred to Activity

A diet high in silicon would benefit patients exhibiting the following symptoms: flabby flesh; dizziness with inclination to tumble forward; chilly sensations in neck and head, washing over the body in waves; agitation from motion; longing for rest; failure of cranial sutures to close in children; appearance of large, fleshy warts; unsightly scars as an aftermath of boils; rosy patches on the skin; slow healing of wounds and inclination toward pus generation; intensified skin eruptions from sunlight; skin affictions due to malnutrition; formation of skin afflictions due to malnutrition; formation of subcutaneous tissue into small nodules; putrid and skin nerves; partial paralysis or numbness of body parts; rattling and misplaced feeling of bones; stenotic body canals; chilly sensations in areas on left side of body; chills which migrate through the body; low heat generation; preference for sleep over work, activity or motion; sweating from minimal exertion; extreme thirst after midnight but not before.

Enervation and Exhaustion

Enervation and aversion to exertion call for abundant silicon. Hand tremors, limb convulsions, itching soles of feet, exhaustion of flexor joints and feeble joints all require silicon foods.

Additional Symptoms Calling for Silicon in the Diet

Additional symptoms include debility of ligaments; discomfort when riding; pulsation in cerebellum or lumbar plexus; gout of certain vertebrae; faulty breathing resulting from temper, passion, banter, singing, even reading; soreness of lung lobes; catarrh and mucus which is thick and tenacious; shortness of breath; larynx spasms; enlarged thyroid gland; husky voice; cowardly behavior; tender breasts; feebleness of limbs; mental fatigue; bloody milk; lumpy subcutaneous tissue; fetid foot perspiration; painful hemorrhoids; nausea from intercourse; pain and tenderness of genital organs; premuature ejaculation; lumpy feces; swollen or lumpy glands with pus formation; yellowish complexion; enlargement of liver; hardened pylorus; fitful heartbeat; fickle or absent appetite; ticklish tip of tongue; pus generation in roots of teeth; dental caries; sensitivity to chilling air currents; dry, parched lips which may become scabby; hardening of cornea; soreness with contraction of retina; itching ears; chilled tip of nose; swelling, dryness of nasal membranes; curdlilke earwax; sensitive scalp; scabby neck; stinging, tingling, itching of neck or other body parts; sensitivity of brain to shocking or jarring vibrations; soreness and pain in tophead; head congestion causing flush of cheeks or alternating yellowish hues in face; night sweats of head and face and less frequent sweating at other times; disinclination for brain labor; melancholy; idea that death is near or that a fatal disease is imminent.

Treatment of Silicon Deficiency

The above symptoms, all of which should be recognizable by competent professionals, require liberal quantities of silicon in food or food-supplement form.

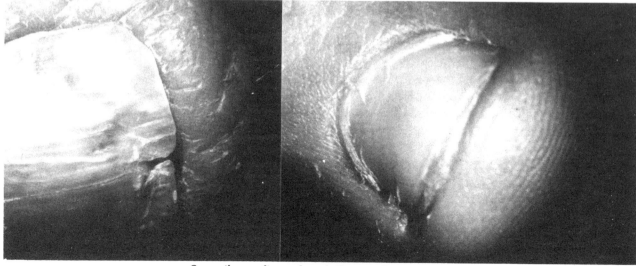

Our nails are alive and need silicon, calcium and zinc.

HIGHEST SILICON FOODS

Oats and barley head the list of silicon foods. More concentrated supplemental sources are rice polishings, rice bran syrup, kelp, oat straw tea and alfalfa tablets. These and other good food sources are listed below.

It is important to note that all refined starches and carbohydrates (i.e., white flour, white sugar, white rice) are nearly devoid of silicon because the outer skins and hulls, which contain silicon, have been removed in the refining process. Nuts, seeds, grains and cereals have a generous supply of silicon in their outer coverings.

Alfalfa broth and tea	Marjoram
Apples	Millet
Apricots	Nectarines
Asparagus	Oats
Bananas	Onions
Barley	Parsnips
Beans	Plums
Beets and beet greens	Raisins
Cabbage (red, common, savoy)	Pumpkin
Carrots	Rice (brown and wild)
Cauliflower	Rice bran and syrup
Celery	Rice polishings
Cherries	Spinach
Corn	Sprouted seeds
Cucumbers	Strawberries
Dandelion greens	Sunflower seeds
Dates	Sweet potatoes
Figs, dried black mission	Tomatoes
Grains	Turnips
Greens (mustard, turnip, etc.)	Watermelon
Horseradish	Wheat bran
Kelp	Wheat germ
Kohlrabi	Whole wheat
Lettuce (leaf)	

SILICON MENUS

Veal joint broth, barley muffins, steamed asparagus tips, steamed beets and beet greens, fresh strawberries topped with well-beaten egg whites which have been sweetened with fruit juice concentrate.

Cheese sticks, nut and seed butter, dates, peaches, watermelon, bananas, grapes, cherries, alfalfa-mint tea.

Fruit omelette topped with rice polishings, wheat germ, sunflower seed meal; revived prunes, revived figs, blueberries or gooseberries, goat milk.

Steamed rye or yellow cornmeal topped with flaxseed meal, almond meal, rice polishings, wheat germ; baked apple, nectarines, soft-boiled eggs, grape juice.

Mixed green salad with cucumbers, avocado, leeks, cauliflower, alfalfa sprouts, lentil sprouts, celery, tomatoes, shredded beets; steamed brown rice (or baked sweet potato), steamed parsnips, steamed mustard greens, vegetable soup, alfalfa-leaf tea, tomato dressing.

Corn on the cob (or cornbread or baked potato), barley and green kale soup; leaf lettuce salad with sprouts, dandelion greens, cucumber, shredded carrots, shredded beets, shredded turnips, fresh green peas, sundried black olives, cauliflower, cherry tomatoes; steamed kohlrabi, steamed cabbage; avocado and horseradish dressing with kelp seasoning; oat straw tea.

SUMMARY OF SILICON

GENERAL CHARACTERISTICS

"Magnetic" element

Nearly colorless, odorless, tasteless

Silica a compound of silicon, oxygen

Silicon type = Sillevitic type

SILICON IN THE HUMAN BODY

Lends rigidity, firmness, elasticity, toughness to bones, teeth, tendons

Found in all tissues, particularly resistive tissues

Reinforces membranes, walls, linings, ligaments, nails, skin

Increases alkalinity of body

Aids transfer of nerve impulses

Vital for healthy hair, nails

Helps retain body heat and electricity

Increases vigor, energy, strength, resistance

SIGNS OF SILICON EXCESS *(Characteristics of Sillevitic Type)*

Optimism, cheerfulness   *Spontaneity*
Graceful, agile, quick movements   *Unpredictability*
Overactive intellect   *Speech and finger dexterity*
Overconfidence, innocence   *Restlessness, constant activity*

SIGNS OF SILICON DEFICIENCY

Alternating sleepiness/sleeplessness   *Fatigue, strengthlessness*
Nervous stomach   *Depression*
Low body temperature   *Slow healing power*
Mental strain   *Weakness in ligaments*
Acrid foot perspiration   *Falling hair*
Sensitive nerves   *Cracking, swelling joints*
Skin abscesses, scabs, scales   *Intensified gout symptoms*
Husky voice   *Phosphates, amber urine*
Involuntary urination   *Sexual weakness*
Tender spine

HIGHEST SILICON FOODS

Oats   *Rice polishings and bran*
Barley   *Kelp*
Nuts, seeds   *Cereals, grains*

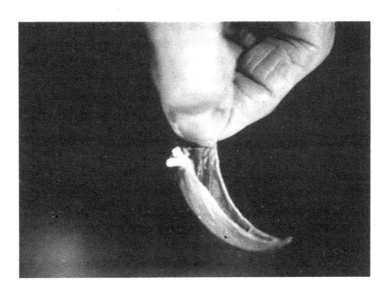

The resilience in an eagle's powerful talon is due to its high amount of silicon.

fifteen

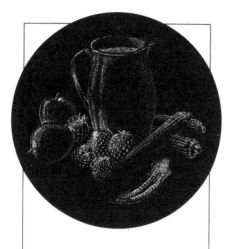

Sodium, the "youth" element

As I have mentioned before, there are four biochemical elements that I have used most successfully in my practice: calcium, sodium, silicon and iodine. By adding extra tonics and supplements, I have been able to do the greatest amount of good with these four, which are always lacking in the average patient who comes to me. Above all, sodium is the element I am most successful with because I deal with so many cases of arthritis and general acid conditions. In fact, almost the entire American nation and the world at large is suffering from diseases caused by sodium hunger. Dyspepsia can best be cured by teaching the farmer to supply sodium to the soil, and the homemaker to use foods where the sodium has not been lost.

Doctors measure a patient's age by the suppleness of the joints. and such suppleness is attributable to sodium, the "youth element," which keeps us youthful, pliable, limber and active. Without good activity, we do not feel like playing or working—a direct consequence, for instance, of calcium deposits. A healthy person is constantly testing the body's limits in running, dancing, etc., and these vigorous activities are impossible without the proper sodium balance in the body.

Sodium's importance is widespread in the body. It keeps calcium and magnesium in solution, and is active in the lymph and the blood. Biochemical sodium, iron and chlorine make the blood salty and favor the generation of electromagnetism. Lack of sodium results, not only in hardening, stiffness, rheumatism and gout, but also gallstone and bladder ailments. Fevers, heavy physical work, Turkish baths, excitement, temper, brain work, pregnancy, menstruation, spleen functioning, fibrous tissue and cartilage, all call for sodium salts. Additionally, sodium foods should be eaten when digestion is poor, when infants vomit and when frontal headaches appear.

Sodium and Arthritis

When a joint becomes hard, most doctors recommend a sodium-free diet, not realizing that every disease represents a **shortage** of a biochemical element. If the joints get hard, sodium is lacking. So what do I do? I pour in okra and celery (obtainable in tablets also). All the sodium control foods are needed, including fruits (if

Salt is a drug—not a food sodium. The U.S. Surgeon General's Report says Americans get too much salt. As little as 5 grams a day is too much for some people.

Gout is a sign of sodium deficiency.

Sodium makes calcium more soluble and convertible into bone tissue.

Lymph is high in sodium.

The spleen is a sodium organ.

Goat milk is rich in sodium because the goat is a sodium-type animal.

Whey is the natural food highest in organic sodium, which is different from the chemical sodium in table salt (sodium chloride). Sodium is normally stored in the joints and gastrointestinal system walls. Depleted of sodium, joints pick up calcium deposits, the stomach becomes hypoacidic and bowel elimination may become underactive. Whey is the best food for arthritis, rheumatism, digestive conditions and for dissolving cholesterol.

326

they have matured properly; not picked green), which ripened by the sun—a sodium star—have a goodly amount of sodium. However, because ripe fruits are difficult to obtain, I recommend we get our sodium primarily from vegetable sources.

I estimate that 30% of my arthritis cases get well; 30% show improvement; the remaining 40% get no results whatsoever. Some patients come too late and some have problems beyond repair. Still others do not follow the program instructions. Thus, there are many reasons for lack of good results. I should also note that I do not see quick results in my very serious cases. It takes at least 3 months for even a minimum sodium reserve to be replenished in the body. In direct contrast, at times there are astonishing recoveries. For example, there was the television repairman who had not been able to use his arms for one year, but by taking 18 okra and 18 celery tablets a day, he regained the use of his arms in a couple of weeks! These supplements are the highest sources of sodium other than whey (goat whey is the best).

Problems with Acid

Sodium is stored in the stomach wall first and secondly in the joints. Whenever we find joint trouble, there is also stomach trouble. Note that sodium neutralizes acidity in the body, by taking care of stomach and bowel disturbances such as gas and excess hydrochloric acid. But sodium is also needed for a deficiency of hydrochloric acid. Thus, whenever a patient has an ulcer, sodium is beneficial, whether we are speaking of hyperchlorhydria or hypochlorhydria.

Generally, when people lack hydrochloric acid, they lack sodium. Hospital tests have found that 85% of patients over 50 lack hydrochloric acid, perhaps because at that age we stay away from milk products a great deal. Now all the oldest men of the world I have visited drank clabbered milk. Of course, normally the stomach uses hydrochloric acid to clabber milk; thus, for people lacking hydrochloric acid and the digestive juices to get the nourishment out of milk products, clabbered milk can be used with wonderful results.

For good health, along with the joints, the stomach and the lungs, the lymph glands must be in good working order, and in them we find an additional sodium storehouse. A certain type of person holds excessive sodium in the body and stores it in the lymph glands.

Potassium-Sodium Balance

In some cases, we have to reduce the sodium intake, if, for example, excessive weight is a problem. Here we use potassium broths instead of sodium foods and broths. (See potato peeling broth in potassium chapter.) Potassium helps drain the acids, rather than neutralize the acids as sodium does. Sodium intake is lowered as a temporary measure only, because removal of sodium entirely would lead to stomach troubles, arthritis, rheumatism and joint disturbances.

Dr. Percy Robinson has mentioned that the high cancer mortality increase in Japan, especially at the end of the 19th Century, was due to an upset in the balance between potassium and sodium. He mentioned that the Japanese, of course, had a great deal of salted fish as part of their daily routine in eating. When this salted fish was cut down in their diet, there was a drop in cancer.

This is possibly one of the reasons that Dr. Gerson, in his treatment of cancer cases, used more potassium and cut down on the sodium. To know what is necessary for a proper balance would be a tremendous factor in the prevention and cure of disease.

Few people are free from stomach problems, so we need a goodly amount of sodium. Stomach problems—including lack of hydrochloric acid—are probably one of the first considerations in every patient.

Sodium Foods

Dr. Rocine stressed that we should take milk only from a young and healthy animal with lively joints, because the milk is representative of the whole body of that animal. A young animal gives the greatest amount of sodium in its milk. I might add that I have seen the sick practically raised from the deathbed by the use of warm raw goat milk. Goats are a part of my life due to the wonderful work I have done with raw goat milk. It has been important in my own health, and comes from a very limber animal, a sodium animal.

The goat is a browser, not a grazer like the cow, and more intelligent than the cow. A cow has a greater calcium content in the body and in the milk. I suggest you read more about the merits of goat milk in my *Nature Has A Remedy*, Chapter 19, in which my knowledge of goats and goat milk—stemming from Dr. Rocine's teaching—is developed. Also go over the list of sodium foods and do not neglect to examine the charts giving sodium contents of foods. A person in need of sodium should know which foods have the most, and how to add these foods and tonics to the diet. A good sodium reserve is essential in order to get well and keep well.

In our sanitarium work, we have used sodium in the form of whey, especially goat whey. While, usually, I do not believe in advertising any company, I must say that wonderful results can be obtained with a goat whey product available from Briar Hills Dairies in Chehalis, Washington. Their product, called Whex, is very high in sodium and has tremendously aided my patients. Additionally, for my arthritis patients, I recommend raw goat milk and black mission figs—a fine tonic.

Another remedy, coming from Dr. Rocine, is to use egg white beaten to a froth as a topping for a broth. It should be consumed slowly, and will add sodium to the stomach wall by coating the stomach to prevent irritation by hydrochloric acid. This remedy does not cause

the deficiency normally associated with raw egg whites. Sodium is also found at high levels in most salad vegetables—but the average person does not eat enough salads.

Finally, veal joint broth should not be overlooked when sodium is needed. It is rich in sodium and excellent for glands, stomach, ligaments and digestive disorders, as well as helping to retain youth in the body.

Veal Joint Broth

Use a clean, fresh, uncut veal joint and after washing in cold water, put into a large cooking pot; cover half with water and add the following vegetables and greens cut up finely:

Small stalk of celery

1-1/2 cups apple peelings, 1/2" thick

2 cups potato peelings, 1/2" thick

1/2 cup chopped parsley

2 beets, grated

1 large parsnip

1 onion

1/2 cup okra (use canned if you cannot get fresh; or 1 tsp powdered okra)

Simmer all ingredients for 4 or 5 hours; strain off liquid and discard solid ingredients. There should be about 1-1/2 quarts of liquid. Drink hot or warm. Keep refrigerated.

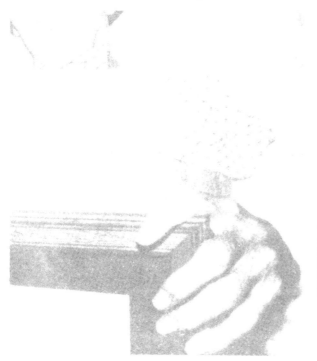

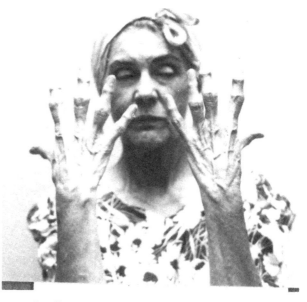

Swollen joints in arthritis mean calcium has come out of solution in the blood and deposited there. Dried goat whey (Whex) and vitamin C are needed to bring calcium back into solution.

SODIUM
"The Youth Element"

GENERAL CHARACTERISTICS

Sodium, which bears the symbol Na (natrium), is silvery-white, brilliantly lustrous, alkaline and positive in electrical charge. Its atomic weight is 23; specific gravity, 0.972. Sodium has a powerful affinity for oxygen and oxidizes rapidly in air (but less rapidly than does potassium). The combustion of sodium and oxygen produces a yellow flame.

"Sodium is found in almost all water bodies and virtually every type of soil."

Sodium Found in Water and Soil

Sodium is found in almost all water bodies and virtually every type of soil. Plants and crops cultivated near salty water contain abundant sodium; a gallon of ocean water yields approximately four ounces of common salt, which is rich in sodium. Humidity in the air attracts sodium.

Table Salt (Inorganic Sodium) Not Compatible with Human Body

Vegetables and fruits possess an organic (biochemic), assimilable form of sodium. Common table salt and chemical concoctions contain an inorganic sodium not compatible with the human body. The sun, a sodium star, ensures a high sodium content in mature fruit.

Sodium Compounds

Organic sodium keeps calcium in solution in the human body. Organic forms of sodium carbonate, sodium bicarbonate, sodium chloride and other compounds of sodium are important agents in biochemical processes in the body. Bicarbonate of soda, used in food preparation, is a white powder not in biochemical form and therefore not beneficial to the body.

Why is Sodium Called the "Youth" Element?

Sodium was named the "youth" element due to its properties of promoting youthful, limber, flexible, pliable joints. The sodium type (Desmogenic) is known for a youthful appearance into advanced age. The youth-producing characteristics of sodium are transferred to the joints of animals and man. Joint troubles need not manifest in the individual who has a good reserve of sodium, the "youth" element, in the stomach walls and in the joints.

329

SODIUM: ITS ROLE IN THE HUMAN BODY

The functions of sodium in the body are numerous and extensive. A normal man weighing 150 pounds contains in his body two-and-one-half to three ounces of sodium. Free sodium enters the constitution of some individuals more than others—particularly those of the Desmogenic (sodium) type. Sodium and sodium compounds and colloids affect physical as well as brain functions and general metabolism. Calcium metabolism, the blood, the medulla oblongata, secretions, mucus and serous membranes, the throat, secretory glands, the alimentary tract, the synovial membranes, the stomach and intestinal walls, the spleen and pancreas, and albumin metabolism are all influenced by sodium. Osmosis is increased and calcium, albumin and fibrin are kept in solution by sodium.

"Vegetables and fruits possess an organic (biochemic), assimilable form of sodium. Common table salt and chemical concoctions contain an inorganic sodium not compatible with the human body."

Where Sodium is Found in the Body

Sodium is contained in virtually all connective tissue of solid, fibrous makeup: joints, bone tissue, cartilage, ligaments, synovial membranes, liver, spleen, muscles, stomach, brain, blood corpuscles and other body constituents. The liver contains approximately 0.02% sodium salts; the brain, 0.2%; blood corpuscles, 0.2%. Considerable amounts of sodium are contained in cartilage (0.9%), lymph (0.7%), fibrous tissues (0.7%) and the synovia (0.8%).

Functions of Sodium Compounds

Sodium, which is highly alkaline, contributes to the alkalinity of the lymph and blood. Sodium phosphate is found extensively in the tissues of carnivorous animals. (Sodium bicarbonate works with sodium phosphate.) Sodium carbonate is more extensive in herbivorous creatures and is necessary for normal fat metabolism, breaking down neutral fats into fatty acids and glycerine; in cooperation with pancreatic juice it attracts and holds fat. Sodium bicarbonate is found in organic tissue salts in the pancreatic juice; pancreatic juice also contains amylopsin, a ferment which aids in converting starch into maltose in the small intestine. Intestinal juice, according to laboratory analysis, contains sodium carbonate, mucin and proteins; it is brown and has an alkaline reaction.

"Organic sodium keeps calcium in solution in the human body."

Value of Sodium Bicarbonate

Organic sodium bicarbonate is favorable to the throat tissues, tissues of the nasopharynx and larynx and other similar tissues when catarrhal congestions are present; its solvent action helps remove catarrhal pus. Bronchial mucus, catarrh and thickened secretions on canal walls are combatted by sodium bicarbonate; stomach and intestinal walls are favorably stimulated. When urine or the stomach is acidic, when the bladder and/or kidneys develop concretions (deposits), when the bladder becomes catarrhal or any part of the body develops catarrh, an alkaline sodium diet is indicated.

Diabetes Related to Sodium Lack

A diet and tonics rich in sodium carbonate and bicarbonate (organic) are in demand when gout manifests. Diabetic acidity, subacid blood, stomach catarrh and diabetic coma tendencies call for sodium foods. If sodium is not present in sufficient amounts, calcium deposits form in the body.

Value of Sodium Phosphate

Sodium phosphate from food sources is favorable to gastric and intestinal ailments accompanied by stomach acidity, sour perspiration, acrid eructations, parasites, colic and a yellow-coated tongue. Sodium phosphate enables carbonic acid (carbon dioxide) to be expelled more effectively from the lungs; it allows lactic acid to split and moisture to be freed. Sodium phosphate is present in all solids and fluids of the human organism, helping to maintain their alkalinity, especially in lymph, blood and tissue fluids.

Value of Sodium Sulphate

Sodium sulphate, as derived from food, reduces dropsy and biliousness; it counteracts scarlet fever, skin diseases, liver enlargement, vomiting, jaundice, ague. It helps control humidity in body fluids, prevents excessive blood humidity, promotes peristaltic action in the stomach and intestines. The biochemic form of sodium sulphate enhances performance of the liver, notably the secretion of bile; it ensures proper humidity levels throughout the body.

Constituents of Saliva

An alkaline medium is necessary for optimum health and performance of all body tissues and fluids; sodium and related compounds—calcium, sodium and magnesium phosphates, sodium and potassium chlorides, sodium carbonate—provide this medium and help form saliva, which is itself an alkaline medium. During a 24-hour period, a normal man secretes 2 to 3 pounds of saliva.

"Sodium was named the 'youth' element due to its properties of promoting youthful, limber, flexible, pliable joints."

Compounds of Bile

The bile contains the following compounds: sodium carbonate (0.93 parts per thousand); calcium phosphate (0.37); sodium phosphate (1.33); potassium chloride (0.28); sodium chloride (5.45); lecithin (0.04); sodium palmitate and stearate (1.36); free fat (0.1); cholesterin (0.54); sodium taurocholate (trace); sodium glycocholate (9.94); and water (977.4). Sodium taurocholate and sodium glycocholate are important ingredients of bile salts. The taurocholate is more abundant in the bile of carnivorous animals, while the glycocholate is found in larger quantities in grass-fed animals.

Contents of Lymph

Lymph salts contain considerable sodium; sodium chloride is present to 0.55% and sodium carbonate to 0.24%. Traces of magnesium, potassium and calcium are also present, along with 3 to 4 percent protein, some fat, sugar and water. Lymph salts also contain a good deal of free oxygen and carbon dioxide.

A Sodium Diet Counteracts Acids

A sodium-rich diet has a pronounced effect upon urine acidity, kidney and liver acidity. (Potassium is another powerful alkalizer.) Organic acids—notably acetic, buturic, lactic and other fatty acids which are products of excessive intake of fatty, starchy foods, meat, lard, margarine, potatoes, oily nuts—are neutralized by a rich sodium diet. In the absence of sodium and potassium salts, fatty acids are likely to form during digestive fermentation. Intake of such fatty, acidic foods results in precipitation of sodium and potassium until these elements are depleted; this in turn facilitates indigestion, fermentation, prostration and other complications. The "unfriendly bacteria" take over the digestive tract when sodium is deficient. Heartburn indicates a need for more sodium, and drowsiness following a meal indicates that digestion is slow and more serious digestive troubles are impending.

Precipitation of Sodium from the Body

Hot, humid weather precipitates sodium salts rapidly; water consumption also reduces them. Extreme physical work demands a liberal sodium diet, as do fevers, sauna baths, extreme excitement, passion, sweating. Self-abuse and self-hatred precipitate sodium as well as brain neurolin and the iron in hemoglobin and reduce the efficiency of nitrogen metabolism. Pregnancy requires liberal iron, potassium, silicon and sodium; menstruation uses much sodium. The spleen, the bile, the gastric secretions, the blood, intestinal and other secretions must have sodium. Calcium metabolism depends on sodium to keep it in solution. Liver, muscle, brain, blood corpuscles, fibrous tissue, cartilage, synovia, blood serum, lymph—in fact, almost all body fluids—need sodium.

Sodium Promotes Alkalinity

Overconsumption of fats, starches, causes fermentation and acid formation; sodium helps relieve these symptoms. Acids, heat and uneliminated waste material join forces to produce a medium for germ life; sodium neutralizes acids and germ life, especially in the intestinal tract, and produces an alkaline medium unfavorable to harmful bacteria, germs and acid poisons. Sodium also sweetens the stomach, destroys mucus, neutralizes acids, stimulates stomach and intestinal walls, disintegrates gases produced in the digestive tract, keeps elimination channels active, makes fluids and secretions and tissues more alkaline and thus unfavorable for germ life, mucus, catarrh, phlegm. Sodium works with "friendly bacteria" (bacillus acidophilus) to maintain favorable flora in the intestinal tract.

"A sodium-rich diet has a pronounced effect upon urine acidity, kidney and liver acidity.

SIGNS OF SODIUM EXCESS

Physical Characteristics of the Desmogenic Type

The Desmogenic or sodium type of individual is the only type who burns sodium faster than it can be replenished. His body is made up of much cartilage, gelatin, strong albuminoid material, phosphate and calcium salts; animal heat, oxygen, fat, starch and sweets are supplied in smaller quantities. His complexion is pale, either yellowish or brownish; his body is lean, lithe, svelte, fragile-appearing, often emaciated, but possessing tough ligaments, capsules (sheaths) and tendons. The body is flexible and lithe and the muscles surprisingly strong; the pale, fragile appearance is deceiving. Connective tissues, ligaments, membranes, power of coordination, motor nerves, cerebellar vitality, solid fibrous tissue, cartilage, skin, hair and the entire motor and vegetative structure are keenly active. Tissue is elastic, soft, but tough and solid in function. The Desmogenic type is ambitious, hardworking, active, high-strung, sinewy; his moods are chaotic. He is graceful, fluid in movement, quick, nimble, skillfull and precise in actions. The tissues are tenacious and

332

muscles keen; gravity perception is exceptional; muscle coordination is responsive and precise.

Diet and Habits of the Sodium Type (Desmogenic)

The dietary favorites of the sodium type are gelatin-textured foods, butters, vegetable phosphates, sodium foods and animal fat. In youth, this type is athletic, sporting, active and energetic. His heat generation and oxidation are relatively low, so a cold winter is damaging and a warm summer favorable. The outdoors, nature, forests and hills are preferred and are favorable to his health. His circle of friends is small and he wants it that way. Rush and speed describe him well: rush at mealtime, rush in work, rush in travel; restlessness in sleep; speed, activity, impatience in all things. He is more animated at night and easily angered in the morning. Force antagonizes him and sympathy makes him sullen; injustice or injury are not forgotten, and he harbors animosity toward the bearer.

Keen Reflexes of the Sodium Type (Desmogenic)

The Desmogenic type is skilled with his hands, whether as a surgeon, mechanic, chiropractor, masseur, draftsman or dentist. His reflexes are spontaneous and lightning quick; he can almost see behind him; his hearing is exceptionally keen; senses and muscles are more rapidly responsive than in most individuals. He is aware of an approaching storm long before it breaks, due to the effect on his blood, joints, tissues and fluids of electrical tension, gases and ferments in the air.

"Heartburn indicates a need for more sodium, and drowsiness following a meal indicates that digestion is slow and more serious digestive troubles are impending."

Disposition of the Sodium Type (Desmogenic)

The wife of the sodium type must brace herself for periodic temper outbursts, possible jealous streaks, occasional bitterness, cruelty and powerful passions which lie just below the surface. He is generally serene, with occasional outbursts, recklessness, sullenness, rebellion, defiance, malice, derision, drinking, money-spending sprees.

Peculiar Hobbies of the Desmogenic

If both sodium and potassium are excessive in the constitution, the individual is inclined toward peculiar hobbies, interests, obsessions, possibly bordering on the cruel or sadistic. He may want to attack people in the dark, kidnap women, steal, take up the study of poisons, explosives, snakes, ferocious animals, bombs or hypnotism; he may go on alcoholic binges. These temptations may, of course, never surface, but the latent tendencies are there.

> ## "The spleen, the bile, the gastric secretions, the blood, intestinal and other secretions must have sodium."

Health and Disease Tendencies of Sodium-Excess Type

The body metabolism and functions of the patient manifesting sodium and potassium excess are cyclical, as are his ailments. Thirst alternates with no thirst for weeks; appetite is ravenous or absent by turns; good health alternates with a spell of serious diseases or illnesses, seemingly for no reason. Ailments, actions, constitution are periodic, extreme and hurried. Moods are variable from happy to gloomy to amorous.

Extremism of the Sodium Type (Desmogenic)

Tendencies toward dishonesty lead to excessive thievery; at the opposite extreme tendencies are toward religious fantacism. If he drinks, he becomes an incurable alcoholic; as a smoker, he is likely to die of tobacco-related cancer; if inclined to drugs, he becomes an addict; if a study interests him, it consumes him, often producing genius.

Female Extremism

The sodium woman is also an extremist. If she objects to marriage, she enters a convent; if she is a religious reformer, she mercilessly persecutes "sinners." If she is happy, she is almost hysterical; if she likes men, nymphomania may result; if she is generous, she will give away all she owns. She may become insanely jealous of her husband, driving him to leave her. Her anger is uncontrollable; study consumes her completely; as a fighter, she is deadly; as a playmate, she is rowdy; she may fast for a month or more; she may take a whole bottle of vitamins or drugs at once; if antisocial, she becomes a hermit; if in love, she smothers her lover or becomes his slave with heart and soul. Hobbies may include birds, dogs, snakes, cats, chickens, rodents or love for the forest, herbs or black magic.

Where Sodium Types are Found

Americans are not often sodium types. The Desmogenic type is more often found in France, Austria, Arabia, Italy, Germany, Japan, Turkey, and among American Indians or Russian Cossacks.

The animal kingdom has its own sodium types in the panther, tiger, fox, wildcat, zebra—all of which are fleet, restless, responsive, keenly instinctive. The plodding, bony ox would be more like the calcium type in man.

The Sodium Type is a Difficult Patient

Sodium types are prone to accidents, injuries, fevers, indigestion, fractures, dislocations, sunstroke, pneumonia—due to intemperate living habits and exposure to extreme weather conditions such as rain, snow, heat, gales. The diseases contracted are difficult to remedy. Sodium intake is great in this type and sodium is needed in great quantities during illness, along with hills and mountains, forests, massage, horseback riding and a diet rich in alkaline elements.

> ## "The body metabolism and functions of the patient manifesting sodium and potassium excess are cyclical, as are his ailments."

Ailments of Sodium Excess

If an alkaline man imbibes excessive sodium through a diet high in alkaline elements, many ailments eventually manifest. The serous glands, synovial membranes, synovial fluid, mucus membranes, lacteals and secretory glands are adversely affected by too much sodium (from drug or food sources); the bloodstream may be affected because the activity of red corpuscles is hindered and the oxygen-carrying ability of hemoglobin partially nullified; anemic cachexia may result. In the fleshy or obese individual, fat metabolism is increased and nitrogen metabolism decreased to the point of developing anemia and alkaline obesity. Sugar metabolism may be increased until it creates a sugar craving. The body may become clogged and congested. Bile action may be decreased, secretion of pancreatic juice lowered, proteolytic power reduced. The system may become overalkaline, precipitating calcium phosphate until it is depleted in the body. Alkalinuria may develop due to exaggerated stimulation of the glycogenic center of the brain, resulting in an abnormal craving for sugar.

Consequences of Overalkalinity

Some types of patients have an overalkaline system under normal circumstances, as do those by whom excessive silicon is consumed. If such individuals continue to take in excessive quantities of high-alkaline foods—foods in which sodium phosphate, sodium carbonate, potassium, magnesium and silicon predominate—the ultimate result is alkaline cachexia or alkaline diseases.

Overalkalinity is a Rare Occurrence

The likelihood of a diet too alkaline is much less common than a diet too acidic. In addition, the average person produces many acids through daily living and thinking. Few patients have a constitution so alkaline that excessive alkalinity is a problem. Acidity complications are much more difficult to correct than are those arising from overalkalinity.

SIGNS OF SODIUM DEFICIENCY

Mental Symptoms of Sodium Deficiency

Hot, arid climates increase sodium requirements and often contribute to sodium deficiency. The mental symptoms of sodium deficit are decisive and pronounced: a patient suffering from sodium hunger becomes melancholy, depressed, quarrelsome, provocative. His nervous system is inflamed and overheated; his memory is faulty, thinking difficult, recall incomplete. He is apathetic, dull, unintelligent, disinterested, averse to study, to speaking and to society; his nerve control is

334

poor and judgment undependable. Darkness brings apprehension, particularly to the female patient, though she admits her fears have no logical basis; she is critical, antisocial, sorrowful, sleepy, restless, slow to comprehend, particular; she complains of weakness, a weighty feeling, drowsiness following a meal; she bursts into tears with the slightest provocation; her mind and passions are dark and negative. The sodium-impoverished man finds it nearly impossible to master intellectual subjects; his mind is forgetful; reasoning, debates and reading are difficult for him; public speaking, teaching, lecturing are taxing; he stutters; he is overtaken by sensations of dizziness, apathy, animosity, sadness, melancholy; he declines social invitations, exercise and pleasurable pursuits; wife, home, vocation, friends seem unimportant. Crying babies or children, arguments of others, traffic noises, household noises (diswashers, vacuum cleaners, mixers, etc.) disturb his nerves and brain centers.

Strange Dreams of Sodium-Deficient Patient

In times of sodium hunger, dreams are unsettling, strange, even fear-inspiring, as in dreams of war, violence, beasts, pits of snakes, storms, floods, death, destruction, corpses. However, if great misfortunes actually strike the world or the individual, they matter little to him.

Sodium deficiency manifests in sleeplessness between the hours of one and five a.m. At this time, the brain is very active; because brain and nerve force are thus wasted during the early morning hours, the individual is tired, depressed and irritable upon arising. Insomnia is the result of scattered squandered brain and nerve force.

"The likelihood of a diet too alkaline is much less common than a diet too acidic."

Unfavorable Mental States of Sodium Patient

Mental states resulting from sodium deficiency include anxiety, fears, malancholy, restlessness, craving for something unidentifiable (as in expectant mothers who are using large amounts of sodium salts for the baby). When sodium, particularly sodium carbonate, is deficient, thinking becomes difficult; there may be mental stupidity, poor concentration, inability to comprehend fully, difficulty hearing, aversion to society, vague fears, dislike of people, sorrow, hypersensitivity, irascibility, temper flare-ups, greedy tendencies, vindictive inclinations, depression, fatigue, unsteadiness, a dull feeling in the forehead, restlessness, inability to relax due to anxiety. Fatigue spells force the individual to rest at intervals; though he prefers physical activity, he needs to allow his brain to recuperate.

Depression, A Sign of Sodium Deficiency

Sodium poverty contributes to severe mental despondency, nervous irritation, hysterical outbursts, headache, dizzy spells, defective eyesight, insomnia, melancholia (a feeling of personal demerit, dejection); psychological and physiological exhaustion. The nervous system and brain are agitated, irritated; the individual is occasionally tense with intervening periods of cerebral atonia or uneasiness, depression, gloominess, provocation. The patient thinks himself worthless to himself and to the world. He may fantasize about imaginary maladies and fear he has incurable afflictions. Valor, objectives, determination, faith in self and others disappear. He complains of feebleness, listlessness, tiredness, laxity of nerves, tendons and brain. The female patient says she feels helpless, dejected and childish. Internal organs feel flabby, out of position or loose. Exertion seems futile, life meaningless, the smallest effort too great. The female patient sinks to hopelessness and becomes a hypochondriac. Although lack of sodium is not directly responsible for such afflictions as hysteria, neurotic tendencies, chlorosis, melancholia and depression, lack of it does contribute to these psychological states and a high-sodium diet may be of benefit.

Sodium Aids Peristaltic Action

Sodium and sulphur foods have a great influence over the intestinal tract and its related glands; they are able to increase the peristaltic action of the bowel. Also subject to the influence of these two elements are the liver, pancreas, skin, sexual system, nerves, brain and cerebellar function, nerve temperature, nerve well-being and vitality.

Sodium is Needed for Good Digestion

Organic sodium carbonate enhances digestion and stimulates activity of the stomach walls. Oxygen in the blood and carbon gases found in the body are benfitted by it; with it, decomposed protein by-products are more effeciently eliminated. The vital, chemical and sexual functions are improved.

Sodium Needed by Those Who Live in Hot, Dry Climates

Sodium is precipitated at an alarming rate during hot summer weather, in dry climates and in harsh sunlight; consequently, nerve heat and inclination to heat stroke and nervous prostration are likely. Residents of torrid, dry climates and those who work in intense heat and sunlight should include high-sodium foods in their diets.

Sodium Helps Prevent Emaciation

If sodium is deficient, digestion is disturbed, gas is generated in the intestinal tract, the liver becomes fevered and sluggish and bile secretion is sluggish. Hot gases may be produced by the liver, having an unfavorable power over peristaltic action. Meat decomposition in the stomach results in gas generation; the same is true of decomposition of starches, sweets, proteins and sulphur foods. The eyes develop blue rings; complexion becomes muddy or claylike; the slim patient becomes emaciated, wrinkled, aged-looking; the stout patient becomes obese and ill.

"Organic sodium carbonate enhances digestion and stimulates activity of the stomach walls."

Dangers of An Acid-Producing Diet

A diet made up of cabbage (sulphur), polished rice, white bread, biscuits, coffee, tea, chocolate, hard-boiled eggs, fried eggs and other refined and processed foods results in acid production, gas formation, fermentation and decomposition in the digestive tract. Food sodium must be liberally supplied or serious ailments develop: pus sacs form all through the body; teeth decay; the liver enlarges; the spleen is adversely affected; mucus membranes become congested with catarrh; skin is feverish and dry; menses are late; circulation is sluggish during the night; head congestion results in excruciating morning headache; the face turns crimson, becomes hot and dry or earthy; the countenance is apprehensive; facial skin shrinks and wrinkles; great thirst results from a heated stomach. The patient cares nothing for solid food. Gums soften and pyorrhea and inflammations set in; breath is offensive; pus may form at the roots of teeth; stomach walls generate catarrh; saliva secretion is reduced to almost nothing and has the unpleasant taste of blood. A diet high in sodium, potassium, chlorine and silicon is called for.

"Food sodium must be liberally supplied or serious ailments develop...."

Pains Due to Sodium Deficiency

Pain may develop in the small of the back, along with trembling, nerve fever, headache, extreme thirst, lip blisters, chills, debility, indigestion, poor appetite, sluggish colon, ballooned bowel, bilious tendencies, poor vision, pimples, eczema, falling hair, scorching or pounding headache. Digestion is poor and emaciation increases in spite of food intake. Numerous ailments manifest as the condition worsens, including neuritis in the arms, pain in sides, enlarged heart, cardiac complications, rheumatism, throat afflictions of a rheumatic nature, deafness, muscular rheumatism, dizziness, stiff and painful tendons, gout and sciatica due to acidity.

Lack of Sodium in Children

A child who lacks sodium is prone to flu, croup, throat disorders, diphtheria, black diphtheria, spinal meningitis; the latter produces pain and inflammation in the base of the brain, lower backhead and near the ears. The liver is tender or enlarged, causing pressure against nerves and nerve nets around it and making the outside of the body near the liver very sensitive. Sleeping on the left side or on the back may be uncomfortable. This child is susceptible to germs, gases, acids and ferments produced in the body.

Nerve Problems of Sodium Deficiency

Further sodium-deficiency problems include stupidity, weak eyesight, paralytic complications,

convulsions or twitch in nerves or muscles and undermining of nervous system and brain activities. Liberal sodium chloride in the diet improves these conditions, as well as bowel elimination.

Potassium Requires Liberal Sodium and Chlorine

A person eating foods high in potassium must also have plenty of sodium and chlorine in the diet. As livestock grazing during summer months need rock salt because they get such a high percentage of potassium in grass, a man with a diet high in potassium demands large quantities of sodium and chlorine; this is because every ounce of potassium excreted from the body precipitates 50 to 60 ounces of sodium.

Prolapsus Due to Sodium Shortage

In times of sodium poverty, internal organs are prolapsed and feel loose or displaced. Headaches may bore through the brain; abdominal muscles become sore; the tongue turns white and yellow, moist or dry and rough. Strength, power, vim, ambition and nerve force are abnormally lowered.

"A person eating foods high in potassium must also have plenty of sodium and chlorine in the diet."

A Hypothetical Case of Sodium Deficiency

Consider the typical hypothetical case of sodium starvation in a female patient. Let us say her diet consists chiefly of ice cream, coffee, tannic acid tea, white bread, cooked vegetables, puddings, pies, fried foods, pancakes, biscuits, fried eggs, bacon, doughnuts, chocolate, catsup, beef full of hormones, sausage, greasy soups, canned foods filled with preservatives and chemical additives, pickles, white sugar foods, condiments, sauces, pastry—all devitalized, demineralized, devitaminized and processed "dead" foods. Our case is a secretary, who sits all day at a desk, typing in a dark, stuffy, depressing office. Her complexion fades, her eyes become fatigued and dull, her energy drags; she experiences nervousness, weakness and pain throughout her body; depression, dyspepsia, catarrh, shaking and extreme exhaustion eventually develop; life becomes meaningless and death is longed for to end her misery. Eventually emaciation, anemia, exhaustion, poor sight and hearing, obsessive fears and phobias will take possession of her. Her memory fades until her work can no longer be performed satisfactorily. Then begins her "doctor shopping," attempting to find a solution to her multitude of problems—all because of sodium lacking in the diet, along with oxygen deficiency, poor and anemic blood, lack of tissue salts. With the proper diet and biochemical elements supplied, this woman could have accomplished many great things instead of feeling herself to be a failure.

Headaches Due to Sodium Hunger

Lack of sodium salts in the body causes restless nerves, pain in the eyeballs, pain in lower backhead or tophead with throbbing sensations. Throbbing may be felt in the abdominal area as well. Dryness, localized heat, head inflammation or fever and inflammation elsewhere in the body while extremities are chilled, distorted body heat and thermal control—all result from low sodium salts.

Hot Climates Precipitate Sodium

Laborers in hot sun and arid climates lose body oils, tissue salts and fluids rapidly, resulting in brittle bones, hardened and stiff joints and ligaments, dry and wrinkled skin, due to depletion of sodium salts. Resulting tendencies include meanness, irascibility, vindictiveness and a generally hard-to-please attitude.

Stiffness of Joints, Tendons and Fibrous Tissue

Blood consistency is influenced by sodium. Blood and nerves suffer if sodium is short in the body; the energy level is low; eyesight declines and glasses may be required. Eye muscles and the optic nerves do not have proper elasticity; glasses offer only temporary solutions. Cold dampness is very hard on the body, as moisture and wind rob heat from the body with resulting sore, quivering, stiff joints, nerves, tendons and muscles. Eyelids twitch, sting and become weakened because the vital energy of the eyes is lacking. Sodium shortage causes stabbing pains and disrupts generation of nerve force throughout the body. Chiropractic and osteopathic treatments are needed because joints stiffen, tendons draw up, fibrous tissue stiffens and nerves are under pressure or stress but lack tone.

Catarrh Prevalent in Respiratory System

Catarrh is generated in many parts of the body when sodium is lacking, particularly in nasal membranes, nose, throat, bronchial tubes, mucus and serous membranes, lungs. Aches develop in the base of the nose, malar bones, muscles, throat, nasal passages and in many other parts of the body. The blood cannot maintain its proper alkaline balance when sodium, a highly alkaline element is deficient.

Gas Pressure Symptoms

Production of gas and pressure facilitate colic attacks, gas centralization, ballooning of certain parts of the bowel, flatulence, constipation and poor peristaltic action. Gas pressure may be experienced on the kidneys, other organs, nerves or stomach plexus, causing pain convulsions. Often heart disease, uterine complications, kidney disease are suspected and are the incorrect diagnosis when there is such pressure from gas. The reproductive organs are highly sensitive and sore when sodium is needed. Food causes unpleasant fullness in the stomach, gas generation and heat. Digestion is disrupted and cold water is needed for relief. Food digests improperly and ferments, causing belching, burping, gas symptoms, even nausea or vomiting after a meal. The appetite vanishes. The smallest meals produce discomfort; the stomach may contract excessively, causing poor digestion and a weighty, nervous feeling in the stomach.

Abnormal Pulmonary Function

The lungs and breathing patterns are often abnormally altered when sodium is depleted, causing asthma, chest tightness, sneezing and the common cold. Such a patient is predisposed to diphtheria, throat catarrh, croup, even pneumonia, as lack of sodium prevents proper expelling of carbonic acid and fatigue end-products. The pulse rate may become erratic and the bloodstream inconsistent in flow and volume because oxygen is deficient.

Nerve Ailments and Acid Generation

Acid generation results from sodium shortage, which is harmful to nerves and results in acid neuritis, nerve aches and debility. The body from hips downward feels fatigued; nerves are painful; colds develop easily; muscles are sore and stiff; the

337

blood circulates slowly; behavior is malevolent; mind and nerves are restless; nostrils are ticklish; there is an aversion to bright sunlight, din or commotion. Further symptoms indicating a need for sodium include puffy eyelids, stinging face, freckled skin, toothache, extreme sensitivity and soreness in periosteum and bones, bloodless complexion, salty taste in mouth, parched tongue, mouth blisters, coughing and dry throat in the morning, thirst following a meal.

An Array of Symptoms

The sodium patient rests less at night because his body manifests more aches and pains at that time, yet much sleep is needed for the brain and nervous system. The first part of the night is more restful than early morning after two o'clock. The patient's breathing apparatus is irritated by smog, dust, smoke and other particles foreign to clean air. His vision seems clouded and he wipes his eyes often to try to clear it. His skin may develop a gluey dampness which then disappears. His arteries stiffen; blood circulates poorly and its quantity is subnormal; the spleen is sluggish, feverish or inflamed at times; secretions are scanty and poor in quality; muscular power is reduced; feet and hands are chilled, damp and clammy or feet may be chilled and hands hot, or hands and feet may be chilled while face is flushed and feverish. Muscles of the neck are stiff; ribs are painful; arms and lower legs may have convulsions or become stiff or useless.

Heart Disturbances and Falling Hair

This patient may be diagnosed as having gout as a result of gourmet dining, but he is actually suffering from sodium hunger and deficiency of other tissue salts. His legs and feet are numb, stiff and weighty. Tendons of the popliteal spaces become drawn and stiff; calves of legs cramp; sides of feet sting unless bathed in cold water; ankles swell; traveling pains shoot rapidly here and there; itching in ears and perineal areas is bothersome. Gout symptoms are intensified by cold dampness, chilling winds which affect stiff, drawn tendons. Massage has a momentary benefit but pains soon return when sodium, magnesium, potassiuim chloride and silicon are still deficient. Heart disturbance may be noted; emaciation sets in; dyspepsia with flatulence develops; gouty pains are worse during the night. Skin is sore, hair falls, the scalp is sensitive, catarrh invades the throat,

albumin is found in the urine, digestion is poor, nitrogen metabolism becomes defective, kidney disturbances arise, and the life force is lowered. Even bones of the cheeks may become tender; muscles bruise easily; the breath is offensive. Blisters, vesicles, tiny ulcers, hives, herpes, bloody saliva, appendicitis, gastritis, tonsillitis, dental caries and miscellaneous other disorders manifest. The constitution has low recuperative ability.

Symptoms in Female Patients

A female sodium-deficient patient suffers from the above problems, with added complications in the female organs and sexual system. She often craves unusual or artificial foods; cooked sulphur foods are eaten with resulting gas formation; fatty foods cause heartburn; sugary foods, starches and meats magnify complaints. The epigastrium is sore and internal organs below it may be hard. Peristaltic action is poor; hemorrhoids develop; urination becomes painful or difficult; urinary tubes constrict due to sodium chloride shortage.

Classic Symptoms Recognizable by Doctors or Nutritionists

The doctor or nutritionist should watch for classic symptoms of sodium deficiency, which are numerous: weak voice, hoarseness, joint stiffness, tender cervical glands, insufficient bile secretion, stiff and sore hip and shoulder joints, crippled lower legs, shortened step. Former minor movements of fingers become difficult or clumsy because joints, motor nerves, tendons are stiff and unreactive. Raising of arms may produce pain or numbness; riding in cars or trains is unpleasant to nerves and the body in general, particularly in the female patient.

"Beauty and charm are possible through the proper balance of sodium, iron, potassium, silicon and chlorine in the body."

Reduced Muscular Function in Males

A male sodium-deficient patient loses athletic skill, muscular efficiency and work ability; motor apparatus is less responsive than previously. Lower legs may give off a gummy substance. Arms feel like lead; feet fall asleep easily; bone joints crack because snyovial fluid and sodium are lacking. Sodium shortage in a boy causes chorea, deficient blood, mild rheumatism, but not gout.

Female Charms Vanish

A woman patient is likely to submit to surgery. She has much suffering and misery, may become hysterial and consequently makes a poor marriage partner. Feminine charms vanish, as do other pleasant qualities of a good wife; she becomes a stranger to her husband.

Elements Promoting Beauty and Charm

Beauty and charm are possible through the proper balance of sodium, iron, potassium, silicon and chlorine in the body. Lack of sodium causes a pale, muddy, ashen complexion with no color. Lack of sodium in women may cause crying spells, morning irritability, bad temper in stuffy, sultry weather; warm rooms cause her to gasp for air and rush to open windows. Tenderness and pain manifest in regions of the spine, neck and other places; hands and fingers may become numb and painful by turns.

Further Symptoms of Sodium Deficiency

In case of a low or nonexistent sodium reserve, appetite becomes whimsical. Tympanitis, quarrelsomeness, digestive tract catarrh, wasting disease, parasitic inflammation of the mouth (thrush), chronic salivation, mouth ulcers and catarrh of mouth, nose, throat, intestines, stomach, bladder, uterus, membranous surfaces develop. Scorbutic complaints, diseased mucus membranes, skin complications, hiccough, morning sickness, belching, nausea, flatulence, flushes, uterine trouble and many bacterial problems of skin or the digestive tract may manifest. Deficient blood, due to lack of sodium, may facilitate pubic itching, vaginal abrasion, vulvar eczema, tender nipples, spells of hysteia, suppuration, chronic rheumatism, production of phlegm, acidity of the urinary apparatus. Symptoms of tuberculosis are prevented by a good reserve of sodium in the body, by building immunity, natural defenses and vital energy.

Bacterial Growth Becomes Profuse

Gastric fever, acid production, gout, cholera infantum, germ propagation, toxin formation and chronic disorders difficult to reverse and correct may result from sodium starvation. Oxygen deficiency and resultant anemia and shortness of breath, even asthma, may develop when sodium is lacking because toxins are allowed to form; they attack the hemoglobin- and oxygen-carrying ability of red corpuscles. There may be menstrual disruption, faulty bile secretion, deficient gastric secretion and resultant indigestion and bowel sluggishness. Stone formation, hardening, ossification, calcium deposits, chronic rheumatism, poor hearing, faulty vision and other "old age" afflictions may arise. Germ and bacterial growth is so profuse that the intestinal tract is overwhelmed by harmful agents which destroy the ratio of "friendly bacteria" in the colon. (The colon should have 85% "friendly" bacteria.)

From Mild Itching to Severe Brain Disease

Itching, sore corns, tendon tension, painful elbow tendons, dysmenorrhea, rheumatism in shoulders and arms, cramping calves and feet, spleen inflammation, sore and enlarged liver, inability to retain urine, difficult urination, itching rectum, headache directly above the eyes are further symptoms. If the sodium reserve is utterly exhausted, the ailments are chronic; sodium hunger results simply in a milder form of symptoms. Germ life, toxins, bacteria, parasitic life are allowed to flourish in the body when sodium is lacking and, as a result, many chronic diseases are given an opportunity to undermine the constitution. The blood, heart, kidneys, body tissues, even the brain, may become diseased.

Symptoms Vary Greatly

Many symptoms of sodium hunger or starvation are evident to the trained doctor, nutritionist or nurse. Sodium is called for in delayed digestion; in vomiting of infants; when gout or rheumatism are troublesome; when there is frontal headache, vertex stiffness; bloating, poor vision and when reading small print is a problem; in times of mental confusion and uncertainty; when the sense of smell is faulty; when the nose is congested with catarrh; when dampness causes discomfort or the patient is susceptible to drafts; when symptoms are pronounced on some days and nonexistent on others; when skin eruptions are plentiful; when complexion is mottled and muddy; when drowsiness is a problem during the day; when warm rooms cause the feeling of a weight on the head; when there are heart troubles; when the saliva tastes salty; when joints make cracking sounds; when spots appear on palms of hands or on skin; when face is fevered, tongue parched, skin dry and feet icy; when tendons are drawn and stiff; when the body feels bruised for no apparent reason; when tendons feel shrunken and cramped; when the stomach produces uncomfortable gas; when icy drinks cause aches; when abdominal organs feel hardened and the stomach feels as tight as a drum; when the skin crawls; when urine odor changes and its specific gravity is altered; when women have menstrual troubles; when insufficient saliva is secreted; when hydrochloric acid is deficient and stomach ulcers develop; when the patient is depressed following meals or icy drinks; when digestion of starches, sugars, fats and meats is delayed and poor; when sulphur foods cause gas; when the stomach burns and develops ulcers; when young girls are irritable and prone to tantrums for no obvious reason; when the tongue becomes coated; when depression is excessive; when a child has a fickle appetite; when a

patient is bothered by morning sickness, agitated nerves, flabby muscles or fatigue. When any part or combination of these symptoms manifests, a high-sodium diet is indicated.

Sodium for Diabetics

In cases of diabetes or diabetic coma, sodium is indicated in heavy supplementation, in conjunction with other important alkaline food elements. Such vegetables as celery, okra or greens such as watercress are valuable sources of sodium when it is crucial to the health of the patient.

Treatment of Sodium Deficiency

When plenty of sodium is available in the diet, results are favorable. Memory, long life, social enjoyment, accomplishments, youth are enhanced; pain is minimal; health is generally excellent. Sodium and other alkaline salts are invaluable to health.

It is important to know what the symptoms of sodium deficiency are and what foods and tonics benefit the patient suffering from such symptoms. A list of high-sodium foods and sodium menus follows.

Although many whey drinkers seem to have enjoyed the beverage, whey was drunk more for its reputed therapeutic benefit than for its taste. Holsinger found that the earliest mention of whey was in the 5th century, B.C., when Hippocrates, the Greek physician, prescribed it for an assortment of human ills. Physicians continued to prescribe whey through the centuries. "There are few fluids more salutary, and better adapted to prevent and cure the diseases of the human body than whey," wrote Dr. Frederick Hoffman, physician to the King of Prussia, in 1761. In the mid-19th century, there were over 400 whey houses in Western Europe which offered something called a whey cure. During a cure, the ingestion of up to 1,500 grams (52.2 ounces) of whey per day was prescribed for ailments ranging from arthritis to liver complaints. At Ischl, a famous Austrian spa, the whey cure took the form of a whey bath, which was claimed not only to calm the nerves but to soften the skin. It was particularly popular with women. As late as the 1940s, some European spas were still offering a whey cure.

HIGHEST SODIUM FOODS

Veal joint broth and powdered whey (cow's milk or goat milk) are highly-concentrated sources of sodium. Goat milk or whey and black mission figs are a superior sodium combination (and this is also a champion arthritis remedy). High sodium foods include:

Apples	Kale
Apricots, dried	Kelp
Asparagus	Lentils
Barley	Milk, raw
Beets and greens	Mustard greens
Cabbage, red	Okra
Carrots	Olives, black
Celery	Parsley
Cheeses	Peas, dried
Chickpeas, dried	Peppers, hot red, dried
Coconut	Prunes
Collard greens	Raisins
Dandelion greens	Sesame seeds
Dates	Spinach, New Zealand
Dulse	Strawberries
Egg yolks	Sunflower seeds
Figs	Swiss chard
Fish	Turnips
Goat milk	Veal joint broth
Horseradish	Whey
Irish moss	

Fair sources of sodium include other cabbage, water chestnuts, garlic, peaches (dried), radishes, broccoli, brussels sprouts and cashews.

SODIUM MENUS

Broiled whitefish, steamed beet greens, steamed carrots; leafy green salad made with celery, okra, black olives, shredded carrots and beets, parsley, radishes; roquefort dressing; glass of half carrot juice and half raw goat milk.

Spinach omelette, Spanish-style sauce, steamed okra, steamed turnips; leafy green salad made with dandelion greens, parsley, watercress, shredded beets, carrots, turnips, black olives, radishes; egg yolk, tomato and garlic dressing; celery stuffed with sunflower or sesame seed butter; veal joint broth.

Split pea soup, steamed brown rice, steamed brussels sprouts, steamed Swiss chard, cole slaw with pineapple, celery stuffed with cashew butter, leafy green salad, black olives, whey drink.

Raw cottage cheese (goat milk cottage cheese preferred); steamed rye cereal topped with revived raisins, figs, prunes (chopped); plain angel-food cake with nut butter (sweetened with grape concentrate); goat milk.

SUMMARY OF SODIUM

GENERAL CHARACTERISTICS

"Youth" element   Found in most waters and soils
Alkaline   Sodium type = Desmogenic type
Oxidizes rapidly

SODIUM IN THE HUMAN BODY

Active in the body fluids, organs, connective tissues
Contributes to alkalinity of lymph, blood
Promotes excretion of carbon dioxide
Essential to liver, pancreas, spleen
Stored in stomach wall, joints
Helps prevent blood clotting
Increases osmosis
Counteracts acidity

SIGNS OF SODIUM EXCESS *(Characteristics of Desmogenic Type)*

Keen reflexes

Always in hurry

Accident proneness

Overalkalinity (very rare)

Cyclical ailments

Tendency toward extremism

SIGNS OF SODIUM DEFICIENCY

Calcic gout

Catarrh

Bloating, flatus

Poor eyesight

Murky complexion

Dry skin, tongue

Cracking joints

Stiff tendons

Difficulty digesting sweets, starches, fats

Restless nerves

Delayed digestion

Daytime drowsiness

Lack of saliva

Lax muscles

Mental confusion

Frontal headache

White, coated tongue

Fatigue

Sensitivity to drafts

Offensive breath

HIGHEST SODIUM FOODS

Veal joint broth

Powdered whey

Goat milk

Black mission figs

If it wasn't for the neutralizing power of sodium in the walls of the stomach and bowel, they would be eaten away by the powerful acids, enzymes and digestive juices secreted as foods are eaten. Sodium keeps calcium in solution in the blood, keeps joints and ligaments supple and feeds the friendly bacteria in the bowel. Sodium in the blood helps regulate the fluid balance in the body, and the nerves use sodium and potassium to relay electrical nerve impulses.

Our bodies can't use the sodium from inorganic table salt or other similar inorganic sources such as sodium bicarbonate. Instead, we must have the sodium from foods such as whey, celery, okra, cabbage and so on.

Whex, a dried goat whey, is the most concentrated source of organic sodium.

343

sixteen

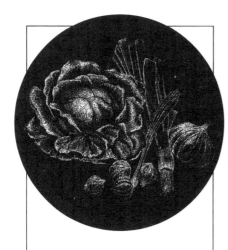

Sulphur charges the cerebellum with blood and increases blood tension.

Psoriasis can be a sulphur hunger symptom.

Except for scabies, sulphur in the diet helps correct skin diseases.

Dark rings around the eyes may indicate sulphur deficiency.

Foods containing sulphur combined with foods high in magnesium and phosphorus are important to the nervous system.

Redheads get the color of their hair from sulphur, and their familiar temperaments are largely a result of the sulplhur in their body chemistry.

Sulphur, the "heating" element

Sulphur, the "heating element," is a volatile agent that drives impurities to the surface of the skin and produces heat within the body. Along with phosphorus and manganese, sulphur is a brain and nerve element. One of the cardinal rules I recall from my studies with Dr. Rocine is that when a person eats brain and nerve foods, in order to drive their nutrition to the brain cells a sulphur vegetable should be added to the meal. Having onions, cauliflower, broccoli, brussels sprouts or any other sulphur vegetables, along with lecithin foods, makes a good brain and nerve combination. Sulphur also forces lecithin to the brain and nervous system.

Sulphur vegetables are known as winter vegetables, because they can withstand the cold, bitter weather. Sulphur creates this stamina. However, many of these sulphur vegetables in the raw state can cause excessive gas in some people as can some of them when cooked. This problem can be avoided if the vegetables are prepared by steaming at low heat instead of boiled in water. Steaming preserves the balance nature intended, causing less flatulence.

The sulphur type of individual (the Exesthesic) holds a good deal of sulphur in the body. This impetuous element can create an explosive temper and fiery, eruptive emotions. It makes this type excitable, over-anxious and apprehensive; disappointments are more severe and more outwardly expressed. In short, emotions tend to be more volatile and dramatic. Sulphur contributes to a flushed face from blood rising to the surface and to a racing blood and hotheaded temper. There is much sulphur in the redhaired person and in many blonds, perhaps accounting for the origin of the slogan, "Blonds have more fun."

The "It" Girl—A Classic Sulphur Case

In the 1930s, one of the most popular movie stars in the United States was Clara Bow, called the "It" girl. A sulphur "volcano," always ready to explode, it seemed this beautiful, talented young woman was cast in films as a sultry seductress, who lived in the fast lane of life— singing, dancing and partying all the time. Off the screen, her life seemed very much like it was on screen—fast and exciting.

For several years, she lived on her nerve supply, burning the candle at both ends and getting very little sleep. At the age of 30, she burned out, using up the last of the chemical reserves that supplied energy to her mind and body. Years later, I found out that she had never encountered anyone who could tell her what chemical elements she needed for repair and rejuvenation.

Clara Bow spent the rest of her life trying to regain her health. She married a very physical man who owned a ranch in Nevada. But, with all the nice things she had, she could only regain her health back in part.

Countering Excess Sulphur

It is possible to counteract overconsumption of sulphur with magnesium and chlorine-rich foods. In balance, sulphur is the great expeller of impurities. It cleanses and heats the blood, and works best when taken with phosphorus or protein foods. Besides purification, it lends itself to versatility and adaptability. Sulphur hunger, or deficiency, indirectly affects the emotional side of the mind, producing irritability, tendency to hysterical outbursts and extreme impatience and touchiness.

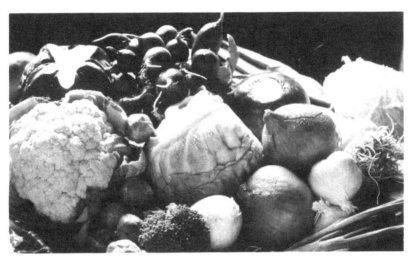

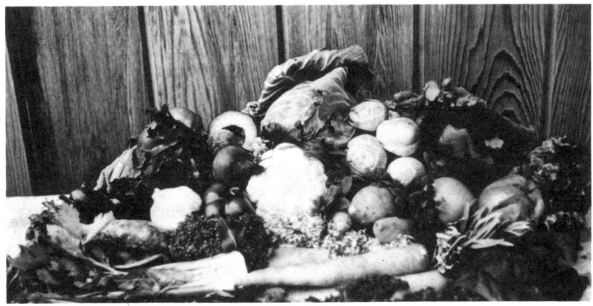

Sulphur vegetables. The brain and nerves need a certain amount of sulphur to function efficiently. Eggs are also high in sulphur.

SULPHUR
"The Heating Element"

GENERAL CHARACTERISTICS

Sulphur, known as the "heating element," is also called brimstone. It is described as a nonmetallic, smoky, combustible, acidic, volatile, restless element found in clay beds and with certain metals, as in sulphates and sulphides. Volcanos contain much sulphur. Sulphur forms compound with hydrogen, oxygen and chlorine and combines also with other elements. Its color is lemon yellow; it does not conduct electricity. Its atomic weight is 32; specific gravity is 1.99. It is not water soluble. It is tasteless but has an offensive odor when burned. The "heating element" is distinctive in that it is able to unite with all metals and most nonmetals, tends to form crystals and exists in many diversified forms.

Manufacturing and Medical Uses of Sulphur

In manufacturing, sulphur is used in gunpowder, in vulcanizing, in making metals and sulphuric acid. Sulphuric acid is formed by the oxidation of sulphur in air and moisture. In medicine, sulphur assumes many forms and is often used as a refrigerant.

Sulphuric Acid and Hydrogen Sulphide

Pure sulphuric acid is described as a dense, oily, acidic, corrosive liquid which disintegrates animal and vegetable materials when in the presence of heat. It combines with alkaline agents and separates most acids from alkaline counterparts. It has a great attraction for water; this union produces heat. Chemistry and medicine alike depend greatly upon sulphuric acid. Tissue damage—especially to mucus membranes—occurs through sulphur administration; the stomach and throat are burned and great thirst results. Alkalis are neutralized, water extracted and albumin precipitated by sulphur; collapse and suffocation can result. Blood alkalinity is destroyed and normal removal of carbonic acid hindered. In the event that sulphur is administered for prolonged periods of time, anemia and emaciation develop. Hydrogen sulphide, a poisonous gas, can be generated in the body by overconsumption of sulphur foods or sulphur drugs.

"Sulphuric acid is formed by the oxidation of sulphur in air and moisture."

The outcome is detrimental to body functions, especially to the red blood cells, as the gas destroys the oxygen-carrying ability of red corpuscles by disorganizing iron in the hemoglobin of the blood. If sulphur foods are overcooked, taken in indigestible form or overconsumed, hydrogen sulphide may be produced; the same may result from food decomposition.

346

Food Sulphur Preferable to Drug Sulphur

The drug form of sulphur (sulfa, sulphates and sulphides) may cause adverse reactions in some patients; but food-derived sulphur does not cause abnormal or unfavorable reactions. Drug sulphur is apt to be transformed by the alkaline secretions into certain sulphides which are expelled through the lungs, kidneys and skin, whereas the organic (food) sulphur is easily assimilated into the body.

Problems Due to Sulphured Fruits

Sulphuring of foods, especially of dried fruits, is commonplace. Such sulphur is cumulative in the human tissues and results eventually in autointoxication. Serious illnesses and even diseases may be due to sulphur-treated foods.

SULPHUR: ITS ROLE IN THE HUMAN BODY

A man weighing 160 pounds contains about 4 ounces of sulphur in his body. Sulphur's main food compounds are potassium sulphate and sodium sulphate. Free sulphur is used by the body hourly. Sodium sulphate enters the body in food form and is manufactured within the organism by decomposition and oxidation of proteins.

"Chemistry and medicine alike depend greatly upon sulphuric acid."

Keratin Contains Sulphur

Keratin, an agent found in all horny tissues such as nails, hair, feathers, epidermic layer of skin and cornea of the eye, contains a large percentage of sulphur. It is a combination of many complex proteins, but it differs from proteins because of the large amount of sulphur it contains.

Sulphur Influences the Liver and Other Organs

Sulphur is known to have important influence upon the liver, promoting bile secretions; it also affects the cerebellum as a mild hypnotic, aids in production of protoplasm, and affects the skin powerfully. Certain organic impurities are propelled to the surface of the skin because of sulphur's action upon internal organs. By nature, sulphur is volatile, revolutionary, explosive, compulsive, expulsive. It acts as a roaring internal holocaust, producing surface explosions and eruptions, heat and organic gases. Internal heat and metabolic gases are increased in liver nerves, sex brain and reproductive organs. When sulphur is liberally present in the body, sulphur heat and organic gases evaporate rapidly through the pores of the skin. This congests capillaries, veins, skin and nerve tissues. Pimples and skin eruptions are the results. The skin is warmed by sulphur; waves of heat pass over the skin increasing nerve function and adding a pink tint to the skin.

"In the event that sulphur is administered for prolonged periods of time, anemia and emaciation develop."

Sulphur Affects Every Cell

The activity of sulphur reaches each minute cell, enabling it to eliminate toxic substances through agitation. Each and every drop of blood, nerve fiber and cerebral neuron is affected. The action is a paradox of hypnosis and revolution; its action is slow, yet accumulative. It resembles a volcano, driving gases, toxins, germs to the surface for expulsion.

Sulphur Enhances Beauty

Like iron and fluorine, sulphur is a beauty ambassador and a youth promoter. A diet supplying the normal quantity of sulphur helps ensure youth and beauty.

Sulphur Affects the Hair

Sulphur enters the hair to the extent of about four percent. The hair color is a general indicator of the amount of sulphur present: the lighter or more blond the hair, the more likely sulphur is to be present; the amount of sulphur is reduced by degrees from golden to black hair. Individuals having curly hair are also apt to have more sulphur than do straight-haired people. Hair color and curliness are not, however, infallible barometers of sulphur content in the system. (It is also interesting to note that a thyroid gland pigment has an influence on hair color.) Red-haired and curly-haired people tend to possess sulphur-like hot tempers and to be somewhat fickle, changeable, hypersensitive, difficult to please; their moods of anger and congeniality run in close cycles. Sulphur consumption in these types is substantial. However, in some cases the hair robs most of the sulphur from the rest of the body, giving a false impression of sulphur consumption. In addition to the hair, sulphur enters other horny tissues, the skin, flesh, liver, fluids, and even perspiration. Sulphates are almost entirely eliminated through the kidneys.

"Serious illnesses and even diseases may be due to sulphur-treated foods."

Sulphur Regulates Nerves and Temperature

When a normal reserve of sulphur is present in the body, nerve impulses are properly regulated and normal nerve temperature is maintained; proper temperature is also ensured in sensorial brain centers, sexual nerves and plexuses, spinal reflexes, nerves of the liver and kidneys, vasomotor system, optic centers, heat centers, Meibomian glands and oily secretions such as perilymph, cerebrospinal fluid, endolymph, neurolin, gonoblastic fluid and so on. The sulphur balance within the body must be correct for neurological and psychological health. If sulphur consumption is high, the patient is probably versatile, emotional, adaptable, flexible, but not strong. Excessive sulphur in the body promotes cell diffusion, strength and tenacity of tissue, ability of the brain to carry on continued activity, toughness, wiriness, strength, durability of bone and muscles. nerve heat, tone of nerve impulsion, nerve tension, reflex response, impressionability, emotionality, idealism and romanticism are intensified.

Sulphur Necessary for Egg Production

As we have said, sulphur is essential to the function of each cell. It is necessary for developmental and neurological processes. It functions in the protection and construction of protoplasm in male and female reproductive functions—specifically in the egg yolk and the ovum. Life in the ovum or the egg yolk (fertile) is guaranteed when sulphur is in good supply; without sulphur, chickens could not be hatched nor babies born.

Sulphur Responsible for Link Between Soul and Matter

Sulphur is responsible for the sensations of soul communication with the physical world. It ensures thought and emotion through support of and channel of soul expression and nerve force. This element works with phosphorus, serving as a channel linking the soul and brain and soul and sensory-physical functions. Through the nerves and psychological faculties, sulphur links the soul with matter—the physical world; if sulphur were removed from the organism of man, the soul could no longer communicate with the world of matter. While phosphorus is the fuel for thinking, impulses and emotions, sulphur is the communicative, controlling and magnetic avenue for thought action, nerve impulses, soul intelligence, telepathy, sensorial transmission and emotive transferral. If sulphur is over or under supplied, disturbances are likely in thermal, psychological, isothermal, communicative and psychoconductive functions. Lack of sulphur has repercussions in physical and sensorial activities, life, nerve and soul functions.

"Sulphur is known to have important influence upon the liver, promoting bile secretions; it also affects the cerebellum as a mild hypnotic, aids in production of protoplasm and affects the skin powerfully."

The Sulphur Type (Exesthesic)

Sulphur excess produces a distinctive type of individual. Female sulphur types are characterized by ovoid head, oval faces; soft, warm, delicate rosy-red skin; elastic, wiry, wavy, thick, golden, flaxen or light-brown hair; soulful eyes of glittering, magnetic, intelligent, blue-gray or light hazel hue;

348

complexion color changes as often as the weather, like the sulphur element itself. This woman is emotional, intense, luxury-loving, versatile, electrical and magnetic in touch, imaginative, tall and beautifully proportioned, high-strung, eruptive in feelings, graceful in movement, stately beautiful, firm of joints, tidy and selective.

Sulphur Waters Not Recommended

Sulphur waters are not recommended for improving health. Consumption of much inorganic sulphur water can result in anemia, nervous disturbances, unfavorable habits and atrophy of vital organs. When sulphur is provided in suitable quantities, in food form, nerve communication, bile flow, emotional expression, hair growth and other vital body functions are favored. Drug sulphur, inorganic sulphur and sulphur mineral waters are not favorable to the human machine.

SIGNS OF SULPHUR EXCESS

Characteristics of Sulphur Type (Exesthesic)

A major characteristic of the sulphur-excess individual is a fitful condition of the nerves and mind. This condition affects mind, feelings, disposition, personality, encouraging moody, spasmodic outbursts of actions; these actions resemble the properties of the element sulphur. Responses range from happy to morbid and venomous to excited; life is at one time a rose garden and at another a pit of snakes. Individuals whine, rage, love, loathe, hope, despair; at one time they are optimistic, at other times pessimistic, determined, courageous, selfish, careless, enterprising, wishful, distrustful, self-condemning, ecstatic, cowardly, charitable, independent, dependent, miserly, liberal, serene, kindly, emotionally excited, hateful, congenial, cheerful, exclusive, selective, hostile, vindictive, forgiving, grudging, remorseful, uncertain, friendly and countless other contradictory characteristics. They belong on the stage; if they are not there, the world is their stage. They can change in the flash of an eye from loving and purring like a kitten to scratching like a wildcat.

Emotions Intensified

The movements and attributes—mental attitudes, physical activities, pain sensations, symptoms, proclivities, diseases—of the sulphur-excess patient are spasmodic, vigorous. Sense perceptions are enhanced, but intellect, motor impulses, will, cerebellar energy are not. Emotional response is intensified, as are nerve transport, nerve and brain catabolism, thermal sensitivity, sensitiveness to odor, gases, fumes found in the air.

Male Sulphur Patient Changeable

The masculine sulphur patient changes from amorous, loving, passionate and romantic to cold, indifferent, uninterested and depressed. After this phase, a total change occurs; the pattern is repeated again and again.

"The activity of sulphur reaches each minute cell, enabling it to eliminate toxic substances through agitation."

Patients Slow, Depressed in Morning

Morning brings sullenness and depression; warm, confining rooms create irritability and sluggishness; in the morning hours, body functions are torpid; a heavy morning meal causes indigestion and oppression all day. These patients do not come alive until about 11 a.m. or noon; prior to that time, they are irascible, cranky and difficult to please; their workday begins late but they work late.

Volatile Nature of Sulphur Type (Exesthesic)

Sulphur-excess individuals are capricious, sensitive, spasmodic, meticulous, finicky and, on occasion, volatile. At one moment they are angelic, at the next, demonic, angry, impulsive; characteristics change rapidly; personality and emotions are variable; they detest brain labor; they are fond of mountains, breezy air, motion, life, childlike fun, frosty air; idealistic moods alternate with frequent irritation; moods are chaotic; disposition is transformed rapidly from happy to sorrowful, from vivacious to lazy, from relaxation to agitation and temper flare-ups, from sprightliness of mind to listlessness; they are foul-tempered, peevish and resistant by turns and nerves are easily vaulted into a panic state. Irritation is displayed toward their marriage partners; in their heart and soul they mean no harm and expect others to overlook readily their outbursts of temper which only reflect their active emotions. Mental work is taxing; sensations of pain are like needles when walking or from a sudden jarring; blood rushes to the emotional centers in the brain and to the internal vital organs, producing coldness in extremities.

Results of Sulphur Overconsumption

If sulphur is consumed with indiscretion the results may include dry hair; glittering, shivering, unsteady pupils; expression of anxiety on the face with infrequent merriment; false pride with hypersensitivity to public opinion; fever and burning face; headache resulting from emotional stress. Another symptom is a ferric taste in the mouth; generation of hydrogen sulphide gas disintegrates iron in red corpuscles of blood; iron in hemoglobin of blood is transformed and ferric property causes the iron taste in mouth; red corpuscles are unable to transport enough oxygen for blood and tissue purposes. There may be a yellowish tongue with whitish coating in the center; hot and putrid breath; craving for high-sodium foods, chocolate, juicy food, tart drinks, sour, cooling, mucilagenous liquids or tonics, greens, strong tea, vegetables, beer (because it may soothe symptoms in suffocating weather), or vinegar which seems to soothe gastrointestinal colic due to gas pressure. Hunger spontaneously grows extreme and symptoms are magnified if patient does not eat; in a few hours symptoms are again agitated; rapid pains stab various parts of the body and brain; head develops splitting headache; diarrhea develops in torrid weather.

Complaints of Female Sulphur-Excess Patients

Women patients suffering from sulphur overuse develop such symptoms as love of electrical storms, fondness for cold wind blowing on face in bedroom; air is craved, especially in mountains where a cool breeze blows and oxygen is readily consumed; extreme cold is soothing; feverish sensations in various parts of the body occur along with cold feet and hands; occasionally soles of feet burn; menstrual cycle is erratic; all functions, sensations, nerves, symptoms, maladies, moods, tastes, etc., are fitful and convulsive. There may be poor memory; querulous behavior; occasional numbness and weakness in finger joints, fingers, eyelids, elbow joints, knees and ankles; tender knees; cold knees for long periods. She finds warm rooms suffocating.

Electrical Storms Calm Her Nerves

Reclining agitates her sensory nerves; sitting causes nerve tension and flatulence; conversation tires the brain, resulting in exhaustion and irritability; standing forces blood to the spleen, liver, heart, causing pain in these organs; arising in the morning is difficult because eyes do not want to open; rising is attended by headache; shaking impacts cause neuralgic pain; dizziness manifests from climbing; turning, rocking, dancing, vibration, sudden descents, rolling motions and watching moving objects facilitate dizziness. Any body pressure attacks weak spots, especially the ankles; worst pains manifest at sunrise; patient gains energy in evening, but tiredness is still bothersome. She enjoys unhampered movement in open air and breeze; watching billowing clouds, observing thunderbolts, staying outside in a rainstorm placates her nerves and emotions.

> "A diet supplying the normal quantity of sulphur helps ensure youth and beauty."

She is an Enigma

Nerves, mind, ganglia, thoughts, habits, moods, preferences, emotions, personality, temperament and wants are made capricious by excess sulphur. Spells of love and devotion alternate with indifference; wants, likes, dislikes, tastes, loves change often; tastes are spasmodic; everything about her is variable and chaotic; like sulphur she is eruptive, acid, eccentric, allotrophic, unstable, inconsistent; doctors are mystified by her; she is an enigma to friends and loved ones; childlike behavior ensues when she does not have her way, and then she returns to her former self again.

Inconsistency and Inconstancy

Nerve transmission, when influenced by sulphur in excess, is not consistent; dispersion is imbalanced; functions are chaotic; symptoms, afflictions, fevers are interrupted and then recur; at one point recovery seems accomplished and then there is a relapse into fevers for many days; disposition is inconstant; symptoms elude patient and doctor; diagnosis is a dilemma. Perspiration may take on the smell of sulphur; sulphur-carrying foods such as cabbage, cauliflower, horseradish, sprouts, turnips, radishes, onions, leave an aura of sulphur for days.

Excess Sulphur Harms Digestion and Blood

Excess sulphur attacks the cells, skin and sex function by disrupting digestion; damaging assimilation; generating hydrogen sulphide gas; undermining red corpuscles; engorging capillaries; developing unsightly pimples; turning skin red, crimson, pale yellow, muddy, then red and irritated, even rough like sandpaper.

"The sulphur balance within the body must be correct for neurological and psychological health."

Constrictive Complaints Are Common

Constrictive complaints are common to the sulphur-excess patient; so are psychosomatic pains, corrosive discharges, skin eruption due to engorged capillaries, bloating and unpleasant feelings resulting from sulphur gases and acids attacking the body. Sulphur exerts a volatile effect upon skin, skin capillaries, secretions, making them putrid, rank and excoriating, congesting dermal and subdermal structures and resulting in eczema, rose rash, psoriasis, face flushes, faintness and acne.

Identical Symptoms from Excess of Food or Drug Sulphur

Food or drug sulphur in excess have identical effects. Constricted nerves; stinging sensations; contracted throat and chest; congested veins; aching head; sensory nerve pressure; agglutinated tissues; congested organs; bloated stomach; stinging palms and soles of feet; congested portal system; torrid, acrid discharges; feverish skin; sulphuric eyelids; spasmodic symptoms; stringy, frothing mucus; convulsive symptoms and functional ailments; burning carbuncles or boils; changing body temperature; acid and toxic secretions; irregular appetite; choking; belching; hysterical spells; depressive pains; menstrual dysfunction—all indicate intemperate use of sulphur.

"A major characteristic of the sulphur-excess individual is a fitful condition of the nerves and mind."

Effect of Vaccinations on Sulphur Patient

It is interesting to note that the sulphur patient is immune to many diseases; vaccinations "take" only occasionally. In other individuals, fluorine and manganese may be broken down by inoculation and certain essential liver, blood and tissue salts destroyed, culminating in undermined resistive power, lowered oxidation, weakened vital functions, reduced bone metabolism. But these have a minimal effect upon the sulphur patient. This patient is not susceptible to tetanus, tissue disintegration, paranormal growths, vaccinosis, necrosis, gangrene, hydrophobia, blood poisoning or other maladies related to vaccine viruses which penetrate blood, fluids and tissues of the body.

Sulphur Excess Affects Many Functions

Superfluity of sulphur consumption disrupts assimilation, resulting in emaciation, temper fits, faint spells, night sweats of nervous origin, fever, itching and scratching. Other indications are dry and hard stool similar to burnt sulphur; temperature in nerves, liver, uterus, spleen, heart rises; emotional waves rip through nerves causing intense pain and burning sensations. Women become sullenly melancholy, hysterical, agitated; vibratory rate in some nerve and brain cells is magnified causing tension, pressure, compression; sulphur by-products and toxins in gas form are generated causing nerves to be adversely affected; oxidation is hampered; breathing, heartbeat, nutrition and digestion are undermined; discharges become acrid; lips turn brown; throat becomes foamy; liver becomes congested and agitated; nerve centers are enfeebled; there may be dizziness, sleepiness, muscular debililty, brain lethargy; expensive and agonizing operations may be indicated due to growth of fibroids in muscular tissues; blood clots develop; blood takes on darkness and congestion, especially in liver, cerebellum, uterus; hair roots become inflamed so that hair falls; heart is under stress; iron in blood is neutralized which damages oxidation; manganese and magnesium metabolism is disrupted and nerve impulses become convulsive.

"...sulphur patient is immune to many diseases; vaccinations 'take' only occasionally."

Patient Wants Cold Breeze on His Face at Night

A proper reserve of sulphur insures uniform temperature and regulates nerve impulses, but too much or too little sulphur upsets the functions of the body. Sulphur is an unsuccessful heat conductor for muscular electricity, but it intensifies nerve, brain and liver heat with resultant nervousness, peevishness, oppression, stasis in eliminative channels. After retiring to bed, the patient suffers discomfort due to insufficient oxygen in the room or overheated condition of the body so that body vapors and heat are imprisoned in the body; surface capillaries are engorged; pores close up; sulphur vapors are locked into the body so that internal liquids or solids are speedily transformed into gaseous form; heat production in nerves, brain and liver is multiplied. At night, the sulphur patient leaves feet uncovered because they are feverish; he wants a cold breeze blowing on his face; icy air, outdoor air, cold baths, frosty winter days are preferred because cold and wind touching the skin raises oxidation, promotes evaporation and radiation of sulphur gas through the skin pores. Icy water absorbs sulphuric acid and sulphur fumes more than warm water does; thus, cold water baths are favorable to sulphur patients. Other favorable agents are cold outdoor air, trips to the mountains, skin ventilation, cold showers. Because cold showers and chilling air increase skin ventilation, extremities must be protected. Massage, deep breathing exercises, body motion, skin ventilation dispel gases and reduce the temperature of nerves and skin, clear stuffiness, relieve throat contortions and general disturbances.

"A proper reserve of sulphur insures uniform temperature and regulates nerve impulses, but too much or too little sulphur upsets the functions of the body."

Autointoxication A Danger

Hydrogen sulphide generated by intemperate use of sulphur foods results in self-poisoning, autointoxication of the system which instigates blood complications and sulphur poisoning symptoms. Man is susceptible to poisonous hydrogen sulphide in the air, its symptoms including faintness, vertigo, convulsions, shaking, blood deoxidation due to its union with iron in the hemoglobin of red blood corpuscles; this nullifies the blood's power to carry oxygen.

Blood Problems of Sulphur Patients

Sulphur-indiscreet patients are hungry for oxygen, lacking in blood salts (hypoalonemia), lacking in blood (hypoemia), anemic since sulphur acid and gases reduce blood salts and cripple oxidation. A blood test, however, does not reveal the condition; the blood count may be normal, but the red corpuscles are unable to carry iron. Each of these patients is anoxymic to a mild degree. The overuse of sulphur foods, taking of drug sulphur and sulphuric acid poisoning have similar effects on the body; sulphur gas is destructive to brain cells and nerves and results in sleepiness, mental confusion, skin rashes, red urine possessing hematoporphyrin (a hematinic property from the red corpuscles). There may also be feebleness, meager albuminous urine, diarrhea, paresthesia, scirrhus, colic, degenerative liver changes, ataxia, degeneration of heart and kidneys; anemia or blood deoxidation, dark stools, brain autointoxication and nerve toxicity.

352

Harmful Effects of Excess Sulphur are Cumulative

The ill effects of sulphur are cumulative; toxic effects are retained in the body after sulphur itself is expelled. If the dietetic intake of sulphur is excessive, headache the next or third day may result. Eventually prolonged overuse of sulphur can cause body tremors, eructations, stomachaches, stinging of mucus membranes, strangury; dry, sluggish tension or hyperemic conditions of the cerebrum of the liver, uterus, spleen, cerebellum; burning coryza, swelling of throat and roof of mouth (palate), consuming hunger with gas production in the digestive tract, torrid flatus, crippled movement with heaviness and pressure, exhausted limbs, inclination to erotic habits due to excitement of sex brain and sexuality; hysterical, neurotic behavior. Other manifestations are suffocating sensations; chilled arms, hands, knees and feet with infrequent burning of soles of feet; disrupted lymph production; damaged blood; congested organs; tumors; boils, painful pustles, skin breaks on forehead; pustules on top of head; eruptions on neck, on genitals or under armpits.

Sulphur Reaches Man's Deepest Parts

Manifestations and symptoms of sulphur overuse may be modified, but they are similar whether the problem is caused by excessive sulphur foods, sulphur medications, sulphur poisons and gases, tissue disintegration or autointoxication from sulphur. Sulphur reaches the deepest part of man—the vital life force of each cell and the magnetic force of life—creating havoc in blood, blood salts and the oxygen function.

SIGNS OF SULPHUR DEFICIENCY

Deficiency Symptoms Resemble Excess Symptoms

In times when sulphur is deficient, the effects are noted in the emotional nature, possibly indirectly. Sulphur-deficiency symptoms resemble those of sulphur excess.

Sulphur Poverty Causes Irritability

Sulphur poverty produces emotional irritability, love of change and diversity, inclination to hysterical scenes, volatile eruptions of emotions, accompanied by inordinate impatience and hypersensitivity. The personality is altered; finger muscles become spasmodic; there is craving for chololate, sweets, ginger ale, even beer; nerve impulse transport is agitated; nerve pressure increases causing difficulties with blood vessels. There may be dizziness; aversion to talking and reasoning for extensive periods of time; throat weakness; craving for vigorous pressure or massage; disinclination for gentle massage and light touches; difficulty in swallowing. Enterprising spirit may lack strength and courage against adversity; pulse is brief and quick; there is a tendency to sleep late in morning and stay up late at night.

"The ill effects of sulphur are cumulative; toxic effects are retained in the body after sulphur itself is expelled."

Female Patient Has Marital Troubles

The female sulphur-deficient patient usually meets trouble with her spouse due to her temper, ill humor, impulsiveness, rashness, contempt, peevishness, querulous nature—unless her husband is extremely forgiving, easy-going, tolerant and loving. Insignificant things worry her excessively; she is hypersensitive about everything; she lacks appetite in the morning and is unable to digest food at that time; some days bring energetic well-being and others, indisposition; ankles are feeble and knees usually chilled; skin is soft and flawless; skin color changes several times a day; temperature changes are impressive; atmospheric gases and fumes are irritating. Contraction, pressure, aches and tension plague her; epigastric region is tender; alimentary tract is bothered by gas generation which enters nerve and brain matter causing irritation and resulting in irritable moods, hysteria, chaotic behavior and convulsions.

Fresh Air is Craved

Sulphur deficiency facilitates extreme nervous irritation attended by a stuffy sensation. Eyesight and speech are altered; speech faculty may be temporarily lost; vocal cords become soft, dry, inflamed and filled with hard mucus; there is an inclination to stretch lower limbs; feet are restless, especially when patient is under scrutiny of many people and nervous system and motor nerves are under more stress; standing motionless removes restlessness but blood flows to internal organs and to the emotional brain faculties. The patient is compelled to lie down because of weakness and prefers a dark, silent, cool room; head feels congested, as do liver, spleen, feet; gasping for breath in sultry environments or in warm rooms forces one to rush to open doors and windows for fresh air; heat and oppression are unbearable; strong light is adverse to brain, nerves, general well-being; there may be super-sensitive nerves, irritable temperament, agitated moods, fickle wishes; sense of odor is acute unless sinuses are congested with dry catarrh; cold showers are refreshing and soothing; morning brings tiredness; eyelids seem feeble and eyes are difficult to open in the morning; there is general sluggishness in the morning because of internal congestion caused by oxygen shortage; nervous system, sensory nerves, portal system, colon, liver, spleen and male genitals are sources of difficulties.

"Sulphur reaches the deepest part of man—the vital life force of each cell and the magnetic force of life— creating havoc in blood, blood salts and the oxygen function."

How Hydrogen Sulphide Causes Ailments

Hydrogen sulphide causes most of these infirmities for six major reasons: (1) intake of sulphur was too great in the past; (2) sulphur is improperly assimilated; (3) sulphur foods are improperly combined with other foods; (4) digestive tract, tissues and secretions are acid, producing more gas and acid unless sulphur foods and antacid foods are combined; (5) sulphur acid and gas reduce oxidation; blood salts are dissipated, sodium reserve lowered and carbonic acid improperly expelled; (6) excessive phosphorus is dismantled in the brain and the by-products create more acids which precipitate magnesium and clog the body with waste material that accommodates germs and germ toxins; these aggravate ailments even further.

Inherent Mystical Nature and Love of Beauty

The sulphur-deficient patient may exhibit heart weakness; excessive bladder contractions resulting in frequent urination; cramps in pubic, uterine, ovarian and epigastric areas (females); brain unable to perform in culture, study, work though these avenues are attractive; perverted idealism; anemic complications; anoxemia; spasmodic and premature menses; cerebellum pain; falling straight downward; aversion to small towns, miserly men, uncouth and crass people, literary triteness; inclination toward Oriental philosophy, mental healing, astrology, palmistry, autosuggestion because of inherent esthetic and mystical nature. Wrists, ankles, small of back, fingers are feeble; steady and prolonged work is impossible without frequent rest periods; work is hard but little is accomplished because it is chaotic, spasmodic and disorganized; temporary speed, emotional turmoil, fuss and absentmindedness manifests in work unless many rest stops are allowed with fresh air, movement, variety and alternations; eye muscles are usually weak. The establishment, rules and regulations are abhored; a time clock is disliked; a systematic and unyielding manager is not cared for; spinal centers and cerebellum are undergoing stress. Such a patient is at home with art, culture, refined interests, high ideals, classic beauty and platonic love. Continual work is impossible without rest, fresh air, activity, variety and change since tiredness overcomes quickly but recuperation is rapid. Alcoholic beverages flush eliminative organs.

Craved Foods Increase Problems

Salads, greens, tart desserts, magnesium vegetables, berries and fruits are favored, but there is a craving for sweets, common tea, starch, creamy dishes cleverly prepared—which only aggravate the troubles; personality is refined and sensitive but nerves and brain cells are irritated by acidity in tissues and by sulphur gases, leading to unrefined and crude behavior, peevish temperament, strange wants, quarrelsome tendencies, spasmodic love and unintentional irascibility. This patient possesses extreme pride, great sensitivity; head feels vacant or weighted; complexion may be pale rose or slightly ruddy due to capillary congestion and nerve irritation at the surface of the skin.

Will is Weak; Emotions Rule

The downfall of the sulphur-deficient patient is an uncontrollable temper due to nervous irritation and lumbago; nerve control is lacking so temper is difficult to control; will is weak and erratic or absent; emotional impulsiveness rules; limbs tremble; top of head is pressured; domestic duties are disdained due to attendant dirt, heat, smoke, gas, fumes; thoughts are disorganized and knowledge not utilized; bell-like noises occur in the ears; throat is extremely sensitive to atmospheric fumes and impurities; fumes have a stifling effect; heat enfeebles and produces nausea; breezes are invigorating; immense work is exhausting; moisture is relieving; medium light is elating, while strong light enfeebles the brain; candy, sweets, desserts, sugar are transformed into gas in the body adding to symptom severity; apprehensions, spouse difficulties, failures are almost unbearable; divorces are likely.

Mind is Faster than Tongue

The sulphur-depleted patient is impressed by vibrations of dead and living people; mediums, psychics, seances interest them greatly because of their own high-strung, nervous, tense, nerve-sensitive, idealistic and mystical tendencies. Tongues cannot keep pace with the mind; under excitement, the tongue has special difficulty keeping up with the mind and emotions causing garbled speech, hysteria; energetic work for extended periods of time is disagreeable; sentiment makes them stubborn but reason is more flexible. If this patient trusts someone, the patient is under his power; susceptibility to kindness is keen. Perfumes and aromas are pleasing; self-pity from alleged neglect causes much complaining.

Moods are Eccentric

This patient is typified by eccentric moods: melancholy, touchy, careless, exhausted, obtuse, joyful, envious, playful, nervous, irritable, amorous, sympathetic, agitated, depressed, lonely, shy, faint, feeble by turns. He shows contempt for people of other nationalities and aversion to noise, long-winded sermons, and fear of snakes; distance, time, movement, equilibrium, efficiency, speed, momentum, physics, are not clearly interpreted; point-blank interrogation provokes him. Romanticism is appealing, especially devotion from lover, attention from celebrities, spouse; but affections are fickle; self-interest is so great that others are forgotten. Travel, pastel colors, stylish clothing, successful and renowned men, opulence, breezes, water, harmless fun in the hills appeal to the female patient; energy fails quickly so rest periods are essential. Equilibrium, gravity, perception and motion are distorted; at times it seems impossible to go further; hunger weakens one spontaneously and strangely; refined, platonic love is important; sympathy riles but is craved; perspiration has a sulphur smell and its acidity may stain clothing, bedding or handkerchiefs brown, yellow, brownish yellow; sexual system is under tremendous stress and this facilitates hysterical and chaotic behavior; skin is hypersensitive.

> *"In times when sulphur is deficient the effects are noted in the emotional nature, possibly indirectly."*

Youthfulness Important to Sulphur-Deprived Patient

Both men and women sulphur-poverty patients are extremely concerned about appearance and retention of youth and beauty; clothing, beauty treatment, charm courses and general appearances are very important.

Altitude of 2000-4000 Feet Ideal

These patients demand a high altitude, moist climate—ideally an elevation of about 2 to 4 thousand feet—for improvement. If elevation is excessively high—10 thousand feet or above—the ailments are aggravated. Dryness can also be unfavorable.

Salts Not Assimilated Well

Vegetable salts are not assimilated properly—especially magnesium, silicon, sodium, manganese, calcium, iron, chlorine, iodine, potassium—so the body lacks most of these essential elements; metabolism is faulty; blood is anemic; metabolism of fats, sweets, proteins is disrupted; there may be mild anoxemia, ataxic manifestations; body gases and acids attack the tissues most of the time. Reflex control of ankles, knees, lower legs is convulsive, showing mild ataxia of lower limbs; joy alternates with unhappiness; irritation and quarrelsome tendencies appear often; emotions are constantly under stress.

Sulphur Hunger Follows Sulphur Excess

Excessive sulphur consumption precedes sulphur hunger because sulphur is not available in large quantities in the average diet. The body normally holds a reserve of sulphur, but if the body becomes starved for sulphur that reserve is rapidly depleted. A certain type of person is more susceptible to sulphur hunger, but any type may suffer this condition. Remember that sulphur deficiency resembles sulphur-excess, but the symptoms are not identical.

Symptoms and Maladies of Sulphur Deficiency

Sulphur-poverty symptoms and maladies are numerous: burning pains, venous congestion, faint states, relapse of illnesses, nervous anxiety, extreme tactile sensitivity, nerve unsteadiness, stinging headache, neurasthenia, heart flutter, nervous perspiration in the middle of night, globus hystericus, chaotic appetite, aches in pit of stomach, stiffness, spasmodic functions, skin irritation; stomach has gnawing sensation with gigantic appetite; appetite must be indulged immediately for feeling of well-being, but an hour later there is again discomfort. In specific regions of the body temperature does not rise; palms burn; soles of feet, eyes or scalp burn. Feet may be chilled in daytime but soles of feet burn at night or feet alternately become heated and chilled.

Brain Damage Possible

Functions are irregular; menses are irregular; kidneys are disturbed and occasionally dark rings appear under eyes; heart palpitates; eyesight changes from good to defective by turns; there are tumors, abscesses, skin breakouts; psoriasis, pimples, pustules, dermatitis, rash, hives, heat rashes alternate; there may be cardiac complications; falling hair manifests. The grey matter (neurons) of the brain generate excessive heat; if this condition stretches for years, brain may be permanently damaged; insanity results from

permanent neuron damage in the cortical brain areas.

Old Wounds Act Up

Sulphur deficiency encourages eruptive disorders, spontaneous fevers, pharyngeal catarrh, scanty secretions, heteroplastic interstices in tissues, dry hemorrhoids, chronic dry catarrh of digestive tract, trouble with portal system, liver engorgement, weakness in motor nerves, finger tendons, joints; throbbing neuritis, uterine disturbances, ovarian contractions, headache, nervous irritability, gravel, chronic bladder catarrh, dry skin, liver dysfunction. Other sulphur hunger tendencies are problems with old sprains, scars, wounds, fractures, injuries; pulmonary catarrh, urinary complaints, benign scrofula, dandruff, torpidity, mucus membrane catarrh, acne, nerve aches, gastro-intestinal catarrh, nervous agitation, emotional problems.

Weaknesses are Profuse

One may experience throat inflammation, follicular tonsillitis, carbuncles, rosacea, cerebellar dysfunction causing staggering walk or inability to direct physical movement, trembling legs, spasmodic muscles, weak knees, chilly knee joints; there is greater proclivity to kidney inflammation, motor, static and thermal ataxia, numerous optical illusions, anxiety, prostration, extreme itching, furuncles, putrid secretions; all are sulphur shortage indicators. Nervous irritation is likely to cause difficulties during the menopause. There may also be unfavorably-altered pulmonary function; generation of yellow pus; scabs, ulceration of eyelids; chronic and perodic catarrh culminating in seven to ten days, then subsiding and beginning again in about a week; red tip of nose; danger of fractures; black spots on face; swelling, puffiness of neck, ankles, face, hips, thighs.

Reproductive Functions are Damaged

Ailments may be of psychological or physical nature when sulphur is in deficit. The brain, nerves, ganglia, sex organs, generative secretions and vital forces need to be nourished and their normal functions insured against psychological, physical, spiritual disorders. If sulphur is lacking, the sex brain and reproductive functions are damaged. Ovarian weakness, neuralgia, lower limb weakness, pruritus vulva, clitoris hypertrophy, labia minora enlargement, enlargement of fluor albus, cervical catarrh, voluptas impotence, organic impotence, lack of libido, frigidity, sterility, symptomatic impotence, orgasmus retardatus, orgasmus precox, psychological impotence may result.

Sexual Weakness May Be Inherited

In the event the parents suffer sulphur deficiency, the offspring inherit a weakness in the sexual system. This may cause sexual irritation, abnormal growth, improper sexual development, perversion tendencies, neuroses, psychotic sexuality. Other manifestations are inflammation of glands, irritation of glands, nerve tension, pruritis, itches, swellings, congestion; one brain faculty is hyperemic, another chemic; other brain faculties are under stress; sexual fluids are unfavorably changed and the soul is ill—all of which breed perversions. Mental sex functions are abnormally altered, as are the soul quality and reproductive activities. There is a predisposition to erythema, red neuralgia, red vision, arterial plethora, esophagalgia, esogastritis, softening of the esophagus due to excessive stomach acidity; sense of discernment is dulled. Perimetritis, emotional eccentricity, exocolitis, eruptions of chin, soreness of mouth corners, swelling and bleeding gums, sore throat, vocal cord difficulties, sloughing of palate arches or of tensor palati muscles or palatine glands—all herald lack of sulphur.

"Like calcium-excess patients, sulphur-deficient patients complain of dryness in the body—but from different origins."

Tastes Become Perverse in Extreme Cases

Complete sulphur exhaustion may culminate in sexual weakness, marital quarrels, divorces and feelings of wretchedness due to irritation of organs, vital centers, fluids, nerves and sex force, acidity of digestive tract, nerve acidity and acidity of secretions and genitalia. Other eventualities include vaginal disease, vulvar inflammation, uterine irritation, ovarian inflammation; inflammation of uterine tubes, lumbar plexus and various sexual plexuses which may precipitate psycho-sexual

unconcern or abnormal dislikes. It may end in love of the perverse, sadism, masochism, vaginal atresia, mammae degeneration, motor aphonia, momentary throat constriction causing mild and transitory suffocation or thoracic discomfort.

Body Dryness A Problem

Like calcium-excess patients, sulphur-deficient patients complain of dryness in the body—but from different origins. The dessication of sulphur patients is attributed to congestive, neuropyretic, pyocytic and inflammatory dryness due to lack of organic tissue salts, lack of sulphur, lack of oxygen. Dryness occurs in glands, capillaries (especially at the skin surface), digestive tract, throat, spinal centers, psycho-sexual brain centers and throughout the sexual system. Extreme fevers are likely in the respiratory system which do not necessarily climax as pneumonia or other lung diseases but are quite serious. Alveoli are often dry and inflamed; mumps, typhoid fever, intestinal complications are likely; chin becomes rough and dry and a rash develops on it; organs become dry and congested, inflamed; catarrh and congestion of the bowel, transient stomach problems, stasis of organs, delayed digestion and elimination, arthritic aches occur; fingers and joints become so numb that objects are easily dropped; mental centers in brain become dry, partially paralyzed, anemic; memory fails; fever occurs in the nervous system precipitating nerve moisture so nerves are subject to high pressure, tension, irritation; skin is rough, scaly, dry; mucus membranes are feverish and dry; reproductive system is tense; nerves are spasmodic; menses are irregular; personality is changeable; temper may become hysterical, wants fickle, mind confused, organs anemic, tissues deficient of certain biochemical elements; ganglia are in state of irritation, stress and disquiet.

Surgery May Not Correct Problems

Other striking sulphur-shortage symptoms are relaxation of pelvic organs, build-up of blood in head, altered perception of gravity, weaving sensations, uterine and ovarian cramps, soreness and stiffness, capillary congestion, depression, miscarriage, headache, sinus abscess, pernicious anemia, intestinal cramps, bladder complications, frequent urination; ganglionic network, sensory nerves and vaso-motor systems are usually implicated. Surgery is probable, but not necessarily successful. Sensations of congestion, oppression are common, as are uremia, throat conditions, discharges; hepatic, renal and passive congestion; chlorotic disorders; mesenteric and intestinal lesions due to putrid, arid, catarrhal and inflammatory conditions of the colon. Oily lubricants necessary to the eliminative organs and bowel are lacking; as are tissue salts and bile salts. Venous diseases and venous wall complications arise. The child-bearing years are diminished; menopause arrives early; it may be complicated by mental derangement, dry catarrh, irascibility, throat irritation, diarrhea during hot weather, gloominess, erotic fantasies, emotional stubbornness, crying and envious spells, coughing, hysterical outbursts, intermittent nerve transmission, nerve stress, passive congestion, sluggishness in portal system and other disturbances.

Needed Salts are Rapidly Precipitated Out of Body

In the sulphur-short patient nerves, ganglia and psycho-sexual areas of the brain are damaged; nerves suffer; ganglia are irritated, canals arid, secretions scanty, walls and membranes acidic. Antacid and basic tissue salts are in demand for restored alkalinity but are speedily precipitated. The patient complains of backaches, nervousness, nervous respiration, morning melancholy, erotic sexual activities, fickle friendship, perverted idealism, gruesome love, attacks of indigestion, pains and aches, nervous aphonia. Whims are transient; everyday life seems disgusting; functions are chaotic, faculties confused, complaints abundant; nervousness, extreme tears and temper proliferate.

Serious Consequences of Sulphur Lack

The sulphur-deficient patient is not easy to identify. Symptoms are transient, sometimes indirect, variable, circumstantial, subjective, liable to other influences; some appear in consequence of other abnormalities in the body. The doctor, nurse, nutritionist, parent may notice sulphur-shortage signs including morning depression and evening happiness; irritation from trivialities; remorse following temper rages; soft, dry, velvety butanemia skin with a pigment resembling sulphur; tension attended by numbness and congestion; desire for sensationalism; morbid idealism; late rising and late retiring at night; appetite which is minimal until noon; perversions of sex and love; strong thoughts

of and inclination toward obscenity; gruesome fantasies; interest in travel, air, fun in the hills. Storms, rough water, cold showers are pleasant; tissues, canal walls, organs, eliminative channels, skin capillaries, capillaries in glands, liver, kidneys, colon, veins, heart, eyelids, cerebellum, heart walls are dry. Also exhibited are extreme cramps during menstruation, but not prior to or after; aversion to cooking, odors, fumes, smoke, heat, kitchen work; spasms in spleen, liver, kidneys, eyesight, heart, digestion, voice; chaotic love, desires, whims, plans, apprehensions, will; unreasonable irritation with flare-ups of temper; mind which works faster than tongue, with attendant screaming, hysteria, crying, vocalized resentments; extreme need for rest, fresh air, movement, fun during working hours, showing that functions are chaotic; emotional obstinence regarding rules, laws, regulations, duties, discipline, reason, love, necessities; perspiration with acid odor of sulphur; acid sulphur odor in secretions, discharges, expectorations, breath, body or eruptions; corrosive discharges that are liable to stain clothing, linens or handkershiefs brown, yellow or deep brown; rage, obstinancy, maltreatment of others one moment replaced by remorse immediately afterward; build-up of blood in emotional centers of the brain; granulated eyelids; eye irritation; falling hair; dry hair and itchy scalp in hot weather or evening; red and glossy nose tip; swelling and dryness in some body areas such as chin, gums, eyelids, liver, inner throat, spleen, uterus, attended by pulsations in the dry area; putrid saliva; burning throat; partial constriction of respiratory tubes causing distress and red and inflamed face with desire to scream from irritation.

Possible Symptoms Are Many

The patient looks young, healthy, rosy-skinned but is wretched, achy, congested, upset and complains that channels of elimination are all clogged, plethoric, sluggish or filled with stiff mucus; food is distressing; eating prior to 11:00 a.m. distresses and food remains undigested all day; morning produces lethargy, sluggishness, obtuse inclinations; sleeping late in morning is preferred; if late rising is impossible, patient is miserable, sluggish, depressed, obtuse, irascible, difficult to please and moods prevail; urine is putrid and greasy; vulvar itch with stinging sensation is attended by menstrual and hemorrhage complications, possible strong hatred for sexual activity. There is near mania for outdoors, open doors and windows, chilly

358

wind and frosty air touching face, neck, chest, skin, without which patient feels suffocated, choked, feeble; if this is not available a patient will develop convulsions, nerve spasms, temper tantrums, hysterical outbursts, epileptic seizures, nervous symptoms, constant throat discomfort. Further complications include disturbance of colon, stomach, nerves, liver, spleen, cerebellum; stomach is continually acid causing gas production and intermittent indigestion; feet, knees, hands are generally cold, but soles of feet burn frequently due to congestion; cold food, baths and bare feet after retiring are preferred; walking, effort, movement, apprehension, emotion, excitement cause rush of blood to neck and back, producing stiff nerves in these regions; falling straight down occurs occasionally; faint states come and go without reason; fever manifests in brain, heart, nerves, liver, kidneys, spleen, uterus; high temperature, hot rooms, warm beds, cause congested sensation with red face, weak eyes, obtuse senses; flesh seems dry, clogged and swollen; sulphur-based freckles appear; skin erupts in many ailments with fever on occasion; hot temper accompanies nervous explosions, bruised egos, inflamed nerves, touchiness, irascibility, volatile moods and feelings, hypersensitive extreme emotions. Odors, gases, fumes annoy the patient excessively, and may seem stifling; response is trigger-fast but fickle; pornographic literature is enjoyed at night. All indications are for a diet rich in sulphur, magnesium and specific vegetable salts which can cool, relileve and placate nerves, brain, blood and organs of the body. Also foods possessing specific oily substances are in demand.

Female Patient is Not Vindictive

The female sulphur patient is quick to start an argument, but she is not vindictive; in the end she cries and begs; excessive conversation creates a hoarseness; she perspires little; her skin is frequently feverish and arid.

Symptoms Which Indirectly Point to Sulphur Lack

Many symptoms are indirectly indicative of sulphur poverty: pressure and tension pain with contractions; weight in head, spleen, liver, epigastric area, liver, heart; weakness in ankles, wrists, joints, knees; extreme susceptibility to heat; depression and oppression during hot weather; contraction with cramping in ovaries, uterus, bladder, peritoneum,

appendix, mesentery or other body areas; blind faith in mental cures and suggestive therapy; continual desire for different foods; fickle whims, wishes, dress, plans, furniture choices, recreation preferences; ailments, symptoms which seem to be unfounded; bleeding, itching, yellowish, putrid eruptions. A milk diet causes acidity, nausea, vomiting, cramps in abdomen and general intensification of symptoms; spontaneous hunger pangs are concomitant with feelings of faintness, but about an hour after eating, symptoms are magnified. There may also be constipation; chills that move upward; internal pressure which seems to shoot toward surface of the body; pains that move downward; burning feet; irritated nerves; lack of perspiration, but feverish skin and inflamed nerves due to partial capillary or arterial congestion; convulsive sensations, facilitating the sensation of a steel vice constricting head, arms, thoracic area, heart or other area; disrupted heart activity when altitude changes rapidly. Intense concentration is fatiguing; light is uplifting; strong light is enraging. All of the above are secondary or indirect signs of sulphur exhaustion.

"If sulphur or any other deficient element is not replaced, health is an impossibility."

Symptoms Are Often Elusive

Other transient symptoms are failure to assemble and utilize knowledge, thoughts, resources adequately; great awareness of departed persons; patient alleges that husband or wife and others neglect him or her; he or she attacks those thought to be. guilty of neglect without meaning animosity; mental conditions are chaotic; there is excessive aversion for anything lengthy, droning, uninterrupted; symptoms are difficult to fathom and elusive; distaste is exhibited for strangers, foreigners, heat, noise, torrid weather, commotion; equilibrium and gravity perception are faulty; extreme fatigue, feebleness and listlessness force patient to recline often because he feels he cannot proceed another inch without collapsing; articles are mislaid or lost easily; lack of concern for others is due to preoccupation with self; blood floods to emotional areas in brain and attacks membranes of ear which results in ringing, clanging, buzzing, humming sound; numbness occurs along with aches from vibration of cars, trains, planes; partial clogging of optic nerves accompanies great weakness of eyelids, even eye inflammation.

Dislikes Are Pronounced

Other symptoms include rectal afflictions; dropsy; conversation, study, emotion, anxiety, passion, excitement aggravate troubles; mounting stairs or climbing hills cause heart palpitation because greater oxygen is necessary; minimal effort results in depression and pulmonary oppression; tension occurs in back of head, upper back, neck with pain and weakness in small of back; patient is inclined to recline on stomach; doctors often diagnose patient as having "imaginary ills;" there is a predisposition to hysterical epilepsy; nervous perspiration occurs nightly on chest but dissipates rapidly upon awakening; patient makes determined plans and deviates as soon as they are made; sexual activities become perverted, and there is a dislike for normal sexual acts; smells are disgusting, noise disruptive and nauseating; fumes, gases and heat are felt to be stifling; the patient resembles a steaming pressure cooker; water relieves, soothes him; hurry causes him turmoil; a prolonged sleep refreshes and facilitates near recovery; cold compresses to head and hot compresses to body are used; sense of hearing, sight, smell, thought processes, reflexes are keen but objective mind is confused; moving downward causes heart palpitation; nausea results

from movement of trains, buses, cars, ships, airplanes; spontaneous movement causes mental chaos. Such are transient sulphur-deficiency symptoms.

Treatment of Sulphur Depletion

A number of requirements are indicated in times of sulphur depletion: (1) a sulphur-rich diet; (2) a diet abundant in magnesium, nitrogen, iron, sodium, manganese, potassium silicon, chlorine, iodine, calcium; (3) a diet rich in phosphorized fats, oily fats for good bowel elimination; (4) icy air, outdoor activity, laxative foods, cathartics, cold compresses to head, heated compresses to abdomen and small of back; understanding, compassion, devotion, tenderness, tranquil friendships, balmy and cool climates, ocean topography, forests and hills, massage, polarity treatment, breezy and humid weather, horseback riding in the mountains, moderately high altitude (2 to 4 thousand feet) and supervision by a competent physician or nutritionist. A female sulphur-deficient patient requires guidance by a watchful individual, residence in the hills, scientifically constructed menus for her demands.

Each Patient is Different

Each patient is different and his or her needs must be considerd. If sulphur or any other deficient element is not replaced, health is an impossibility.

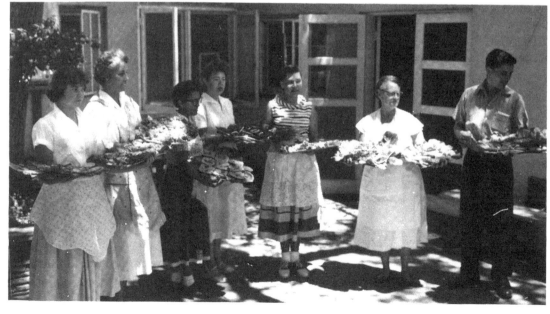

I have found that a variety of foods is the most important health law. Only variety ensures that we get all the essential chemical elements.

HIGHEST SULPHUR FOODS

The highest sources of sulphur are kale, cabbage, cauliflower, horseradish, brussels sprouts and watercress. Cranberries are also an excellent source. The primary sources of food sulphur are:

Asparagus
Avocados
Black currants
Brazil nuts
Broccoli
Brussels sprouts
Cabbage
Carrots
Cauliflower
Celery
Chervil
Chestnuts
Chickory
Chives
Corn
Cucumber
Dill
Figs, dried
Filberts
Globe artichoke
Horseradish
Jerusalem artichoke
Kale
Kohlrabi
Leeks

Lettuce (leaf)
Lima beans
Marjoram
Mustard greens
Oats
Okra
Onions, dry
Parsnips
Peas, fresh green
Potatoes
Radishes
Red currants
Salsify
Savoy cabbage
Snap beans
Sorrel
Soybean, dried
Spinach
Swiss chard
Tamarind
Thyme
Tomato, ripe
Turnips, white
Turnip greens

361

SULPHUR MENUS

Muesli, goat milk, sliced peaches, bananas, apricotsa, papaya, marjoram tea.

Broiled veal, steamed cauliflower, steamed broccoli; tossed salad of mixed greens, shredded beets, carrots and turnips, avocado wedges, tomatoes, celery, dandelion greens, watercress, cucumbers, dill, leeks; avocado dressing, mushroom sauce.

Tomato juice and cod roe, barley and green kale soup, baked potato or corn on the cob; goat butter; sour cream and chives; steamed asparagus; steamed brussels sprouts; mixed green salad; pumpkin pudding.

Cheese sticks; raspberries, loganberries, cherries, strawberries, coconut milk sweetened with grapes; rye crackers; filberts, brazilnuts, raisin-stuffed, baked apples.

SUMMARY OF SULPHUR

GENERAL CHARACTERISTICS

"Heating" element

Unites with all metals, many nonmetals

Sulphuric acid used in chemistry, medicine

Sulphur type = Exesthesic type

SULPHUR IN THE HUMAN BODY

Promotes flow of bile
Builds hair, nails, skin
Stimulates egg and sperm production
Warms skin

Regulates brain heat
Beautifies complexion
Drives impurities to surface
Stimulates, regulates nerves

SIGNS OF SULPHUR EXCESS (Characteristics of Exesthesic Type)

Fitfulness, changeableness, inconstancy
Intensified sense perception
Depression, slowness in morning
Falling sensations, dizziness
Changeable symptoms

Moodiness, volatility
Intensified emotions
Shallow breathing
Intolerance of warm rooms
Forgetfulness

SIGNS OF SULPHUR DEFICIENCY

Symptoms resemble excess symptoms
Impulsiveness
Jerkiness, fitfulness
Stormy emotion
Mysticism, love of beauty
Body dryness

Irritability
Great temperature changes
Worry
Craving for fresh air
Weak will
Aversion to early rising

HIGHEST SULPHUR FOODS

Kale   *Cauliflower*
Horseradish   *Watercress*
Cabbage   *Chervil*
Brussels sprouts

seventeen

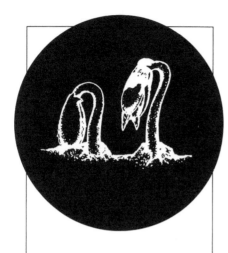

Biochemists at the University of Wisconsin have found that laboratory chickens fed supplements of garlic, ginseng and barley had lower cholesterol levels than those fed a normal diet.

Prince Charles of Great Britain, as well as many other members of Britain's Royal Family, prefer natural healing methods rather than the drug-oriented approach to treatment. Queen Victoria, in 1755, was the first British monarch to rely on homeopathic medicine.

Wounds heal 40% faster when people take a gram of vitamin C daily, according to Dr. Sheldon Pollack of Duke University, who recommends 250 mg after each meal and before bedtime.

Biochemistry: The chemistry of living things; the science of the chemical changes accompanying the vital functions of plants and animals.
— *Taber's Cyclopedic Medical Dictionary*

Biochemical notes

I express my appreciation for permission to use research data by Sivad BioResearch Co., Inc., Madison Heights, MI 48071.

The following biochemical notes show that doctors have been interested in the chemistry of man and aware of the problems caused by deficiencies for some time. However, the approach of Western medicine has been one of "bits and pieces" rather than looking at the whole man, his diet and lifestyle, and determining what is needed for balancing over the long term. Occasional identification of a deficiency and prescription of a temporary mineral supplement is not sufficient in the great majority of cases to balance the chemistry of the body.

In reviewing the notes that follow, keep in mind the need to take an integrated wholistic approach to prevention or treatment. We find that 99% of the patient is on the other end of any symptom, and we must take care of the whole person, not just the symptom.

Iron deficiency anemia occurs frequently in women during reproductive years because of menstruation and pregnancy. Most arthritis sufferers are anemic. Men and children can suffer the effects through chronic blood loss, poor absorption and poor diet. Signs and symptoms include weakness, fatigue, pallor, palpitation, headache, tiredness, shortness of breath and moderate cardiac enlargement. Fingernails show longitudinal ridges; vague gastrointestinal complaints such as distress, fullness and constipation. Tingling or numbness of the hands and feet are also experienced. Iron given with B-12 and liver is effective in regenerating hemoglobin; high intake of vitamin C with iron, B-12 and liver improves utilization. Stool softner combined with this formula helps constipation.

People who complain of cold hands and feet are generally anemic.

Low iron intake in food is partly due to lower average caloric intake, refinement of foods and the declining use of iron cooking utensils. There are an estimated 6 mg iron per 1000 calories of food intake.

It is easy to see why anemia is so widespread since the daily requirement in adults is 10 mg of absorbed iron. Absorption of iron from food usually ranges from 5-15%. There are probably several million women deficient with a lesser amount of men also deficient.

Simple anemia suggests the need for more iron in the diet. The problem may be one of absorption however. When 50 to 200 mg of vitamin C is taken before meals, the amount of iron absorbed is sometimes tripled. The iron is chelated in the stomach by the ascorbic acid. Meat and fish or other proteins enhance iron absorption by the same mechanism in the presence of adequate HCL.

A 1% amount of magnesium strengthens bones and teeth and prevents osteomalacia, curvature of the spine and tooth decay. The teeth of carnivorous animals are about 5% magnesium phosphate which enables them to crush and grind bones of their prey.

Recent tests indicate that magnesium integrates with calcium. The effects are not simple chemistry of ions but some deeper-seated conditions and reactions by which interrelations of the two nutrient elements exhibit effects in specific quantities as "balance" of which the soil is one of the cases commonly exhibiting itself.

Manganese, often in short supply in civilized diets, is necessary to the skeletal enzyme system of the body. The effects in man and animal when deficient include impotence, skeletal and postural defects, liver, kidney and pancreas malfunctions. Manganese added to the diets of M.S. and Myasthenia Gravis sufferers aid in neuromuscular control.

Manganese improves elasticity and strength of ligaments and muscles by activating blood phosphatases, which improve tissue utilization of calcium to build intracellular ground cement.

Manganese deficiency linked to epilepsy seizures.

Potassium depletion most often caused by diuretics and poor diet.

Potassium is essential for normal heart rhythm, other muscular contraction, normal nerve activity, glycogen formation and energy and normal pituitary function. Symptoms of deficiency are muscular weakness, malaise, vague muscle and abdominal aches and pains, tachycardia, hypertension, rapid respiration, dry mouth, low gastric acidity, constipation and dehydration.

It has been found that 50% of deaths from heart attacks are due to potassium deficiency instead of blood clots.

Trace minerals in soil of iron, calcium, selenium and chromium favorably affect longevity of residents.

Over half a million people over 40 years of age are walking around with asymptomatic vertebral fractures. Backache is the most common symptom of this disorder.

Trace element chromium, deficient in the American diet, is due to refinement of foods. Chromium added to the diet enhances glucose utilization and it plays an important role in liver synthesis of fatty acids and cholesterol.

Children suffering from hyper- or hypo-glycemia were relieved of symptoms by oral doses of chromium.

A link between heart attacks and hardening of the arteries and the American diet of refined foods has been found. Chromium and zinc are lost in refining process, and are needed by the body to prevent these diseases.

Chromium is a very essential element in the body because it combines with the cell membrane and insulin to allow glucose to move across the membranes.

In the absence of insulin or chromium, the effectiveness of glucose transport from the blood into body cells is diminished. When this mechanism of glucose transport breaks down, the body shows the first signs of diabetes.

Zinc is important to the body as a carrier to get rid of waste carbon dioxide in the same way as iron is important in transporting oxygen from the lungs to the blood cells.

Whole wheat and peas are main sources of chromium, while whole grains and meat are the best sources of zinc.

When there is a deficiency of chromium, it takes twice as long for insulin to remove glucose from the blood. Chromium deficiency is a major factor in the development of heart disease.

Manganese is not a mere trace element but a precious metal as far as the economy of the body is concerned. It has been shown to catalyze formation of thyroxine. Manganese is probably involved in the formation of thyroxine in the thyroid gland, because this organ has a particular ability to store manganese and manganese injection has been shown to cause increased oxygen consumption. It is found in Nova Scotia dulse.

Best food sources of chromium are those which have received little or no processing such as whole wheat bread, fish, shellfish, meats, fowl and brewer's yeast.

The rationale of zinc therapy for vascular disease was based on a study that body zinc levels were about 30% of normal in patients with atherosclerosis. Correcting zinc deficiency has improved patients' tolerance for exercise and there is improvement in mental processes. Cancerous patients were reported to have low zinc levels.

It has been found that one month of zinc deprivation produced gray or oily hair or loss of hair, growth retardation and prevention of sexual maturation and gonads.

The need for zinc is world-wide and its deficiency is considered only secondary to nitrogen deficiency among soil fertility problems.

Magnesium regulates vital actions within cells; it affects the health of muscles, nerves, the brain, kidneys, liver and other organs. These normally contain a high concentration of magnesium and without it, their function is impaired.

Magnesium is especially important as an activator of enzymes through which we use protein and vitamins. It also helps the utilization of potassium. Magnesium starts the chain reaction in the body to metabolize food.

Magnesium is important for proper muscle function and lack of it can cause muscle irritability or tremors.

Chelation is the natural process of building an amino acid fence around a metal so that it is available for absorption in the digestive tract. The metals being chelated or "coated" with amino acids, are quickly and easily absorbed.

Zinc is involved in the production and function of several sex hormones. Severe zinc deficiency has been shown to cause male sterility. A zinc deficiency may result in smaller sex organs, possibly due to inadequate gonadotrophin.

Gonadotrophin is a hormone which has a sexually-stimulating effect on the sex glands of both male and female. Sufficient levels of this sex hormone are produced only in the presence of adequate zinc.

The production of sperm, spermatogenesis, could not take place without a large amount of zinc. Not only is zinc involved in the production of sperm, the development of primary and secondary sex organs and sex drive, but it also is involved in every phase of the female reproductive process.

Research indicates that the body must convert most forms of swallowed zinc into an amino acid chelate form before it can be utilized. Unless zinc is in an amino acid chelate form, it has no biological effect on the body and your body would be just as zinc deficient as if you were not getting any at all.

Oral zinc has achieved dramatic cure in Crohn's disease patients with associated low zinc levels.

Vitamin A deficiency causes four different problems: loss of vision due to failure of rhodopsin formation in retina; defects in bone growth; defects in reproduction (lack of sperm formation in the male and failure to carry through to normal birth in female); keratinization of tissues.

A worthwhile quote from Westchester Medical Bulletin: "The simple uncomplicated term, human kindness, is not even heard in clinical conversation. The best and most modern health care is defective if it is lacking in this simple element of human kindness. One may call it empathy, sympathy, compassion or any other term, but it is essentially that crucial element of humanness that we dare not take for granted."

Selenium and vitamin E function together in preventing oxidation of fats, including cardiovascular disease. Evidence indicates the possible anticancer value of selenium as well as its value against other chronic diseases.

PABA (Para-AminoBenzoic Acid) influences intestinal bacteria enabling them to produce folic acid which aids in the assimilation of pantothenic acid, prevents vitiligo, a depigmentation of hair.

Adrenal exhaustion has become widespread by the millions of persons suffering from "stress diseases" and by the number of illnesses for which physicians now give cortisone.

Insomnia, a common cause of fatigue that interferes with sexual expression is the inability to sleep well. Severe insomnia has been induced in volunteers made deficient in vitamin B-6. Insomnia together with sleepiness throughout the day occurred in subjects deficient in pantothenic acid.

The lack of pantothenic acid alone causes faulty digestion producing food allergies in varying degrees.

Eighty-one percent of all back pain is due to muscle weakness or inelasticity.

Muscle heating to relieve muscle spasm can be valuable in enabling a patient to exercise. The most common cause in the elderly is abdominal muscle weakness. Depression is a frequent factor, producing poor posture, sleep difficulty and sexual inadequacy. Emotional problems were an important cause also.

Eight out of a hundred people have emphysema, a condition of gradually increasing rigidity of the cells in the bronchial tree and chest with breathing difficulties. Vitamin A deficiency is a contributing factor. Vitamin A releases a proteolytic enzyme which tends to soften the matrix of the cell tissues.

The Popliteus muscle shares its lymphatic drainage with the liver and gallbladder and the addition of bile salts will frequently aid.

Acidophilus products seem to support the tensor fascia femoris where it is found weak in recurring knee problems as it shares its lymphatic drainage with the large bowel.

Restoration of normal intestinal flora and increased synthesis of B complex in the body is accomplished with massive niacinamide-niacin intake, which can be compared to the effect of an infusion of Lactobacillus Acidophilus.

It has been found that much fatigue and weakness called "aging" arises simply from a diet depleted of potassium.

Four factors required for an active enzyme system are vitamins, minerals, amino acids and unsaturated fatty acids.

In the body, vitamins act as catalysts in the enzyme system. An enzyme is composed of a vitamin, a mineral, an amino acid and a phosphate radical. Trace minerals are essential to the enzyme system of the body metabolism.

It has been proven that liver impairment exists in the obese. Weight reduction was associated with reduction in liver impairment.

Many chronic ailments have less to do with fatty diet, smoking, etc. than tension. Nutrients depleted in stress situations are: Protein, vitamin E, riboflavin, choline, pantothenic acid, vitamin A, unsaturated fatty acids and vitamin C. Stress makes nutritional needs skyrocket.

Magnesium deficiency can cause parathyroid failure. Parathyroid output is low even in low serum calcium states. Administration of magnesium resulted in parallel increases in parathyroid output and serum calcium levels.

Cooking in iron, copper or badly tinned vessels causes destruction of ascorbic acid.

Mashing or whipping potatoes and keeping them hot destroys their ascorbic acid rapidly.

Chopping vegetables before or after cooking destroys a considerable amount of ascorbic acid, particularly if a steel or metal knife or chopper is used.

Shredded lettuce loses 80% ascorbic acid in one minute.

Restaurant, cafeteria and army meals usually contain little ascorbic acid because of the long time elapsing from the peeling and preparation of the vegetables to their appearance on the plate. The hot plate and steam table cause rapid inactivation.

Better eating habits could improve dramatically the dental health of 95% of our population, who suffer with chronic tooth decay or gum disease.

Alcoholics with withdrawal symptoms have low blood levels of magnesium.

Kidney stones recurrence may often be prevented by adequate intake of magnesium.

Muscle contraction depends upon the availability of both calcium and magnesium.

Too few physicians treat arthritis as a long time illness, leaving the patient unsupervised during periods of remission.

Rheumatoid arthritis mainly affects the synovial and other joint structures, but no tissue is exempt; muscles, serous membranes, spleen, bowel, tendons and sheaths, central and peripheral nervous system all can be affected.

Magnesium within the body is an electrolyte more accurately termed a magnesium ion.

Magnesium affects enzymes. It starts the enzymes working. Enzymes cause the food to be utilized.

Neuromuscular spasms were relieved by increased magnesium intake in 9 patients.

Irritability, dizziness, poor muscle coordination and muscular weakness were observed in hypomagnesemia.

Potassium deficiencies result in cardiac, liver and kidney lesions.

Potassium is essential for normal heart rhythm and nerve activity. Deficiencies result in decreased pituitary and adrenal function along with tachycardia, hypertension, rapid respiration, gastrointestinal toxicity and constipation.

Deficiency of vitamin B-12 might lead to functional impairment of the adrenal cortex or the anterior lobe of the pituitary gland either as a result of the general debilitating effect of the deficiency or because vitamin B-12 is actually necessary for proper function of the glands.

Zinc was used in a well-controlled test on dwarfs who were also deficient in gonadal development. Growth was rapid. Also sex functions were restored and intelligence levels were enhanced.

The nutritional evaluation of the patient is as important as any other aspect of the total evaluation.

It is reasonable to assume that nutritional deficiencies of all grades exist and do not necessarily appear as the florid evidence of the classical deficiency diseases. The deficiencies may begin early in life and continue for long periods of time. They may contribute ultimately to an illness without themselves becoming identified as the cause of or even related to the illness.

Arthritis is characterized by faulty calcium metabolism and poor glandular secretion. Arthritics commonly complain of gas and belching due to protein putrifaction. The use of HCL supplies a natural hydrochloric acid source to aid in calcium solution, protein digestion and clears up the gastritis.

Marked reduction in incidence of epilepsy convulsions have been reported by regular use of HCL in generous dosage. Availability of glutamine and arginine is increased.

Lack of gastric hydrochloric acid is often a basic cause of stubborn anemias. This is probably more likely with older patients, arthritics and in pernicious anemia. As a result ingested proteins are not digested into components necessary to build hemoglobin and red blood cells.

Hydrochloric acid restores normal acidity so natural secretion of insulin in diabetics can maintain its activity. Insulin is only active in acid. Lipotropic effects of HCL is also helpful.

Most cancer clinics use hydrochloric acid routinely—cell ionization and detoxification is aided.

Hydrochloric acid aids breakdown of protein complexes (allergens) which otherwise may go through the liver into the bloodstream, thus causing congestion.

HCL aids natural gastrointestinal action, normalizing the flora.

Apparently the brain cells of mentally-disturbed patients accumulate indoles, indicans and other toxic materials which interfere with normal brain function. HCL aids in their more complete digestion and removal. Clinical results have been excellent.

Protection of the nervous system against convulsions is an important function for vitamin B-6.

Potassium has value in picking up pituitary output and prevents depression of the parasympathetic nervous system. Potassium is highly concentrated in the cells of cartilage and muscle.

Benefits of low dosage estrogen replacement include prevention of osteoporosis in the elderly. In a group of women who had undergone hysterectomies treated this way, it was found to successfully prevent osteoporosis.

Irradiated Ergosterol (vitamin D-2) is a very toxic, unnatural, growth-promoting steroid hormone which induces unnatural mineral deposits throughout normally soft tissues of the body. The addition of this hormone to milk significantly increases its toxicity and vitamin D milk may be a significantly contributing factor in the development of many chronic adult illnesses.

Freedom from back pain depends not only on exercise and adjustments to restore muscle tone, but also on ample intake of chelated manganese.

Manganese has been shown to catalyze formation of thyroxin. The thyroid gland stores manganese and manganese injection has been shown to cause increased oxygen consumption.

Twenty-five percent of advised surgery could not be justified. The operations involved were hysterectomies, dilation and curettage, various breast operations and gallbladder removal.

Manganese deficiency in pregnant women may be a factor in giving birth to epileptic children, according to research in Canada.

Loss of taste and smell can be due to poor thyroid function. The function is involved along with zinc ion which is bound to a protein involved in taste bud function. Some drugs which interfere with utilization of zinc or which lower thyroid activity or illnesses with these actions can be the cause.

Most heart attacks occur from deficiency of the cardiac minerals, magnesium, potassium and zinc.

Necrosis of the heart, kidney and liver occur with deficiency of magnesium and potassium.

Sedatives interfere with calcium metabolism. Increasing the intake of natural vitamin D-3 tends to counteract these effects. Phenobarbitol and dilantin could aggravate convulsions in epileptics.

The amino acid arginine increases the number and mobility of sperm in some men. Arginine has been considered a nonessential amino acid, yet it is indispensable to normal protein synthesis. Deficiency of the amino acid first effects those tissues in which mitosis is frequent, such as testicular tissue. Arginine deficiency may result from poor diet, malabsorption or abnormal requirements on the gland.

Combining vitamin A with vitamin E enhances assimilation. Vitamin E also prevents oxidation of the A.

Vitamin A is now believed to participate in at least 5 distinct metabolic reactions. Abnormal fingernails indicate a need for additional vitamin A, as well as protein.

When vitamin A is undersupplied, cells of skin and mucus membrane die quickly and accumulate, providing ready food for bacteria.

Weight reduction usually leads to a fall in the plasma level of uric acid. It is possible for the obese patient with mild hyperuricemia and infrequent attacks of gout to be adequately managed by weight reduction.

Weight loss is associated with relative hydration, which has a dilutional effect on uric acid.

Television tubes emit X-rays harmful to the pituitary gland; hence, produce emotional and physical problems especially noted in youngsters. The same rays are also given off by fluorescent lighting with similar results.

Most vitamin A materials are rapidly neutralized in people working under fluorescent lights.

Vitamin E biochemically feeds the pituitary. When used in a vitamin A formula, it helps protect the A from destruction.

The pituitary is the master gland controlling glands in the endocrine system.

Television sets are shielded in front so viewers six feet or more away are protected, rays are emitted from the sides and back.

The pituitary gland needs and uses magnesium in the regulation of other glands. It is also involved in parathyroid function, adrenal output (as can be seen in deficiencies by twitchings and convulsions) and thyroid function.

Magnesium, as the key mineral in the Krebs cycle, is involved in close to 100 various enzymes.

Research at the Mayo Clinic indicates that supplementation with bile salts can dissolve gallstones.

Atherosclerosis is responsible for most heart attacks and for the chest pain called angina pectoris.

In atherosclerosis, the passageway through the arteries becomes roughened and narrowed by fatty deposits that harden into patches along the inner lining of the artery.

Coronary thrombosis is what most people mean by a heart attack. When a clot (thrombus) cuts off the blood supply to a section of heart muscle, the result is a heart attack.

Shingles (Herpes Zoster) responded dramatically with ribonucleic acid daily.

Ample intake of sulphur bearing natural amino acids seems to prevent accumulation of metabolic toxins in brain cells.

A combination of two vitamins and another common food substance could possibly protect humans against many of the harmful effects of smoking and heavy drinking. Vitamin

C is one of the vitamins; the second is thiamine known as B-1. The third substance is cysteine, a common compound found in most high protein foods.

Patients receiving aspirin therapy should be given ascorbic acid on a supplementary basis.

Potassium supplementation may be indicated for athletes engaged in long-term repetitive exercise. Progressive reduction of serum potassium levels during training are interpreted as a possible detrimental effect on muscular function.

Potassium supplements in heart disease are superior to any other treatment.

Regular exercise often improves the health and the adverse symptoms disappear for diabetics, particularly among mature-onset diabetics. Use of formulas to normalize liver function can also help them.

Refractory anemia of the iron-deficiency type may be the result of chronic blood loss in patients receiving regular aspirin therapy.

Vitamin A reduces risk of stress ulcer. Increased intake of vitamin A preserves the function and normal growth of mucus cells in the gastrointestinal tract; thus preventing the occurrence of ulcers in many stress situations.

Only 7 out of 60 medical schools offer nutrition courses and those are more likely to be incorporated into other courses than taught as an individual science.

Aging may now be considered to result from an accumulation of defective protein molecules within the cells, for test tube experiments show changes in ratios of protein to DNA and in concentrations of various enzymes.

Chelated magnesiums carry a negative charge so they do not adhere to the negative charged cells of the stomach wall. They pass readily through stomach tissues into the bloodstream.

Women who use oral contraceptives are twice as likely to develop gallbladder disease as those who don't. Gallbladder disease may have something to do with the hormone estrogen.

Humidity and exercise can cause a strain on the body as temperature rises. Often essential electrolytes such as magnesium or potassium are lost. These are important for normal muscle activity, especially for heart muscle action and rhythm.

Obesity is a prevalent health problem, at every age, in both sexes, and at every economic level in the USA today. A person is generally considered to be obese if he weighs more than 20% above the average for his age and height. The greatest increase in weight occurs in the 20 to 30 age group.

Obesity and overweight are not considered to be a cause of death; however, they are closely associated with increased mortality from other conditions. Statistics reveal that overweight people are more likely to develop certain diseases and die at a younger age than people of normal weight.

Diabetes mellitus is becoming a leading cause of arthritis. Liver malfunction which is thought to contribute to poor calcium utilization, is also considered a principle reason.

Gallstones are formed from cholesterol in patients who lack enough bile acid to keep the cholesterol suspended. There are about 300,000 gallstone operations performed yearly.

Lactobacillus acidophilus is a nonmotile organism normal to the intestine of humans.

The bacterium creates a distinctly acid stool. The acidity produced is believed to aid in the absorption of calcium and the bacterium enhances the intestinal synthesis of B vitamins. Some forms of arthritis respond dramatically to normalization of the flora.

Clubbing of the fingers has been linked to colitis and a deficient acidophilus.

A severe form of arthritis called ankylosing spondylitis has been reported as associated with colitis and deficient acidophilus.

The widespread use of antibiotics results in many intestinal upsets and liver malfunction due to loss of the intestinal flora. Colitis, constipation, diarrhea, gingivitis, cold sores, perianal itching.

Upset of the intestinal microbial equilibrium can occur from diverticulosis, dieting, aging, fatigue, menses, upper respiratory infections, alcohol, emotional stresses and extensive dental procedures.

Obesity increases surgical risk; is a hazard in pregnancy; prevents self-care in arthritis and increases fracture risk in the aged; places a greater load on the heart and circulatory system; and increases the work in breathing. Reduction in weight to normal levels increases the likelihood of success in treating the above.

Liver impairment in the obese is a basic cause of uncontrolled hunger and rapidly falling blood sugar.

Conditions of spasm and calcification of muscles of digital arterioles and skin areas seem to respond to vitamin E's beneficial effects on circulation and softening of the tissues. The action of vitamin E as an antioxidant is valuable to cell membranes and intracellular organelles which contain lipoproteins.

Aging "turns off" protein synthesis. Aging causes patients to lose their ability to provide the enzymes necessary so RNA can help build new tissues.

Selenium and vitamin E function together in preventing oxidation of fats. Nutritional inadequacy of selenium is thought to underlie various chronic diseases caused by such oxidation of fats, including cardiovascular disease.

In areas where selenium intake is low, death rates from hypertension-related disease, including stroke, are up to 300% higher than in selenium-rich areas.

Selenium has proven essential as an antioxident working in partnership with vitamin E for more complete biological activity.

High blood pressure is relieved in animals by supplemental selenium.

Animals deficient in selenium fail to reproduce because sperm cells cannot be formed without this mineral.

A combination of selenium and vitamin E has been used in veterinary medicine to treat canine arthritis. Veterinarians report dramatic success.

Zinc protects against lead poisoning. Increased zinc intake sets up a process in the intestinal area inhibiting lead absorption.

Zinc is of great importance in the functioning of the pancreas. It is a necessary factor in the male genital tract, especially the prostate gland, the eye and other organs. The pancreas needs zinc for the normal synthesis of insulin.

Zinc in the cells control various body processes through association with enzymes. It is found in greatest proportion in the hair. Next comes the prostate gland, then kidney, liver, muscle, aorta, heart, pancreas, spleen, ovary, testes, lung, brain and adrenal.

Canning depletes zinc. Refining of flour reduces zinc contents in white bread as compared to whole wheat.

A zinc deficient diet produces irreversible damage to the male reproductive organs of rats and significant but reversible damage to the esophagus in the same animals.

Injections of zinc concentrations brought recovery of the esophage area in 124 hours but did not improve the condition of the damaged male reproductive organs.

A very mild zinc deficiency caused as many as 50% of animals to be deformed at birth. Some were fatal causing as many as 30% of the animals to die within 7 days. Phytate, a form of phosphorus present in many foods, tends to block zinc utilization from the diet. Unfortunately many natural foods are rich in phytate.

Drinking aggravates the problem. Alcohol tends to flush zinc out of the system.

Zinc is helpful in the management of rheumatoid arthritis.

The need for zinc is world-wide and its deficiency is only secondary to nitrogen deficiency among soil fertility problems.

Zinc is essential in advanced or inoperative vascular disease, alcoholism, atherosclerosis, diabetes, occulusions, stenosis.

Zinc deficiency attributed to dwarfism, dermatitis, disruption of extrous cycle.

Zinc is essential in healing of arterial injuries, improvement in mental processes, upper respiratory infections. Cancerous patients are reported to have low zinc levels.

Zinc deficiency prevents incorporation of phosphorus into liver cells, interfering with nucleic acid metabolism.

Zinc is a precious metal for pregnant mothers. The babies from mothers deprived of zinc were smaller and had smaller-than-normal brains.

RNA weekly injections more than doubled the lifespan of rats.

Zinc is readily displaced by cadmium, which interferes with certain enzyme systems requiring zinc. Cadmium in kidneys in relation to zinc contributed to the cause of high blood pressure.

Foods rich in selenium are organ meats such as liver and kidney, marine seafoods and whole grains grown on high selenium soils. Fruits and vegetables (with the exception of garlic and mushrooms) contain very little.

Professor Jackson, University of Minnesota Department of Anatomy, has shown that rats fed 155 days on an 80% cooked food diet revealed an increased pancreas weight of 20-30%. It is known that Filipinos and Malays, due to their daily rice intake, have a pancreas 25-50% larger than the average.

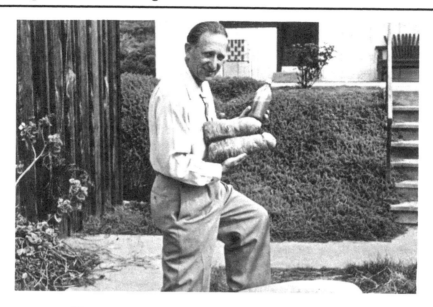

We grew some of the largest carrots anyone had ever seen.

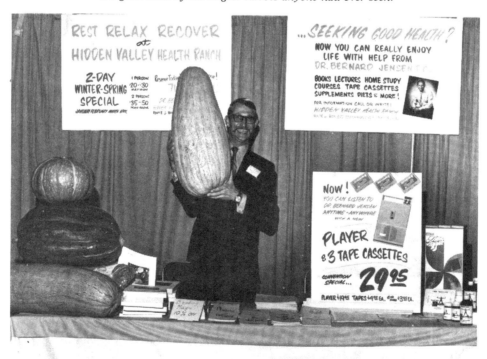

Arthur Jensen, my son, displays one of the gigantic squash that grew from the rich black soil of my Ranch. This was at the National Health Federation Convention in Los Angeles, California.

eighteen

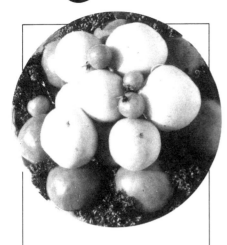

Trace elements

There are many new trace elements which have been discovered and investigated since Rocine first began expounding the virtues of the sixteen major chemical elements. These newly discovered trace minerals are just as important as the sixteen basic elements, but are not required in the same amounts for body processes.

We must consider the trace elements as well as the major elements. Successful work has been done with new trace minerals in the past few years, treating symptoms discovered to be caused by their deficiency in the body. Some of this information is included here to show the value of newer trace elements in the human body.

Trace Elements

Aluminum. Biochemic aluminum, as found in human and animal tissues, is integral to good health, but its specific functions are, as yet, undetermined. A distinction must be made between the biochemic and chemical forms. The latter is easily absorbed and forms residues in the body, especially in the arteries. Aluminum cooking utensils are the chief source of chemical aluminum residues and many doctors advise against the use of aluminum utensils, as a precautionary measure. Other possible sources of undesirable aluminum are baking powders, some bleached white flour, children's aspirin and false teeth.

Chemical aluminum has a weakening effect on the entire digestive tract. It also damages the efficiency of vitamins in the body.

This element—aluminum—exists in nature in compounds with other elements, never in the free form.

Approximately 50 to 150 milligrams of aluminum are found in the body of an adult male or female. The daily intake of aluminum is estimated to be 10 to 100 milligrams or more.

Symptoms of excessive aluminum, biochemical (food form) or chemical and drug form, include constipation, nausea, skin problems, colic, lack of appetite, convulsions in leg muscles, profuse perspiration, fatigue or lack of energy. A poisoning, indicated by motor paralysis and localized numbness is accompanied by fatty degeneration of kidneys and liver. The nervous

In New Zealand sheep became paralyzed when they fed on range depleted of cobalt. The problem was solved by adding 3-4 founds of cobalt to the acre.

Selenium—helps prevent cell breakdown. One study showed low levels reduced enlarged muscle tissue around the heart. Another study showed it aided healing of connective tissue, reducing muscle discomfort and aiding mobility. Recommended intake is 50-200 micrograms/day, as advised by the Food and Nutrition Board of the National Academy of Sciences. Food sources are considered the best method of intake; i.e., seafood, kidney, liver, meats, dairy foods, fruits and vegetables.

To know your foods, their chemical makeup and their activity in the body is to be able to eliminate deficiency symptoms due to disease.

system and digestive tract undergo unfavorable changes in an effort to eliminate the foreign and harmful substance.

Arsenic. The chemical form of arsenic is a widely-acclaimed poison. However, in food form, arsenic is essential for proper human nutrition. Traces of arsenic are found throughout the body in varying quantities and are concentrated mostly in the liver. The liver seems to store this element and releases it into the bloodstream, as needed. Arsenic is released to the blood during menstruation and during the fifth and sixth months of pregnancy and also in cases of cancer.

More research is needed into the function of arsenic in the human body. In spite of the fact that arsenic is closely correlated with human physiology, its precise role in the human body is still not explained by biochemistry.

Beryllium. This trace mineral is known as an agent in neon signs, electronic equipment, some alloys including steel, bicycle wheels, common house products and fishing rods. As an industrial agent, it endangers the breathing apparatus of those coming in contact with it and permanent lung damage is possible (scar tissue and fibrosis).

The effects of beryllium on the human body are detrimental, especially as it destroys the reserve of magnesium (the "relaxer"). Vital organs are attacked by beryllium because the bloodstream often deposits it in them. The body's enzyme activities are disrupted by beryllium to a considerable extent.

Boron. Boron is known to be an essential nutrient for plant growth. Experiments disclose that plants could not grow properly without boron, even when all other necessary nutrients were present. Boron is believed to influence calcium utilization by plants. Due to its universal presence in soil, boron is acknowledged as an integral part of plant and animal nutrition. Its specific purpose in the human body is not yet known.

Bromine. Although it has been found constantly present in the blood, little scientific data is available on bromine. Manic-depressive psychoses are characterized by a lowered bromine level in the blood to about half the normal amount which remains low until improvement in the patient is evident. The bromine level is altered during menstruation. The growth-monitoring portion of the pituitary gland contains seven to ten times the bromine concentration of any other organ. Bromine levels vary markedly with age. After age 45, the bromine level begins to drop and at age 75, only a trace remains, if at all.

Sea plants such as kelp and dulse contain traces of bromine, as do mussels, sea water and animal glands. Further research will divulge the role of bromine in the human body.

Cadmium. The necessity of cadmium for health of the human body has not been determined. It is toxic to all body processes. It is associated with zinc and bears many similarities to this element. Zinc is believed to act as a policing agent to keep the cadmium from harming the body.

Cadmium is present, primarily, in refined foods such as white flour, white sugar, polished rice. It is also found in the air due to industrial pollution. Soft water usually contains higher quantities than hard water. Coffee and tannic acid in tea are high in cadmium which is another reason for avoiding them entirely.

Cadmium and zinc are stored in the liver and kidneys. A zinc deficiency is often accompanied by an excess of cadmium in the system. (The normal ratio of cadmium to zinc in whole wheat, for example, is 1 to 120.) It is estimated that the average daily ingestion of cadmium is 0.2 to 0.5 milligrams (according to dietary differences). Cadmium has a cumulative toxic effect in the body. A sufficient reserve of zinc counteracts cadmium's detrimental effects.

Recently, researchers determined that cadmium is a factor in hypertension (high blood pressure). Tests revealed that the urine of patients with high blood pressure symptoms is abnormally high in cadmium. Cadmium may also be linked to heart complications.

Currently, no information is available regarding the effects of cadmium deficiency. Benefits to health have likewise not been established.

Chromium. The blood contains approximately 20 parts of chromium per one billion parts. A Recommended Daily Allowance of chromium has not been established. The daily chromium absorbed by adults is approximately 80 to 100 micrograms. There is no known toxicity.

Absorption of chromium is difficult and the body holds only about 3% of the intake. The kidneys, spleen and testes are the principal storage organs for chromium. Trace amounts are also found stored in the heart, lungs, pancreas, brain. Some enzymes also contain traces, as does the RNA factor. The kidneys excrete most of the chromium. Elderly individuals are unable to store as much chromium in the body as are younger people.

Enzymes that are implicated in the metabolism of glucose, for energy and for the formation of fatty acid and cholesterol compounds, are stimulated by chromium. The performance of insulin is enhanced by chromium, enabling more efficient transfer of glucose to cells. It vies with iron for carrying proteins. The formation of protein and RNA compounds is influenced by chromium. No data dealing with excess amounts of chromium in the body are currently available.

Chromium deficiency has a pronounced effect on the body. Soil of American farms is deficient in chromium. Other countries are rarely found to have chromium-deficient soils. The refining of starches and carbohydrates also robs food of its chromium supply.

According to current research, chromium deficiency is believed to be a factor in atherosclerosis. It also is implicated in amino acid metabolism in conjunction with insulin. A deficiency disrupts the insulin function, resulting in extreme glucose intolerance in diabetics and a stunted growth rate.

The blood balance of chromium aids in regulation of sugar levels in the blood. Good sources of chromium are corn oil, cloves and other spices, whole grain cereals, clams, meat. Traces are found also in fruits and vegetables. Brewer's yeast offers a good supplemental source of chromium.

Cobalt. This element has been established as a necessary constituent of human nutrition. Cobalt is an important agent of vitamin B-12 (cobalamin). They are an important team in the human body.

Many enzymes of the body are stimulated by cobalt. The performance of red corpuscles, especially, and other body cells as well are normalized by cobalt.

The human body does not easily assimilate cobalt. What is absorbed is excreted chiefly through the kidneys. Red blood cells store cobalt, as does plasma. Smaller amounts are stored in the kidneys, liver, pancreas and spleen.

A Recommended Daily Allowance has not been established since the amount needed is extremely small. The average daily amount obtained from the diet is about 5 to 8 micrograms.

Excessive cobalt in the body is believed to attack the thyroid gland, causing its enlargement or toxicity.

Cobalt deficiency is possibly responsible for symptoms inherent in pernicious anemia and a stunted or retarded growth rate. Prolonged cobalt deficiency may result in irreversible nerve damage.

Cobalt has been proven an effective agent in pernicious anemia (to be used only under strict medical supervision) by building red blood cells. The blood and circulatory system, in general, are both benefitted by cobalt. It increases the assimilation of iron.

A strict vegetarian diet is in danger of lacking sufficient cobalt (and B-12). The best sources of cobalt are raw milk, goat milk, apricots, meats (especially liver and kidneys), oysters, clams, sea vegetation.

Copper. Traces of copper are present in all body tissues. It is a partner in the formation of hemoglobin and red blood cells because of its ability to increase iron assimilation.

Many enzymes responsible for disintegrating and building tissues contain copper. The amino acid tyrosine is converted into a dark pigment that gives color to skin and hair. Protein metabolism and general healing functions are influenced by copper. Synthesis of phospholipids requires copper. They are the necessary ingredients of myelin nerve sheaths which form a protective covering for nerve fibers. Vitamin C oxidation is improved by copper and it joins forces with vitamin C for producing elastin, a major constituent of the elastic muscle fibers of the entire body. It is also integral in the formation of RNA (ribonucleic acid). It may be destructive to vitamin C in the body; however, according to Adams and Murray in *Improving Your Health with Niacin*.

About 30% of copper taken into the body is utilized. It is absorbed through the walls of the stomach and small intestine. Fifteen minutes after being taken into the body, copper is absorbed into the bloodstream. Wornout copper is eliminated chiefly through the bowel and in bile. Minute amounts are expelled through the kidneys.

Tissues of the body store the largest portion of copper. It is found most concentrated in the liver, heart, kidneys and brain tissues. To a lesser extent, the bones and muscles contain copper but they house about 50% of it due to their percentage of body makeup.

The Recommended Daily Allowance of copper is set at 2 milligrams for adults. It is estimated that the normal daily intake of copper is from 2.5 to 5.0 milligrams and at least 2 milligrams per day are essential. About 200 to 150 milligrams of copper are found in the human body.

Excess of copper is not commonly known because a small percentage is assimilated. The larger percentage is eliminated. Wilson's disease, an uncommon genetic malfunction, is attributed to paranormal copper metabolism, causing the liver, brain, kidneys and corneas of the eyes to hold excessive copper.

Copper deficiency is rare. Low levels of copper in the blood of children suffering iron-deficiency anemia, edema and kwashiorkor are found occasionally. Copper shortage is characterized by general feebleness, oppressed breathing and skin eruptions or sores.

Copper is a partner of iron in the formation of hemoglobin. This partnership aids the correction of anemia. Edema is prevented by the proper balance of copper in the body, especially in children. Disorders which are possibly improved by copper are anemia, osteoporosis, baldness, bedsores, edema.

The best food sources of copper are liver, whole grain cereals, almonds, green, leafy vegetables and dried legumes or beans. Sea food is a good source of copper, in general.

Germanium. Germanium is one of the most dynamic new discoveries in the realm of trace elements that are necessary for the optimum nutrition of man. This amazing element raises the level of activity of various organs by enabling them to attract more oxygen. Germanium is responsible for bringing more oxygen to the body as well as expelling volatile and harmful pollutants and germ life or rendering them harmless. As a semiconductor of electricity, germanium helps correct distortions in the electrical aggregate of man's body. Dr. Azuhiko Asai, of Tokyo, Japan, the discoverer of the nutritional properties of germanium, attributes all diseases to a deficiency of oxygen in tissues and body fluids. Germanium brings life-giving oxygen to the body.

Organic germanium has proven successful in dealing with pathologies including asthma, diabetes, hypertension, cardiac insufficiency, inflammation of maxillary sinus, neuralgia, leukemia, softening of brain tissues, myoma of the uterus, neurotic disorders, nephritis, hepatic cirrhosis and various cancers (breast, lung, bladder, larynx) according to the research findings of Dr. Asai.

The best sources of organic germanium are garlic, ginseng, aloe vera, comfrey, chlorella and all chlorophyll-rich foods.

Lead. Today, lead poisoning has become increasingly common. Lead is an extremely toxic trace mineral, responsible for toxic reactions in the body when present in amounts in excess of one or two milligrams. One part per million lead is equivalent to nearly one milligram in two pounds of food.

Algin, a constituent of kelp has been found successful in combating lead poisoning. Liquid chlorophyll is also beneficial.

The body assimilates lead with difficulty, but the alarming prevalence of lead in the atmosphere, cosmetics, hair dyes, water pipes, automobile exhaust, cigarette smoke, lead based paints, lead laden cooking utensils and containers, lead glazed pottery and even moonshine whiskey, makes it an increasingly serious problem. It is absorbed through the skin pores and the digestive tract; from here it enters the bloodstream and is deposited for storage in the bones and the soft tissues of the body, especially the liver. The body can successfully eliminate lead up to certain saturation levels. The above listings, in addition to deposits of lead in plants and vegetation next to busy roads, are serious sources of lead poisoning.

Symptoms of lead poisoning include abdominal colic, myelopathy (pathology of the spinal cord), encephalopathy (malfunction of the brain).

No data is available regarding organic lead and its role in the human body, if any. It is not currently known to have beneficial effects in the body.

Lead poisoning is counteracted by calcium, calcium chloride and vitamin E as well as the previously mentioned agents.

Lithium. Lithium, a mineral found in some rock formations and in the ocean, may have a connection with mental stability. Although it is harmful in excess, small amounts of lithium may be useful in treating depression and alcoholism. The average daily intake is about 2 milligrams per day; however, it is still classified as a trace element "nonessential to human nutrition."

Mercury. The atmosphere contains considerable mercury, especially due to industrial use of mercury and its compounds. Mercury has no known necessary function in the human body. Occasionally mercury is found in measurable amounts in inland fish from waters polluted by mercury from industrial use.

Chemical mercury poses no real threat to the human body. Its compounds methyl mercury and ethyl mercury are dangerous, however. Agriculture and industry use massive quantities of methyl mercury in pesticides, fungicides, chemical by-products and end-products of chlorine, and as mercury vapor from smoke stacks. These chemicals are detrimental to the central nervous system if imprisoned in tissues for considerable lengths of time.

An adult averages about 0.5 milligram mercury intake daily through foods. Mercury chloride is a poison; 500 milligrams have lethal power.

Subacute mercury poisoning is identified by excessive salivation, stomatitis and diarrhea; also Parkinsonian shaking, vertigo, moodiness, irascibility, depression, melancholia. Brain damage may result from the assault of methyl mercury on the central nervous system. Methyl mercury poisoning is indicated by symptoms of vision and hearing impairment, loss of mental ability, uncoordination.

Mercury is found in the liver. It is not injurious to human health in the normally-absorbed quantities, but in the drug form it will injure the kidneys.

Molybdenum. Nearly all tissues in animals and plant life contain molybdenum. Xanthine and oxidase, enzymes which help draw iron from its reserve stores in the liver, must have molybdenum for their function; oxidase is also essential for oxidation of fats in the body.

Tiny traces of molybdenum are found in the human body; it is absorbed from the digestive tract and eliminated through the kidneys. The liver, bones and kidneys store molybdenum.

Molybdenum is not found in many common foodstuffs; thus there is no Recommended Daily Allowance. The estimated daily need is only about 100 mcg. Signs of toxicity include diarrhea, anemia and stunted or retarded growth.

Excessive molybdenum is believed to precipitate copper reserves.

Prevention of anemia may be a function of molybdenum; the liver is involved. No deficiency signs have been found to date.

Nickel. Large quantities of nickel are present in the human body. Its function in the human body is not clear, but it is an essential trace mineral for the nutrition of man. Nickel acts as a catalyst in the hydrogenation of vegetable oils such as corn, peanut and cottonseed oils.

Nickel is more concentrated in the pancreas than in any other organ. It is more widely distributed than cobalt in human tissues. It comes largely from whole grains and oysters. More study is necessary to learn about the role of nickel in human nutrition, as its biological function is not as yet known.

Selenium. Selenium is an essential trace mineral which enters the body in exceptionally small amounts. Only about three millionths of an ounce enter the human constitution. Vitamin E works with selenium in metabolic functions and in the assurance of normal body growth and fertility. It is a youth element in the sense that it encourages tissue elasticity by delaying oxidation of polyunsaturated fatty acids that can promote hardening of tissue proteins. It is an antioxidant which naturally reduces retention of toxic metals in the body.

The Recommended Daily Allowance of selenium for an adult is minute; only five to ten parts per million is toxic to the human body. Its toxicity is a result of an inclination to replace sulphur colloids and compounds and hinders the performance of certain enzymes. Cases of selenium toxicity have been reported in areas having soil rich in selenium. Excessive selenium can cause hair loss, fever, dermatitis, paralysis.

Muscles and other tissues contain tiny traces of selenium. The liver and kidneys hold four to five times that amount, though still extremely small. The kidneys are responsible for eliminating selenium; if it is found in the stool, it has been abnormally absorbed.

A selenium deficiency may contribute to premature aging, since when present it preserves tissue elasticity. Most of the soil in the United States is deficient in selenium; this may contribute to such problems as high blood pressure and infertility.

A diet containing protein and the correct dosage of selenium are beneficial in dealing with kwashiorkor (a protein deficiency disorder).

Good sources of selenium are bran and germ of cereals and grains, broccoli, onions, tomatoes, tuna, asparagus, mushrooms. Meat, eggs, nuts, milk products and seafood are fair sources of selenium. The amount of selenium in vegetables depends on the selenium available in the soil in which they were grown.

Tin. Due to its profuse use in the canning industry, tin has recently gained considerable publicity. Tin is found in many human tissues. It seems to be concentrated in the suprarenals (or adrenal) glands and occurs in measurable amounts in the liver, brain tissues, spleen and thyroid gland.

The mucous membrane of the tongue also has considerable tin. The biochemical and metallic or mineral form of tin have not been proven detrimental to the human body.

Vanadium. Vanadium is a trace mineral necessary to the adequate nutrition of man. The vanadium level in the human organism is difficult to measure; about 90% of imbibed vanadium is excreted through the kidneys. Due to its presence in such microscopic amounts an overdose is easily possible.

The circulatory system needs vanadium for proper regulation. Excessive cholesterol deposits in blood vessels are prevented when vanadium is present in the brain in sufficient quantities. Cholesterol buildup in the central nervous system can be combatted by vanadium.

The best sources of vanadium are fish, seafood, kelp and some vegetables. Gelatin and bone meal are good sources when from animals

that are not themselves deficient in vanadium. It is possible that it can be inhaled directly from the air.

Zinc. Zinc follows iron in quantity in the human body. About five grams of iron are found in the body to 1.8 grams of zinc.

The upper part of the small intestine absorbs zinc. It is expelled chiefly through the bowel; a very small quantity is eliminated through the kidneys. The greatest percentage of zinc is stored in the thyroid, pancreas, liver, kidneys, bones and voluntary muscles; it is also stored in parts of the eyes, in the prostate gland and spermatozoa, skin, hair, nails (finger and toe) and in white blood corpuscles.

A high consumption of calcium and phytic acid is believed to curtail assimilation of zinc (this specific source of calcium and phytic acid is in certain grains). If this is the case, zinc intake should also be increased to maintain proper balance.

Zinc's functions in the human body are diversified. It enters the proper assimilation of vitamins and their proper functions (notably B complex). Some 25 enzymes needed in digestion and metabolism, even respiration, depend on a proper supply of zinc. Carbohydrate digestion and phosphorus metabolism are influenced by zinc. The synthesis of nucleic acid calls for zinc for proper formation of different proteins in each cell. All-around growth and normal development of sexual organs and the reproductive system, and proper function of the prostate gland require sufficient zinc. It is found in insulin and is also a constituent of the enzyme which disorganizes alcohol.

In addition, zinc has been found beneficial in proper healing of burns and wounds. The synthesis of DNA (dioxyribonucleic acid) which is entrusted with the genetic code necessary for duplication of each cell—needs zinc; DNA contains all inherited traits passed on to the next generation.

The Recommended Daily Allowance of zinc is set at 15 milligrams. The allowance is upped to 30 milligrams during pregnancy and to 25 milligrams during lactation. The average diet contains from 10 to 15 milligrams of zinc.

Compared to many trace elements, zinc is much less toxic (poisoning is possible from eating foods stored in steel galvanized containers). If the assimilation of zinc is excessive, coppper metabolism is disrupted; this results in improper and incomplete iron metabolism. Iron and copper are precipitated rapidly from the liver if zinc intake is overbalanced. Vitamin A is also required in larger amounts when zinc supplements are added to the diet.

Zinc deficiency may result from an unbalanced diet. Alcohol consumption flushes zinc reserves out of the liver; it is excreted through the kidneys. Extreme fatigue may be attributed in part to zinc deficiency; tendency to infections, injuries and dulled awareness may indicate a shortage of zinc. Lack of sufficient zinc may cause retarded growth, delayed sexual development and extremely slow healing of wounds. Atherosclerosis may be facilitated partly by zinc, copper and vanadium deficiencies.

Cadmium, a toxic trace mineral, contributes to a zinc shortage. Cadmium is stored in the body when zinc is not present; high intake of cadmium increases the tendency toward zinc deficiency. Zinc intake must be increased to combat the detrimental effects of cadmium.

Sterility and dwarfed stature are attributed to zinc deficiency. Abnormal or pathological changes take place in the prostate when zinc is lacking. The prostate gland contains the highest concentration of zinc in the entire body (males).

Alcoholic cirrhosis demonstrates low levels of zinc in the blood; the same is true of other liver pathology, ulcers, heart attacks, mongolian idiots and cystic fibrosis. Pregnancy and oral contraceptives also reduce the level of zinc in women.

In leukemia and Hodgkin's disease, zinc is precipitated at an alarming rate.

Symptoms of zinc deficiency include excessive fatigue, loss of natural taste sensitivity, loss of appetite and poor growth.

Cholesterol deposits are dissolved by zinc, in combination with other factors. Atherosclerosis is benefitted by zinc. Healing of internal injuries is speeded up by zinc; any arterial injuries are more rapidly healed with zinc. Still other external wounds heal more rapidly due to zinc.

Infertility and sterility are prevented and corrected with zinc and other elements combined. The sexual system develops properly when a zinc reserve is in the body. Hodgkin's

disease and leukemia may be benefitted by zinc. Cirrhosis of the liver and alcoholism call for zinc. Diabetes is aided by zinc because it helps properly regulate insulin in the blood and promotes the proper release of glycogen from the liver as needed. Combined with insulin, zinc helps maintain the proper blood sugar level. Tests have shown that the pancreas of the diabetic patient contains half the normal quantity of zinc.

The liver of an infant contains more than three times the amount of zinc found in the liver of an adult. This suggests that zinc is stored in the infant's liver before birth as in the case of iron and copper. Mother's milk contains the highest percentage of zinc immediately after giving birth. For a period of ten to fifteen days, there is a sharp drop in the zinc level, and then it levels off to a uniform quantity.

A zinc deficiency produced in test animals proved the need for zinc in human nutrition in 1935. But its specific functions are still somewhat vague.

The best sources of zinc in foods are mother's milk, cow's milk, goat milk, brewer's yeast, whole grain cereals, high protein foods, wheat bran, wheat germ, pumpkin seeds (one of the best sources). Unrefined and unprocessed foods contain more zinc.

Other Trace Elements

Casesium, rubium, strontium, silver, gold, titanium, tritium and traces of nearly all other metals have been detected in human tissues. Their role in human nutrition is not yet known in many cases. More research is indicated. However, more information is being formulated rapidly.

Don't underestimate the vital role of trace elements in the health of man. Make sure they are obtained from food sources. While not everything is known about all the functions of mineral elements, we have presented them knowing that many are very important in the normal functioning of our bodies.

We hope it will also convince you that the addition of a few chemicals to the soil, as is the general practice in our country, is not enough— the soil must be prepared according to the laws of nature.

Tests and Experiments with Minerals

Calcium

1. A bone meal food, rich in calcium, was used with dramatic effectiveness to build resistance to arthritic conditions and symptoms. (Drs. Frank and Heppner, as reported in Wade, *Magic Minerals: Key to Better Health,* 1967, p. 34).

2. Calcium, in combination with vitamins D and F, counteracts symptoms of menopause, such as hot flashes, leg cramps, night sweats, nervousness and irritability, according to Adelle Davis. (Reported in Wade, *Magic Minerals,* p. 145).

Iodine

1. The relationship of iodine to basal metabolism was studied at the University of Oregon Medical School. During pregnancy, the basal metabolism rate was found to be higher than normal. When iodine was administered, the rate returned to normal. In fact, if the basal rate was low, iodine raised it, as well as *vice versa.* Mothers who received the iodine also felt better during pregnancy and had little difficulty nursing. Apparently, more iodine is needed during pregnancy than at other times. (Reported in Rodale, *The Health Builder,* 1957, pp. 513-514).

2. An Icelandic scientist found a link between iodine, thyroid functioning and hardening of arteries. From some 2,000 autopsies, he discovered that Icelanders, whose diet includes abundant iodine, have smoother aortas and lighter (in weight) thyroid glands than do Austrians who live in goiter regions. When iodine is deficient, the thyroid gland swells and blood vessels tend to harden; it is not known how this process works. *(Science News Letter)* as reported in Rodale, *The Health Builder,* pp. 512-513; see also *Lancet,* the *British Medical Magazine,* July 1959, for similar findings).

3. Sodium iodine was used with good results in treating herpes zoster (shingles). Two grams in 30 cc of water given intravenously every other day was found to be effective in relieving symptoms. (Beck, 1953; *Beers,* 1939; Ruggles, 1931—as reported in Rodale, *The Health Builder,* p. 671).

Magnesium

1. Over a six-week period, a pregnant woman, who had passed 8-12 kidney stones during previous pregnancies, was given 500-1500 mg magnesium daily. She passed no kidney stones during the pregnancy during which she took the magnesium. (Kohler and Uhle, as reported in Rodale, *Complete Book of Minerals for Health,* 1962, p. 78).

2. There seems to be a relationship between the magnesium content of soil and certain causes of death. M. L. Robinet of the French Academy of Medicine says that deaths due to cancer and suicide are more frequent when the soil in the area is poor in magnesium. Deaths due to senility are more rare in those areas. (Reported in Rodale, *The Health Builder,* pp. 545-546).

3. Magnesium tablets were beneficial in reducing or eliminating troublesome nocturnal urination due to prostate gland problems. (Dr. Joseph Favier, as reported in Wade, *Magic Minerals,* p. 138).

Phosphorus

Calcium-phosphorus balance in the body is disturbed by refined white sugar intake. Blood tests showed that there was no change up to two hours after eating a quarter pound of chocolate candy; but 2-1/2 hours afterwards, the phosphorus level in the body dropped 0.5 mg. (Melvin E. Page, DDS, *Degeneration-Regeneration,* 1949, p. 190).

Potassium

Potassium is closely related to the functioning of glands which are affected in cases of diabetes. When potassium is given to patients with **milk,** their blood pressure and blood sugar levels fall. Potassium broth is helpful in bringing patients out of diabetic coma. (Rodale, *The Health Builder,* pp. 695-696.)

Vitamins

Talk about vitamins is on the tongue of nearly every dietitian, housewife, doctor and groceryman today.

Vitamins commanded attention first, it seems in 1794 when citrus fruits were found to prevent scurvy. To date, science has isolated eleven vitamins (not to mention the many sub-vitamins in the B complex) and will probably find many more in the years to come. Vitamins work with minerals in our bodies and help in many ways to build and maintain a healthy body.

Natural foods contain all the vitamins that have been and will be discovered. Some diseases are the result, at least partially, of a vitamin-starved diet. When the body is deprived of vitamin-rich food, disease is much more likely to occur. It is the quality of foods that counts—not the quantity. Vitamins essential to the body are best found in natural foods, preferably raw and certainly unprocessed.

Vitamin A

Vitamin A. Fat-soluble; antiophthalmic. RDA 5,000 I.U.

Conditions Caused by Lack of A. Loss of weight and vigor; loss of vitality and growth; loss of strength and glandular balance. Susceptibility to infection. Eye infections, night blindness, poor vision. Poor digestion, emaciation; acne; diarrhea, nephritis; rough, dry skin.

Conditions Controlled by Vitamin A. Makes tissues more resistant to colds and catarrh, especially in respiratory organs, sinuses, ears, bladder, skin and digestive tract. Increases blood platelets. Promotes growth and feeling of well-being. Fights infection and bacteria. Important to health of eyes, bones, teeth, skin tissue.

Foods Rich in Vitamin A. Green, leafy vegetables and yellow vegetables; spinach, chard, leaf lettuce, cabbage, tomatoes, carrots, peas, sweet potatoes, endive, beet greens, mustard greens, brussels sprouts, celery, yellow squash, butterfat, egg yolk, whole milk, fish liver oil, cheese, bananas, apricots, peaches, melon, cherries, papaya, avocado, mango, prunes, pineapple.

Stabililty. Cooking temperatures do not affect A very much, but it is destroyed by heat in the presence of oxygen, by overcooking, by high temperatures and by excessive light.

Storage. Stored in the body but depleted quickly under strain and/or stress.

Vitamin B. All B complex vitamins can be cultivated from bacteria, yeasts, fungu or molds. Known B vitamins include B-1 (thiamine), B-2 (riboflavin), B-3 (niacin), B-6 (pyridoxine), B-12 (cyanocobalamine), B-13 (orotic acid), B-15 (pangamic acid), B-17 (laetrile), biotin, choline, folic acid, inositol, PABA (para-aminobenzoic acid) and pantothenic acid. All B vitamins are water-soluble and anti-neuritic.

Conditions Caused by Lack of B. Nervous exhaustion, loss of growth, loss of reproductive function, loss of appetite; beriberi; polyneuritis; intestinal disorders, fermentation, faulty nutrition and assimilation, indigestion, convulsions, soreness and pain; slow heart beat; impaired secretion of insulin; fatigue; dull hair, dry skin, acne.

Conditions Controlled by Vitamin B. Improves absorption of food and normalizes the brain and nervous system by increasing metabolic processes; maintains muscle tone in intestinal tract. Promotes health of skin, hair, eyes, mouth, liver.

Foods Rich in Vitamin B. Yeast, egg yolk, whole milk, lean beef, liver, kidney, asparagus, peas, spinach, tomatoes, turnip greens, mustard greens, chard, celery, carrots, potatoes, cabbage, beet greens, cauliflower, leaf lettuce, broccoli, onions, peppers, grapefruit, lemons, oranges, bananas, pineapple, apples, melon, peaches, avocados, grapes, prunes, dates, cherries, pears, whole grains, almonds, walnuts, chestnuts, Brazil nuts, pecans, all legumes.

Stability. Ordinary cooking does not affect B, although high heat destroys it, as does soda used to keep vegetables green.

Storage. Stored in the body in limited quantities so must be replaced daily.

Vitamin B-1 (Thiamin). RDA 1.4 mg for men, 1.0 mg for women; or 0.5 mg per 1000 calories ingested.

Conditions Caused by Lack of B-1. Fatigue, loss of appetite, heart and nerve trouble, gastrointestinal disorders.

Conditions Controlled by Vitamin B-1. Needed for metabolism of carbohydrates. Fosters good muscle tone and growth. Preserves health of nervous system; provides pep; stabilizes appetite.

Foods Rich in Vitamin B-1. Yeast, yogurt, whole wheat and wheat germ, other whole grains, sprouts and seeds, potatoes, barley, wild rice, lean meat and organ meats, shellfish and fish roe, almonds, beans and peas.

Stability. Foods should not be overcooked or oversoaked. Cooking water should be drunk.

Storage. Stored in the body in limited quantities; must be supplied daily.

Vitamin B-2 (Riboflavin). RDA 1.6 mg for adults.

CAUTION
Overdose can kill infants!

Conditions Caused by Lack of B-2. Dermatitis; sores and cracks in the mouth; retarded growth; eye disorders; digestive upsets.

Conditions Controlled by Vitamin B-2. Carbohydrate, fat and protein metabolism; cell respiration; formation of red blood cells and antibodies.

Foods Rich in Vitamin B-2. Mustard and other greens, wheat germ, yeast, yogurt, organ meats, soybeans, broccoli, mushrooms, nuts and seeds, fruits, parsley.

Stability. Destroyed by light.

Storage. Must be supplied daily.

Vitamin B-3 (Niacin). RDA 1.8 mg for men, 13 mg for women; or 6.6 mg per 1000 calories ingested.

Conditions Caused by Lack of B-3. Nervous disorders, mental illness and schizophrenia; dermatitis.

Conditions Controlled by Vitamin B-3. Needed for metabolism, for digestive system and for health of skin and tongue.

Foods Rich in Vitamin B-3. Whole grains, bran, wheat germ, rice polishings, organ meats, nut butters, almonds, apricots, soybeans, broccoli, squash, melon, seafood, fish roe, yogurt, mushrooms, seeds, alfalfa.

Stability. Water-soluble so affected by cooking, but more stable than B-1 or B-2.

Storage. Stored in the liver.

Vitamin B-6. RDA 1.8 for men, 1.5 mg for women; or 0.2 mg per 100 mg of protein.

Conditions Caused by Lack of B-6. Nervousness, anemia, weak muscles, dermatitis, mouth problems; oversensitivity to insulin.

Conditions Controlled by Vitamin B-6. Carbohydrate, fat and protein metabolism; balance of sodium and phosphorus in body; formation of blood antibodies.

Foods Rich in Vitamin B-6. Wheat germ, bran, whole grains, organ meats, nut and grain oils, molasses, egg yolk, honey, rich polishings.

Stability. Fifty percent destroyed by overcooking, oversoaking or overwashing. Consume the cooking water to preserve benefit.

Storage. Excreted within 8 hours.

Vitamin B-12. RDA 3 mcg for adults.

Conditions Caused by Lack of B-12. Nerve damage; neuritis; brain damage similar to schizophrenia. Pernicious anemia.

Conditions Controlled by Vitamin B-12. Important for healthy bone marrow; needed for red blood cells; necessary for metabolism of carbohydrates, fats and proteins. Fosters nerve and mental health.

Foods Rich in Vitamin B-12. Liver, kidney, yogurt, cheese, eggs, soybeans, fish and fish roe, whole wheat, kelp. Plants in the United States contain very little B-12 due to soil.

Stability. Destroyed by light, excess acid, excess alkali.

Storage. Stored in blood, bone marrow, glands.

Vitamin C. Water-soluble; antiascorbutic; antioxidant. RDA 45 mg for adults.

Conditions Caused by Lack of C. Tender, swollen gums and joints; poor health, faulty nutrition; loss of appetite, loss of weight; scurvy; irritability; poor complexion; loss of energy; irregular heart action, rapid respiration, poor digestion; reduced hemoglobin; reduced secretion of adrenals; cataracts; hemorrhage, bruising, nosebleeds, slow healing of wounds.

Conditions Controlled by Vitamin C. A marvelous health promoter, as it wards off acidosis. Helps heal wounds, fractures and scar tissue. Strengthens blood vessels.

Foods Rich in Vitamin C. Oranges, lemons, grapefruit, limes, melons, berries, apples, pineapple, cabbage, tomatoes, spinach, peas, broccoli, rutabagas, collards, brussels sprouts, celery, parsley, endive, watercress, turnips, cucumbers, cauliflower, radishes, strawberries.

Stability. Least stable of vitamins. Destroyed by heat, cooking, low temperatures, oxidation, exposure to air and light.

Storage. Not stored in body. Must be replaced every day.

Vitamin D. Fat-soluble; antirachitic. RDA 400 I.U. for adults.

Conditions Caused by Lack of Vitamin D. Rickets, soft bones and teeth, lack of body tone; fatigue, respiratory infections, irritability, restlessness; constipation, ptosis, prolapsus; retarded growth; inadequate calcium absorption; instability of nervous system; dental caries.

Conditions Controlled by Vitamin D. Facilitates absorption of calcium and phosphorus from foods and is a great bone builder. Guards against tuberculosis; regulates mineral metabolism; stabilizes nervous system and heart action.

Foods Rich in Vitamin D. Fish oils, cod liver oil, halibut liver oil, halibut, sardines, fish roe, egg yolk, butter, milk, green leafy vegetables grown in sunshine.

Stability. Heat and oxidation do not normally affect D; however, very high temperatures may injure it.

Storage. Stored in the body in limited amounts. Greatest source is sunlight; ultraviolet rays change ergosterol into D.

Vitamin E. Fat-soluble; antioxidant. RDA 15 I.U. for men; 12 I.U. (women).

Conditions Caused by Lack of Vitamin E. Sterility, loss of adult vitality; unhealthy nervous system; rupturing red blood cells; muscular weakness.

Conditions Controlled by Vitamin E. Essential in reproduction. Aids lactation, menstrual disorders, miscarriage, dull mentality, pessimism, loss of courage; protects red blood cells; prevents blood clots; promotes healing of wounds.

Foods Rich in Vitamin E. Milk, cottage cheese, wheat germ; vegetable oils such as olive oil and soybean oil; green, leafy vegetables, yellow corn, raw fruits.

Stability. Heat and oxidation do not affect E.

Storage. Stored in the body in limited amounts.

Vitamin F (Essemtoa; Unsaturated Fatty Acids). Fat-soluble; growth-promoting; RDA not established. Men need five times more than women.

Conditions Caused by Lack of Vitamin F. Stunted growth, sexual immaturity; brittle or falling hair, baldness; loss of appetite; skin disorders, eczema; varicose veins; nervousness; brittle nails, dandruff, diarrhea.

Foods Rich in Vitamin F. Liquid vegetable oils, whole grains, yeast, eggs, root vegetables, fresh spinach, fruits, nuts, orange juice.

Stability. Long cooking and light destroy F.

Storage. Stored in fat cell tissue.

No ailment is more common among middle-aged males than prostate trouble. By age 50, 20% of American men have enlarged prostates and by age 60, over 50% have it. Zinc deficiency has been linked to prostate trouble.

The proposed ban on saccharin will increase tooth decay because people will eat more sugar and brush less frequently, dentists warned the Food and Drug Administration. The Academy of General Denistry and the toothpaste industry both decried the FDA's proposed ban, which would outlaw 90% of the current uses of saccharin. An Academy spokesman said that without saccharin, toothpastes and fluoride treatments won't taste good.

nineteen

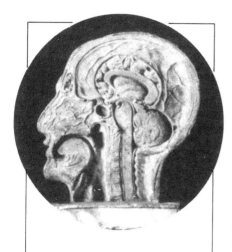

Rocine's temperaments

In 1796, Dr. Francis Gall of Austria discovered the connection between mental faculties in the brain and the temperaments through which they were expressed. All modern forms of character reading are based directly or indirectly on Gall's discovery. He and his student, Spurzheim, originated and expanded upon the Mental Motive and Vital Temperaments in their writings, stimulating the interest of many others in further developing the study of temperaments.

One of the outstanding researchers of the human temperament was Dr. Jacques, who published a book titled *Jacques' Temperaments* in which four basic character types were proposed: the Sanguine, Lymphatic, Billious and Nervous temperaments. In the wake of his work, Dr. Mary O. Stanton, in the 1800s, researched and wrote about five basic systems: the Vegetative (or Vital), the Thoracic (corresponding to Jacques' Sanguine), the Muscular, the Osseous and the Brain and Nervous System.

V. G. Rocine was familiar with the works of all these people and read them with interest. His work in nutrition and homeopathy, however, gave him a quite different perspective. By 1908, he had come to believe there were twenty distinct temperament types.

Many years of experiments and observations led Rocine to the understanding that different persons, due to inherent temperament, metabolic disposition, mental activity and predominant faculties, use the basic chemical elements at different rates, producing chemical imbalances in the body which correspond to distinct types of temperament. He identified twenty basic chemical types with associated temperament types.

Rocine believed there was no such thing as a "normal" metabolism. All persons were imbalanced in some respect, due to a faster or slower rate of utilization of one or more of the main chemical elements in the body. A chemical type, in Rocine's system, is never a balanced man, and that is what, in his view, produced deviations from the "standard" temperament.

The "standard" man in perfect health, for example, would have a perfect balance of the chemical elements, all being used at a harmonious rate of metabolic function. If we assume the standard man has four pounds of calcium, and we discover a man who has eight pounds of calcium in his body, then we can identify him as a

Calciferic Chemical Type with an Osseous Temperament. His mind, faculties, disposition and tendencies all show the influence of calcium. The nature of calcium or lime is slow unfoldment, strength, endurance, persistence and positiveness. This, then, is the key to understanding the nature, disposition and character of a man who uses calcium more than other elements.

If we know this, then we can more easily understand how to take care of a calcium person's diseases, ailments and symptoms. We can change his diet after determining what elements are in short supply in his body and whether this is because they are lacking in his diet or being used up faster in his body. We also look at what elements may be excessive in the diet, because excess can also produce symptoms.

The science of Chemical Types, in short, allows us to understand and systematically use nutrition to bring out the highest possible level of well-being in each person we take care of—including ourselves. It helps us to know and understand the talents, dispositions, characters and health requirements of each person we take care of.

For years, I have been interested in human nature and the mental activities of man. The research and discoveries of V. G. Rocine fascinated me and opened many doors to understanding. I began to compare one man with another, one woman with another. "Why are they different?" I asked myself. Even among trees of the same type on my Ranch, I could see differences in strength, growth rate and hardiness. The inherent qualities, the genetic makeup of living things seemed to be the key to understanding how to take care of them.

Animal breeders have understood the importance of genetic inheritance for many years. Cattle, horses, sheep and even dogs and cats have been bred to bring out certain qualities. Cattle are bred to give more milk. Horses are bred for speed, endurance, agility in ranch work (the Quarter horse, for example). Cats are bred for longer, silkier fur, for shorter ears, for faces of certain types. A certain disposition can be brought out in a horse or other animal. And, it is generally realized that breeding for what we consider a strong quality may also bring out an undesirable weak quality with it.

Of course, we can't experiment with human beings. But we do know from studies of the Royal Families of Europe, where intermarriage was once common, that characteristics of intelligence, sensitivity, perseverence, authority, bravery and so forth can come out of the genetic inheritance—as well as weaknesses such as hemophilia, poor lung structure, thyroid troubles and so on.

Through my studies with V. G. Rocine and Judge Jones, I could see clearly that each person was different and you had to take care of each one differently. I began to understand how there could be such a thing as a natural gift for music, for mathematics, for crime, for mechanical work. One of my sons can take a watch apart and put it back together perfectly. I wouldn't dare try that. Yet, we encounter people who have unique outstanding gifts in some area so often that we know they exist.

At times, people seem to "burn out" certain mental faculties through overwork and poor nutritional habits. Business and corporate executives are a prime example. When an executive must work 10 to 16 hours a day with exactness, seriousness, critical and analytical thinking, the search for success can lead to mental exhaustion or breakdown. Motion picture stars are known to have a similar problem with "burn out."

Among the thousands of patients I've treated, I've noticed a few with exceptional appetites. Science has found a brain center called "the appestat," and I wonder if people with hearty appetites are not designed to have a heavier body. I've wondered about those who would rather read than eat—what kind of body are they meant to have? Would the phosphorus and calcium tend to be used up more in the brain than in the bone structure? These are interesting questions.

The personology work of Judge Jones has been verified in my experience, and I find it consistent with Rocine's work. I know that many mental faculties show up in facial features. Those with sharp chins, I have noticed, have heads that are enlarged significantly in the upper area, and these are idealists, people who tend to be spiritually-minded. We also find people who are physical-minded, parental-minded and sex-minded. When we have an overly sexual person marrying an underly sexual person, many difficulties arise. Sex-mindedness can lead to infidelity.

I am convinced after all this time that as our soul emerges into expression in a physical body, from the time of conception onward, our body attracts the nutrients it needs to become structured according to our mental qualities. Notice how many musicians—Liberace, Frank Sinatra, Stowkowski—have the big, bell-shaped ear. Music has powerful, mind-touching vibrational qualities, and I recall a case in which a boy who had been in a hospital 90 days in a state of coma, came out of it when a great violinist played at his bedside. Was the right chord touched in that boy's brain?

In acupuncture, there are points on the ear which are used to stimulate vision and liver function. A court room artist who has observed thousands of jurors over the years, has stated that the shape of the ears tells much about the personality. The creases on the ears of President Ronald Reagan are said to reveal a tendency to hide his personality. The ear lobes of film star Clint Eastwood and former California governor Jerry Brown are small, indicating considerable indifference to those around them. It is possible that we have much to learn from the human ear alone.

Eyes are revealing. There are loving eyes, analytical eyes. There are people whose eyes are so cold, harsh and hostile that we wouldn't want to meet them on a dark street at night. They seem to reflect a mental tendency that triggers a reaction to get away from them.

I sometimes wonder if there is really such a thing as a highbrow or lowbrow? I wonder also if criminal tendencies can be observed and measured in terms of physical characteristics? I wonder if the high cheekbones observed in Indians, nomadic tribesmen, immigrants and others reflects a love of travel?

When we see such obviously inherited features, we can't help wondering if there are not mental attributes that shape the physical body. I have occasionally pondered over whether there are ways to feed the mind differently and I have pondered over whether fasting is the best way of getting rid of toxic materials in the brain which may be impeding the expression of mental qualities, or may be perverting them. Are people starving for foods that make them feel good?

For jobs that fit their temperaments and talents? For spouses that complement their personalities? For climates and altitudes that bring out their best?

There's a little poem that goes like this.

Carbon Copy
He has his mother's eyes, his father's chin,
His auntie's nose, his uncle's grin,
His great-aunt's hair, his grandma's ears
His grandpa's mouth, so it appears—
Poor little tot,
Well may he moan.
He hasn't much
To call his own.

—Richard Armour

I have encountered a research survey that claims over 90% of the working people in the United States are mismatched to their jobs. The same report claimed that job misfits tended to goof off for up to two-and-a- half hours during an 8-hour work day.

V. G. Rocine often emphasized that an "evolved" phosphorus was needed to feed the brain and mental faculties. He believed that phosphorus derived from animal sources was vibrationally higher and more evolved than that obtained from plants. Phosphorus, we have seen, is called the "light bearer" in its work of bringing light to the mind. It is lecithin that carries the phosphorus and keeps it in the right proportion, while cholesterol gives us the brain-force and power to think accurately, clearly and well.

When Rocine told me the phosphorus from meat fed the combative faculties, I didn't believe him at first. Yet, I have watched the heavy meat eaters, and I believe there is something to Rocine's idea. It seems contradictory to point out that Hitler, Stalin and Mussolini were vegetarians, but the question is, what would they have been like if they ate meat? Certainly, they are no credit to vegetarianism, but it is entirely possible that meat would have brought even harsher qualities out in them.

I sometimes wonder if we could go to the nuts, berries, fruits and vegetables to develop

386

more spiritual qualities or idealistic qualities, and it is an equal challenge to find out the best foods for the competition-minded athlete who is interested in strength, speed, reaction time and winning over his competitors.

When we stop and think about the calcium man, is it possible that we could help him broaden his temperament by holding back on the calcium he seems to draw to himself and utilize so completely? These are things to think about.

The day is coming when everything known about human nature will be put into a computer. Then, many of our complex questions can be answered. Man can see as little as a 50th of an inch, perhaps, but a computer coupled to an optical scanner can see down to thousandths of an inch. When we fill the computer's memory banks with "micro-information" about man, we will be able to make correlations and draw conclusions never before available to science and the healing arts. This is the reason I've been interested in Rocine's temperaments, Judge Jones' personology analysis of facial features and the study of mental faculties.

My diet programs have been worked out with these things in mind. In taking care of any health problem or condition, we must take the whole person into account. Personality and temperament simply can't be separated from the chemical makeup of the person, on the one hand, and the soul expression on the other. The healing process requires changes at the spiritual level, the mental level and the physical level. The patient may need to forgive his wife for an old hurt, change jobs to give expression to a mental faculty which has been held back and change his diet to supply depleted elements. This is why I say health is a way of life.

In my work, iridology has proved its worth a thousand times over by revealing, through the structure, color and markings of the iris, which organs and tissues are chemically depleted. When the diet is corrected, and other appropriate changes are made in getting enough exercise, rest, fresh air, sunshine and recreation, we can see white healing lines coming into the dark areas of the iris that revealed chemical deficiency in the first place. Unless changes are also made at the mental and spiritual levels, however, nutrition can't do the whole job.

Depending on background and training, few persons can be expected to understand and use the wholistic approach right away. So, we start with the role of the chemical elements in nutrition. We start by understanding that each person is made up primarily of 16 chemical elements, that the quantity and disposition of the elements in the body corresponds to the basic 20 temperament types discovered by Rocine, and that taking care of the deficiency or excess among these elements allows change to take place at the mental and spiritual level.

We all understand that cells in the body are dying and being replaced every day. We can, therefore, understand that the rate of replacement and the quality of the new tissue depends upon the nutrients available for rebuilding. To become free of disease, to achieve high level well-being, we must give the mind and spirit the best possible physical vehicle to work through.

The ultimate goal for each person is to understand what type he or she is, what mental faculties are available for use and development, then to begin walking upon the path of life that makes the fullest use possible of all gifts and abilities while recognizing and taking care of inherent weaknesses and the limitations of each type. We need to understand how and why we act, think, work, react, play, marry, reject, reflect, initiate, oppose and feel in terms of who we are.

Well-being is not simply a matter of getting the right treatments in chiropractic, osteopathy or any of the other healing arts. It's not a matter of going into the latest diet fad or getting the body toxin free. It's not a program of vitamins, minerals, fresh juices or vegetarianism. Instead, we must realize that man is a multifaceted being, expressing in action what is in his mind, body and spirit—his particular human nature.

According to a study by the Harvard University Energy and Environmental Center, pollution kills as many Americans each year as the entire Korean war.

---

twenty

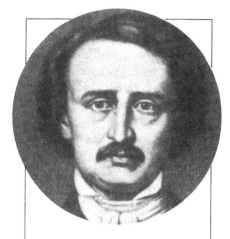

The 20 chemical types

A temperament is a system of organs, functions and faculties adapted to carry on the processes of life.

The four temperaments work in conjunction and yet each is separate and the significance is that each has its particular effect upon talent, disposition, character and state of health of the individual.

The body size of man depends upon his temperament and constitution.

There are many chemical types and, in some persons, the type can't be determined. Yet, every type needs all the basic chemical elements and trace elements. If one does not learn the types, he should learn the symptoms of the lack of each chemical element.

In the previous chapter, we discussed how Rocine discovered and elaborated upon the 20 temperament types of people. In this chapter, we will bring together and summarize Rocine's system, definitions, analyses, discussion and comparison of the 20 types, starting with the 4 main divisions of types.

Mental Temperament Types are four in number, all using phosphorus and sulphur mainly in their makeup: Neurogenic—Neuro (nerve), genic (produce), nerve-producing); Nervi-Motive means combination of nervous and motive temperaments; Exesthetic: Exe (out), esthesic (feelings)—one who expresses feelings; Pathetic: Pathos (emotions), ic (relating to).

Muscular Temperament Types or those people who are quick, active and adaptable; Desmogenic: Desmo (band), genic (producing), the ligamentous structures; Marasmic: Marasmos, Greek meaning lean, emaciated; Myogenic: Myo (muscle), genic (producing).

Osseous or Bony Temperament Types or those who are large in bones, slow and hardworking; Calciferic: Lime-carrying; Isogenic: Iso (balance or harmony) in temperament; Sillevitic: Sil (silicon), levis, Latin for light or easy (in motion); Barotic: Baros (Greek) meaning heavy.

Vital Temperament Types or those who are fleshy, rotund, full in body build: Carboferic: Carbon (sugar), feric (carrying); Hydripheric: hydrogen (water) carrying; Nitropheric: Nitrogen-carrying; Oxypheric: Oxygen-carrying; Lipopheric: Lipo (fat) carrying; Pallinomic: Pallas (wise) omen (destined).

Pathogenic Constitutions or those who are born with a predisposition to disharmony and disease (which can be overcome, however, by understanding and developing vitally); Atrophic: A (not) trophic (nourish), or not able to digest food and nourish the body easily or sufficiently; Medeic: Greek word Medea (Magic or able to enchant), so named because the first man of this type whom we studied was a magician, although all are not magicians, of course; Pargenic: Para (wrong), genic (birth) or tainted by birth.

We have: Four Mental Temperament Chemical types; Three Muscular Temperament Chemical types; Three Bony Temperament Chemical types; Six Vital Temperament Chemical types; Three Pathogenic types which give us the Twenty Chemical types of people.

The Temperaments

In order to properly understand the Chemical Types of People, it is well to recognize that man possesses four temperamental systems of the body, i.e., Mental, Vital, Muscular and Bony or Osseous.

A temperament is a system of organs, functions and faculties adapted to carry on the processes of life. Every man, woman and child possesses the four great body systems: bones, muscles, vital organs and brain, including the nerves. The reason that some people are large and others small is because the large people build the more bulky systems of the body, i.e., the bones, muscles and vital organs excessively, while the small people build the brain and nerves which are the smallest part of the body. It is therefore ridiculous for one to try to make himself the same size as another. "Which of you, by taking thought, can add one cubit to your stature?" says the Bible. Each temperamental type may keep himself or herself the normal weight and size, according to his height and type but more than this, he cannot do and remain healthy and normal or beautiful.

The Vital System consists of all the vital organs: lungs, heart, liver, stomach, circulatory system and the functions of secretion, absorption, nutrition, respiration and other vital functions, all carried on by the centers in the brain and spinal cord. The processes of life and death are carried on by this system. The individual who builds this system above the other three systems, builds a body like Illustration No. 1.

The Osseous or Bony temperament is the system of locomotion, consisting of the bones or skeleton of the body, solid membranes, nails, teeth, protective coverings, the motor centers in the brain and spinal cord. It is the framework of the body; it leads to action, protection, locomotion, greater internal functional energy, executiveness, strength, endurance. If it were not for this temperament, man would be compelled to remain in one spot all his life, like a jellyfish, unless moved by wind or wave. The bones in the lead give the man a rugged, angular appearance. He is slow, positive and patient. See Illustration No. 2.

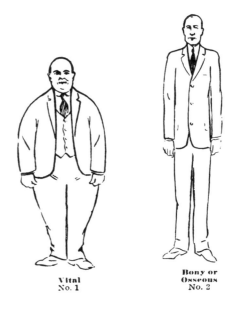

Vital
No. 1

Bony or
Osseous
No. 2

The Muscular System consists of the muscles, tendons, ligaments, hair. This system gives speed and strength combined, quick, jerky movements, grace and love of action. He is the most versatile man. Mentally he is alert, able to sum up things at a glance, practical and balanced in judgment. It is this inherent state of mind that enables him to build muscles in the lead, instead of other parts or systems of the body. He is oval in body, face and head, as shown in Illustration No. 3.

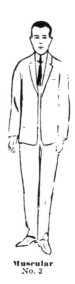

Muscular
No. 3

389

Most of the neuric functions are carried on by the Mental Temperament, such as intellection, emotion, hearing, seeing, tasting, smelling, perception, reasoning, memorizing, understanding, speech, attention, etc. He is the smallest in the body of all the temperaments, but his head is large and his nervous system active. Illustration No. 4.

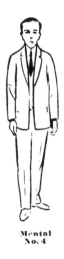

Mental
No. 4

The four temperaments work in conjunction and yet each is separate and the significance is that each has its particular effect upon talent, disposition, character and state of health of the individual. Temperament is innate and each person is born with a tendency to develop such a body. From these four temperamental divisions, which are fundamentally chemic in structure, we build our system of the Nineteen Chemical Types of People.

Brain and Nerves or the Mental Temperament utilize and call for phosphorus and sulphur.

Bones, teeth, nails and solid structures throughout the body require calcium, fluorine and silicon, mainly.

Muscles call for potassium, sodium and chlorine.

Vital System develops from the elements oxygen, hydrogen, nitrogen and carbon.

Key to Temperaments and Chemical Constitutions

Introduction. Classification, general explanation, induction and systematic presentation of a subject always favor students in their studies. This classification presents, in brief space for easy reference, the science of the temperaments, so that students may obtain a "bird's eye view" of temperamental knowledge; and by comparison and contrast, be able to learn more easily and remember more clearly than would otherwise be possible.

Definition. A temperament is a system or systems of organs, functions and faculties.

Subdivision. (1) Vital Temperament (2) Muscular Temperament (3) Osseous Temperament (4) Mental Temperament. These are the four basic temperaments. A combination of the Muscular and Osseous strongly in the lead is called the Motive temperament.

Comparatively few people are of the temperament only strongly in lead. Most people are of a combination of two or more temperaments in the lead, such as Mental-Muscular, Mental-Osseous, etc.

Mental Temperament. This temperament consists of the brain, nerves, ganglia, nerve plexuses and skin. Or it is represented by the central nervous system, the ganglionic system and of membranes containing nerves, nerve ends, nerve buds; also, by the nerves and nerve ends in the skin.

Muscular Temperament. This temperament consists of about 528 muscles, also fascia, tendons, cords and ligaments.

Osseous Temperament. This consists of the bones, joints, nails and teeth, which form the framework of the body.

Vital Temperament. This consists of the vital organs and the vital fluids; or those organs, functions, faculties and systems concerned in blood manufacture and elimination—as, for instance: the lymphatic system, the circulatory system, the sexual system, the digestive system, the respiratory system, etc. In other words, such organs as the heart, lungs, stomach, liver, kidneys, spleen, intestines and others; also secretions, blood and lymph.

Arrangement. Each temperamental classification is set forth under subjects and headings as follows.

The Body. That part of the human anatomy known as the torso contains all the organs, the main vital organs between the neck and the lower limbs.

The Extremities. Comprise (1) the lower limbs, the organs of locomotion; (2) the arms, hands and fingers, which are the organs of execution, skill, dexterity and technics.

The Face. The face is the map of the mind and soul. It reveals thoughts and feelings representing passing mental states, also long continued past action of mind and soul.

The Head. That part of man that contains the brain or the organ of intelligence, emotion, thought and impulse.

General Construction. Here we take into consideration the chemical consistency of the cells, also the general form of the body.

Tendencies and Characteristics. This describes the talent, genius, emotions, passions, appetites, impulses, inclinations, predilections and traits of character peculiar to each temperament.

Chemicals. Under this heading, we point out which those body chemicals or chemical compounds are, which predominate in a certain type or constitution and how chemical elements influence thought, emotion, talent, character, study, health, disposition, love, etc.

Constitutions (Chemical). Under this heading are shown the various temperamental, chemical, anatomical and pathological "types" of man; so that you may know and understand types of man, types of patients, laws of affinity by reason of types; also the difference between type and type from various viewpoints.

Constitutions (Diseased or Pathogenic). Under this head, we describe from a hereditary, toxic, narcotic or congenitally diseased viewpoint how diseased types of men differ, one from the other; how hereditary traits of character appear; how soul qualities are altered under pathogenic and toxic agents.

THE CHEMICAL CONSTITUTIONS
The Vital Temperament Constitutions

	Temp Comb.	Chemicals in Lead	Shape of Face	Distinguishing Peculiarities
CARBOFERIC	Vital	Carbon (Sugar)	Conic, full moon shape.	Small bones (sugar), flabby tissues; sickly. Subject to paralysis, prostration, dropsy. Nervous; timid.
HYDRIPHERIC	Vital	Hydrogen (Water)	Conic, dbl chin, large lower face.	Great cell communication and delicacy. Lacks solids (salts) in blood and tissues. Acts when acted upon. Silent, latent.
LIPOPHERIC	Vital or Vit-Ment	Fats	Full, lge, circular, long.	Skin appears white, but is oily, greasy. Flesh is hard. Stature often short. Limbs tapering. Feet short and sore.
NITROPHERIC	Vital	Nitrogen Carbon Hydrogen, Oxygen	Full, circular, square.	Dark complected. Dark-white skin. Tender, brittle tissues. Nitrogen leaves tissues soon. Sores, burns, etc. heal slowly. Tendency to tissue decomposition. Affinity for oxygen and gelatin. Exclusive in association. Deep, mysterious, mediative. Mild.
OXYPHERIC	Vit or Vit Harmon.	Oxygen, Pot.,Iron	Large, square	Short lived. Excitable, emotional, lively, wonderful affinity, cumulative, sudden, full-blooded, loves freedom.
PALLINOMIC	Vital-Fibrinous	Alb, Calc Nit, Gel	Square	Harmonious temperament. Neutral sex type. Complexion pale, muddy. Large feet, tense tissue, strong black hair. Wide mouth.

The major source of man's sulphur comes from food protein combining one of the four sulphur-containing amino acids—cysteine, cystine, taurine and methionine.

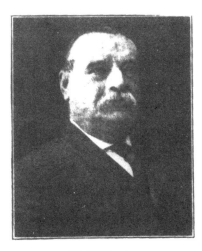

Hydripheric

Grover Cleveland was not realy a sociable man nor a good mixer. He would sit in a boat alone for hours day after day and fish.

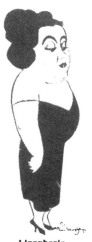

Lipopheric
Cartoon, Courtesy of "Chicago Topics"
Typical body outline of the Lipopheric.

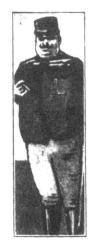

**King Carlos
of Portugal**

Lipopheric
A Gormand King

King Carlos of Portugal Stopped in Mad Eating Career.

Lisbon, Sept. 23.—King Carlos of Portugal, the royal gormand of Europe, has been halted in his mad gastronomic dissipation by order of the court physicians, who fear that he will become the victim of fatty degeneration of the heart.

It is said that King Carlos has of late been outdoing even his royal predecessor, King Charles V. of sixteenth century fame, who was accustomed to eat six enormous meals each day.

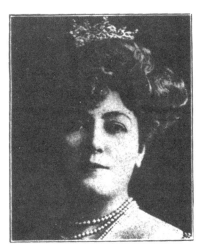

Carboferic
Lillian Russell
The Most Beautiful Actress of the '90s

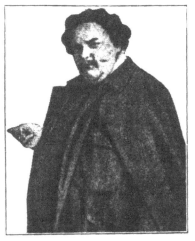

Hydripheric
Gilbert K. Chesterton
English writer and poet, said to possess a keen sense of wit. Note the heavy ponderous body and the little soft hand.

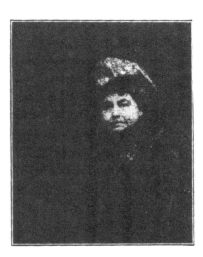

Nitropheric
Mrs. Woodrow Wilson

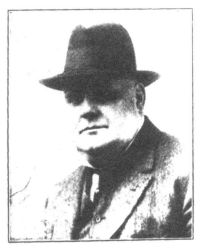

Oxypheric
Tom Lewis

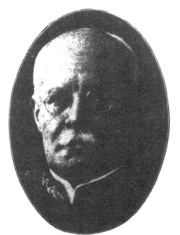

Pallinomic
Maj. Gen. Hugh L. Scott
Former Chief of Staff in U. S. Army

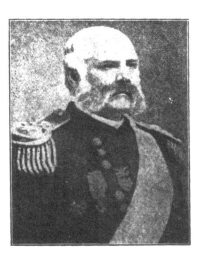

Pallinomic
Late General John McAllister Schofield
Of the United States Army.

392

THE CHEMICAL CONSTITUTIONS

THE MENTAL TEMPERAMENT CONSTITUTIONS

Constitution	Temp. Comb.	Chemicals in Lead	Shape of Face	Distinguishing Peculiarities
EXESTHESIC	Ment-Mus. or Ment-Vital-Mus.	Phosph., Potassium. Sulphur, Magnesium	Oval, shapely. Proportionate. Beautiful.	Proportionate, slender build. Soprano voice. Small liver; poor oxidation. Generates electrical ferments because of excessive sulphur consumption and great nerve action. Hysterical tendencies. Generous to strangers. High toned, emotional. Loves culture, flattery, station, wealth, distinction, personal tidiness and influence.
NERVI-MOTIVE	Mental-Osseous.	Phosph. and Calc.	Circular, square	Small people. Long extremities. Intensity in mental functions and physical organs. Appear like neurogenic people. Very wilful.
NEUROGENIC	Mental or Mental-Osseous.	Phosphorus.	Pear shaped, upper part large; lower part small	Forehead hot, body cold and moist. Head proportionately large; feet long, slender; hands small; shoulders sloping. Sunken stomach, chest, cheeks. Appears old.
PATHETIC	Ment-Vital or Vit-Ment	Phos. and Carbon ep.	Even, shapely, rosy, beautiful.	Feminine build and characteristics throughout. Tender, soft tissue. Chronic neuritis. Face fairly full.

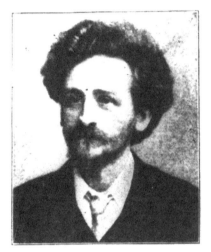

Neurogenic
JAMES ALLEN
Author of "As a Man Thinketh"

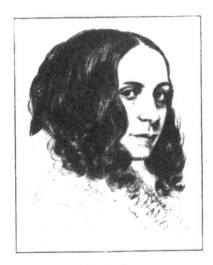

Pathetic
ELIZABETH BARRETT BROWNING
Poet.

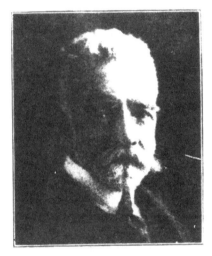

Nervi-Motive
HENRY CABOT LODGE

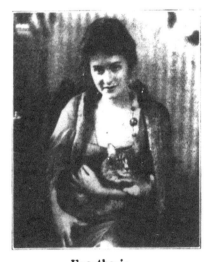

Exesthesic
ELSIE FERGUSON
If she knew sulphur, the "soulful" element, she would know herself also.

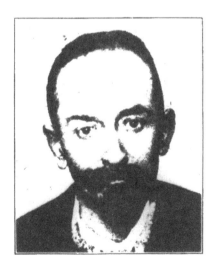

Neurogenic
GEORG TCHITCHERIN

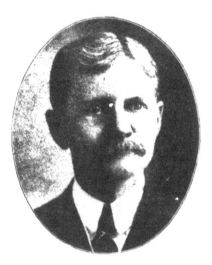

Nervi-Motive
VICE PRESIDENT THOMAS R. MARSHALL
(With President Wilson)

393

THE CHEMICAL CONSTITUTIONS
THE MUSCULAR TEMPERAMENT CONSTITUTIONS

Constitution	Temp. Comb.	Chemicals in Lead	Shape of Face	Distinguishing Peculiarities
DESMOGENIC	Ligamentous. Mus. or Ligamentous-Ment.	Sodium, Cartilage, Calc.,Pot.	Wide, square or long narrow.	Pale skin, bilious. Great muscle and ligament strength. Compact tissue. Great motion ability; athletic and pugilistic tendencies. Tendency to chronic diseases, low state animal heat.
MARASMIC	Fibrinous-Mental.	Fluorin, Chlorin, Phosphorus, Calcium, Potash.	Small.	Organic elements lacking. Very short and lean; extremities long. Wide head. Dark brown, murky brown, muddy brown, yellow brown, green, coppery-green or black-yellow complexion. Dense tissue and fiber; compact, elastic, solid, strong, wiry. Wonderful endurance and hardihood. Appears weak and sickly. Brain and muscles efficient. Corresponds to choleric or bilious temperament. Poor nutrition. Loves heat; dreads cold. Masculine sex type.
MYOGENIC	Mus Ment or Harmonious.	Fibrin.	Oval or oval square.	Oval or egg-shaped head. Skin brown-red. Hair fluffy, thick. Neither very positive, nor very negative; neither fat nor lean, tall nor short, fleshy nor lean. Loves outdoor life, motion, action.

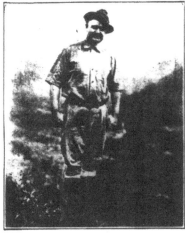

Myogenic
GEORGE WATKIN EVANS
Former prospector of the Klondike rush. Today he has an international reputation as a consulting coal mining engineer, one of the highest authorities on coal fields in western North America.

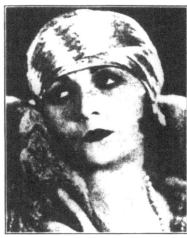

Desmogenic
POLA NEGRI
Emotional tragic movie actress.

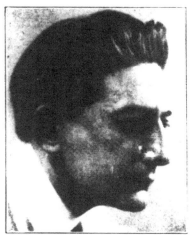

Desmogenic
JOHN DECKER
whose imposing title as The Caricaturist of the Cruel Line has helped mold public opinion and "turn the tide of Destiny" in individual lives.

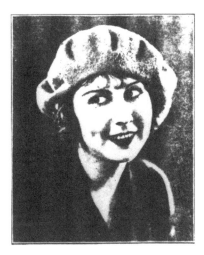

Myogenic
DOROTHY DALTON
The athletic screen star prefers to play the Wild West and Northern scenes, wear rough clothes and have dogs and horses around.

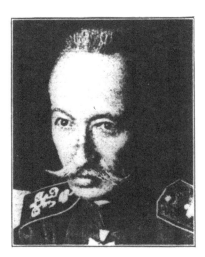

Marasmic
GENERAL ALEXEL BRUSILOFF
Commander in Chief of Russian Armies, 1917

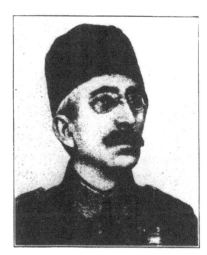

Marasmic
MOHAMMED VII
Sultan of Turkey, 1918

THE CHEMICAL CONSTITUTIONS
THE OSSEOUS TEMPERAMENT CONSTITUTIONS

	Temp. Comb.	Chemicals in Lead	Shape of Face	Distinguishing Peculiarities
CALCIFERIC	Osseous-Mental or Ment.-Oss.	Tricalcium phosphate	Long, narrow, angular, rectilinear.	Large parietal, small in front of ears, in upper temples, in back head and in centro-horizontal forehead. Sunken cheeks. Mas. body and mind; lean, bony and angular. Thin chest, square shoulders.
ISOGENIC	Osseous-Ment.-Vit. almost equal.	Calcium, Phosphorus, Organic elements.	Large, full. Appears lean compared to body.	Feminine body, masculine head. Short extremities; long torso. Usually rather fleshy. Hands large, firm. Kidneys weak; liver and bone functions sluggish. Tendency to calcium ailments or chronic diseases. Poor memory in general; good in matters of learning and understanding.
SILLEVITIC	Oss. Ment. or Men.-Os.	Silicon.	Small, long, sq.	Alkalinity; quick pulse. Activity in bone function. Suppleness, agility, nimbleness. Speedy.
BAROTIC	Os. vital.	Vital elements Calcium Sulphur	Large and heavy cheek bones.	Slowness, latency, strength.

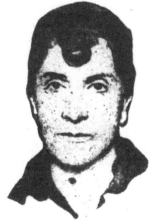

Calciferic
MRS. ROCKEFELLER McCORMICK

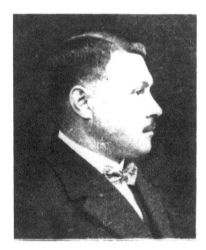

Barotic
See last page for description. Note large face, cheekbones and circular head.

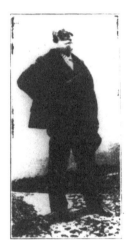

Isogenic
JOHN BURROUGHS
The Great Naturalist and Author

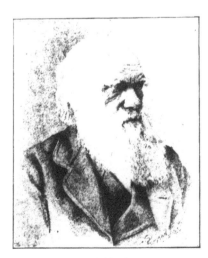

Calciferic
CHARLES DARWIN

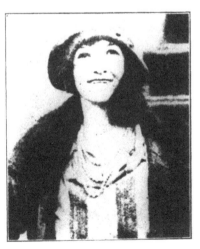

Sillevitic
VERA, LADY CATHCART

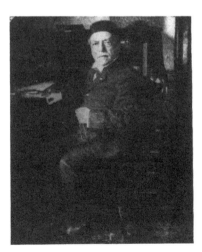

Isogenic
SAMUEL GOMPERS
The Great Labor Leader

THE CHEMICAL CONSTITUTIONS
THE PATHOGENIC CONSTITUTIONS

	Temp. Comb.	Chemicals in Lead	Shape of Face	Distinguishing Peculiarities
ATROPHIC	Mental-Osseous or Oss.-Ment.	Phosphorus and Calcium.	Long sq., or rec- tilinilar; angu- lar, thin, lean.	Bony, long extremities, heavy joints. Long, heavy, narrow, even fingers. Large ears, prominent nose. Large forehead, small backhead. Head is flat, but wide. Slender, tubercular, intellectual.
MEDEIC (not chemical)	Muscular Osseous or Osseous- Muscular- Mental.	Potassium, Phosph., Calcium. Miasm.	Square angular, or square tri- angular.	Pivots on the Medeic miasm. Appears old when young. Hair gray at 35; Sex type always masculine. Lean. Anatomical build similar to dwarf, only larger. Arms and legs long. Sharp features. Skin is dark, faded, bluish pale, blue yellow, always dark and apparently shriveled. Rest, darkness, cold wind, moisture and malaria aggravate. Cold baths make him sick. Hot baths improve him.
PARGENIC	Osseous- Vital; or Vital- Osseous.	Carbon, Pargenic taint, Organic elements, Calcium.	Puffy. Usually square and large.	Syphilis, pus, germ impurity from meat, fish and pork are principal causes of his diseases. Very heavy set, voluptuous in appearance. Large abdomen, heavy hips and limbs; brittle bones; large, square hands; coarse, bushy hair; wide head; heavy cheeks; large shoulders and chest; puffy skin; sensual eyes; thick nose, neck and lower backhead. Brain action slow but ponderous. Obesity.

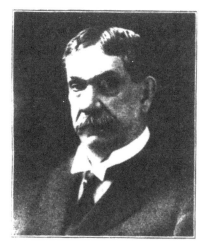

Pargenic
JOHN G. BATTELLE
Executive, Iron and Steel Mfg.
Industries

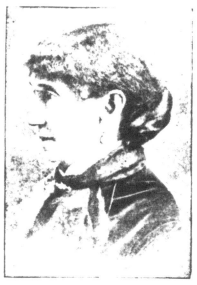

Atrophic
MARY JANE HOLMES
Noted Novelist

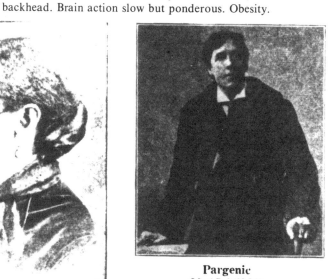

Pargenic
OSCAR WILDE
He is described by biographers as being tall and of great corpulence, having
a high cred- complexion, with fleshy,
plump hands.

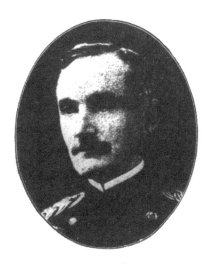

Atrophic
MAJ. GEN. H. P. McCAIN
Adj. General of the U. S. Army During
World War

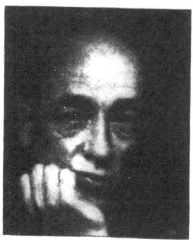

Medeic
JAMES STEPHENS
Irish Poet

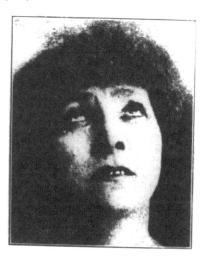

Medeic
SARAH BERNHARDT
Tragedian. One of the greatest act-
resses.

THE MENTAL TEMPERAMENT CONSTITUTIONS

Prominent Faults

Exesthesic. Has great irritability, but is well meaning. Fussy, impatient, spasmodic, strong temper. Subject to mental confusion, nerve storms and even brain storms. She is strongly inclined to quarrel with her husband, and, although true as steel, her marriage almost always ends up in the divorce court. She is proud, extravagant, jealous, aristocratic, full of dislikes, hard to please; obstinate at first, then yields.

Nervi-Motive. Hypersensitiveness; hyperesthesia, great wilfulness and obstinacy; fault-finding and quarrelsome, especially with nearest relatives. Intolerant in the home. Suspicious of others. Excessive physical sensitiveness of nerves and organs. Punishes in a passion, then cries.

Neurogenic. Dislikes work. Inclines to self pity and despair. Depreciates, then exhalts self alternately. Wants stimulants. Very restless, exclusive, impractical. Exaggerates. Visionary, imaginative, idealistic rather than sentimental. Extravagant, domineering in creed. Sarcastic; but so sweet about it that it is not discovered until later.

Pathetic. Lacks will power and concentration. Dislikes studies, and is unable to learn mathematics.

Prominent Virtues

She is faithful and true; loves culture, literature, personal neatness, study (yet she does not generally have sufficient ability to carry on studies extensively). She appreciates noble, honorable characteristics; takes great interest in the rising generation; has a keen sense, appreciation and judgment of ethics. Her love is periodic; she may love today and not tomorrow. She has a pleasing accent and refined manners.

Very neat, tidy, orderly, systematic, industrious and versatile. Self sacrificing to those in whom mostly interested. Hates interference. Very speedy. All faculties acute.

Great ability to fight the desires of the flesh. Loves sacred things, also spiritualism, evolution, the occult, oriental philosophy, romance, nature, magnetism and conventionalism. Tends to religion, imagination. Is idealistic and has wonderful intuition. Has ability for fine arts, dress reform, aerial invention and everything pertaining to the air.

Is sociable; can associate with all classes of people. Has angelic manners and disposition.

THE MUSCULAR TEMPERAMENT CONSTITUTIONS

Prominent Faults

Desmogenic. Is cynical at times. Has occasional spells of seriousness, temper and pessimism. Has a restless and choleric disposition; has a tendency to anxiety, hatred, fault-finding and gossip. May roam everywhere. Lacks literary judgment and is poor in spelling and in expression. Very intolerant; may punish on provocation. Very good, then suddenly very bad. Very suspicious, sly and jealous. Bold, reckless, unconventional. Usually fails in matrimony.

Marasmic. He is interested in hypnotism, is wily like a serpent, has many dog-like characteristics. He hides his plans, is sedentary, spasmodic, distant, indifferent, cold in manner, pessimistic, sly, unsociable, morose, cowardly, panicy, cynical, critical, treacherous and cruel. Always a failure in matrimony. Sometimes kills wife. Sometimes a bigamist. Wise and sarcastic; dictator.

Myogenic. Lacks mental concentration, especially on abstract subjects. Does not have many faults. Too many-sided, and has too many irons in the fire. He is rubber-like in his ways; can do things with a double meaning. Lacks self control at times. May be reckless, wilful, exacting, cranky. He may sow wild oats when young.

Prominent Virtues

Very devoted. Understands heat, pressure and color changes. Good judge of fire, heat, clay, metal, oils, gas, explosives; a good landscape gardener, mining engineer, good judge of pottery and fire-clay work. The Chinese and Japanese are mainly Demogenics. Are good detectives, jugglers, hunters, cowboys.

He is witty, comical, skillful, a great worker, studious—great in gardening and in glass arts. He is slavish to employers, but treacherous to others. Many Chinese and Japanese are Marasmic. Very able men, druggists, surgeons and military men, philosophers, teachers and speakers. Surprisingly strong and wiry. Does good work especially at night.

Usually harmonious throughout; even tempered, sociable, genial and pleasing in disposition; he has ability in many ways. Has strong judgment, love and fidelity. Understands people and how to deal with them; can adjust himself to all conditions; has excellent judgment and observation; has ability to arbitrate; is not aggressive, but is always ready. Can adjust his muscles, nerves and senses to all mechanical work.

Laughter—Prescription for Health. Laughter, according to medical researchers, reduces stress, helps relax the body, increases levels of natural pain killers and neurotransmitters in the blood and may help lower blood pressure.

THE OSSEOUS TEMPERAMENT CONSTITUTIONS

Prominent Faults

Calciferic. He is hard to please, indifferent, stern, unforgiving, fault-finding, distrustful, skeptical, blunt, unpolished and perhaps cruel. He is greedy of power. Domineering in executive lines. Dogmatic and compulsory. Believes too much in force, fist and might. Not well balanced. Does not rest or believe in recreation. Positive in body and head; hence must deal with inanimate things.

Isogenic. Usually has weak parental love, hence is not very sympathetic. He is skeptical, hard and could even be stern and cruel. Storms are slumbering in him. He has many feminine characteristics or weaknesses; hence can be led into trouble and difficulties, at which times he may sacrifice money and health. The world considers him an "easy mark"; hence he must fight for his rights. Patiently endures until his patience is exhausted, then he resents further trouble. Makes a good general.

Silivetic. Will not yield to impulse. He is changeable in plans, views and in disposition; a spendthrift in traveling. Heedlessness, visions, levity, undue familiarity, innocent self deceit, falsification, hyperbolism and phantasy are his prominent faults.

Prominent Virtues

He has great endurance, good reason, judgment and will power; loves truth and material facts; he has capacity and desire to work and study; he believes in work and in accomplishments. He has intellectual and executive ability in science, philosophy, engineering and mechanics; he is studious, quiet and serene; optimistic in questions of principle, nature, results, law, God, forces and authority. Otherwise, he is pessimistic and impatient.

He is honorable, good natured until aroused, patient, benevolent, sentimental and serious. His disposition is seemingly phlegmatic; has strong tendencies to mental and physical habit making. He is interested in science, usually relating to man. When once interested in a certain direction he goes on in spite of opposition. He is unyielding—a brother to eternity. He can be killed, but never conquered. He is an experimentalist, and is interested in results. He has strong will power, good judgment and practical ability. Has an analytical and analogical mind. Usually he has great success and enterprise in later life.

He is industrious, benevolent, optimistic, pleasing, winning, lively, friendly, sympathetic, charitable, hopeful, enthusiastic, adaptable and stimulating.

THE PATHOGENIC CONSTITUTIONS

Prominent Faults

Atrophic. He prefers solitude, is unsociable, irritable, hard to please, gloomy in disposition, easily offended, gets angry and remains angry; is unforgiving, faultfinding, wilful and reckless of himself and others. Slow to anger, but stays angry; has a critical disposition, stubborn notions, ugly moods; highly sensitive.

Medeic. His disease makes him worse at night; he is better while in motion; he is contrary, sullen, vindictive, stoical, reclusory, sensational, tragic, revengeful, wild, malicious, jealous; interested in blood, dissections, battles, scenes, sensations and murder. His mind runs to crime, obscene subjects; is subject to insanity, paralysis, motor contraction, kleptomania, arthritis, convulsions and sexual diseases. He is fond of poisons, stimulants, morphine; he does shocking, humiliating things and is a great outlaw. Premediatates crime. His wit hurts. He is a failure in matrimony. May kill his wife. Thinks all people are bad. He is part saint and part devil.

Pargenic. He is fond of sports, eating and drinking. He is awkward, stupid, sulky, forgetful, cross, suspicious, coarse, blunt, shabby, distrustful, depressed and cynical. He has a dark, morose disposition, fixed moods, a secretive nature, many delusions, a polygamic mind, an excessive appetite. He is a free lover, marries to be supported. Has heavy headaches; is subject to insanity, has suicidal tendencies, is physically sterile; has lust germs, and is a sexual degenerate, at times.

Prominent Virtues

Has reasoning capacity, understands abstract subjects. He is quiet, studious, serene, patient in enterprise or hard studies. He has engineering tendencies and a constructive mind. He loves principle and honor. He is resigned, accurate, steady in work, scientific and constructive. Brilliant and intellectual, but gives out account amativeness giving out.

He is sometimes a wonderful prophet and evangelist; a great fanatic when religious; punishes and kills if you do not believe also. He is witty; sometimes liberal, then parsimonious; a wonderful genius in certain lines. He is great in spy-craft; a good cavalry man and an artillerist. Fresh air and vigorous work improve him. Very shrewd due to taint.

Learns slowly, but makes good use of what he does learn. He is wonderful in revivals; has great influence over others; he is a great veterinary surgeon, a great breeder of animals, a specialist in sex diseases, a great demonstrator, good in general merchandise and commission business.

THE VITAL TEMPERAMENT CONSTITUTIONS

Prominent Faults

Carboferic. She is awkward, complaining, inactive, lazy, sleepy, negative, dependent, extravagant, fretful. She worries, sometimes weeps. Favorite among men until married, then husband is disappointed. Not born for hard work; no energy. Unsteady, undecided, often gloomy; sometimes commits suicide. Full of fear and distrust. Nervous system collapses.

Hydripheric. He has insane tendencies to stay at home; is jealous, worries over love objects; is negative, inhibitive, dreamy, conservative. He has an excessive appetite, and hates strangers. Self hypnosis.

Lipopheric. Craves wines, fats, pleasures and dissipation; is sportive, flirtatious, frivolous, lazy and hypocritical in association. Extravagant in dress to win hearts and tempt opposite sex. Has a loud voice and a piggish aspect. Does nothing for husband. Innocent expression; fat; mercenary mind.

Nitropheric. He is absentminded, seemingly indifferent, suspicious, procrastinating, gloomy in murky weather and imperious; he is timid, sleepy and fearful in darkness; he cannot forget nor forgive. Silently jealous. Gloomy in heat. Solemn in disposition; slow to reveal himself. Easy.

Oxypheric. He is impatient, excitable, autocratic, explosive, stormy, wordly, lustful, polygamic, impulsive, passionate, restless and hilarious; he has culminating periods, is full of plots, excessive in eating and drinking. Lies, but means no harm; he needs tropical climate. He is a poser and bluffer; never carries out his threats; likes intrigue. Never confesses a wrong.

Pallinomic. He has a poor expression, an awkward movement and sedate manners. He is simply good, but good generally. Never a social success. Found mainly among working class. Dependent independence. Very jealous, strong feelings. Depressed and has depressed moods. Heavy walk; penetrative eyes.

Prominent Virtues

She is quiet, genial, poetic and sentimental. Loving in times of prosperity; but not otherwise. Born to be petted and humored. Harmless, well-meaning; has excellent traits. Loves innocent pleasure and fresh air.

Has delicate finger technique, wonderful olfaction. Fidelity, monogamic and platonic love, passivity, purity, politeness, good temper, kindness and peacefulness are among his virtues. Patient disposition.

Pleasing disposition, tactful in dress and expression, genial, persuasive; has a laughing, ringing voice. Has a conversational talent and is a leader among prominent people.

He is patient, resigned, forebearing, toward loved ones, tactful in association with others, magnetic, controlled and economical. Dislikes changeableness; has a mind for regulation, retention and suppression. True as steel. Good worker. Cannot tolerate familiarity. Sympathetic. Controlled, good, sentimental.

He is liberal, generous, hospitable, adaptable, progressive, demonstrative. He is a "live wire"; a great orator, an executive, constructor and a promoter. Not revengeful; holds no grudge; avenges as he goes along or leaves the people alone. Enthusiastic, hopeful.

He has high domestic virtues; practical religion, business reliability; reason, judgment, enterprise, industry; and business management. He is skillful in technique, in manufacturing dressmaking, leather goods, textiles, soft metals, nursing and jewelry. A great lover of home.

NOTE

In the Motive Temperament or motor (moving) part of the body there are in reality three parts; i. e., bones, ligaments, muscles.

This leaves the ligaments unaccounted for in the classification of Temperaments given in this book.

We find that those people who have the ligaments in the lead are different from the people who have the other motor systems in the lead. In the animal creation, the ox represents the bony temperament; the bear represents the muscular; the tiger, the cat, and all the animals of the feline species have ligaments in the lead or they belong to the ligamentous temperament.

The only Chemical Type having the ligamentous temperament is the Desmogenic

These people are small and very strong, because they are dense and compact in tissue structure.

They have a short, wide face and a small chin.

This temperament develops from Sodium.

NAME OF CHEMICAL ELEMENT. PROPORTION OF THESE CHEMICAL ELEMENTS IN PERSON WEIGHING 160 LBS.	FOODS RICH IN THESE CHEMICAL ELEMENTS	NORMAL FUNCTIONS OF THESE CHEMICAL ELEMENTS	EFFECT OF EXCESSIVE CHEMICAL CONSUMPTION OF THESE ELEMENTS	CONSTITUTIONS IN WHICH CHEMICAL CONSUMPTION OF THESE ELEMENTS IS EXCESSIVE	CONSTITUTIONS IN WHICH THESE CHEMICAL ELEMENTS ARE DEFICIENT
(A)	(B)	(C)	(D)	(E)	(F)

PREDOMINATING CHEMICAL CONSUMPTION OF MENTAL TEMPERAMENT CONSTITUTIONS:

(A)	(B)	(C)	(D)	(E)	(F)
IODIN ¼ oz.	Smoked salmon, Artichokes, Grapes, Pears, Irish moss, Whole rice, Tomatoes, Onions, Potato skin, Green peas, strawberries, pineapple.	Prevents auto toxins from injuring the brain. Increases brain activity.	Emotionality Excess oxidation; over stimulates sexual appetite.	Nervi motive.	Neurogenic, Pathetic, Carboferic, Nitropheric, Lipopheric, Atrophic, Pargenic.
MAGNESIUM 3½ oz.	Almond nuts, Citric fruit, Rye, Grape fruit, water cress, Endive, Tart apples, Barley bread, spinach, lettuce, rye food, orange marmalade.	Neutralizes phosphorous products; Regulates bowels; calms nerves and brain. Relaxes muscles, makes blood alkaline.	Diarrhea. Brain and body stupidity.	Exesthesie, Neurogenic, Oxypheric, Pallinomic.	Exesthesie, Neurogenic, Desmogenic, Isogenic, Oxypheric, Pallinomic, Marasmic, Medeic.
MANGANESE ½ oz.	Almond nuts, Walnuts, Greens, Chestnuts, Parsley, chives, dill, peppermint leaves, romaine, pignolias.	Adapts nervous system to darkness. Communication of the white fiber of the brain. Nerve and brain tonic.	Neuralgia Excrutiating pains.	Nervi-motive, Desmogenic, Marasmic, Myogenic.	Nervi motive, Neurogenic, Desmogenic, Marasmic, Myogenic, Carboferic, Nitropheric.
PHOSPHORUS 2 lbs.	Egg yolk, Fish; beechnuts, barley, Wheat, Bran bread, prunes, blueberries, cherries, gooseberries, meat, black bass, clam broth, lobster broth, oyster broth, crab meat.	*Bone and brain metabolism.* Stimulates all bodily functions.	Spendthrift, Phthisis, Brain decay, deficient bone metabolism. Feeble mindedness, Hydrocephalus.	Exesthesie, Nervi-motive, Neurogenic, Desmogenic, Marasmic, Some Isogenics, Oxypheric, Atrophic, Medeic.	Neurogenic (excess consumption) Carboferic (Deficient phosphate metabolism)
SULPHUR 3¾ oz.	Horseradish, red and white cabbage, Radishes, Figs, cocoanut, cauliflower, cucumbers, potatoes, peas, turnips, head lettuce, shrimp.	Stimulates; grows hair.	Fitfulness, Hyperesthesia, Temper, nervous hypertension.	Exesthesie, Nervi-motive.	Exesthesie, Carboferic, Nitropheric, Pargenic.

PREDOMINATING CHEMICAL CONSUMPTION OF MUSCULAR TEMPERAMENT CONSTITUTIONS:

(A)	(B)	(C)	(D)	(E)	(F)
CHLORIN 1¾ lbs.	Ham, meat, cocoanut, Roquefort cheese, Salt, Meat, lentils, meat juice, ripe olives, sun dried olives, German prunes, herring, cheese, salted nuts, cocoanut, beech nuts, goats' milk, Swiss cheese.	Promotes purification; aids secretion. It is the laundryman in body. Overcomes fat, prevents constipation and aids the stomach in its functioning.	Dechlorination of blood and tissues; defective albumin metabolism; growth of germ life, excessive nerve heat. Generates anger and revenge.	Nervi motive, Isogenic (old), Carboferic, Hydripheric, Lipopheric, Nitropheric, Oxypheric, Pallinomic, Atrophic.	All (except Marasmic; and sometimes in him account excess consumption). Badly needed by Carboferic, Hydripheric, Atrophic.
POTASSIUM 3¼ oz.	Dried Olives, bitter Herbs, Teas, Salads, Greens, Vegetables, Cereals, Peaches, spinach, potato skin, peas, carrots, bitter nuts, bran bread.	Stimulates activity, tissue oxidation, gives energy to heart, lungs and muscles. promotes sleep; Laxative.	Prostration, Paralysis, Impulsiveness.	Exesthesie, Nervi-motive, Desmogenic, Marasmic, Myogenic (some) Oxypheric, Medeic.	All constitutions. except Myogenic.
SODIUM 3 oz.	Celery, Okra, Gizzard, Carrots, Pistachio Nuts, Smyrna figs, spinach, strawberries, ripe olives, beets, egg yolk, goats' milk cows' milk, salt.	Promotes secretion, excretion of carbonic oxide; *alkalinization.* Curative in nature.	Auto intoxication; growth of germ life; indigestion. Hatred, Malice.	Desmogenic, Pallinomic, Medeic.	All constitutions. except Myogenic.

400

NAME OF CHEMICAL ELEMENT. PROPORTION OF THESE CHEMICAL ELEMENTS IN PERSON WEIGHING 160 LBS.	FOODS RICH IN THESE CHEMICAL ELEMENTS	NORMAL FUNCTIONS OF THESE CHEMICAL ELEMENTS	EFFECT OF EXCESSIVE CHEMICAL CONSUMPTION OF THESE ELEMENTS	CONSTITUTIONS IN WHICH CHEMICAL CONSUMPTION OF THESE ELEMENTS IS EXCESSIVE	CONSTITUTIONS IN WHICH THESE CHEMICAL ELEMENTS ARE DEFICIENT
		PREDOMINATING CHEMICAL CONSUMPTION OF OSSEOUS TEMPERAMENT CONSTITUTIONS:			
(A)	(B)	(C)	(D)	(E)	(F)
CALCIUM 4 lbs. (Tri-calcium phosphate)	Milk, cheese, cabbage, lemons, undistilled water, Egg yolk, limes, walnuts, cottage cheese, halibut, shredded wheat biscuits, rhubarb, currants, apricots.	Bone making, cell vitalization.	Ossification, calcic ailments, falling sickness.	Calciferic, Isogenic.	Neurogenic, Pathetic, Carboferic, Hydripheric, Lipopheric, Nitropheric, Atrophic.
FLUORIN 3¾ oz.	Cartilagenous broth, goats' milk, Cod liver oil, Roquefort cheese, oats, Oatmeal bread, mackerel, oysters, Swiss cheese, river water.	*Bone cementation*, construction of solid membranes; destructive of certain species of germs. Stimulates bones and spleen.	Bone disease, Brittleness of bone; *bone defects*; *abnormalities.*	Marasmic,	Marasmic account excessive consumption; All vital constitutions; Atrophic account low oxidation; Pargenic account taint.
SILICON 1¼ oz.	Oats, barley, lentils, figs, Oatmeal bread, oatmeal muffins, oatmeal mush, barley bread, olives, spinach, red cabbage, figs, lettuce, rye food.	*Alkalization*; sexualization; *tonicity*; growth and repair of teeth, nails and hair. Ligamentation. Stimulates brain, nerves and entire system.	Hyperbolism, Speculation, excessive energy and work.	Sillevitic.	Sillevitic account excessive consumption. All constitutions especially vital and Atrophic.
		PREDOMINATING CHEMICAL CONSUMPTION OF VITAL TEMPERAMENT CONSTITUTIONS:			
CARBON 45 lbs.	Sugar, starch, sweets. All sweet foods, Pastry, cake, glucose preparations, polished rice, tapioca, sago.	Construction of Vital system. Protoplasmic in function.	*Obesity;* auto-intoxication. Lack of organo-metallic salts; *stupidity;* poor bone production because sugar uses up the calcium salts.	Pathetic (some) Isogenic (some) Carboferic, Nitropheric, Pallinomic, Pargenic.	Nervi-motive, Neurogenic Desmogenic, Marasmic, Calciferic, Sillevitic, Atrophic Medeic,
HYDROGEN 15 lbs.	Water, juices, juicy greens, vegetables.	Elimination, *perspiration, osmosis, cooling processes, nerve conduction, secretion, circulation.*	Hydric *obesity,* eczema; weakness; excessive action in nerve and brain cells.	Hydripheric, All diseased people having a lack of silicon, sodium, calcium and potassium salts; and in times of low oxidation.	Marasmic, Calciferic, Medeic.
NITROGEN 2 lbs.	Meat, peas, beans, lentils, air. Chuck, lean flank, kidney, lean mackerel, muskellunge, pickerel, scallops.	Regulation. Prevention of excessive heat production.	Phlegmosis, excessive conservatism, timidity, acidity, lack of oxidation.	Nitropheric, All phlegmatic people.	Exesthesic (because of generation of sulphur gas which interferes with oxidation), Oxypheric, Atrophic.
OXYGEN 89 lbs.	Air, water, Carbohydrates, horseradish, onions, greens, watery vegetables, Peppers, spices, condiments, rhubarb, most all other foods, more or less.	Oxidation, respiration, excretion of carbonic oxide, vitalization; growth, repair.	Sensuality, drinking habits, mental and physical excesses.	Myogenic (some) Oxypheric.	All constitutions, except Oxypherics and some Myogenics, are low, or very low in oxygen.
		CHEMICAL NOT AT THE FOUNDATION OF ANY TYPE OR CONSTITUTION			
IRON 2 oz.	Beets, Lettuce, wild blackberries, spinach, prunes, strawberries, German prunes, bran bread, head lettuce, shredded wheat biscuits, red currants, black currants, pears.	Oxidation of the blood, sexualization, generative functioning.	High blood pressure, plethora, hemorrhages, stupidity, hebetudinous senses.	Myogenic (some) Oxypheric.	All diseased people. Sadly lacking in Neurogenic, Pathetic, Carboferic, Atrophic.

The Neurogenic Constitution

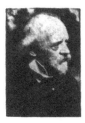

Hall Caine

The body size of man depends upon his temperament and constitution; that is, as to whether bones, muscles, the vital system or the nervous system is in the lead in activity and growth. When the life force lives and is active more particularly in the nervous system, the man or woman does not grow large but remains short in stature and small in build, because the nervous system is the smallest part of the human constitution. This is why some people are naturally small, slender and petite; they belong to the mental or nervous types of people.

The Neurogenic Type is highly conscious, so much so that he is constantly noticing things around him until his brain is in a sort of whirl. His attention is caught by everything he sees and by everything he hears. He wears himself out completely each day and must have sufficient rest and sleep in order to get his supply of nerve energy for the next day. He has no bank account of nerve force, but lives up each day's supply, unprepared for any emergency caused by shock, sickness or extra work. He needs much sleep because his nerves are so active when he is awake, on account of phosphorus acting on them.

This man is apt to be an extremist. He is actuated by speculative tendencies and interested in speculative and idealistic philosophy. He has a very lively imagination and is a natural born optimist. He has plenty of faith in suggestion, but often has less faith in work, effort, diet and matter. He is fond of idealistic reading, idealistic systems of diet, such as raw food diet, fruit diet, meatless diet (because of killing), and so on.

He has more ambition and optimism than he has strength and power. His blood rushes to his brain and produces over-activity of the higher imaginative intellect and of idealistic emotions. These people are highly keyed-up, particular, fine, exclusive and eager to know the future. They often receive revelations from the unseen forces regarding man and his destiny. Excitable moods are followed by faintness. Joy is excessive; mental attitudes are extreme, varying, sudden and spasmodic. Optimism, speculation, hope and expectation are excessive. They have a natural appreciation and understanding of doctrines, creeds, miracles, psychic phenomena and religious philosophy. They feel that they are qualified to teach and tell others what to do in the world of mind, thought, creeds, idealism, ethics.

They often study excessively, neglecting health, nutrition, sleep, exercise, until they are exhausted and sick. They live in a world of fancy.

When phosphorus unites with stronger elements, it leads to genius and practicality; but when phosphorus predominates among the chemical elements, the man is impractical.

The Myogenic Constitution

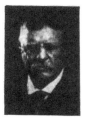

The type most favored at birth for a healthy, successful and happy life is the Myogenic. He is the most human of all the types, understanding the weaknesses and temptations of human nature.

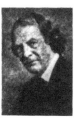

Theo. Roosevelt   **Elbert Hubbard**

It is the type that makes a very liberal use of potassium in the chemistry of the body. Wherever there is sufficient of potassium (an alkaline element) there will also be a liberal use of oxygen in the body, and as oxygen calls for iron in abundance, we have potassium, oxygen and iron, a wonderful trinity for optimism, courage, action, joy and health.

The Potassium Type is "the salt of the earth"— and if the salt lose its savor (health and usefulness it is only through wicked and deliberate waste and debauchery of inherited health qualities, in his case.

He is quick intuitive, tactful, diplomatic and mirthful. Charles Schwab is a splendid example of this Type. Strong, positive, aggressive, hard-working, but emotional, sympathetic and known as a "good fellow." This is typical of the best side of the Potassium Type.

They love to eat, drink and be merry and unless they have a balance of the controlling faculties, they are sure to over-do and so ruin their careers through the sins of commission.

The mental faculties of these people run to approximate harmony. Environment does much to influence the faculties to inharmony, especially when the natural faculties are near to balance. When the faculties are strongly uneven or unbalanced, some being strong and some extremely weak, as is the case in the man of genius, environment has very little effect on him. Environment has a strong effect on the Potassium Type, because of his adaptability.

The face of the Potassium Type flushes easily from exercise or excitement. In the blond of this type, the complexion is sanguine or reddish brown or red white-brown. In the brunette it is sanguine dark brown. The skin is warm to the touch and adheres closely to the muscles, it is usually more hairy than the skin of other types of people.

Their faces are wide-oval, features rather small and harmonious, their heads are wide and oval in shape. Their manners are animated and responsive and they are usually good talkers. Their talent turns toward commercial life for they are very practical and like to make plenty of money which they quickly spend. Some are professional athletes, while others are only amateurs but all are ardent supporters of athletics. This is their hobby. Some of our best writers and authors belong to this Type, as for instance Shakespeare, Jack London, Rex Beach and Elbert Hubbard.

402

The Nervi-Motive Constitution

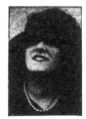

Gloria Swanson

The Nervi-Motive type of people are so intensely emotional, volcanic and dogmatic that they appear to have a thousand talents to the superficial observer, but their talents pivot mainly on courage, practicality, hard work and painstaking accuracy in what they do. They study rules, laws, systems, efficiency methods, and they never forget the money side of a proposition.

It is very difficult, almost impossible, for anyone to understand Nervi-Motive people unless, indeed, they live with them for a long time. They hide their real nature from the public. They are either silent and talk very little (as our President Coolidge), or else they talk a great deal (especially the women of this type) and hardly ever say what they really mean unless, indeed, they are scolding in the privacy of home. To strangers they are most pleasing and gracious.

They are very hard to please, but great workers. They have energy and tenacity which they get from the calcium in their makeup; while the explosive temper and irritability come from sulphur, and this element, combined with phosphorus, which is also active, give them a love of the beautiful, a strong desire for money, luxuries and a high position in life. They like to rule through money, possessions and position.

They accept responsibilities and worry regarding the present, are concerned about the future, uneasy about business and success, loans, interest, rents. They have grievances about neighbors, trouble about themselves and are full of vexations and fears about a thousand and one insignificant things that very early seam and line their faces with thousands of shallow wrinkles and produce a troubled expression.

At one time this type is congenial, liberal, accommodating; at another time uncivil, cross, rude or abusive, perhaps for seemingly no reason at all. He is a man of moods, uneven in disposition. Now he is patient, then impatient. Now he believes, then he doubts.

They possess good judgment, usually, with regard to profit and loss, buildings and money making, economy, politics, law, administration, management. Their minds gravitate towards power and wealth.

In general appearance they are short and spare in build, having a face that is square, or long and square and triangular at the chin, or it may be long pyriform in shape. They do not look happy, but have a tense, almost worried look.

They are economical, industrious, good managers and wiry, enduring in a physical sense and usually live to be quite old.

They are often found among statesmen, politicians, lawyers and wealthy property owners. They are usually talented people, more or less handicapped by poor health and low vitality.

The Nitropheric Constitution

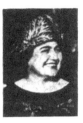

**Nitropheric
Mrs. Woodrow
Wilson**

The Nitrogen Type, being governed by the element nitrogen, and nitrogen being the wet blanket that subdues oxygen, it may easily be understood that the Nitrogen man is the direct opposite of the Oxygen man in appearance, nature, disposition, talent and state of health. The Nitropheric is the large, rather fleshy brunette, quiet, subdued, but nevertheless the manager and dictator. He is cold, distant, inhibitive and indifferent. He is repressive and represents inertia or control in human nature. He is strong but negative, still and controlled. In disposition he is secretive and never speaks his mind directly, though at times he can be bitingly sarcastic. He is a manager, preventing leaks and losses in business or in the home.

The Nitrogen man is calm, controlled, haughty, distant and independent. He is a natural born aristocrat. He seeks high positions so he can keep out of the hurly-burly of common life and living. He draws apart from the noisy, the uncouth and the vulgar.

The affinity of nitrogen for other chemical elements is distant, hence the slightest jar will shake it free, for nitrogen seeks freedom. So long as it is absolutely necessary for the Nitrogen Type to mix with the people for the purpose of gaining success, wealth and position, he does so, but longs for the time when he may withdraw. A certain wealthy woman now living in the most aristocratic section of Chicago, thirty years ago was helping her husband in a very humble way to get a start in the business world. They made money easily and comparatively quickly. Today they live in a mansion, but she is very rarely seen. She never mixes in society, possibly because she cannot reach the highest notch, nor does she cultivate many friends. Her children and her husband constitute her world and they are as devoted to her as slaves to a queen. She loves them and they love her, but she is cold and proud. To all other relatives and friends, as well as the people at large, she is distant and as cold as a Siberian frost. She tolerates only those who adore her, and these she holds in allegiance through her self-control, her stately personality and wonderful calm and poise, backed up by a tremendous will and haughty, sarcastic temper, ready to gleam in her deep eyes at the slightest provocation. Her disapproval manifests itself in greater frigidity of manner, cold looks, veiled or cutting sarcasm expressed in a low, controlled tone of voice, and a tendency to disappear until she is sufficiently placated by the humility and repentance of her subject.

Nitrogen has power to attract the dark pigments from plant food. The Nitrogen man is always dark in complexion. He is a brunette type, with a beautiful skin, satin-like in quality and very white. Never does his face show color except in the lips. The hair is usually smooth and shiny, like a raven's wing.

The Isogenic Constitution

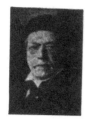

Isogenic
Samuel Gompers

This type combines equally the positive and negative qualities. When inactive, the Isogenic man is negative, bashful and timid; but once aroused can perform hard physical labor or mental work for long periods of time without rest or change. He never desires to change, always wanting to continue his work until he obtains the planned result. Like General Grant, he says: "We will fight it out on this line if it takes all summer."

The Isogenic brain acts slowly at first, gathering power gradually and persistently until it reaches a maximum, when by reason of its own momentum it can scarcely stop.

Isogenics are not tall, but heavy set and weigh heavily in proportion to size of body. They are compact and stiff in tissue. The hands are hard and bony, the bones cushioned with flesh. They are more lean in face than in body, have a large masculine face, long and wide, especially from eyes to mouth, large cheek bones, angular neck and well developed jaw.

Most everybody feels comfortable around the Isogenic Type. They appear strong, quiet, controlled and interesting. They are not really sociable nor sympathetic, but people give them credit for being both. They are phlegmatic and peaceful in mind until aroused, when they may become stormy and dangerous until the trouble is all over, when they sink back into the same peaceful state of mind until again disturbed. They will not yield to danger nor disaster; are restless when aroused, but slow to anger. They appear easy and good natured, more sociable and more negative than they really are. This *seeming* physical strength and self-repose enables them to attract and get other people to *work for them*. They work hard themselves and insist on hard work from everybody around them. They believe in practical efficiency. They aim to be just to all and can conduct business honestly, dealing with all classes of people successfully.

The Isogenic is a marrying man and marries early in life. Love never loses its attractiveness for him and he may remarry even at 80 years of age. He has wonderful recuperative powers, but once his vitality is exhausted it is seldom regained. The Isogenic is steady, regular and conservative in habits, a family man who enjoys simple living and long life.

They are not good-looking men nor women, but attractive nevertheless, clever and tactful when dealing with people, and natural-born character readers. They have strong feelings and emotions, with a powerfully active intellect. Even if this type has neither money, friends nor education, they rise above every disadvantage and succeed as educators, scientists or public benefactors.

Among the best known great and successful men and women who may be classed as the Isogenic Type are Thomas Paine, Lloyd George, Thomas Edison, Marshall Field, Jane Addams, George Eliot, Edna Ferber, Samuel Gompers and Queen Victoria.

The Exesthesic Constitution

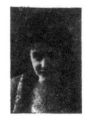

Exesthesic
Elsie Ferguson

If variety is the spice of life, the Sulphur Type is the spiciest individual of all the types, for her moods are constantly changing. Sulphur is used up in temper, anger and excitement. It is the predominating element in the person who is governed by impulse and sensitiveness. The Sulphur Type is a feminine constitution generally, though many of the "matinee idols" belong to this type. They are beautiful in face and coloring, and harmonious in body contour, symmetrical in feature. They have a thousand charming and fascinating qualities, and some have as many irritating qualities. They have beautiful, fluffy, or wiry, luxuriant hair, usually blonde and rich in color, yellow, golden reddish, auburn or chestnut brown. Occasionally we find an Exesthesic brunette.

They usually have long arms, limbs, neck, feet, hands, fingers, face and bodies. Their heads are long and oval in shape, as is also the face and the body itself. In fact, they are harmonious in bodily build. They are refined and cultured in appearance, though sometimes they may carry a haughty, distant, exclusive expression. They dress well, have excellent taste; they may sing, play and act. They are versatile, adaptable and able to entertain. They are full of sentimental emotion, sympathetic but very fussy.

The principles that underlie the ailments of the Sulphur Type are:

(a) Electrical ferments.
(b) Nerve intensity.

Exesthesic people are healthy, but not really strong and robust. For this reason they usually overdo and may become sickly if they work too hard in an unfavorable and inharmonious environment. Happiness makes them well; they live more in the mind than in the body. People of this type should give themselves the right environment, for they are more affected by environment than other types. They should live near the forest or near the ocean. They need outdoor exercise and motion, travel, and a diet rich in vegetable salts and phosphorized fat. They need association with people who are pleasing; they must exercise the platonic love affections, and they should avoid those whom they dislike and who irritate them.

Sulphur is the agent of soul expression. "No phosphorus, no thought," says the German philosopher. He might as well have added, no sulphur, no sensation, no soul communication with body and matter, no sense, no life, no soul expression.

In most Exesthesies, all faculties of feeling, emotion, intensity are in the lead.

In talent they are artistic and they are also interested in public work. They are able in music, drama, literature, painting, rural art, interior decorating, commercial or domestic art, writing, expression, literary side of business, secretarial work.

Mary Roberts Reinhardt belongs to this type and many magazine writers and artists.

The Calciferic Constitution

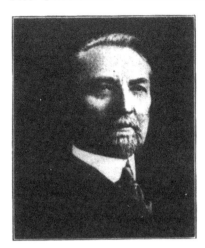

John W. Tayler
Attorney and Real Estate Broker

The Calcium man is the type who teaches us the *labors* of earth and not the *arts*.

Calcium is the rock in man and when it predominates in the human body it gives us our heavyweight men of genius. They are the men who undertake the great big jobs, the hard work, such as discovering the laws of gravity, the principles of electric lighting, the Darwinian theory of evolution, the invention of the automobile, etc., etc. History has produced some massive men of calcium, such as Thomas Carlyle, Thomas Edison, Woodrow Wilson, Ralph Waldo Emerson, William E. Gladstone, Charles Darwin, Henry Ford, John D. Rockefeller, Erickson, the inventor, and Abraham Lincoln.

Thomas Carlyle loved his wife and revered her memory, but in the words of Elbert Hubbard, "he never rushed to pick up her handkerchief. He could not bow gracefully nor tell funny stories, nor play the mandolin, but he was a great man. His touch was not always gentle nor was his voice low, but on his lips was no lie, and he forsook all to follow truth. When he took time to bring the ponderous machinery of his intellect to bear on a theme, he saw it through and through. His was a masculine mind."

This was a typical calcium nature. Thomas Carlyle was Scotch. A great many calcium men are found among the Scotch and Swedes, and among Americans of the pioneer type.

The Calcium man is undemonstrative and seemingly indifferent. He stands still and says nothing; he is passive until he is strongly aroused. He is silent and indifferent even when it is a question of self-protection or of vindicating his own actions. He is patient, strong and slow. He is like stone in structure, stubborn and set in disposition, strong and willing when it is a question of hard work. He is awkward in movement. He is sturdy, patient, enduring, grim and willful. He does not show his capabilities until he is opposed. A man like Abraham Lincoln, the Samson of the Civil War, was, so to speak, a living, breathing, humanized rock. This is true, perhaps in less degree, of all men in whom calcium is the leading element.

He may be a surgeon or a lawyer or executive. He is usually the master and boss, wherever he is. He is not always great, of course, but those of this type who are great lead in originality of thought. All of the imitators come after them.

The Pathetic Constitution

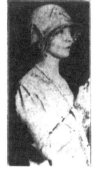

This type is found among both sexes, but most usually it is found among women. She is the "old-fashioned girl," so-called, sweet in disposition, sympathetic, very affectionate. Mrs. Browning, the poetess, is one.

Lillian Gish

When the three elements—carbon, hydrogen and phosphorus—unite as predominating factors in the organism of man, it is difficult to assimilate the organo-metallic salts, because will power and internal functional energy is lacking. The mind of the Pathetic woman is so sentimental that her chemistry is one-sided. She lacks will power, power of concentration and power to metabolize the stronger or metallic chemical elements for body structure. Hence the tissues are flabby. She has very little working capacity except along the lines of very light physical or mental work. Yet she appears so healthy that every physician will not hesitate to pronounce her a perfect specimen of health. If the chemistry of her body is not balanced she will suffer from nerve complaints and from chronic diseases later. In order that she may take up the calcium and other bone and muscle-building elements, her tissues must be recharged with will power. She seems harmonious in body build and beautiful in appearance. Her manners are pleasing, her disposition is sweet and her mind loving, but she has no reserve motor energy, no matter how large she may be nor how healthy she may appear. She possesses a passive determination, in favor of her strong emotions which may be mistaken for will.

If the salts of iron, calcium, silicon, magnesium, chlorin, sodium and potassium are not taken up (and when the sentimental faculties are in the lead) it is evident to the most superficial thinker what the final results and consequences of such unbalance, mentally and physically, would be. Lastly, chronic ailments arise with which medical science seems to be unable to cope. The indicated cure of such a patient would necessarily be in the direction of will building, physical exercises and scientific diet.

The Pathetic woman is a soul companion for the one who appreciates her. She possesses the qualities of fidelity, mutuality, sympathy, grace and beauty, but she lacks working ability, strength, courage and resolution. She is a peacemaker and a home decorator. She is naturally polite, cultured, refined, gracious, even when poor and untrained. Breeding is as natural to her as athletics is to a monkey. She does not need to attend a seminary in order to become a lady of refinement and culture. Refinement is in the soul, in the disposition; it is inherent. Educational refinement is a very thin veneer. The Pathetic lady is inherently refined because of her type, chemistry, faculties and soul. She could not be coarse, crude, ugly and abusive, however much she tried. The faculties of refinement and culture are all strongly in the lead in her mentality, and chemically speaking she has those compounds that result in fineness and softness of body structure and refinement of soul. Her very chemistry favors faith, hope and love. Her influence is in her tears and not in her will.

405

The Desmogenic Constitution

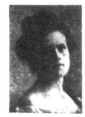

A Young Actress

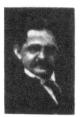

Desmogenic
Sydney Flower
Promoter

The Desmogenic is the Sodium type. Sodium in the chemical laboratory of the body builds ligaments, or the bands that hold bones firmly attached at the joints, producing that flexible strength necessary for the most efficient use of the bones. This is the chief use of sodium in the body and it is the reason also that the Desmogenic Type is so strong in motor development and also strong in the will section of the brain, for it takes strong impulses to extract sodium from food.

He is small, compact, wiry and pale-faced, and looks insignificant, yet is surprisingly strong. He loves action and he is like a living vegetative dynamo.

From the combination of chemical elements, the complexion of these people is extremely pale or greenish pale. They are slender or delicate looking, lean, often emaciated, but remarkably strong in ligaments. Flexible as a reed, lithe as a panther, possessed of wonderful strength of muscular tissue, they are enduring and tough in structure, although they look pale and delicate. They have a very wide space between the cheek bones and from ear to ear, though the lower face and jaws are sloping and narrow. The women sometimes are more fleshy, but they also possess this wiry, muscular strength and pale skin.

The Sodium man is an extremist. He is a specialist in some line, his likes and dislikes are very decided. If a girl of this type doesn't care for men she becomes a nun. If she likes men she may become an adventuress. If she is liberal-minded she will give food, clothes, money or anything she may have to anyone who is in need. Economy in this type may develop into parsimony. As a student he may study himself into the grave. Whatever he does he does thoroughly. He is prone to do things by spells and rushes, but at the same time is secretive, inhibitive, able to use other people when they do not know they are being used, for he is never really sociable, but self-centered, cool and calculating. When angry he loses all control, and when he fights he may kill. On the other hand, when he makes up his mind to control himself, he is very controlled and patient, but only up to a certain point, when he falls into a terrific rage. If he loves, he is devotion itself and very jealous. He is always going to extremes because his mind and motor equipment are like a dynamo of energy and he responds with heart and soul.

Our most dangerous criminals, strongest pugilists and relentless, aggressive business executives belong to this type, also some of our greatest reformers and inventors. Jack Dempsey and Jimmy Britt, pugilists, belong to this type. Billy Sunday, revivalistic whip; Marconi, inventor of the wireless; Irene Castle, noted dancer; John Decker, famous cartoonist; Galli-Curci, the great opera star; and Marshal Ferdinand Foch, are Desmogenics.

The Oxypheric Constitution

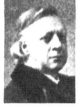

Oxypheric
Henry Ward
Beecher

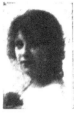

Oxypheric
A Young Mother

The Oxypheric Type is one of the most aggressive and at the same time executive types of men. He is red-faced, warm-blooded, with a heavy, thick neck. He has a deep, thick chest. His feet and hands are relatively small. Has strong muscles, but in a physical sense is lazy. He makes his living usually through his scheming and smooth tongue. He is a great success as a salesman and organizer, negotiator and promoter.

Big, blustering, dictatorial, good-hearted, generous, polygamistic in instincts, loud, outspoken, his anger flaming out like lightning streaks, then gone. Terrible in anger, but forgiving, tender, warm, magnetic.

The Oxypheric Type likes all foods containing oxygen in abundance, such as onions, radishes, tomatoes, etc., and these foods have a highly stimulating influence upon the brain. He practices deep breathing and takes a great deal of outdoor exercise, swimming, riding, etc., thereby increasing the oxygen supply and adding to his physical discomfort without knowing it. This is the cause of his predisposition to disease and ailments. These foods may produce serious ailments in this type through their combined properties and action in the stomach, as they contain oxalate of lime and a trace of oxalic acid. By eating such foods his system becomes overloaded with oxy-acid, oxalate of lime and oxygen, both organically and functionally. Such a diet and habits produce mental hilarity and arouse the emotions and passions until they become difficult to control in a man in whom free oxygen consumption is great. They produce urinary troubles, gout, gravel, kidney ailments, hardening of arteries, etc., in this type.

If the Oxypheric Type understood himself and would practice self-control, it would be the easiest thing in the world for him to keep well, for the processes of oxidation are perfect and heat is never lacking in his body.

They are as a type very apt to be imprudent in regard to food and habits, and when sickness does overtake them it is usually their own fault, the result of wrong diet or excesses in diet and habits. They must avoid over-heating foods, such as highly seasoned and oily foods, sweets, fats, oxygen and sulphur vegetables, bananas, potatoes, meats as a rule else the blood, brain, liver, bowels, kidneys, nerves, may at last become overheated and plethora may develop because too much blood is made. Figuratively speaking, such a patient is on fire. He is a healthy-sick man, and when he is sick he is acutely sick, burning up with fever and almost unbearable pain. Such a man when he knows his chemical type can easily keep himself a perfect specimen of health. But, paradoxical as it may seem, some of the things that are health producing for other types are the things that make him sick, such as an abundance of fresh air and exercise and an exclusive vegetable diet.

The Lipopheric Constitution

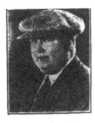

Lipopheric
Walter Hiers
Jovial, wholesome
comedian of the
movies. Knows how
to make everybody
laugh.

There are eight different and distinct causes of avoirdupois but there is only *one* "fat" Type. Hydrocarbons mainly, are absorbed in this Type to make them heavy.

Fatty tissue is a compound of carbon, hydrogen and oxygen, the proportion of oxygen being insufficient to convert the hydrogen into water. Adipose tissue is composed of fat lodged in the meshes of aureolar tissue, well supplied with blood vessels and lymphatics, but having no nerves. Hence fatty tissue is nerveless or dead tissue. Such tissue is hard and oily.

Individuals of this type have a large central body, oily hair, fleshy neck and a voluminous chest. The skin is white, smooth, somewhat hot and dry.

They have short arms, small fat hands, short tapering fingers, heavy thighs and short legs tapering down to very small feet. The face is circular and very fleshy in the lower part; they have a heavy double chin and a small fleshy nose. There is a pronounced fat ball on the cheeks and at back of neck. They carry the head well back and look at people with laughing, sparkling, flirtatious eyes. When healthy, they have a good deal of red color in cheeks and lips, and the hair has a rich bronze or reddish tinge, whether they be dark or medium dark in complexion.

They are jolly, free and familiar in manners, usually loud in speech and always strongly attracted to the opposite sex. Very fond of pleasures of the flesh—eating, drinking, social amusements, gay life and travel. They are especially interested in the mystic Oriental countries. Their religion as well as their pleasures, are of the senses.

They are very changeable in moods—cheerful, social, affectionate; then are depressed or angry. They are, however, always inclined to show their best side to strangers. They are naturally dictatorial. They scold without being angry. They are quarrelsome, but mean no harm unless they are deeply offended.

These people are noted for their pleasing, social, gracious manners in public. They are magnetic; they are adventuresome and daring. They are more selfish than usual and when they find that they cannot use people, often throw them over without compunction.

They love luxury, clothes of very fine fabrics, cars, pleasures, jazz music, darkened rooms, mystery, heavy colors, sensuous perfumes; they indulge in cryptic sayings and suggestive speech. They avoid the daylight, figuratively, and direct expression. Most of them, especially the men of this type are strongly polygamous.

They are haughty, prefer to have servants to do their work and live in extreme luxury. If they have to work, they plunge in vigorously and work very fast to get it out of the way. They possess wonderful executive and managing ability, when they exercise it, but they are always extravagant; they are good schemers and planners. Usually they are physically indolent.

The Atrophic Constitution

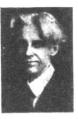

Atrophic

The Atrophic Type have a large head, especially large forehead or intellect, weak vital powers, tall and slender build, unable to increase weight, are characterized by long arms and legs, long neck, long hand and fingers with convex nails; long angular face, more or less sunken cheeks.

Atrophics are ever eager to learn, study and understand, loving books, science, philosophy, literature and sometimes mechanics—better than they love humanity, sport or recreation. When the youth of this type are frivolous, seeking excitement and gay life, they become reckless, undermine their overestimated vitality and soon go to the grave.

Natural born bookworms—these Atrophies read and study while others sleep, being fond of late hours. Their habits, once fixed, remain unchangeable for years until suddenly they change them only to persist just as strongly in a new direction, whether in religion, occupation, study or tendencies. Their diseases are chronic, their headaches may persist for years, suddenly cease, when some new pathological complication appears, only to go on as unceasingly as the former headaches.

They are slow in bodily movements and speech but vigorous in thought and study. Their brain substance is fine and compact like gold. Sometimes they are brilliant but usually low vitality defeats them. If an Atrophic is happy and satisfied with his associates and environment he is stronger in vitality but cannot endure gloom and unhappiness.

Being a sedentary worker, his work should not over tax the body. They should never live in a basement. Creative planning and detail work is the directing tendency of their talent for these careful accurate workers generally choose scientific, literary, philosophical or mechanical pursuits. Though brilliant and intellectual are not as a rule successful among people. Positive, aggressive, they make enemies and are indifferent about it.

In the Atrophic type the cause of tuberculosis is not germs and miasms as much as a weak physical brain, a poorly constructed circulatory system, malnutrition, poor oxidation, poor circulation and elimination, active nerves and brain. When vitality is low the Atrophic lacks calcium phosphates, blood salts, phosphorus, and generally does not reside in the proper climate, altitude and temperature. This constitution is naturally weak in the medulla (chest brain), limited in the functions and powers of respiration and oxidation—unable to secure sufficient oxygen for tissues and blood because of a too weak action of the lungs, cannot eliminate the impurities of the system.

Breathing increases the life forces. Man can live 40 to 60 days without food, but not more than 2 to 4 minutes without oxygen. Proper breathing can stimulate the feeble. The vital principle is in the heart, lungs and medulla of the brain. People weak in the medulla are weak in digestion and lack the essential lung area and oxygen-holding capacity in the air cells of the lungs. Thus the blood is not duly oxygenized.

407

The Carboferic Constitution

Note the sleepy, lethargic, dull expression of Edward VII. of England. When compounds of carbon are in excess, the body is flabby in tissue, the mind is dull, lethargic, sleepy. This is how Edward VII. became in his later years when the element carbon was allowed to predominate to too great an extent and this is what caused his death. It was said that he was in an almost constant sleepy state and could not finish his dinner without nodding. London is not a good climate for a Carbon Type. Edward would have enjoyed better health had he lived in the Highlands of Scotland or of Wales, or anywhere where the altitude was high and the air rare, and where excess carbon products could be burned up constantly instead of allowed to accumulate in the system.

Carbon as a chemical element is very abundant in all vegetable life, constituting about one-half of the entire vegetable kingdom. It is very susceptible to the presence of the vital impulse; therefore, the individual who has an affinity for and who loves carbonaceous food is bound to become bulky in bodily build. No method of reducing in the world will help them unless they give up sweets and starchy foods.

The system in the fleshy Carboferic Type is full of carbon products—acid and gases. They lack free oxygen. The causes of their ailments and weaknesses are:

Weakness in the will areas of the brain; laziness; lack of tissue salts; too much self-pity; too great exercise of the faculties of emotion and sympathy; too great an inclination to sit in a hammock, read novels and eat candy; excess of sugar in the system; carbonic products; saccharic gases.

Whatever the Carbon Type suffers from, the underlying cause is always the same, namely, acid.

If several of the blood salts are lacking and there is an excess of carbon, acid formation takes place. These acids, decomposition products, gases, have a bad effect upon many of the functions of the body. They affect nerves and brain, and make them dull and sluggish; they affect the circulation, heart, kidneys, liver, spleen, pancreas or some other part or function, depending upon the general condition. All Carboferic people are very fond of sweets and starches, and the more they eat of these the more fleshy they become. The Carbon Type is always a blonde or medium in complexion, usually blue-eyed with blonde hair, or light brown or mouse-colored hair.

They have a circular head, a circular face, regular features, tall, heavy, fleshy bodies, stately in bearing, and they have a still, passive countenance. They are friendly and convivial, love eating and pleasures. Carbon builds beauty, especially in youth; but the beauty soon fades unless one knows how to care for the beauty and prevent excess weight. They are more or less clumsy in movement, but are poised, seemingly controlled, though internally they may quiver with fear, for they are one of the most negative types of all.

The skin is milk-white and rose-red in youth, but when the carbonic acid gas is present the skin becomes putty-like in color.

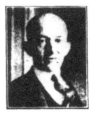

Carboferic
Edward VII of England

The Medeic Constitution

He is the greatest saint and the greatest sinner—the Dr. Jekyl and Mr. Hyde. He suffers great ups and downs, mentally—first gloomy then enthusiastic.

Medeic
George F. Mara
Political Speaker, called "The Human Dynamo."

The Medeic Constitution is dark-skinned, even though he may be light-haired and blue-eyed. They have a very serious expression and are often humorous and witty. They are lean, square-faced, square-headed. The upper jaw is more strongly developed than the lower; the nose usually rather well formed or small; the eyes large or medium; broad forehead; mouth often drawn crooked or one-sided, perhaps pulled down at the corners. They are always slender, with medium-sized body; sometimes deformed, such as the features, arms, legs, teeth, ears or skull sutures. Dwarfs are an exaggeration of the Medeic Constitution, an extreme product of many generations of Medeics.

As a rule, the Medeic Type is weakly developed in the faculties of mateship, though sex instinct is active. They are self-confident, yet at the same time timid. They do not believe much in others and may be disrespectful to people, their beliefs, religions and customs. The mirth faculty is well developed, which is an asset to their naturally morose disposition. They are usually sarcastic and satirical, prone to ridicule the things most people believe sacred. They are quick-witted, sometimes oratorical, dramatic, tragic. Again so genius-like that they are on the border of insanity, as in the case of Nietsche, who was of this type.

They may live their lives in defiance of society's law and order, as did Jesse James, or they may express their genius in poetry (James Stephens, the Irish poet); in literature (Edgar Allen Poe), in music (Beethoven); in satire (Voltaire); on the stage (Richard Mansfield and Sarah Bernhardt); political conspiracy (Richard III. of England, Marat of France, ex-Kaiser Wilhelm of Germany, Hamlet or Aaron Burr), or as a scientist (Steinmetz, or Abrams of "Electronic Theory" fame.)

The geniuses of this type are morbid, gloomy and satirical. In the Medeic, as in every type, are to be found the undeveloped with ugly disposition and criminal tendency. A Medeic feels discouraged and bitter towards all people when sick; liable to divorce his mate without cause or strike his benefactor. In youth they may sow a full crop of "wild oats" or develop a sulky, morbid, contrary nature. Many of this type are found among physicians and surgeons, while the Medeic laborer may work in mines, smelters, refineries and similar places. By right they should live and work in the open, where Nature can better supply the needed natural complements to their characteristic deficiencies.

The Pallinomic Constitution

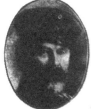

Pallinomic
King William II
Of Wurttemberg

Pallinomic people are different from all other types. Work, practicality, honesty, consistency, will power, courage, seriousness, wisdom relating to this life, and power of decision characterize them.

We know them by their portly appearance; thoughtful expression; large, wide feet; drawn or firm lips and wide mouth; broad, straight back; wide, square and large heads; short, heavy necks; sharp features; small eyes and stiff-jointed lower limbs noticed in their stiff, heavy walk, and by their industrious habits, thrift; penetrating minds, high and noble aspirations and practical judgment.

They have a positive and antagonistic disposition, with stiff, formal, curt, undemonstrative, and simple manners. They lack conversational talent and use a forced, emphatic style with a tendency to clip words and sentences. Their deportment is grave, retiring, almost solemn, and yet they are courageous and independent in spirit.

The Pallinomic possess a pale complexion and are strongly acid in blood and tissues even in youth, causing them to suffer from chronic rheumatism, at which time they have a pasty, murky color. In health the skin is white, pale at the same time, as it is dark in pigment and with a rosy tint. It has that same underlying hue seen in fear and terror. Pallinomic people are courageous, yet they are subject to biliary acids, toxins, fatigue poisons, sick liver, spleen and pancreatic secretions, which produces depressive states of mind, even fears and melancholia, which all have their effects on complexion. Their eyes usually are small and sunken and have a greenish tint.

They usually carry a serene, thoughtful, direct, fearless, penetrative, sharp though honest expression. Their emotions and passions are dynamic when once aroused. They have powerful concentration and self-control, though they are lion-like and thunderous when aroused.

Their features are usually small, sharp and regular though the face is broad and the forehead is wide and square and more strongly developed in the upper part.

The Pallinomic feel strong, even unconscious of their own ailments, and "carry on" until almost ready to die. They live in strength and die in courage; perhaps they do not even know that they are dying. Their vitality does not give out, their physical strength is intact, their mind is dynamic, their judgment is sound, their will is like cast iron, even on the death bed.

They are workers, but seldom physical laborers, because their brain is too large. It is said that "A laborer should have a small brain and large bones and muscles." They are skillful, clever, practical utilitarians, sometimes inventive, executive. They have talent in designing in the useful arts, in drilling, training, contracting, estimating; successful in business, arts and trades. They make good leaders and generals, though they prefer peace.

The Sillevitic Constitution

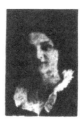

Sillevitic
A Young Actress

Silicon abundantly supplied and utilized in the body makes the blood alkaline and warmer, gives energy to the muscular and motor system and cheerfulness to the mind. These people actually "*feel* their oats." (Oats is a silicon food.) They are strong in muscle and optimistic of mind.

The Silicon girl is lively, light-hearted, loving, unconcerned and heedless. She loves to laugh, dance and sing, but dancing is her favorite pastime. Her face is flushed and fingers and feet are never still. It is as natural for her to be gay and happy as it is for the bird to sing. Whatever happens, she is never gloomy. If sick, unfortunate, neglected or poor, she does not complain. It is impossible for her to worry. It is always summer time to the Silicon Type. She is always slender, but with good-sized bones, rather large feet and bony hands. She has a small face, smiling eyes, bright and glowing. Her hair is luxuriant, glossy and wiry; it may be a rich black or a reddish auburn or golden straw-colored; it is usually curly or wavy.

She may be tall and slender or short and slender, but never *very* short. She is well adapted by nature, disposition and habits to feel at home in stage life. She is free, graceful as a dancer and never timid nor bashful. She can outdo in work and activity a girl of any other type.

This type has been compared to the gazelle or wild goat—light-footed and innocent.

She is likeable and makes many friends and very few, if any, enemies. She possesses a sunny disposition, a smiling and friendly personality, and a tendency to talk incessantly. She makes a very sociable neighbor, but is never clannish. In fact, she has few ties and does not carry the old friends in mind when far away. "*Out of sight out of mind*" holds good with her. She is living in the *future* and in the *present* and forgets the *past*. New friends, new home, new interest—progress and change—this is the life for the Silicon Type. They are thoughtless and changeable, more or less reckless and happy-go-lucky, but very industrious and only at times display a nomadic and tramp-like indifference to conventional life and habits. They are able to work hard and long without depleting their energy; work all day and dance till morning; no type is so able to do this without injury to health and spirits as is the Silicon Type. They are always ready to help others; full of sympathy and accommodation.

Silicon in blood and tissues makes a man jubilant over his plans, enthusiastic and mutual-minded. They want to share their good fortune with others. A man of highly alkaline tissue is speedy and accurate. He can decide instantly and is ready to act at once. Charlotte Greenwood, the actress of "So Long Letty" fame, is a good illustration of this type—tall to lankiness but quick and graceful.

The Pargenic Constitution

The Pargenic Type is known by his voluptuous appearance, puffy cheeks, greasy skin, heavy neck, large lower abdomen, flimsy under lip, thick under eyelids, granulated lids, large chest and shoulders, large abdomen, heavy hips and limbs, large, square hands. He has puffy,

**Pargenic
Samuel Johnson**
Author of the First
Dictionary

hot hands and large feet; his gait is clumsy and awkward. This is especially true in a coarser type and one who has not conquered his innate appetite for strong drinks, cold drinks and a rich diet. In some who have conquered their strong appetites the general appearance is more refined. But even then the incurved face, the massive upper forehead the tall, heavy, ungainly figure, the dark and rather dirty skin are still seen.

The Pargenic has fixed moods. He has still and sulky spells. He may sulk for weeks for no seeming reason. He may sit and listen for some time and say nothing; then, all at once, he arouses and converses in a critical, sarcastic, bitter, caustic and cynical manner. As a rule, he makes no effort to please people and has very few friends, except those he gains through admiration of his mental capacity. He comes and goes when he pleases; acts, speaks, studies and writes according to his own notions, keeping his plans to himself. He is close-mouthed, especially about his own affairs, and people know nothing about his soul life, his internal worries, his struggles with others and with himself, his disappointments, secret plans, silent intentions and repressed emotions. He is morose, abstract in mind. His dislikes are eternal; his hatreds, notions, suspicions, fears, delusions and latent diseases always prevail. He is inordinately conceited and thinks no one so great as he. He feels he is a law to himself and to others all sufficient. He never asks advice. He learns more from his own reasoning than he can learn from books.

He has either a fiery-red or a clay-like or inflamed complexion, a prominent lower jaw and a more or less greasy appearance of face, neck, scalp and hair. He is inclined to baldness in spots, loss of eyelids and eyebrows. Inflamed nail roots may bother him. He has a croupy throat and suffers from bronchial ailments. The alienist in his studies of mental diseases would find this patient very puzzling if he had to deal with him, for he seems rational, yet peculiar. He can reason like a lawyer and we find this type among our best and most prominent lawyers. As a patient the Pargenic complains of shivers in his brain and nerves. He complains of tremendous headaches, unbearable and continuous.

The Marasmic Constitution

The Marasmic Type is based on a high chlorin consumption, with a low, fat, sugar, starch and water metabolism.

This man has an unchangeable mind and a conservative disposition. He has a very dark, even greenish-yellow skin, an emaciated body, sunken cheeks and high cheek bones.

A great many Chinese belong to this type; also Turks and Asiatic people. There are some of any nation, also.

Chlorin combines energetically with the metals and attracts humidity from all bodies, the human body included. For this reason all Marasmics are lean, haggard and heavily wrinkled, and have a very dark skin. Picture a dark, lank Chinese, unsociable, silent, secretive, and you have an idea of the Marasmic Type. He is the very opposite of the Sillevitic and Myogenic types, for he is as pessimistic as they are optismistic.

He is a habit man and sticks to his work without change, rest or recreation. He is willing to work early and late. A work that requires slowness, steadiness, accuracy and long, lonesome hours— nothing but work and monotony — calls for a Marasmic.

People of this type have excellent judgment of art products of a useful nature, of perspective, form, size, shape and methods of application.

He is a stoic because he lacks social feelings or sentiments. He is indifferent to the suffering and appeal of others—unconcerned, unmoved by prayer or tears; but when it is a question of his own personal danger he is a coward and loses his self-control altogether.

He has no interest in humanity. He can be governed through fear so long as he knows there is no escape, but not through love and gratitude. He naturally fears authority.

It is better for him not to come in direct contact with the people any more than he can help. He is not popular. Best for him are independent occupations in which he serves the people without coming in direct contact with them. He should be his own boss. He works according to his own way of doing things. He is not impatient to get away from work —will work night and day, provided he is not interfered with. He may become the butt of ridicule if he works in gangs of men or women. He is dangerous if interfered with too much, but injures his enemy in a treacherous, sly way. He is an industrious, thrifty worker, attends strictly to his own business, and never interferes with anyone. He believes in safety, is economical and sedentary in talent. He makes a very good druggist, chef, watchman, undertaker, taxidermist, running washing, dyeing and cleaning industries, keeper of bath houses, massage parlors, billiard rooms, keeper of museums. He is interested in sciences of the past, past religions, philosophy, mythology. He is peaceable if left alone, but caustic, sarcastic and witty when he takes a strong dislike.

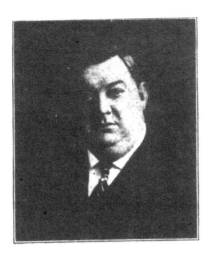

Hydripheric
M. L. Lawrence
Banker and Publisher

We recognize the Hydrogen Type by his seemingly timid, quiet manner; his calm, mild, sad expression. He does not talk much. His body builds largest at the hips and central body as he becomes fleshy. His shoulders are sloping. His flesh is soft, porous, flabby, making him awkward in his gait. His muscles are too watery. His face is large, especially the lower face, under the ears and around the neck. His face is usually inclined to be incurved in profile, with a small, bony formation of chin. His complexion has a waterlike, delicate tint. Like a sponge, he absorbs water until he gradually becomes a walking mass of organized water. His tissues are soft and plastic. He senses the changes in the atmosphere very keenly and can predict the coming storm far in advance.

The ability of hydrogen as an element to penetrate and to leak through matter, even stone walls, is remarkable. It is able to ascend, descend, enter into and go through things with ease—through vegetable fibers and human tissues. This characteristic of the hydrogen man is seen in his mind's action. His mind is penetrative, even though it is something like a London fog.

There is a heavy, foggy moisture in his interior, brain included, that affects his mental understanding at times, and yet his senses and perceptions are keen and his mind penetrates slowly, though surely. His is not a responsive mind nor does he have the power of quick decision; but when he is acted upon he will react slowly and powerfully. If a thought comes to him, he will hold to it until he slowly works out a decision and a solution of any problem. This is the reason that we have a number of famous men among the Hydrogen Type.

Many of our best doctors belong to this type. Hahnemann, father of homeopathy, and Father Kneipp of hydropathy fame belonged to this type.
They dislike to talk and act because they lack oxygen, and it is oxygen that stirs the mind. Things are hazy and obscure in the mind of the Hydrogen man, but he holds on. He bides his time. When in danger he can act very quickly, for the shock clears the fog out of the brain.

They are often able men, but they are serious and inclined to sullenness. They develop criticism and pessimism as well as dependence, because they feel weak and do not like to stand alone, and at the same time they do not trust strangers.

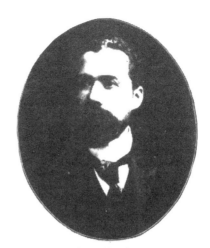

L. A. Vaught
Tall, Slender
Nitropheric

Tall Nitropheric Constitution

There are two types of the Nitropheric, one of which is seldom encountered, i. e., the tall, slender-bodied brunette. He is the most handsome, dignified and poised individual that may be found. He has loose joints; soft, long bones; long, slender hands and feet; a controlled and pleasing personality; dignified bearing. He is about 5 feet 10 inches to 6 feet tall or over. He cares nothing for business, but likes to spend money, especially on books, art, education and training. He is inclined for public service or professional work. He may be a school, college or university teacher or professor, or a surgeon, lecturer, preacher, artist, cartoonist, dress or art designer, lawyer or real estate dealer. He is sure to choose a dignified occupation. He has a large head, high and square forehead, large face, small nose, soft, dark, wavy hair, large dark eyes. His expression is smiling, but distant. He carries his body very straight, almost bending backwards.

The other Nitropheric Type described before, to which Mrs. Woodrow Wilson belongs, is short, stocky in build, more practical and businesslike.

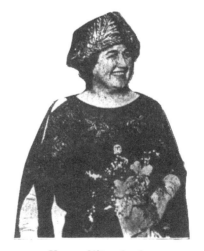

Heavy Nitropheric
Mrs. Woodrow Wilson

The Barotic Constitution

The sleeping lion, the hibernating bear and the passive elephant, all represent strength and latency—and this is what the Barotic Type represents. He is large, slow thinking, slow acting. He is passive until aroused. Large bodies move slowly.

Baros is a word that means heavy. The word heaviness describes this type in every particular. He is serious and ponderous in mind, profound in reason as well as large and heavy in body, slow and awkward in movements. His skill is not in the muscles, bones and nerves of his body, but in his slow moving, powerful brain cells. He is a born executive. This type is rather balanced in the Temperaments, but the bony system is slightly in the lead, with the vital temperament almost equal.

The Barotic is slower than the Calciferic and more clumsy than the Isogenic. He has in the lead the vital chemicals—Carbon, Nitrogen, Hydrogen, also Calcium, with Sulphur. The brain and nerve metabolism is below par and bone and vital metabolism is in the ascendency. Therefore, he is a physical type, but a superintendent of workers rather than one who does the work. No one, not even himself, ever knows his strength until his own exhaust valves open up from terrific emotion or temper, and then he is primitive in his lack of control or restraint. Push the Barotic man until he explodes and then all of the pent-up strength of Calcium, and his powerful cerebellum is back of the outburst. There is a tremendous impulse locked up in this man, waiting to be released.

Physically the Barotic is the largest type. Men of this type are 6 feet 4 inches, up to 7 feet and over, in height, and weight from 225 pounds to 300 pounds and over. Women are not quite so large. His face is large, especially below the eyes; cheek bones are very wide, and the face is broad and flat; the nose large and wide at the wings, the chin broad and long, the lips full and the mouth wide. The eyes are usually small and deep-set and the expression is quiet, passive, good-natured. His skin is dusky, and he may have broken veins in face because his blood is thick and does not flow freely through muscles and solid structures, nor is the drainage of the brain and face perfect. His hands and feet are very large and broad. His shoulders are broad, but the lung development not marked. He always has a heavy appetite for plain substantial food as well as for sweets and starches.

The Barotic man is sturdy, reliable, and possesses good common sense and judgment. He is fair and just unless he is prejudiced by his own dislikes, for he is much disposed to take strong likes and dislikes, and cannot overcome them. He is slow to forgive; meek and docile in his attitude toward others, for he is sadly lacking in self-confidence. He works best under superior leaders, business geniuses, or else for the Government. He does his own thinking. He is slow in school and in psychological tests he would not show to advantage, for the simple reason that he is mentally slow and lacking in powers of expression.

He is not self-acting, but requires external stimuli to call out his slumbering powers. However, he is a mighty man whether he becomes known or not. Much depends upon his environment. Circumstances call him out. Under great stress he becomes great. In times of peace and plenty he is a sleeping genius.

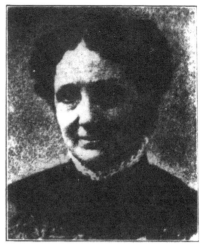

Neurogenic
Mary Baker Eddy

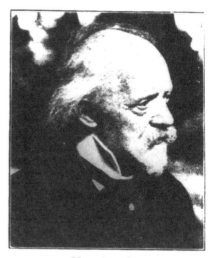

Neurogenic
Hall Caine

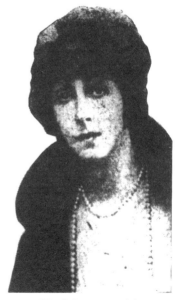

Healthy Atrophic
Duchess of Marlborough

THE TEMPERAMENTS

Body & Extremities	Mental Temperament	Muscular Temperament	Osseous Temperament	Vital Temperament
ABDOMEN	Small, sunken, narrow from side to side and front to back.	Harmonious, proportionate. Full width and thickness.	Medium, flat, wide but lacks depth from front to back.	Large; convex outwardly. Measures 40 to 58" or more.
BACK	Narrow, small, incurved.	Almost straight. Heavy muscles.	Flat, broad, lean, bony.	Full, circular. Long, seat to neck.
BODY	Thin, slender throughout, small in proportion to head; delicately formed, small-sized people. Height 4'8" to 5'8" or more.	Full, proportionate, harmonious. Well Rounded. Weight 150 to 255 lb. Height 5'1" to 6' or more.	Tall, lean, flat, bony, angular. Bony broad hips. Lacks flesh. Tapers from shoulders to feet. Built on principle of a square.	Tapers, hips down and hips up. Long, voluminous, circular. Large hips.
CHEST	Sunken, small insides or in axillary borders. Lacks development.	Large, convex, full in axillary borders. Hairy.	Flat and wide.	Deep, wide, full, circular, fleshy tissue at surface. Voluminous. Long.
NECK	Small; usually from 11" to 14" in size.	Well set, heavy, muscular, fleshy. Short from shoulders to ears. Size 14" to 16-1/2".	Long from shoulders to ears. Bit hollows in neck. Size 15" to 16-1/2". Lean.	Circular, large, size 16" to 19"; wide in sides. Lined with fat. Short, shoulders to ears.
SEX TYPE	Feminine body. Appears masculine when build is slender.	Harmonious; neither large nor small, short or tall. Neutral.	Masculine usually. Always bony.	Always feminine.
SHOULDERS	Narrow, lean, small, delicately formed.	Proportionate, well rounded with muscles.	Lean, bony, broad.	Fleshy. Apparently broad but actually narrow.
VITAL ORGANS	Small, sunken. Out of proportion to height and size of head.	Proportionate, medium.	Small, sunken but less so than Mental temperament.	Large, full, rotund, voluptuous.
ARMS	Relatively long, slender; soft, small bones.	Fleshy, proportionate. Usually hairy and muscular.	Long, bony, lean.	Heavy, fleshy especially at shoulders, but flesh is fatty or watery tissue. Tapers.
FINGERS	Slender, somewhat shiny or transparent. Long.	Proportionate, fleshy, warm.	Long, heavy, bony, lean.	Large, fleshy, broad, tapering. Heavy base. Small bones and joints.
NAILS	Long and thin.	Oval, reddish, well shaped.	Triangular, bent inwardly. Hard, sometimes split; often white indicating poor circulation.	Small, tin, reddish, bent inwardly indicating helplessness in time of emergency.

THE TEMPERAMENTS (continued)

Body & Extremities	Mental Temperament	Muscular Temperament	Osseous Temperament	Vital Temperament
HANDS	Long, small, delicate, narrow, flexible, moist. Grayish or gray-pale, in color.	Large, flexible, warm, red. Usually sun-burned.	Broad, thin, bony, lacks flesh. Every vein and bone shows.	Shapely, soft, large; large at thumb, tapers toward fingers. Considerable tissue. Narrow but thick.
PALMS	Cold, moist, white, indicating anemia; poor digestion, poor circulation.	Rough, warm. Lines long, deep, distinct and red, indicating good circulation and plenty red corpuscles.	Wide, long, warm, thick skin. Whitish lines.	Fleshy, full.
TISSUE	Plastic, like clay. Bones soft.	Flexible, elastic.	Dense, hard, firm, heavy, coarse, unyielding.	Soft, nonresistive. Often fatty or watery.
KNEES	Small, circular.	Medium muscles, rather large.	Bony, lean.	Large, soft, vital.
FEET & ANKLES	Small feet, weak ankles.	Long, narrow, proportionate feet. High insteps. Large but not bony ankles.	Lean, fat, broad, bony feet. Very large ankles.	Small, soft, fleshy, usually short feet. Small ankles.
TOES	Long and narrow.	Proportionate, well formed.	Large, long, bony, stiff, hard.	Short, slender, tapering.
Head & Face BRAIN	Plastic tissue. Very large in proportion to body. Usually developed upwardly. Very large in temples or where hat rim fits. Small in base, lower backhead, crown, in front, behind and above ears. Also usually small in central and lateral tophead.	Evenly developed. Usually oval or egg-shaped. The larger part is posteriorly situated.	Large, compact in tissue. Largest in parietal region, in constructiveness and lower perceptives. Strongly developed behind and above ears. Head is flat, yet wide.	Although the head is large, the brain is small. Heaviest in base, forehead, in front of ears and in anterior tophead.
HAIR	Fine, thin, soft, not very abundant.	Wiry, fluffy, strong, abundant. Sometimes wavy and thick.	Strong and straight.	Fine, soft, often, oily. Clings to head.
HEAD	Large subcoronal. High forehead, weak base, weak around ears.	Even and eggshaped.	Long from front to back. High parietal. Large central tophead and intellect.	Large base and backhead. Broad at ears and in front. Usually circular.
LOBES—Strong	Central section of temporal lobe is strongest.	Even. Proportionate.	Parietal, frontal lobe and posterior temporal lobe.	Base, backhead, anterior tophead and anterior temporal lobe.

THE TEMPERAMENTS (continued)

Head & Face	Mental Temperament	Muscular Temperament	Osseous Temperament	Vital Temperament
LOBES—Weak	Lower backhead. Posterior and anterior temporal lobe. Crown and central tophead, central forehead.	No weak lobes.	Backhead is weakest; then base, subcoronal centro-horizontal forehead.	Crown, posterior temporal lobe, central and posterior top-head.
SKULL	Thin.	Medium in thickness.	Generally thick; thicker in lower central forehead.	Medium in thickness. Very plastic and soft.
CHEEKS	Small, sunken. Short, mouth to eyes, mouth to chin and mouth to ears.	Proportionate, ruddy, sometimes full. Long mouth to ears and from eye bone down.	Long, heavy cheek bones. Sunken mouth to ears. Flat cheeks indicating weak digestion and poor elimination.	Plump. Convex, mouth to ears. Large from cheekbones down. Long, mouth to ears.
CHIN	Small, shapely, harmonious, triangular pointed or rounded.	Pointed but broad laterally. Built downwardly and outwardly. Long, shapely, red. Often padded.	Broad angular, square heavy, sharp bones.	Short, rounded. Fat above and below chin. Narrow, indicating lack of bone development.
COMPLEXION	Pale or pale gray.	Dark red or brown red or ruddy.	Lime white or yellow white or yellow red.	White, rosy or white and oily or white and greasy.
EARS	Small, shapely. Upper part large, rounded, thin. Large concha. Tipsmall often loose.	Porportionate, shapely. Normal position; neither high nor low on head. Red.	Long, large, thick. Low central part strongly developed.	Relatively low set. Lower part is large.
EYES	Keen, active, lively. May have any color. Thin eyelids.	Large, oval. May have any color.	Usually small, sunken, severe. May have any color.	Expressive, pleasing, sympathetic. Usually large. May have any color.
EYEBROWS & LASHES	Shapely, small or slender capilla. Lashes often lacking.	Large, rounded; sometimes extend across root of nose. Long lashes.	Eyebrows, lashes, hair, mustache and beard unruly—sticking in all directions; indicating courage, determination, fight.	Light.
FACE	Small pyriform.	Oval, somewhat long.	Large, square, rectilinear. Long, mouth to eyes. Wide in upper part.	Convex, long. Lower section is long and padded.
FEATURES	Finely chiseled, giving appearance of culture. Usually small, lean yet artistic.	Harmonious in size. Full, fleshy or muscular. Firm tissue.	Angularity, wrinkled cheeks. Sternness.	Almost every feature is broad and convex.

THE TEMPERAMENTS (continued)

Head & Face	Mental Temperament	Muscular Temperament	Osseous Temperament	Vital Temperament
FOREHEAD	High, somewhat square or large. Wide in temples. Prominent and overhanging.	Harmonious.	Angularity in central lower and lateral lower sections. Heavy deep lines between brows.	Convexity. Sometimes bony in central and centro-horizontal sections.
JAWS	Small, short. Slope from lower ears to chin.	Fleshy, ruddy. Developed outwardly and down. Lower jaws heaviest at chin.	Always square. Lean. Sharp angles and long, giving squareness to upper face or forehead. Square from head to foot.	Short, fleshy (not bony at all). Appear large, but are made up of flesh or fatty tissue only.
LIPS	Lips thin, colorless or whitish or white and blue because of anemic condition. Lips sometimes shriveled.	Lips well developed. Fleshy part usually thick. Seemingly well under control.	Lips long, straight. Upper lip flat and tight, indicating determination. Under lip usually larger.	Lips short. Upper lip usually large. Inner part of lips in center protrudes, indicating appetite for food and drink.
MOUTH	Mouth, thin, small, feminine.	Medium and harmonious.	Wide, straight. Angles down indicating pessimism or gloomy mind.	Small, medium width, full, voluptuous.
NOSE	Shapely; often sharp and pointed. Bridge often sharp.	Harmonious in size and proportion. Reddish.	Large, bony, often long. Tip often develops downward, denoting mental depression or serious mindedness. Upper part sometimes developed. Sometimes middle part is, indicating executive power and determination. Sometimes lower third is developed, indicating aggressiveness.	Small, incurved. Usually wide and broad. Tip is large and fleshy.
TEETH	Small; often decay. Heavy dental bills. Bone growth and bone repair defective because of low oxidation and brain and nerves absorbing the phosphorus.	Not overly large. Fairly strong.	Large, broad, white, strong. Sometimes brittle because of lack of silicon and phosphorus or because of excessive quantity of calcium in bones and teeth.	Small; dentification poor; teeth building material lacking, namely: calcium, silicon and fluorine.
WRINKLES & LINES	Almost lacking due to lack of will power and because of an idealistic mind. Some long wrinkles in forehead, indicating humanitarianism.	Face is sociable. Practically none.	Heavy wrinkles somewhere; sometimes on nose running downward or across nose, or in midcheeks, indicating opposition or combativeness.	None. This is a temperament of pleasure and appetite hence no wrinkles nor lines.

General Construction	Mental Temperament	Muscular Temperament	Osseous Temperament	Vital Temperament
BLOOD	Usually anemic. Sometimes watery.	No deficiency. Well supplied with blood salts.	Blood salts always sufficient. Blood sometimes watery. White corpuscles sometimes lacking.	Blood too rich, fatty. Blood salts often lacking.
BONES	Thin, small, sharp, not cushioned with fat. Lightweight.	Proportionate in size. Well established with flesh or muscle.	Very heavy in scale; large, long; tissue compact.	Lightweight; small, soft.
CHEMICALS IN LEAD	Principally phosphorus and its compounds.	Protein, potassium, fibrin, albumen.	Phosphate, especially tricalcium phosphate, silicon, fluorine.	Carbon, oxygen, nitrogen, hydrogen or organic elements.
FAT	Fat metabolism defective in body. Fat principally in brain and nerves.	Fat metabolism excellent but not excessive.	Fat metabolism lacking in both body and brain.	Fat and sugar metabolism excessive because of strong appetite and love of pleasure.
JOINTS	Small, weak, almost lacking especially in fingers and toes.	Harmonious, flexible.	Heavy, hard, stiff.	Small, soft, fairly flexible.
LYMPHATICS	Inactive; often subject to serofula.	Excellent.	Fair condition. Sometimes sluggish, especially in atrophic.	Excessive in action and development, leading to obesity.
MUSCLES	Fine, delicate, weak.	Large, flexible, yielding, active; great tensification and relaxation.	Large, slow, sometimes unresponsive.	Weak, flabby. Tissue is fatty, watery, sugary—not muscle.
NERVES	Quick, responsive, nervous, over impressive. Nerves starved account excessive phosphorus products in system.	Active, normal in innervation.	Heavy, slow, sometimes unresponsive.	Nerves of body and physical senses very active. Cranial nerves less active. Motor nerves do not respond to any great extent.
PHYSIQUE	Body thin, head large. No stamina or endurance.	Harmonious.	Tall, angular, built on principle of a square.	Plump, rotund. Appears voluptuous.
SKIN	Moist, thin, fine, fair; sometimes cold or gray.	Warm, dry, brown.	Thick, rough, unresponsive, yellow white.	Fine, oily, soft, sometimes greasy. Floral.
TISSUE	Plastic.	Elastic.	Dense, hard.	Soft.

Recent medical studies are indicating a correlation between calcium balance within the body and psychiatric depression.

Tendencies & Characteristics	Mental Temperament	Muscular Temperament	Osseous Temperament	Vital Temperament
DISEASES	Nervous, mental.	Rheumatic.	Calcic, tubercular.	Cardiac, paralytic, congestive.
DISPOSITION	Exclusive, finicky.	Pleasing, sociable. Lover of outdoor life.	Mechanical, scientific, cold, cruel, combative.	Good natured. Complains sometimes.
EXPRESSION	Highly intelligent.	Ready, pleasing, sociable.	Reposeful, studious, earnest, positive.	Negative, sociable, dependent, voluptuous.
GESTURES	Lively.	Physical.	Slow, heavy, angular.	Easy, negative.
HABITS	Psychotic and neurotic. May dissipate.	Active, wants motion. Sleepy in mornings.	Psychopathic. Man of nature; desperate; dissipating. Accurate.	Indolent.
HANDSHAKE	Very light.	Hearty but short.	Hard, positive.	Negative.
LONGEVITY	Shortest lived.	Medium longevity.	Long lived.	Short lived.
MIND	Idealistic, particular, lively, responsive.	Pleasing, sociable, versatile, interested.	Executive, military, mechanical.	Social, rural, domestic, associative.
TALENT/ VOCATION	Artistic.	Traffic, transportation, railroading.	Engineering, warfare, mechanics, mathematics, science.	Catering, training, business, superintending; using others.
VOICE	High keyed.	Base, emphatic, yet sociable.	Harsh, husky, strong, positive.	Tender, shiny, tremulous, sentimental, high pitched.
WALK	Lively.	Easy, quick, elastic, graceful.	Slow, ponderous—like an ox.	Light; short steps.

The Mad Hatter Syndrome. In the 1930s, the wool industry used mercury salts for sizing and the strangely behaving workers who had absorbed toxic levels of mercury became known as "mad hatters." Finally, the cause was traced, the use of mercury was discontinued and "hatters" behaved normally again. Like mercury, lead can produce a variety of mental and nervous symptoms, leading to such mistaken diagnoses as hyperactivity or schizophrenia. Little is known about the behavioral effects of cadmium, except that an increased sensitivity to pain may occur. During an outbreak of cadmium poisoning in Japan, victims called it the "ouch-ouch" disease.

twenty-one

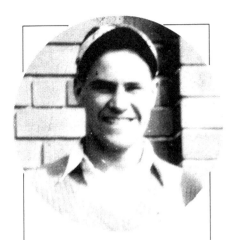

Joe B., a boxer friend of mine, was a Myogenic type. Notice the jaw.

The Myogenic type is congenial, expectant, level-headed, inspired and excitable.

The Desmogenic type is animated, expressive, vehement in gestures.

The Medeic type is highly creative, talented and clever.

The Marasmic type is hardworking, honest and dependable.

The muscular types of man

Myogenic, desmogenic, medeic, marasmic (eldic)

Sketch of the Muscular Temperament Types

The four temperaments: Mental, Osseous, Muscular and Vital, were categorized long before the time of Dr. Rocine. But the development of the twenty chemical types is credited to him.

In speaking of "temperament," reference is made to the characteristics of the human body, not to mental attributes.

Four chemical types make up the Muscular temperament classification. The most representative type is in the **Myogenic** in which potassium is the leading element. The amount of flesh on the bones is exactly right. The body is perfectly proportioned and height ranges from five to six feet. The countenance is pleasant, amiable and sociable. Dr. Rocine considered the Myogenic type to be the most physically balanced of all the twenty types.

The **Desmogenic** type utilizes considerable sodium, as well as the muscle-building powers of potassium. Sodium is valuable to the tendons and joints as a strengthening and elasticizing agent. The strength of the Desmogenic type rivals that of the Calciferic (calcium) type. Height varies drastically in the Desmogenic, from short to rather tall. Like the Sillevitic type, the Desmogenic is limber and speedy. The hands of this type are large and pliable. The face is widest at cheekbone level. The expression is alert and strained.

Potassium phosphate dominates the **Medeic** type, contributing to muscular efficiency and development as well as mental proficiency. Potassium promotes excellent muscle development and phosphorus gives responsive mentality. Height ranges from short to tall. As in the Desmogenic type, hands are limber and pliable. The face and head are elongated and narrow. The eye expression resembles that of the Desmogenic—alert and strained.

The **Marasmic** or **Eldic** type is dominated by chlorine. The effects of chlorine are drying and emaciating. Height varies from about five feet to less in some individuals. The nature is antisocial or secluded. The Oriental races are the chief counterparts of the Eldic type. Water absorption is faulty and starch assimilation deficient. This type should concentrate on weight building.

THE MYOGENIC TYPE

Definition

"Myo" means muscle; "genic" means producing. Myogenic, therefore, means a type in whom muscle development is pronounced.

Classification

Muscular temperament. Combinations may include Muscular-Vital, Vital-Muscular, Muscular-Mental (less frequent). Vital-Muscular type is sturdy and generally Oxypheric; Muscular-Mental is slim, speedy and highly intelligent; Mental-Muscular is generally nervo-fibrous and Exesthesic; other variations exist.

Leading Element

Potassium.

General Characteristics

The Myogenic constitution is caused by a combination of heredity, a muscle-building diet, the cerebellum, mental faculties favoring muscle metabolism and fibrin in lymph, blood and tissue. However, the muscular system of the Myogenic is not necessarily strong. The system is balanced, neither acidic nor overly alkaline. The general appearance is youthful with ruddy-brown complexion, vivacious, happy, outgoing, pleasant, congenial, entertaining, tending toward fleshiness, resembling the Oxypheric type overall. The body is generally well proportioned; chest is large, arms elongated and slim; muscle development overshadows bone development; weight and build are in proportion.

The countenance is lively, vigorous, sunny, shining, open and inviting. Poise is maintained under any circumstances and face does not reveal true state of emotions or mind. This is an active type because vitality and nerve force are high; muscular energy is almost boundless; the individual is always ready for action. Popularity is great, although this is not the universally magnetic type (Sillevitic). Gestures are active, flexible, mobile; gait is elastic, striding, easy. Voice is amiable, gentle, clear, of medium pitch; pronunciation is good.

Perception of people, speed, motion, commercialism is good. Memory for motion, human traits, personalities, behavior, events, conversations, localities and information gained through sight and hearing is excellent. The Myogenic type is inclined to be sociable, commercial, migratory, transient, experimental and variable; tendencies are on a major scale. Mental faults include poor concentration, sympathy, little will power, changeable nature, liberalism.

Head and Facial Features

The head and face are regular and in ideal proportion. Cheekbones slope; cheeks are moderately rounded; features are balanced and pleasing. Hair is often wavy, full bodied, thick, heavy and dry; color ranges from blond to light brown to dark. Mouth is medium sized; lips are balanced; until about age 50, this type looks youthful; few wrinkles appear.

Physical Exterior

Height: Ranges from five to six feet.
Weight: Around 160 pounds (more in the tall, athletic Myogenic).

The body is very muscular and well proportioned. Physical characteristics include: average-sized abdomen; strong ankles; average arm development; well-proportioned back, concave at waist; normal chest expansion; long feet; average-sized hands, slightly long, soft, pliable, fleshy; medium-sized hips in men, larger in women; small-boned knees with average strength; average development of legs; long, medium-sized neck; sturdy build. General physique is well proportioned, balanced, masculine and dignified. Skin pigment is brownish or ruddy or crimson; complexion of hair is brownish; there is much body hair. Skin is warm, sensitive to weather, light, air and externally-applied agents. Thighs are normally developed and muscles prominent; shoulders are heavy and muscular; torso is proportioned to legs; waistline is of average measurement, set in middle of torso.

Physical Interior

Interior characteristics are as follow. Efficient digestion; weak veins; more active arteries; controlled emotion and passion, preventing high blood pressure, nerve and brain pressure; elastic, flexible bones of average length or small, slim and supple; efficient though not powerful circulation; normal glandular function and development; normal, efficient intestinal tract; underdeveloped joints; exceptionally good lacteals; subnormal but active kidneys; efficient liver; active lungs; normally-functioning lymphatic system; superb muscular development and activity; active, efficient pancreas; above-average respiratory system; normal secretions; good digestion; excellent protein digestion and absorption (for muscle development); normally active spleen; average but not highly efficient tendons; above-average throat development and function. This type rarely becomes obese; stoutness is due to muscle development. Nerves are healthy and function normally; the Myogenic is not nervous; sensory nerves are sensitive; nerve impulses are normal and even, though optic nerves may be feeble and easily disrupted.

Five Senses

Vision is generally poor due to small optic centers in the brain. Touch perception is excellent and very sensitive; hearing is acute under many conditions; sense of smell is normal; taste is normal in regard to substances, excellent in regard to quality.

Metabolic Functions

Breathing is exceptionally good; elimination efficiency is average; metabolism is normal, protein metabolism above average to perfect. Nutrition is good, notably for albumin and muscles; perspiration is normal; oxidation of blood and tissue is superior; sexual system is very well developed; pulse is strong and rhythmic.

Mental Characteristics

The Myogenic type is congenial, expectant, level-headed, inspired and excitable. He understands human nature and has an eloquent tongue. Optimism is the general tone; pessimism is rare; he is comforting and cheerful to others, persuasive but seldom overbearing; his concern for others is genuine. He is sociable, extremely curious, candid and open, rarely indecisive, inclined to changes of all kinds, rarely persisting in one subject long enough to cover it thoroughly. The Myogenic is idealistic, exhalted; he has a profound love for nature. He is able to relax at will and to charm others into giving him desired favors.

Brain Faculties

Strong Faculties. Cerebellum, alimentiveness, amativeness, bibativeness, parental love, friendship, language, form, conjugality, locality, comparison, human nature, constructiveness, size.

Weak Faculties. Firmness, combativeness, continuity, self esteem.

Brain Itself. Faculties are generally balanced with no faculties exceptionally weak but some very strong. The mind is under considerable influence of protein, cerebellum, motor energy, manganese, oxygen, potassium, social and commercial faculties. Faculties dealing with people are active; there is more activity in morning and daytime than in the evening (near sunset the blood flows away from the brain, resulting in drowsiness). Cerebellum is large compared with cerebrum.

Talent and Career

The Myogenic type is an avid sports fan and often an athlete in his own right. Salesmanship and public relations are ideal endeavors, as are positions as travel agent, office manager, tour guide, radio announcer, news or sportscaster. The most effective talent of this type is in persuading and comforting others; his amiable nature and congeniality help to soften competitiveness and commercialism.

Biochemistry and Diet

Leading biochemical elements are potassium, sodium, manganese, protein, glycogen, myo-hematin, fibrin or albumin. Elements most often excessive are potassium, iron, nitrogen and sometimes oxygen. With the exception of iodine, elements are seldom deficient. This type is so balanced that sickness should be rare. Calcium, chlorine and fats are metabolized less efficiently than are other elements, but the constitution is not likely to suffer. The body chemistry of the Myogenic is neutral, neither acidic nor alkaline. He is able to assimilate potassium readily and, in fact, prefers foods high in potassium. He makes a successful vegetarian because of his excellent digestive ability and protein assimilation.

Appetite is normal and a reliable guide to proper nutrition because abnormal cravings are rare. Suitable foods include those high in manganese, potassium; nuts, vegetable proteins, vegetable starches, greens, berries. Intake of dairy products, fish, meats should be minimal. Vitamin supplementation is suggested. Good health comes easily if this type uses discretion and reason.

Additional Requirements

A pleasant, cool, breezy climate with plenty of fresh, pure air and ozone benefits the Myogenic. Exercise should be moderate, light and enjoyable; the individual tends to overestimate his strength and endurance. Country or outdoor living, domestic tranquillity, adequate and restful sleep are suggested. Manganese-rich foods are indicated if nerves are troublesome; vegetables should predominate in the diet.

Common Ailments

Ailments and diseases likely to afflict the Myogenic include acute illnesses, bone disturbances, cardiac problems, concussions, hemorrhages, hernias, neuroses, optical problems, septic disturbances, subacute disturbances, toxic accumulations, tumefaction, traumas. He may contract fevers such as malaria or develop complications of the liver, kidneys, blood, mesentery. Other diseases and possible disturbances when vitality is low include congestions, accidents, heart disease, heart failure, athletic and sports injuries, enlarged liver, complications from overeating, plethora, rheumatism, insomnia and skin eruptions. Overall, however, this is an exceptionally healthy type.

Inherent weaknesses in the Myogenic type include inclinations to recklessness, athletic excesses or accidents and overeating. Health problems are preventable by temperance in eating, limited drinks and tonics, a dry sodium diet, less rigorous participation in sports and athletics. The Myogenic enjoys good health even when abusing his body but is not generally long lived; his lifespan is average. Influenza finds him an easy target in spite of his strength.

Special Notes

The Myogenic is the "muscle man" who loves active sports. Of the twenty types, he is the most balanced, physically and mentally.

THE DESMOGENIC TYPE

Definition

"Desmo" has to do with band-ligaments; "genic" means producing; thus, desmogenic means holding (bones) together with ligaments.

Classification

Motive-ligamentous temperament. Combinations of Motive-Mental; Mental-Motive; Ligamentous-Mental; Ligamentous-Motive-Mental.

Leading Element

Sodium.

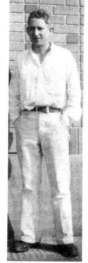
Dr. Jensen, a Desmogenic.

General Characteristics

The system of the Desmogenic is usually acidic because oxygen is deficient, the liver spasmodic, elimination poor and gelatin excessive. The muscles respond instantaneously to the dictates of the Desmogenic mind; the manner is positive, critical, poised for action, scrutinizing, restless, agitated. The body is usually slender, sometimes emaciated; may seem haggard and care-worn or haughty and discontented. This type is animated, expressive, vehement in gestures. The constitution seems iron-clad, but the health may collapse all at once under extreme stress. The nerve force is powerful and prolific. The body gives the appearance of invincible strength, elasticity, resistance, speed. The voice is often deep, resonant, commanding, generally pleasing unless angered, in which case it becomes rough and hoarse. Balance is excellent, step sure and graceful. Manners are plain, ideals practical, passions intense. Sixty percent of Desmogenics are male, forty percent female.

Head and Facial Features

Area of forehead above eyes is widest (region of perception); upper part of face is more narrow. Mouth is generally small, lips thin and taut. Eyes are expressive and alert. Skin tone is deceptively pale. Face may be devoid of expression and emotion at will. It often has deep wrinkles, or a network of fine wrinkles. It is short and wide at cheekbones, widest at level of ear opening. Cheekbones are prominent, cheeks sunken, ears low, brows horizontally straight. Hair is usually brown or dark. The face may be oldlooking or wrinkled and pale.

Physical Exterior

Height: Five to six feet.
Weight: Between 120 and 185 pounds.
The body is athletic, sinewy, compact, muscular. Cords, joints, tendons are strong and elastic; ligaments and muscles are generally powerful and nimble, quick to respond. Exterior characteristics include: well-developed ankles; long, powerful arms; broad, muscular back; square shoulders; flat, concave chest (except when fleshy); long feet; short fingers, usually straight and bony (taller types have longer fingers); square-oval hands; broad hips; well-developed and powerful knees; long neck. The body gives the general impression of endurance and wiriness, athletic ability. The skin tone is usually dark, denoting soberness. Skin color ranges from pale to clay brown. If sodium is lacking, the skin may be dry, brittle, cracked. Thighs are muscular, strong, sinewy, efficient. Waist is small and set either low or high.

Physical Interior

Interior characteristics are as follows. Strong arteries and weak veins; normal blood pressure; blood pale or bluish; subnormal oxidation; thin blood resulting in easy bleeding; medium-sized, compact, pliable, elastic bones; concave abdomen; medium-sized heart; subactive intestines; medium or small glands, sluggish or overworked; small kidneys; small liver, often overworked or sluggish and somewhat chaotic in activity (major problem); mediocre-to-fair lymphatic system function; superior membranous system; superb muscle power; usually subnormal pancreas; weak spleen; normal secretions unless sodium is deficient; powerful, tough, wiry ligaments; tendency toward emaciation; strong, efficient, massive, elastic joints; poor respiration due to sodium and chlorine deficiency; powerful, resilient nerves; tremendous nerve impulse, causing tendency toward motor nerve tremors; tendons resembling steel-coiled springs; dry, parched throat; swollen tonsils due to lack of sodium salts.

Five Senses

Senses of hearing and smell are keen; taste is often subnormal; touch is normal or subnormal; eyesight is normal and sensitive to strong light.

Metabolic Functions

Breathing, oxidation and generation of heat are often faulty; gases and toxins generated in the body reduce the capacity of red blood cells to carry oxygen. Eliminative channels are often sluggish. Nutrition is average; the body is not adequately nourished. Pulse rate is slow and erratic. Sexual system is strong but variable with occasional indifference.

Mental Characteristics

Mental attitude is serious, intense, crusading; a pet cause may receive entire devotion. Anger can be revengeful and unforgiving. Literary talent and intense study are rare, but if found in this type, may border on genius. Traits such as frugality and diligence are cyclic. Will power, discipline, sincerity, efficiency are great. The Desmogenic is a good judge of fire, heat, metals, cold, gases, oils, explosives, mechanics, engineering, athletics. He tends to overwork mentally and is an extremist in all things. In youth, his memory is good, particularly for the objective world; distance perception is keen. He can never be forced to do anything against his wishes; his will bends only for highly-respected authorities.

Brain Faculties

Strong Faculties. Cerebellum, destructiveness, approbativeness, often combativeness, self esteem, comparison, constructiveness, spirituality, size, weight, pons varolii, heat center highly-developed in highly-evolved individuals.

Weak Faculties. Bibativeness, acquisitiveness, parental love, conjugality, alimentativeness, friendship, continuity, eventuality, suavity, mirthfulness, hope, often veneration.

Brain Itself. Strongly-developed cerebellum. Any faculty may be strong or weak in the Desmogenic. Destructiveness and muscular brain area are invariably the most powerful.

Talent and Career

Enthusiasm and inspiration regulate talent. Suited for detective work, boxing, strenuous athletics, weightlifting, judo, karate, skiing, team sports, equestrian sports, evangelism, office management.

Biochemistry and Diet

Biochemical elements most active in the Desmogenic type include sodium, cartilage material, potassium, gelatin, calcium, phosphorus, albuminoid material, animal fat. Elements most often deficient in this type are sodium, gelatin, potassium, free oxygen, iron land magnesium. The element most likely to be excessive is sodium, although it may also be deficient due to large quantities being burned and robbed from the blood.

Desmogenics may be hearty eaters, but they appear malnourished or emaciated. Meals are eaten in a great rush, without regard for the needs of health; appetite is unnatural, favoring stimulants, spices, condiments. A diet of fish, fowl, whole grains, nuts, seeds, vegetables and fruits benefits this type. The craving for stimulants and alcohol must be controlled. Good health and vitality can be preserved into old age if the Desmogenic learns balance and learns to capitalize on his talents, energy and zeal.

Additional Requirements

Warm baths are good for the Desmogenic type; massage is also helpful. Climates which are warm, stimulating, with liberal ozone are most suitable. Altitudes between 4000 and 6000 feet are suggested.

An even temperature is best. Beneficial physical exercises include walking, deep breathing, active and demanding athletics or sports. The mind needs deep and disciplined concentration. Because of his extremism, the Desmogenic is likely to have only an average lifespan.

Suggestions for prevention of ill health or correction thereof include much sleep, alkalinity, arid climates, hilly regions, deep massage, joy, love, sunbaths, horseback riding, activity, cheerfulness. Exercise in the outdoors is a must. The bloodcount and alkalinity should be increased; bodily heat should be increased, uric acid decreased, gouty deposits dissolved. Alkaline foods are called for, along with milk and eggs; the stomach must be made alkaline and cooled. Healing ability of this type is low; chronic ailments are likely. Sunstroke and heatstroke should be guarded against. Anger should be curbed as it attacks the medulla and brain faculties. Depression and self pity should be guarded against.

Common Ailments

The Desmogenic is predisposed to such ailments as spontaneous abortion, accidents, alcoholism, arthritis, asthma, biliousness, bladder problems, cystitis, blood dechlorination, devitalization, diarrhea, dropsy, endocarditis, endometritis, eneuresis, feeblemindedness, gallstones, gout, infection, itch, kidney trouble, membranous afflictions, morphinomania, muscular prostration, nymphomania, paralysis, peritonitis, pleuro-pneumonia, pleurisy, pneumonia, rheumatism, stomach trouble, strangury, sunstroke and heatstroke, tonsillitis. Other maladies include cramps, colic, prolonged pain, insomnia, ear congestion or buzzing, hoarseness, muscle spasms, back pain, ravenous appetite accompanied by emaciation, lung congestion, enlarged prostate, aggravation of ailments in damp weather, infantile paralysis, autointoxication, acidity, hemorrhoids, excessive bleeding, paralysis after age 60.

Weaknesses and afflictions are chiefly due to hate, excitement, depressing surroundings, alcohol consumption, negative and detrimental emotions; to deficiency of sodium, silicon, oxygen, manganese, potassium; to excessive bile acids, gelatin, animal fat in joints; to intemperate consumption of sodium, to mineral deposits, autointoxication, acidity, lack of animal heat; to moisture, wind, cold; to overseriousness; to improper diet (major cause).

THE MEDEIC TYPE

Definition

"Medeic" derives from the Greek word *Medea* (of Sanskrit origin) which means magic or able to enchant; hence, the Medeic type is enchanting.

Classification

Mental temperament leads, followed by Muscular and Osseous.

Leading Element

Potassium phosphate.

General Characteristics

General appearance of the Medeic is tall, slim, emaciated but having broad shoulders; complexion is dark, ominous; face is thin, expression sober, sad, mysterious or unhappy; arms and legs are long; shoulders are bent and angular; impression is awesome or fearsome. Hair is dark or black and unmanageable; body seems out of proportion, too thin. Countenance is disturbed, troubled, apprehensive, mirthless; attitude is predominantly unhappy, sinister, threatening, despondent, intimidating, depressed, disheartened, formidable; on occasion, the Medeic may be friendly, open and confidential. Other noticeable characteristics include jerking of head; forceful, spontaneous nervous foot and hand movements; lack of mental tranquillity; deep, harsh, loud, gutteral, sometimes husky or nasal voice; head carried in front of body, giving rushed appearance; heavy steps and stooped body. Ninety percent of this type are male; only ten percent are female.

Head and Facial Features

Head and features are narrow and elongated; complexion varies from dull to muddy to rosy; usually complexion is dark, occasionally medium, rarely light. Expression of eyes is generally hostile, serious, unhappy, attentive, sober, alert. Hair is dry, unmanageable, often bushy, coarse, thick, bristly; it is often black but grays early. Lips are pessimistic, tight or snarling; mouth is turned down at corners and is wide; face often has puckering wrinkles. Cheeks may appear hollow; cheekbones are medium in size, prominent. Features are often homely or plain.

Physical Exterior

Height: Generally medium to tall; rarely taller, however, than six feet.

Weight: Approximately 100 to 150 pounds.

Arms and legs are longer than torso; appearance varies between mental and muscular, making the Medeic a hard type to identify. Abdomen is sunken; ankles are powerful, well developed; arms are very long; back is short and flat; shoulders and chest are broad; chest is hollowed by poor posture, stooped shoulders; feet are large and unattractive; hands are long and slender and seem inflexible, bony, but are actually pliable and soft; hips are narrow and lean with sunken pelvic area; knee joints are well developed. Further characteristics include exceptionally long, slender legs which may be unsteady; long, slim neck; upper spine curved forward; dark skin tone, often with brownish tint; resilient, thin, supple skin with countless spots—nerve spots, liver spots, freckles, brown spots, moles, warts, patches, dots, etc.; tender, sensitive, mottled, dry, wrinkled skin; long, lean thighs; small torso; slim waist set high on torso.

425

Physical Interior

Interior characteristics follow: defective assimilation ability; small abdomen which may be stretched from overeating; powerful, pliable, enduring arteries and veins; deficient blood, low blood pressure, irregular circulation; very pliable, limber bones; elongated bones which are always slender; sluggish fat metabolism and glandular system; faulty heart function; slow intestinal activity; well-developed joints; small, overworked kidneys; deficiency in number of lacteals; wiry, powerful ligaments; small, erratic liver; large lungs (largest vital organ in this type) which are chaotic, erratic; weak lymphatic system; powerful tendons, ligaments, cords (small muscles except for shoulders); sluggish pancreas; deficiency in secretions; medium-sized, erratic spleen; protein digestion more efficient than that of fats, sugars or starches; lack of digestive juices (leanness shows insufficient digestion).

Five Senses

Like other functions, the five senses are periodic and erratic in activity. Vision is normal but there are complaints of eye pain, flashes, spots before eyes, tears; hearing is acute but periodic; olfactory sense varies from good to poor; sense of taste is moderately keen; touch is exceptionally keen.

Metabolic Functions

Breathing is normal though sometimes sporadic; digestion is poor; elimination channels are sluggish; catabolism is excessive and anabolism deficient; nutrition is inadequate; oxidation is below par; perspiration is active; sexual system is weak and affected by mental morbidity, depression.

Mental Characteristics

Autointoxication facilitates chaotic mental states, apprehension, restlessness, even harmfulness. The brain is generally energetic, active, large, though not so large as in some types; large cerebellum accounts for the tough constitution which makes the Medeic type athletic, active, diligent, wiry. Mentality is extremely intense and deep; wit may be caustic and biting, critical; judgment is erratic, changeable, extreme; memory is

periodic, subjective, bizarre, better for criminal activities, violence, disease, danger, injuries. The Medeic has a good understanding of human nature, acting, sports, journalism, moneymaking, leadership. The individual is earnest, often secluded or hermit-like, unpredictable.

Mental tendencies include drama, sensation, cruelty, mistrust, pessimism, neurosis, psychosis, vindictiveness, disobedience, irritability, desperation, evasiveness, seduction, hostility, abuse, rebellion or revolution, fanaticism. The mind lacks self control; lacks understanding of the difference between good and evil or right and wrong; lacks love, sentiment, compassion. The mind is deep, fiery, periodic, energetic; imagination is morbid, suspicious; will power is strong though periodic; reason is often lacking. Individual is predisposed to insomnia, overwork, nervousness.

Brain Faculties

Strong Faculties. **Caution, destructiveness,** conscientiousness, amorousness; moderately strong faculties include weight, size, spirituality, calculation, approval.

Weak Faculties. **Hope, veneration,** friendship, bibativeness, time, self esteem, conjugality, human nature, medulla, eventuality, suavity, vitativeness, alimentiveness, continuity.

Talent and Career

The Medeic type is highly creative, talented, clever. Creative writing is often an area of excellence. Medeics may also be outstanding comedians, actors or actresses, magicians, mediums, cartoonists. Well-known Medeic types include Edgar Allen Poe (poet), Sarah Bernhart (actress) and Humphrey Bogart (actor).

Biochemistry and Diet

Phosphorus is the leading element in the Medeic type and is the only element likely to be excessive. Most often deficient are hydrogen, manganese, carbon and sodium. Appetite is generally good but capricious; stimulants and alcohol may be preferred to foods; narcotics may also be desired, as may condiments and sauces, pepper, animal proteins. Excessive appetite may alternate with starvation. Foods and tonics needed by the Medeic include sassafras, hops, sarsaparilla, clover and other herbal teas, warm foods, veal, fish, fresh vegetables and fruits; energizing foods, vitamin-rich foods, phosphorus foods, predigested foods, sodium foods, lecithin foods, fruit juices and broths. Such a diet must be adhered to in order for health to manifest and for talents to be fully developed. Foods which the Medeic naturally prefer are to be avoided.

Additional Requirements

Warm baths and showers are good for the Medeic type; vigorous, deep massage should follow. A balmy, warm climate is most beneficial; the air should contain much oxygen and ozone. Rest and as much sleep as possible are suggested for this type. Overexercising should be avoided.

Common Ailments

Most common ailments and diseases of the Medeic type include adhesions, alcoholism, anemia, apoplexy, arthritis, astigmatism, atrophy, backache, blood disorders, chills, bowel trouble, chondroma, colic, colds, curvature of the spine, depression, fever, fissures, glioma, headaches, heart failure, hysteria, itch, lameness, mastitis, mastoiditis, catarrh of membranes, miscarriages, ossification, osteoma, ovatitis, paralysis, paresis, pericarditis, pericystitis, periodic constipation, pneumonia, scirrhus, spasms, surgeries. Health is periodic and erratic, due largely to morbid mind. Life expectancy is not predictable; some Medeics reach old age while others die young.

Special Notes

The Medeic is generally wiry, touch, tenacious, stalwart; his vital energy is strong. However, he is constantly besieged by health destroyers, due largely to his inherent pessimism and his body's erratic functions.

THE MARASMIC (ELDIC) TYPE

Definition

"Marasmic" is derived from the Greek words *marasmos* and *marainein*, which mean to grow lean. (The term Eldic refers as well to the Marasmic type.)

Classification

Motive temperament. Fibrinous-Mental.

Leading Elements

Chlorine and phosphorus.

General Characteristics

The Marasmic constitution results from excessive chlorine consumption; unique body chemistry; low metabolism of fats, water and sugar; heredity; an impassive, stoical personality. The Marasmic type mirrors the qualities of the element chlorine. General appearance is withered, emaciated, aged, wrinkled. Bones are small and unpadded; skin is dry, yellow-brown, tawny, soft, wrinkled, appearing almost scarred (as if burned); physique is too slim to be well proportioned. Bones are light, slim without flesh (weight cannot be gained). The Marasmic has dark, thick blood; analgesic nerves; a preservative, conservative, enduring quality; he is small in stature; his poise and composure seem flawless but result from impassiveness and indifference. The countenance is unyielding, frozen, uncommunicative, reserved, remote; no body gestures are used when speaking; feet and hands remain still, head rigid; grace and fluidity are lacking. There is no personal magnetism; often low vitality; erratic nerve force; shuffling walk; low-pitched, nasal, slow, bronchial or nervous voice. Ninety percent of Marasmics are men, ten percent women.

Head and Facial Features

Head is narrow and elongated; lips are tight and thin; mouth is usually expansive; expression is sober and mature, even in the young. Cheekbones are often long and conspicuous, cheeks concave, chin small and sometimes backward sloping; eyes are elongated and sunken; features are of medium size. Hair is dry, matted, unkempt and often falls out; it may be black, brown, gray-brown or silvery, occasionally blond. The face is the most wrinkled among the twenty types.

Physical Exterior

Height: Ranges from short to medium.
Weight: Approximately 100 pounds or more, according to height.
The Marasmic appears similar to other muscular and mental types, leaning toward the muscular. Characteristics include: sunken abdomen; normal-sized ankles; long, slim, bony arms; short, narrow and concave back; broad shoulders and narrow hips (body is wedge-shaped); flat, emaciated, narrow-waisted body; broad but flat chest; long, bony, slim, flat feet; dry, bony, wrinkled, yellowish hands which are medium-sized and thin; narrow hips, thin from front to back; average-sized knees; long, thin legs; small, sometimes long neck. The body is generally plain, unrefined, old-appearing even in youth, dehydrated, wrinkled. The Marasmic is the leanest of the twenty types. Shoulders are wide, thighs small; largest part of body is above waist, in shoulder region; body appears too short for length of legs; especially small waistline is set high on torso.

Physical Interior

Abdominal organs lack development; assimilation is poor; arteries and veins are diminutive but active; blood quantity is low but blood is well supplied with organic salts; blood pressure is generally low; blood is darker than in other types; red corpuscles may be excessively high compared with white. Bones are inflexible, long, slim; ligaments are efficient. Circulation is below par; fat is not metabolized; glands are small but moderately active; heartbeat is regular but heart function is subnormal; kidneys are small, lacteals medium-sized, liver small but usually active, lungs small but active; lymphatic system is feeble. Joints are of normal size; muscles are small but well-coordinated; tendons are slim but powerful. Pancreas is erratic; breathing is active; secretions may be lacking; digestion is weak; venous circulation is weak; throat capacity is average. Nerves are stable; nerve impulses are transferred slowly; this type never appears nervous.

Five Senses

Physical senses are generally poor in the Marasmic type. Vision is often below average (and undermined by drugs); olfactory function is poor; audio ability is good although comprehension is slow; sense of taste is weak or lacking; sense of touch is average. Mental and physical reflexes are slow, as is mental perception of all senses.

Metabolic Functions

Breathing is normal and oxidation average; digestion is poor; elimination is excessive and dehydration a possibility; metabolism is unbalanced, with excessive catabolism and subnormal anabolism. Nutrition is faulty and deficient; perspiration is excessive; pulse rate is rhythmic; sexual system is weak but mind sensuous.

Mental Characteristics

The brain of most Marasmics is slow, ponderous, sluggish. Memory is often excellent for such things as history, the past, secrets, injuries, stories and literature, evils, diseases, wise quotations, colors, mathematics, philosophy. Judgment of time, law, systems, government, practical arts, science, debate, customs, pottery, etc., is good. The individual gives the impression of unconcern, calmness, even apathy, impassivity; he has immense respect for elders and established customs; he is patriotic; he has a feeling of great self worth, prefers functioning behind the scenes, is serene and soft spoken, may be plagued by nagging dread; he is honest and ethical, unemotional, strong willed and tenacious, a hard worker.

The mind of the Marasmic is inclined toward apprehension, obscenity, philosophy, antisocialism, restraint, vindictiveness, frugality, patience, prejudice, conservatism, archaic behavior and preferences, stoicism, melancholy, confinement, strategies, poverty, avarice, nonconformity, seriousness. There may be fondness for stimulants, drugs, narcotics. The Marasmic honors his word but may indulge in petty thievery; he is not averse to cheating in business and lacks respect for others. If mental faculties are aroused they are active; otherwise there is a tendency toward daydreams, imagination, preoccupation, slowness and lack of responsiveness. Life seems to revolve around the inner nature of the individual rather than outer reality. His will power can be strong but is not often called upon; it is shown in endurance, patience, diligence, resignation; old habits are not easily relinquished, nor are modes of dress, customs, doctrines and social etiquette. Behavior is passive, stubborn, secluded, even self important.

Brain Faculties

Strong Faculties. Continuity, caution, inhabitiveness, self esteem, destruction, secretiveness, calculation, casuality, veneration, acquisitiveness, color, firmness, size, weight, constructiveness, conscientiousness, individuality, central posterior cerebellum.

Weak Faculties. Alimentiveness, approval, bibativeness, benevolence, friendship, hope, human nature, imitation, sublimity, eventuality, mirthfulness, parental love, suavity, medulla, conjugality, combativeness, amorousness.

Brain Itself. Inhibitive faculties are overly strong; cerebellum and medulla are small. The Marasmic is strong, stalwart, untiring, persistent, willing to work long hours; the brain faculties suit him for sedentary work.

Talent and Career Abilities

Suited for ceramics, carving, fancy needlework, laundry or dry cleaning work, farming, doorman or gatekeeper, antique dealer, investigation or detective work. He is hardworking, honest and dependable.

Biochemistry and Diet

Leading elements in the Marasmic type include chlorine, its compounds, fluorine and phosphorus. Chlorine and fluorine are commonly excessive; most often deficient are carbon, hydrogen, iodine, manganese, magnesium, potassium, oxygen, sodium. The appetite is chaotic; starvation or fasting alternates with overeating; there may be excessive drinking but lack of moisture retention; stimulants, drugs, narcotics may be craved.

Great quantities of chlorine are required throughout the lifetime of the Marasmic. Suitable foods include milk and milk products, cheeses, gelatin, cod liver oil, oily fish, fruit juices, nut and seed butters, vegetable and nut oils, juicy vegetables. Tiny meals should be taken often; spices, stimulants, condiments, alcohol should be shunned. Diet and nutrition should be studied to improve personal well-being and health.

Additional Requirements

Turkish baths and hot water bathing are sometimes beneficial, followed by deep massage. Warm and humid climates are best; low altitude and abundant ozone are necessary; moderate exercise is advised. An alkaline diet, energizing foods, social interaction, foods which reduce perspiration, development of human sympathy and friendliness, brisk walks, much sleep, avoidance of reclusive behavior, loving comradeship and vitamin supplementation are needed by the Marasmic type.

Common Ailments

Principal afflictions and diseases of the Marasmic type include boils, Bright's disease, catarrh, cholera infantum, diphtheria, phobias, fibroma, glioma, hernia, infantile paralysis, itching hemorrhoids, mental depression, neuroma, involuntary muscle paralysis, spinal defects, priapism, sexual disorders, spinal curvature, bone decay, meningitis, syncope, stenosis.

Special Notes

Most Marasmic (Eldic) types are found among the Oriental races. They are generally honest, ethical, loyal, hardworking, and they contribute much to the good of others.

Crime and Inheritance
   Studies in Denmark by Dr. Sarnoff A. Mednick indicate that genetic factors may increase the risk of criminal behavior.

---

twenty-two

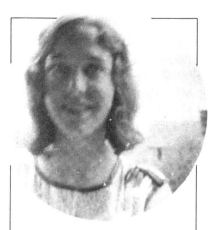

Grace Jensen
Sillivetic Type

The Calciferic type is tall, serious, sincere, meditative; he is light-complexioned.

The first impression of the Sillevitic type is interesting; freedom of movement; amiability; joviality; fun-loving, jesting nature.

The Isogenic is a powerful and accomplishing type, unyielding in will.

The Barotic type is generally strong in mental traits, speech, actions, motions, thoughts and other functions.

The osseous types of man

Calciferic, sillevitic, isogenic and barotic

Sketch of the Osseous Temperament Types

In the Osseous temperament, four classifications exist. The **Calciferic** type is the closest to the ideal characteristics of this category because calcium is the predominant element. Calcium is responsible for a large, bony frame, strong will and rugged bone structure. The calcium type possesses superior endurance, both mentally and physically. Individuals are rarely under six feet in stature; the body has an angular appearance; face is elongated and angular; hands are often massive and rigid. The impression of "bonyness" is the outstanding trait of the Calciferic type.

Silicon and calcium are prevalent in the **Sillevitic** type, a light-boned Osseous type. Tissues are pliable, hair shiny and secretions and tissues alkaline. Silicon types are known for dexterity, deftness, swiftness, vivacity, animation. Their bodies are less angular than those of the Calciferic, but resemblance is seen in the tall stature and slender build. The facial expression is mobile, expectant and optimistic. The body is quite limber and elastic, unlike the other Osseous types, because silicon predominates.

The remaining two Osseous types, Isogenic and Barotic, are characterized by angularity coupled with more flesh and muscle. The **Isogenic** type is much shorter than the Calciferic or Sillevitic but may carry considerable weight; weight is dictated by appetite for starches and desserts. Powerful physical and mental stamina are inherent in the Isogenic type, as in the Calciferic; will is almost unbendable. Arms and legs are slim in spite of considerable weight carried on the torso. The hands are generally massive, powerful and inflexible. Face is elongated and sober.

The **Barotic** type is exceptionally tall and frequently heavy. Height reaches seven feet. This type assumes the impressive strength and iron will of other Osseous temperaments. A great deal of weight can be successfully carried by the Barotic because the bone structure is immense. Hands are large and joints stiff. Facial expression is serious and often impassive. Russians, Swedes, Scots have many representatives of the Barotic type.

430

THE CALCIFERIC TYPE

Definition

Lime-carrying; "calcium" means lime, "fer" means carry, "ic" means relating to. (Lime is actually oxidized calcium.)

Classification

Osseous temperament. Osseous-Mental or Mental-Osseous types.

Leading Element

Calcium (tri-calcium phosphate).

General Characteristics

The Calciferic type is tall, serious, sincere, meditative; he is light-complexioned. The principal complications in his health are hardenings, especially in the joints. He is inclined to overwork and pessimism; he appears old even in youth. His build is bony and angular; he has broad shoulders, deep wrinkles; he may appear malnourished, emaciated, antisocial, overly serious or angry. Yet the Calciferic type is slow to anger, slow-moving, even-tempered, awkward. Nerve force is excellent and life force strong. Voice is powerful, low, determined and loud if angered.

Words which describe the Calciferic type include these: rational, mechanical, technical, protective, scientific, organizational, inventive, reforming, skeptical, critical, military, pessimistic, melancholy, constructive, political, mathematical, materialistic, domestic, sedentary. Will power is strong if vital forces are active; sexual impulses are normal; driving force is powerful; executive ability is keen; mental ability is high; energy is low. Sixty percent of Calciferics are male, forty percent female.

Head and Facial Features

Cheeks are often concave or flat; thick skin produces deep facial creases; chin is square and powerful; nose is prominent, bony. Hair is dry, wiry, thick or coarse, or long and straight; hair color is blond, white-gray or ashen; men often bald in later years.

Physical Exterior

Height: Tall (six feet or more)
Weight: Average for bone structure and slender build.

Exterior appearance is of masculine, yet slim and angular, or bony body type; large bone structure; short torso but long limbs; large, inflexible hands and feet; square hands, blunt fingertips. Body is lean with sunken abdomen; ankles are strong, instep high; arms may be muscular but not fleshy. Back is wide, slender, bony, short; shoulder blades are bony and visible; weakest area is small of back. The body is flat in front and back but wide with broad shoulders and narrow hips; chest is fairly well developed. Hip bones, clavicle, ribs, shoulders, sternum, vertebrae are bony and defined throughout life, unless excessive weight is gained from illness or overeating. Feet are wide, slim, bony; toes are long and unattractive with large joints. Fingers are massive, thick from beginning to tips. Hand is characteristically long but not tapered; tips of fingers are inflexible and blunt or square; the grip is like iron. Knuckles are large, hands dry, chafed and wrinkled; hands give a bony impression; fingernails are ragged, unkempt. Voice is powerful. Neck is slender, long but muscular (15-17 inches). Bone structure of hips is larger than in other types; hip bones are large and wide. Knee joints are well developed; legs are long and strong. Waistline is slim and high on the torso. Skin tone is generally sanguine, sandy, pale or grayish, varying to yellowish, pinkish or pale yellow or dark yellow. Movement is stiff, powerful, deliberate, ponderous; stride is lengthy; bearing is stately; body is stiff or rigid. General physique is tall, stately, powerful, sturdy, earthy, solid and unyielding. The chief characteristics of the Calciferic body are broadness, flatness, angularity, slenderness, squareness.

Physical Interior

Interior characteristics are as follows: poorly-developed digestive system, accounting for lean and bony build; sluggish venous circulation but active arterial; alkaline blood during early life but more acidic later, due to destructive dietary and other habits; inherently alkaline constitution but excessive acids and fatigue products due to extreme use of brain faculties; periodically sluggish eliminative organs; medium-sized, strong heart, unless blood salts are deficient; medium-sized, sluggish intestines, requiring a laxative diet; normally strong kidneys; large, hard, efficient joints; pliable, well-developed, strong ligaments. The liver is the Calciferic type's largest, most vital organ; it may be overworked in purifying blood and neutralizing toxins. Lungs function efficiently and respiratory troubles are rare. Lymph glands are not large or active; their lack of moisture-holding ability results in the dry constitution of this type. The motive system (cerebellum, motor brain faculties, muscles, tendons, ligaments, bones), the system of impelling force and motor impulse, is well developed. The only type to remotely resemble the Calciferic is the Atrophic; however, types such as the Oxypheric, Isogenic, Nervimotive, Atrophic, Pargenic and Medeic often have a strong calcium influence.

The muscular system of the Calciferic is well developed; chest, neck and shoulder muscles are particularly compact and heavy. Nerves are controlled, steady and relaxed; this type appears composed and collected nearly all the time; strength surfaces in times of emergency; emotions are unexpressed. Motor nerves are more efficient than sensory or emotive nerves. Nervousness and panic never bother the Calciferic type. The pancreas is neither large nor efficient; spleen is often overworked; stomach is a weak point.

Five Senses

The five senses are generally below par in the Calciferic type. Ossification affects eyesight after age 45 or 50; tendency is to farsightedness. Sense of touch lacks sensitivity; smell and hearing are duller than in other types; taste is also less developed than in other types. Speech ability is not especially keen.

Metabolic Functions

Respiration is excellent in this type; assimilation of calcium and protein is good but digestion of sugars, fats, starches and acidic fruits is poor. Eliminative channels are sluggish—especially bowel, kidneys, lungs; perspiration is more active. Anabolism (construction or building) and catabolism (destruction and elimination) are unbalanced; catabolism is more active, due to extreme use of mental and physical forces. Nutrition is fair; oxidation is efficient; pulse is rhythmic and powerful. Sexuality is strong and passion is unaccompanied by nervous agitation.

Mental Characteristics

The brain is slow to develop but effective when in full use. Calciferics are good judges of scientific data, the objective world, mechanics, technology, business and mathematics. The activity of the brain resembles that of calcium itself—slow, but gaining in momentum and strength as it progresses. In general, the brain is stable, slow, but active. This type is slow to grasp knowledge; but once information is absorbed, it is remembered. Weak mental characteristics include memorization, dogmatism, lack of faith in the future, lack of hope, lack of emotion, poor memory for names, reckless actions, domination, accident-proneness, excessive use of mind, making of enemies, self-destructive and self-abusive habits, overly high expectations of self and others, inability to control speech when angry, craving for calcium-rich foods and alcoholic beverages, argumentativeness, sexual overindulgence.

The Calciferic has a pioneering spirit, fixed aims and goals; self discipline and self sacrifice are strong in him. He is unemotional and impassive, averse to social functions, particularly in regard to his associates, even tempered and slow to anger. He is interested in facts rather than ideals or philosophy.

Brain Faculties

Strong Faculties. Combativeness, approbativeness, size, weight, firmness, order, calculation, benevolence, veneration, causality, constructiveness, inhibitiveness.

Weak Faculties. Bibativeness, alimentativeness, language, color, eventuality, locality, time, mirthfulness, suavity, hope, imitation, parental love, friendship, ideality.

Brain Itself. Tremendously large cerebellum; smaller medulla; physical excesses should be avoided. Mind is slow but gains momentum, is steady and energetic.

Talent and Career

Suited for construction, scientific research, science teaching, judgeship, civic leadership, law, government office, engineering, architecture, farming, ranching, forestry, carpentry, operation of heavy equipment, accounting, military, truck driving, railroad work, logging, mechanics,

432

hardware dealership. This type is reliable and assumes responsibility readily.

Biochemistry and Diet

This type is intended for health and longevity. Both body and mind are strong; stamina is great. Weaknesses are attributable to excess calcium in the body, lack of sodium, overwork, improper diet (often too dry), poor elimination. Hardening and joint stiffness or arthritis may be a problem, as may sluggish metabolism and elimination. Suggested preventive measures include a diet high in sodium, lower in calcium foods; a laxative diet with plenty of liquids to flush the kidneys and intestines; development of affection; enjoyment of harmless pleasures. Refined carbohydrates, strong seasonings, spices and alcohol must be avoided. The ideal diet would consist of fresh fruits and vegetables, raw milk (preferably goat milk), whole grains, spring water and food supplements as needed. Fatty foods disagree and should be taken only in minimum quantity; obesity leads to serious diseases in this type.

Additional Requirements

Warm baths are more suitable than cold water; moisture, cold air are aggravating. An altitude of 4,000 to 10,000 feet is advised. Exercise should be vigorous to improve internal functions.

Common Ailments

Afflictions likely to develop in the Calciferic type include apoplexy, hardening of arteries, bone tumors, brain shrinkage, calcium deposits, calcic troubles, calcification and ossification, hardening of canal walls, cataracts, chondroma, concretions, contraction of cords, cranial growths, day sleepiness, dull hearing, emaciation, gout, gravel, hardened semen, indigestion, lithemia, phosphatic calculi, swelling joints, thrombosis, urethritis, urinary deposits. In general, illnesses are ocular, sexual, pulmonary, gastric, intestinal, mesenteric, apoplectic, digestive, congestive, rheumatic, chronic, alcoholic, catarrhal, calcic.

Special Notes

The Calciferic type is the longest-lived and strongest of the twenty types.

THE SILLEVITIC TYPE

Definition

"Sil" means silex or flint; *levis* in Latin means light and easy (particularly in motion); "ic" in the suffix means relating to.

Classification

Osseous temperament. Osseous-Mental or Mental-Osseous types.

Leading Elements

Silicon (and calcium).

General Characteristics

The first impression of the Sillevitic type is interesting; freedom of movement; amiability; joviality; fun-loving, jesting nature. The build is slender, tall, often bony; he is agile, nimble-fingered, lightfooted; his mind is energetic; he is unpoised, uncomplicated, natural, informal, graceful, familiar, simple, extroverted, outgoing, lithe, animated. The bones are long, slender, pliable; appearance resembles that of a gazelle or greyhound. The body of the Sillevitic resembles that of the Calciferic but is lighter-boned, more animated, quicker, happier, more supple and agile; the bodies of both types are flat, slim, narrow, bony. The Neurogenic type also resembles the Sillevitic but has a lower nerve force, less nerve energy and tires more easily.

Sillevitics are generally brunette, though some are intermediate and others blond. The countenance is innocent, animated, magnetic, joyful, teasing; the individual is full of jokes, laughter, wit; he is comical, optimistic and entertaining; his nature is unsophisticated. Body gestures are free, easy, energetic, swift, even violent at times; vital energy and life force are almost unlimited. He is highly magnetic, effervescent, optimistic, invigorated, elated, even ecstatic; he is too spontaneous and natural to be poised. His limbs and joints are limber and pliable. His voice is vivacious, energetic, aspirative or breathless, high-pitched, optimistic and vibratory. His movements are staccato, quick, easy. Fifty percent of Sillevitics are men, fifty percent women.

Head and Facial Features

Facial features of the Sillevitic type vary: long, narrow face; short and rounded face with rounded cheekbones; wide, square face with prominent cheekbones; sunken cheeks in long face or regular face. Hair is often shiny, rich, long (lovely in women but less attractive in men); hair color ranges from sandy to sandy-brown, dark golden, flaxen, rich brown; it is often naturally wavy or fluffy, sometimes wiry. Complexion is light, features regular. Lips are normal sized and shapely; mouth is wide and mobile. Face has few wrinkles but may be withered from emaciation.

Physical Exterior

Height: Medium to tall (over six feet).
Weight: Proportioned to slender build and medium to light bone structure.
Exterior appearance is as follows: concave abdomen; powerful ankles; long, slim arms; narrow, concave, masculine back; short, narrow, concave appearance at waist; straight torso and good posture; free body movement; proud carriage; parallel sides of body; shoulders barely wider than hips; small chest, flat in front, narrow from side to side; elongated, narrow, powerful feet with small bones; long, narrow, small-boned, flexible, strong hands and fingers; small-boned, narrow hips which are thin from front to back; medium-sized but strong tendons in knees; slim, small-boned, powerful, wiry, pliable legs; small but powerful neck with slender tendons; lean body, sometimes bony, more fleshy in youth; narrow, small-boned, strong-tendoned shoulders; light, sandy or grayish skin tone; strong, resilient, pliable, healthy skin; small but powerful thighs with active tendons; small waist; high waistline.

Physical Interior

Interior characteristics are as follows: sunken, small abdomen; weak but active assimilation; pliable, strong arteries; excellent capillary action; alkaline blood; deficiency of blood because of slow manufacture; excellent circulation; normal quantity of blood salts; lack of water in blood; pliable, limber, long, slim, diminutive bones; deficient fat metabolism and consequent lack of body fat; small but energetic glands; powerful though small or medium-sized joints; active heart; small but efficient intestines; small but active kidneys; small, active lacteals; medium-sized, powerful ligaments; small but active liver; medium-sized, active lungs; very weak lymphatic system; small but strong bones; small but well-toned muscles; diminutive but active pancreas; healthy and vigorous respiratory system; insufficient secretions; large and energetic spleen; small stomach with active digestion; slim, powerful, retractile, responsive tendons; strong, vigorous, resonant, flexible, effective local cords (may have gift for singing or other music); venous system less strong than arterial; nerves powerful and highly active; swift transfer of nerve impulses; rare nervousness though occasional suffering from nerve depletion or collapse.

Five Senses

Sense of pressure on hands, fingers, arms is keen in the Sillevitic type, making for dexterity in operating keyboards, typewriters, machines and for playing stringed instruments. Vision is excellent; sense of touch is very keen if artistic, refined, creative and intellectual but not so keen if a physical laborer; hearing ability is acute; sense of smell is normal; taste is variable, from keen to lacking.

Metabolic Functions

Breathing is exceptionally good; digestion is erratic; elimination channels are moderately efficient; metabolism is low except in nerves, brain, membranes and tendons; oxidation is powerful; nutrition is defective; perspiration is excessive when hot but thermal regulation is excellent, allowing tolerance to extremes of heat and cold; pulse is strong, rhythmic, often lengthy; sexual system is of average strength and favors conception.

Mental Characteristics

The brain is agile, lightning-quick. Facts are exceptionally well retained if they relate to work or interests; principles, experiences, human nature qualities, figures, accounts, photographs, crafts, precious stones, animal habits, etc., are easily recalled. The mind is optimistic, transient, entertaining, merry, selfless, amiable, familiar, generous. Mental weaknesses include chaotic and excessive speed of tongue and brain; inability to concentrate for a long time; conceit, boasting, exaggerating. Judgment of velocity, motion, balance, momentum, physics is excellent; judgment of human nature, salesmanship, stones or jewels, metals, ornaments, architecture and art, government, domestic arts is good. The Sillevitic type is a "free spirit" who needs to fly.

Brain Faculties

Strong Faculties. Inhabitiveness, approbativeness, firmness, sublimity, individuality, calculation, language, locality, comparison, human nature, imitation, benevolence, spirituality, constructiveness.

Weak Faculties. Bibativeness, secretiveness, ideality, alimentiveness, causality, suavity, hope, veneration, ideality, conscientiousness.

Brain Itself. Large cerebellum; pons varolii larger than in any other type (part concerned with locomotion and connection of medulla to brain proper and cerebellum).

Talent and Career

Suited for situations demanding instant response, quick reflexes, rapid decisions and speed; for active but light sports such as running, track; for dancing, singing, acting, comedy roles. Associates are impressed by the vivacity, gaiety, joy the Sillevitic type feels for life. Thrift is not a Sillevitic quality; overspending is more common.

Biochemistry and Diet

Leading biochemical elements in the body of the Sillevitic are silicon, calcium, gelatin, fibrin, phosphorus, oxygen and manganese; only silicon is likely to be excessive. Carbon, chlorine, iodine, magnesium, nitrogen and potassium may be deficient. Appetite is capricious, variable, unreliable; it may be excessive or completely lacking; eating is rushed; there is a need to drink little with meals, to avoid refined sweets and minimize intake of starches, fats and sugars; only small amounts of liquid should be consumed at one time; foods and drinks high in organic biochemicals are needed. Appetite may be greater than digestive capability, with attendant danger of social overeating; eating habits are chaotic and food selections and combinations are poor. This type can easily overindulge in sweets, desserts, refined starches, pastries; they should avoid canned, chilled, stimulating, additive-laden products. Dietary suggestions include whole grains, goat milk (raw), fish, fowl, game, veal, fresh vegetables and fruits such as papaya, avocado, figs, prunes, raisins, apricots; whole grains, nuts and seeds are advisable. Health is generally well-maintained because of the alkaline constitution and natural optimism. An overly-alkaline constitution calls for heavy vitamin supplementation.

Additional Requirements

Cool showers benefit the Sillevitic type. Massage is not especially beneficial. A cold or cool climate is most suitable, with altitudes from 6,000 to 12,000 feet; ozone is not highly beneficial. Exercise and active sports such as skiing, canoeing, team sports, racing, riding, etc., should not be overdone. Sleep is usually neglected but much sleep is necessary.

Common Ailments

Diseases, conditions and ailments common to the Sillevitic type include accidents (from excesses), alkaline disorders, cerebellar neurasthenia, sudden collapse, degeneration of mucus surfaces, fevers, destructive glandular changes, malnutrition, necrosis, optical illusions, paresis, psychentonia, bone suppuration. Weaknesses result from mental overwork, from too much thinking, muscular activity and nerve activity; for prevention or correction, the mind, muscles, tongue, functions must be allow to rest. Other likely ailments are related to the blood, to lack of blood or water in the body, to excessive water consumption, deficiency of white corpuscles, brain fatigue, hemorrhoids, headache, frequent urination, boils, blisters, cramps, ruptures, pyloritis, fistula, eruptions, etc. If temperance is observed, health is excellent. The mind is strong and not easily undermined. Life expectancy is variable and includes both young and old extremes.

Special Notes

The Sillevitic type is the most popular, charming and magnetic of the twenty types. He or she is attractive, likeable, amiable, happy, optimistic, persuasive and lively. Sillevitic types in the animal kingdom include the antelope, gazelle, mountain goat, deer.

THE ISOGENIC TYPE

Definition

"Isogenic" means evenly producing; "iso" means evenly or uniformly; "genic" means creating or producing.

Classification

The category of Osseous temperament is somewhat misleading; actually, Isogenic is almost uniformly a type of the Osseous, Mental and Vital temperaments. Vital-Osseous-Mental, Mental-Osseous-Vital.

Leading Elements

Calcium (and phosphorus and carbon).

General Characterists

The Isogenic constitution is produced by toxins in the blood which influence the brain and result in strong action, irritability, temper, disgust, negative and pessimistic mental states. The Isogenic is a powerful and accomplishing type, unyielding in will, although others often mistakenly think they can overpower him. The system of the Isogenic is alkaline in youth but acid in old age, due to overconsumption of starches, desserts and fatty foods. The body is often large, well-proportioned, but heavy. The face is leaner than the rest of the body. Appearance is ordinary, even coarse, clumsy, homely; the individual is unconcerned with appearance. A youthful appearance lasts into old age. Bone structure is large and heavy; in later years, the tendency is to fleshiness or obesity. Composure is relaxed and seemingly unconcerned; facial

expression is sober, positive, not stern. Vital energy is high and magnetism sufficient to impress others favorably. In spite of awkwardness, this type seems poised and calm. Strength is shown in the face of confrontation or resistance. The walk is measured, deliberate. The voice is low, quiet, subtle but powerful.

Memory is generally poor; perception is better. Old age may bring absentmindedness. Judgment of proportion, size, distance, quantity, line is good; judgment is balanced and harmonious. Powerful emotions in this type cause drowsiness; sensitivity to criticism or praise; desire for admiration and high position. The individual may be subtly critical and domineering, unforgiving if wronged or manipulated. He lacks domestic concern; prefers solitude; is greatly interested in the opposite sex; fights when necessary; has wonderful powers of concentration; appears dull to others but is not. He possesses a powerful will and great stubbornness. Fifty percent of Isogenics are male, fifty percent female.

Head and Facial Features

Cheekbones are massive, cheeks often sunken or thin; chin is broad, bony, large. The complexion is ruddy, red or yellowish-white; face is elongated, masculine, large, broad; features are large except for small eyes; lips are thick. Hair ranges from blond to medium, even brunette; it is often straight, thin, stiff; in an emotional Isogenic it may occasionally be wavy. Tip of nose may be bulbous and large, showing interest in people; forehead is prominent, particularly directly above the eyes. Facial wrinkles are often deep and straight.

Physical Exterior

Height: Medium (not exceeding six feet).
Weight: 150 pounds is normal; 200 if overweight.

The body is stout with short arms and legs, long torso. Limbs are slim, hands are massive; wrists show heavy bone development; fingertips are blunt and even. Joints are rigid, though not so pronounced as in Calciferic type. Other physical characteristics include large, often fleshy abdomen; large-boned ankles; wide, strong back with stiffness in small of back; thick-set build; medium-sized, bony but not thin face, neck; square, thick, warm, magnetic, heavy, inflexible hands; large-boned, fleshy hips; large knee joints; short, bony legs. The physique is powerful when young, durable with great stamina. Shoulders are sloping, thick and somewhat circular. Skin color is sandy, grayish; its texture is thick, strong, resilient, coarse, warm. Thighs are medium-sized; torso seems large for legs; waistline is large and low on body; bones are stiff, short, massive, stout.

Physical Interior

Interior characteristics are as follows: sluggish circulation; sluggish bowel, liver, lymphatic system and spleen; powerful, active heart; inefficient glands; weak kidneys (in comparison with other organs); subactive lacteals; well-developed lungs; great muscular strength; relatively weak pancreas; good eyesight; shallow breathing and stiff lungs; efficient stomach; strong tendons; poor venous circulation; deficient secretions; strong throat; passive, slow, controlled nervous system. Calcium soothes and controls nerves of this type; carbon dioxide affects the nerves unfavorably.

Five Senses

The senses are not so keen as in many other types. Vision may be farsighted; hearing is likely to be poor; sense of smell is faulty; taste perception is mediocre and appetite not particular (making dieting easy). The sense of touch is sensitive. If the nervous system and creative faculties were stronger, senses would be keener.

Metabolic Functions

Breathing is uniform, strong; digestion is fair to good; eliminative channels, including liver, are defective. Metabolism is excellent until about age 50, when acids, toxins and sluggishness set in. Nutrition is good, especially calcium assimilation; oxidation is low due to lack of sodium and excessive carbonic acid (causing gasping for air at times). Perspiration may be odorous; pulse is strong, regular, uniform when young. Sexual desire and activity are strong; even in old age the Isogenic is highly-sexed, both mentally and physically.

Mental Characteristics

The Isogenic gives the impression of impassiveness and a carefree attitude, but this is misleading. He is fixed in habits, has great mental and physical stamina, an unyielding and clinging manner which shows strength, dependability and endurance. He works hard, seeks knowledge avidly, is independent, creative. He presents the image of the self-made man.

Brain Faculties

Strong Faculties. Amativeness, cerebellum, combativeness, inhibitiveness, conjugality, caution, approbativeness, firmness, weight, size, order, constructiveness, comparison, veneration, benevolence, spirituality.

Weak Faculties. Parental love, bibativeness, ideality, self esteem, continuity, color, sublimity, locality, eventuality, time, tune, human nature, causality, agreeableness, hope imitation.

Brain Itself. Many Isogenic types have a powerful brain; combativeness is highly active; amativeness is one of the most powerful faculties; bibativeness is the weakest. The inherent strength of the brain allows the Isogenic type to toil eighteen hours a day without tiring. Muscular brain is powerfully developed in this type, giving him a strong back, powerful muscles and bones and exceptional stamina. Carbon, calcium and phosphorus affect the brain strongly.

Talent and Career

Strong qualities suit the Isogenic type to education, scientific research, medical fields but not surgery. Isogenics might become homeopaths, chiropractors, naturopaths, herbalists, healers, kinesiologists, chemists, laboratory technicians; some become judges, senators, writers, company presidents, counselors. Well-known Isogenic types include Thomas Edison, Luther Burbank, David Ben-Gurion (Israeli Prime Minister).

Biochemistry and Diet

Leading biochemical elements in the Isogenic types are calcium, phosphorus, carbon and organic elements; calcium is the only element likely to be excessive. Sodium, magnesium and chlorine are most often deficient. The appetite runs to fruit juices, carbonated beverages, champagne, sweet wines; there is little thirst for water. Calcium gives considerable mental and physical stamina and if the individual observes dietary discretion, especially after age 45, good health can be maintained. Suggested foods include whole grains, cheeses, milk (preferably goat milk), fresh fruits and vegetables, fish, sea vegetation. Foods rich in iron, magnesium, sodium, potassium, silicon, natural sweets (fruits) high in sodium, berries and dried foods are recommended; preparation by broiling or steaming is best; a liberal supplement of vitamins is advisable. Oxygen and ozone must be obtained from the air in large quantities. Moderate use of honey is suggested. The Isogenic type must guard against overwork and overindulgence in carbohydrates and desserts (which cause autointoxication and acidity).

Additional Requirements

Warm water favors the Isogenic; deep massage is beneficial; moisture is unpleasant and cold air aggravating. Altitudes ranging from 5,000 to 12,000 feet, rich in ozone, and warm and dry climates are helpful as they attract oxygen and iron to the blood.

Common Ailments

Diseases and ailments of the Isogenic type include apoplexy, boils, Bright's disease, headcolds, diabetes, dropsy, dual personality, flatulent dyspepsia, dysuria, ephidrosis, absentmindedness, hemarthrosis, hip complications, influenza, malaria, paralysis (due to stagnation), periostitis, pneumonia, pytosis, gouty rheumatism, rhinitis, seborrhea, sepsis, insomnia, blood stagnation, liver tumors, typhoid fever, gastric ulcers. Ailments are transient, sometimes chronic; recurring maladies include stiff joints and bones, gouty deposits, liver and kidney troubles, uric acid accumulations, pancreas trouble, poor elimination.

Weaknesses in the Isogenic constitution are attributable to overwork of brain, autointoxication, acidity, deficiency of sodium and chlorine, sluggish liver, poor skin and kidney elimination, lack of phosphorus and calcium due to overactive brain, internal heat contributing to rheumatism and gout, blood and diabetic disorders. This type is slow to mature; consequently youthfulness lasts into old age. Because of their sturdy constitution, they are able to enjoy good health into old age; life expectancy is long and they remain active to the end.

Special Notes

No obstacle is too great for the Isogenic type to overcome when he sets his mind on a goal. His patience, diligence, hardwork and persistence pay off royally.

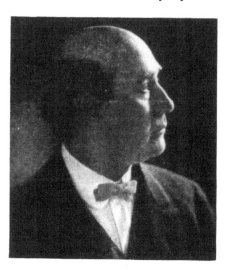

Dr. V. G. Rocine, an Isogenic type.

THE BAROTIC TYPE

Definition

Baros means "heavy" in Greek; the suffix "ic" means relating to, having to do with.

Classification

Osseous temperament.

Leading Elements

Calcium and protein.

General Characteristics

The Barotic type is generally strong in mental traits, speech, actions, motions, thoughts and other functions. The type is identified by simple actions, slow functions, slow and reflective speech, unhurriedness, baritone or low voice which roars when enraged, an iron grip, slowly-aroused temper, patience, energetic moods, forgetfulness, seeming dullness or perplexity, aversion to haste, shy manner, practical perception, silence, poor spelling, slow mind. Other recognizable traits include hidden mental powers, thick-set body, morning sleepiness, large feet, heavy arms, large chest, heavy fingers, heavy legs, large neck, thick hair, big head, large bones, wide face, serious manner, solid build and large cheekbones. The body is proportionate in spite of massiveness; build is fleshy, bony, heavy, vital and muscular. Gestures are repressed, calm, relaxed, quiet, serious, poised. Life force is tenacious and powerful; death overtakes reluctantly. Walk is with long strides and heavy steps. This type is not magnetic. Ninety percent of Barotics are male, ten percent female.

Head and Facial Features

Face is massive and usually fleshy, but firm; chin is strong, large and square; mouth is large and masculine; ears are large, often thick and square on top. Face has a sober expression. Cheekbones are more prominent than in any other type; cheeks are rounded and large. Face is elongated, especially below the eyes, flat, large and wide (indicating great latent power). Features are generally wide, unbalanced, common, unrefined. Complexion may be coarse and rough. Hair is thick, coarse, bushy, unmanageable; color ranges from medium brown to dark; men may bald in later years from excessive study and thinking. Deep creases and lines may appear on the face, denoting powerful will and strong emotions; these are different from wrinkles indicating emaciation.

Physical Exterior

Height: Medium to tall (up to seven feet).
Weight: Heavy because of large bones. (Calcium builds large bones and protein forms the well-developed muscles.)
The body is often so large that it seems disproportioned. Its massiveness causes movement to be slow and deliberate. Bones are well developed. Physical characteristics include: large ankles; elongated, massive and powerful arms; wide, strong, fleshy, straight back; well-developed chest; massive, heavy, bony, fleshy feet; strong, fleshy, bony, massive fingers; wide, thick, bony, inflexible hands; massive, fleshy, bony hips (larger on women); strong knees; long, bony, fleshy, massive legs; large, bony, muscular neck; wide, strong, masculine shoulders; large, forceful, strong, bony, fleshy thighs. Men of this type are large-waisted and women more slender (but still heavier than many other types). Skin is rough, raw, thick, resilient and pigmented—dull, muddy or yellowish-red; skin is dry and rigid on individuals who spend considerable time outdoors.

Physical Interior

Interior characteristics are as follows: large abdomen; good assimilation; efficient arteries; overworked venous system, inefficient in carrying off toxins and impurities; above-normal generation of uric acid; massive, stout, solid, often inflexible bones; excellent circulation; subnormal metabolism of fats, so excessive intake of fatty foods should be avoided; normal glandular function; strong, active heart, good bowel activity unless diet is faulty; subnormal kidney function; average lacteal activity; slightly subnormal liver function; massive and powerful lungs; slightly below-normal lymphatic function; large, solid, powerful, heavy muscles (good protein digestion); well-developed respiratory system; below normal splenic function; good digestion; large, heavy, efficient tendons; good throat development; good vision and strong eye muscles. Nervous system is powerful but susceptible to toxins and acids; motor nerves are most active in the Barotic type.

Five Senses

Vision is usually superior; sense of touch is mediocre or dulled; hearing is average, poor or faulty; taste sensation is dull. In general, the senses of the Barotic type are mediocre.

Metabolic Functions

Breathing is excellent but oxygen absorption is inferior and aeration below average; digestion is superior; eliminative functions need upgrading; protein and phosphatic metabolism are above average; fat, brain and nerve metabolism are subnormal, resulting in stiffness, dryness, rigidity, hardness; nutrition is excellent; oxidation of bones, brain and nervous system is slow; perspiration ranges from copious to inactive; pulse rate is often full, strong, possibly double; sexual system has excellent development.

Mental Characteristics

Judgment is excellent regarding justice, morals, behavior, crime and sentencing, practical living, active sports. Memory is poor, particularly for words and names; recollection of actions and experiences is better. Mental tendencies include confusion, mental sluggishness, lack of forgiveness, self suffering, indifference, passiveness, gullibility, shyness, athletic inclinations, competitiveness, love of nature, inventiveness, constructiveness, experimentation, prejudice, superstition, submissiveness, philosophical bent, religiousness. Mental inadequacies include inability to express self clearly, forgetfulness, poor spelling, slow thinking, enraged outbursts, self condemnation, intolerance of crowds and noise, weak sense of touch, poor sense of smell, alienation from others.

Brain Faculties

Strong Faculties. Firmness, cerebellum, combativeness, conscientiousness, destructiveness, veneration, amativeness, benevolence, constructiveness, caution.

Weak Faculties. Language, bibativeness, eventuality, acquisitiveness, self-esteem; often human nature, tune, imitation, agreeableness, ideality.

Brain Itself. Mind is sluggish unless it receives strong stimulation. The cerebellum (physical brain) oversees functions including physical growth, sexual development, equilibrium, coordination of muscles, strength of heartbeat, physical stamina, heat production, fat and protein metabolism, longevity, neutralizing of gravity; quick readjustment of body during work, motion, activity, exercise; direction of eyes and eye muscles, modulation of tongue when speaking and other vital physical functions; such functions are dependent upon the size and strength of the cerebellum. The cerebellum of the Barotic is exceptionally large, broad, deep but sluggish; it is responsible for the strong and compact body of this type. The mind of the Barotic is powerful, frank, honest, dependable, straightforward; he is plain in manners and reliable.

Talent and Career

Suited for active sports, lumbering, cattle ranching, engineering, architecture, farming, warfare, work with heavy machinery, construction, work with animals, carpentry, masonry, police work, forestry, supervisory roles and strenuous outdoor labor. There is a compassion suiting one for nursing; the Barotic possesses unfailing patience and sincere devotion to helping the needy and ill. Politics are attractive to this type because leadership is important. His self discipline and demands on himself and others are great.

Biochemistry and Diet

Pervading biochemical elements in this type include protein, phosphates, hydrogen, nitrogen, calcium, carbon, sulphur and vegetable phosphorus active in solid tissue. Chlorine, iron, magnesium, potassium and silicon are normally active; free oxygen and animal phosphorus are less active. Bone metabolism dominates that of nerves and brain, which may be subnormal; brain and nerve foods are therefore recommended: cod roe, fish broths, oily fish, egg yolks, fowl, etc. Elements most often deficient in the Barotic type are manganese, iodine, sodium; phosphates and protein compounds are often excessive.

The appetite is always good, regardless of illness or age. Solid foods are preferred, notably proteins and phosphorous foods. Suitable foods include fish, seafood, high sodium foods, fluorine and alkaline foods. Foods which contribute to uric acid formation should be avoided, as should high proteins and phosphates which crystallize in joints and bones. Additional vitamins are not usually necessary. Health is generally excellent.

Foods high in magnesium, sodium, iodine and sulphur are recommended; soups and tonics are beneficial to osmosis. Fatty foods, heated oils, condiments and alcohol are extremely harmful. Beneficial foods include fish, sea vegetation, onions, cabbage and related sulphur foods, watercress, fruits, celery, okra and all fresh vegetables.

Additional Requirements

Outdoor exercise, sauna baths, mineral waters are helpful to the Barotic. Hilly and forest areas are suggested. Carbon dioxide should be at a minimum. Sleep pattern is normal. If the requirements are adhered to, success is possible through determined effort and persistence.

Common Ailments

The chief ailments of the Barotic type are nervous and rheumatic disorders. Diseases do not easily invade this body; if it becomes diseased, this is usually attributed to excessive protein in the diet or to deficiency of sodium and excess of phosphates. Possible maladies include abscesses, forgetfulness, autointoxication, brain complications, mental confusion, congestion, drowsiness, cysts, dull senses, earache, cataracts, rage, painful shyness, calcium deposits or hardenings, lust, impaired or loss of hearing or reason, mania, nerve prostration, nerve toxification, nerve fever, neuroses, paralysis, indifference, rheumatism, swellings, tumors, ulcers, thrombi, varicose veins, vindictive moods.

Weaknesses are principally mental, due to brain congestion and inflammation and unbalanced mental faculties. Corrective dietetics and a suitable climate are recommended. The constitution and general health are superior; the mind is the source of troubles. This type is long-lived, stalwart, vigorous and hardy.

Special Notes

The Barotic type is the tallest of the twenty types.

twenty-three

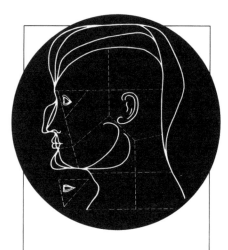

The Oxypheric is known for a youthful and hard appearance, even when aged.

The Nitropheric has low vitality and lack of constitutional fortitude.

The Carboferic type is generally restless and slow moving.

The Hydripheric type appears calm and serene and has a calming influence on others.

The Pallinomic is very diligent, constructively critical and positive in attitude.

The Lipopheric is friendly, well-groomed, vivacious, emotional, unselfish, pleasant and outgoing.

The Pargenic's general mann is unrefined; he has a sensuous nature, an aged appearance.

The vital types of man

Oxypheric, nitropheric, carboferic, hydripheric, pallinomic, lipopheric and pargenic

Sketch of the Vital Temperament Types

Nature follows a plan of classifying and categorizing all things in her realm. The human species is classified into types in accordance with the laws of nature. Dr. V. G. Rocine classified the diversifications found in man into chemical types, twenty in all.

The seven Vital types, as with the Osseous, Mental and Muscular, were determined by observing the workings of the leading elements in the human body. Oxygen colors the characteristics of the **Oxypheric** type, in which it predominates. Human characteristics resemble the characteristics of oxygen in nature. The Oxypheric type is dynamic, explosive, volatile, full of vitality; oxygen in nature may be described in the same manner. This type may be tall or short; chest expansion is great; arms and legs may be slim compared to the stout torso. The face is generally rounded, ruddy, well-padded with flesh. The Oxypheric type is known for a booming voice and unrestrained personality.

Nitrogen pervades the system of the **Nitropheric** type. Nitrogen restrains oxygen. The Nitropheric type mirrors the characteristics of nitrogen: the nature is repressed, suspicious, secretive. Height ranges from short to medium. The complexion is swarthy, dark or olive. Joints are well padded and hands are diminutive but pudgy. The expression is remote and selective.

Carboferic types resemble the Nitropherics, but have a lighter complexion and a different personality. Carbon lends its properties of inactivity, negativity, retention to the Carboferic type. Height ranges from short to medium. Obesity is possible, with more weight gained below the waist. Feet and hands are short and meaty. Joints are concealed under layers of flesh. The face is circular, fleshy and soft. The personality is relaxed, easy-going, calm, but suspicious; generosity is another quality.

A fourth Vital type, the **Hydripheric**, is noted for retaining excess fluids (water) in the body and is thus inclined to obesity. The qualities of hydrogen and water are at work in the body and mind of the Hydripheric individual. Water is a moisturizing, soothing, calming element, as is the hydrogen type. Stature ranges from short to tall. The slim form of youth generally gives way to obesity in later years. Hands and feet are more slender than in the Carboferic type. The face is fleshy and round; heaviness or "extra chins" are likely below the jaws. The expression is sober and pensive; the mind is wise, careful and creative.

The **Pallinomic** vital type is strongly influenced by carbon, weight-building elements, potassium and muscle-making counterparts. The body is more proportionate and its inherent strength greater than in other Vital types. Height is average. The body is stout, well-toned and dense. The face is leaner than in other Vital types; the forehead is prominent. Feet and hands are usually stout and large. The facial expression is attentive and cautious. Pallinomic types are ambitious, domestic, prudent and efficient.

Hydrogen, oxygen and carbon are dominant in the **Lipopheric** type. Carbon turns to fat in this type. This type resembles the Oxypheric (outgoing), the Carbopheric (slow-moving) and the Hydropheric (calm exterior). Height is generally diminutive; the upper chest and torso are thick and heavy. Arms and legs are tapered but stout; face is rounded and well padded. The upper part of the face is narrower, giving a pear-shaped appearance. Disposition is generally joyful and lively. Public service positions and domestic functions are favorably combined—catering, restaurant hosts or hostesses, restaurant management.

The **Pargenic** type becomes obese readily. The bone structure is frequently large and well padded with flesh. Arms and legs range from short to long; both extremes are noted. The torso is ponderous and massive. The Pargenic type is one of the most difficult types to keep healthy, due to susceptibility to autointoxication. The facial expression is serious and melancholy. This is a privacy-seeking, independent, creative, positive type.

According to Arnold Fox, MD, vitamin A drops sharply in the bloodstream during infection. Also, massive amounts of vitamin C compare favorably with antibiotics.

THE OXYPHERIC TYPE

Definition

"Oxy" refers to oxygen and "pheric" means that which carries; the Oxypheric is therefore the oxygen-carrying type.

Classification

Vital and Muscular, with Vital usually dominant. Vital-Muscular or Muscular-Vital with Osseous system are sometimes well-developed, contributing to a balanced temperament.

Leading Element

Oxygen.

General Characteristics

The Oxypheric type is produced by a predominance of oxygen in the system, which causes some faculties to be well developed or over developed and others to lack proper development. The system is usually acidic. This type is known for a youthful and hard appearance, even when aged; a red face; proportionate body but large size and heavy torso; fleshy, well fed, lively, friendly, pleasant appearance. The individual may seem more intelligent, educated, fascinating or professional than he really is. The body is built on double principles of muscular and vital temperaments. The Oxypheric is tall and stout with a stately aura, massive chest and well-developed abdomen; he may be fleshy across the upper back; bones are relatively small; the body matures early; countenance is lively, vivacious, mobile, reactive. He may lack poise and composure because of rash, impulsive tendencies, yet he is fluid, graceful and elastic in movement and gestures freely; feet, hands, body and head are restless, active. Life, energy, vim and vigor are boundless in this type; the presence of an Oxypheric is inspirational, spellbinding, uplifting, optimistic; he possesses much physical magnetism or attraction; his voice is musical, well modulated, pleasing except when his temper flairs, causing it to become rough and severe. Gait is long-strided; the lead is usually taken by the Oxypheric when walking, talking or gesturing. Sixty percent of Oxypherics are men, forty percent women.

Head and Facial Features

The face exudes confidence and self esteem; face and head are large; cheekbones are broad; cheeks rounded, square, broad-square or long-rounded; complexion is ruddy; chin is strong, jutting, often cleft, seldom withdrawn; features are large and youthful. Hair is dry, wavy or curly, full bodied, dull, tangled; it may be light blond or light brown in color. The large head is broad, round or cubic; lower jaw is large and meaty. Mouth is large, pliable and moist (denoting speaking ability); eyes are large and lively. Numerous wrinkles appear with age, along with shallow lines on the face.

Physical Exterior

Height: Medium to tall.
Weight: Approximately 200 pounds.
Chest capacity is large; arms and legs appear slender compared with torso. Neck is short and thick. Abdomen is of average size, lower abdomen often large and puffy. Exterior characteristics include weak ankles; lower arms and wrists which are weaker than fleshy, muscular upper arms; wide, nearly vertical back; weak small of back; excess flesh below neck giving humped appearance; massive, rounded, heavy, elongated torso which gives circular impression; massive, powerful, sturdy, vital, long, deep chest (well developed); small feet compared with legs and hips; small to medium sized; square hands; large, fleshy hips, notably in females; feeble knees; massive, stocky, powerful neck which needs large collarbone; massive shoulder expanse; ruddy, rosy, flushed skin which is very sensitive, dry, coarse with large pores and frequent pimples, warm, itchy; powerful thighs; torso heavier above waistline; waist large and set low on body; stately, impressive, portly appearance.

Physical Interior

Digestion and elimination are active; assimilation is excellent; arteries and veins are active and strong; blood is alkaline, rich, red, plentiful; blood salts are well represented; bones are limber, long or short, small in proportion to body; circulation is excellent and activity keeps blood pressure normal; weight is gained easily, especially around neck, lower face, stomach and chest; glands are active and secretory glands large; heartbeat is poor; intestines are massive, active; joints are generally small; kidneys may be overworked, though strong; lacteals are energetic, numerous, expansive; ligaments lack strength; liver is massive, efficient; lung expansion is massive; lymphatic system is normal and energetic; muscles are well developed, active, energetic, efficient; pancreas is well developed; breathing is deep; secretions are ample; spleen is large and efficient; stomach is efficient, energetic, sensitive to unsuitable foods; throat is large, powerful; tendons are fairly strong. Nerves are healthy, energetic, well guarded, sometimes erratic, controlled with effort; nervousness is more common in the morning and improves when perspiration is profuse; optic nerves may be weak.

Five Senses

Vision is usually not strong; corrective lenses may be required. Sense of touch is sensitive; hearing is acute; olfactory sense is keenly developed (though less so than in the Nitripheric or Hydripheric types); taste is acute. In general, the physical senses of the Oxypheric are keen and active.

Metabolic Functions

Breathing function is superb; elimination channels are active; metabolism, particularly anabolism, is superior; nutrition is efficient; oxidation is energetic; perspiration is copious; pulse rate is powerful and forceful; sexual system is potent, energetic.

Mental Characteristics

The preponderance of oxygen in the system makes this type restless, active, vigorous; sudden actions and impulsive behaviors are likely. The Oxypheric type is joyful, aggressive, optimistic, positive, magnetic, outgoing; he exhibits interest, excitement, faith, hope and adaptability. The mind is active, energetic; circulation to the head is good. Cerebellum and medulla are massive and well developed (accounting for excellent respiratory function). Imagination is prolific though there is a tendency to morbidity and fear of disease. Mental concentration is difficult; secrets are not easily kept; private affairs are often divulged to others. The mind works quickly and is changed often; actions are based on impulse; will power is lacking. Judgment is good in matters of scientific, inventive, theatrical, literary, agricultural, animal breeding or mechanical nature.

Brain Faculties

Strong Faculties. Cerebellum, muscular brain, amativeness, vitativeness, alimentiveness, bibativeness, acquisitiveness, parental love, friendship, sublimity, often ideality, language, weight, size, color, locality, time, tune, eventuality, causality, human nature, constructiveness, hope, spirituality, benevolence, destructiveness, imitation, approbativeness.

Weak Faculties. Secretiveness, conjugality, combativeness, inhabitiveness, sometimes ideality, self esteem, firmness, veneration, conscientiousness, continuity.

Brain Itself. Brain is very active and circulation to head area is excellent; consequently, sleep is often difficult after 4 a.m. Cerebellum and medulla are large, well developed (Medulla is three to four times as large as in the Atrophic or Desmogenic types.).

Talent and Career

Oxypheric is excellent in direct interaction with the public: as promoter of large commercial endeavors; in public relations; as public speaker, singer, entertainer, politician or executive. William Jennings Bryan and Enrico Caruso are examples of the Oxypheric type.

Biochemistry and Diet

Leading biochemical elements are oxygen, iron, potassium, oily material. Oxygen is often excessive; calcium is most likely to be deficient. Appetite of the Oxypheric is capricious and erratic; huge quantities of water and bitter or sour beverages are consumed; females usually have larger appetites than do males, who prefer drinking to eating; appetite is hardy in general and overeating may be prolonged, followed by a hunger strike; highly-seasoned foods, fried foods and rare meats are desired, but these should be minimized or avoided. The most suitable foods are those high in phosphorus, sulphur, chlorine, sodium, calcium, silicon, potassium; greens, broths, vegetables, fish, cooling acid tonics and lean foods are recommended, along with vitamin supplements. Dairy products, fatty meats, fats, sugars, excessive starches, wines, spices, stimulants should be avoided. Skim milk, whey, fruits and vegetables and their juices are beneficial; a vegetarian diet is most helpful to this type.

Additional Requirements

Frequent warm baths are suggested, followed by deep massage. Balmy, humid climates are most beneficial; best altitudes range from 100 to 1000 feet above sea level, with abundant ozone. Outdoor exercise with free and easy motion, such as golfing or horseback riding, is helpful. Sleep is highly recuperative for the Oxypheric type. He also needs a cooling diet; baths to induce perspiration; moisture; ocean voyages; change of occupation; decrease of oxygen consumption; high-calcium diet; sexual and cerebellar activity; pleasant associates; minimal sunbathing; active perspiration without elevation of body temperature.

Common Ailments

Ailments and diseases likely to visit the Oxypheric type include accretion, albuminuria (sudden), arthritis, high blood pressure, brain lag or collapse, extreme fever, sudden flatus, heart disease, hyperemia, extreme nerve pressure attended by psychosis, plethora, psoriasis, sexual disorders. Other possibilities include eruptive, septic, febrile, infectious, sexual, malarial, convulsive, epileptic, neurotic, spasmodic, psychopathic, renal or hepatic disorders—but these are seldom chronic. Fevers, nosebleeds, inflammations, loss of appetite, rupture of blood vessels, vertigo, abscesses, alteration of specific gravity of the blood, hemorrhages of brain or lungs or other membranes may also occur.

This type is intended for excellent health; diseases are usually acute, short in duration, and they often result from excesses. This is the hardiest of the twenty types. Life expectancy is not, however, long, due to volatile nature and attendant excesses; many Oxypherics live only to middle age. Weaknesses in the body of the Oxypheric are generally due to heat pressure, overabundance of oxygen, polyemia, overeating, stimulants, alcohol consumption, poor self-control, excessive amativeness, air pollution. Preventive and corrective measures include self-control; reduction of heat generation; a temperature that encourages evaporation but not heat production or tissue oxidation; bathing for increasing perspiration; sleep; residence near the ocean; an eliminative, cooling diet.

Special Notes

Success in a chosen field is assured if the Oxypheric applies his prominent influential qualities. He is the hardiest of the twenty types.

THE NITROPHERIC TYPE

Definition

The term "Nitropheric" means nitrogen-carrying.

Classification

Vital temperament. Vital-Mental, Vital-Muscular-Mental.

Leading Element

Nitrogen.

General Characteristics

This type is heavy, fleshy, dark eyed, black hair. More than usual weight is carried on the hips and abdomen; chest is large, back straight; central body is largest of the twenty types; obesity increases with age. Nitropherics appear poised, composed, serene, unhurried, stately; they move more quickly as night approaches; their movement lacks grace and fluidity; their countenance is meditative, distracted, pensive but does not mirror their feelings. They gesture little when speaking; hands and feet remain still. Their voices are low, easily strained; they love music but are not good vocalists. The Nitropheric has low vitality and lack of constitutional fortitude; a proud and aristocratic bearing; slow, measured, swinging, straight carriage. Eighty percent of Nitropherics are female; twenty percent male.

Head and Facial Features

The face is full and fleshy, often concave. Lips are shapely. Complexion, eyes and hair are generally dark. Cheekbones are of medium size; cheeks are rounded, especially in the lower section. Features are small and evenly distributed. Hair is soft, wavy, silky, glossy, dark brown or black and generally abundant; nose is small. The face is seldom wrinkled because the mind is not fretful or overly active.

Physical Exterior

Height: Medium to tall.
Weight: Stout to heavy, determined by roundness of body.
The body is well rounded and padded with flesh. Neck is short; there may be a double chin. Abdomen is large; fat often pads the lower portion. Other external characteristics include small, feeble ankles; short arms which are carried regally; large upper arms, tapering in lower arms toward wrists; wide, flat back in hip region; large, corpulent, moist, fleshy body which cannot tolerate tight clothing; large, deep upper chest; tiny, easily-fatigued feet; feverish soles of feet; small, rounded, narrow hands which are nonetheless fleshy; ample, rounded hips; feeble, easily-tired knees; short legs and healthy thighs (often chilled from hips to ankles); sloping shoulders in females, broad and more square shoulders in males; massive thighs; small waist when young, enlarging after age 38; waist set low on

females, higher on males; elongated, heavy torso; dark ivory skin tone; velvety, fine-textured skin.

Physical Interior

The abdominal region is massive and active in function; assimilation is powerful but slow; venous and arterial action is sluggish and individual is subject to varicose veins; blood lacks iron, fibrin and oxygen; circulation is sluggish, particularly in the morning. Bones are soft, small and slim, of medium length. Much fat is carried in lower abdomen and chest regions. Further internal characteristics include well-developed, massive, efficient glands (giving a robust appearance, even during illness); massive but weak heart activity; bowel trouble, such as gas and ballooning; feeble joints; large but chemically deficient kidneys; excellent lacteals; ligaments which lack strength and are often painful; massive, energetic liver which secretes insufficient bile; subnormal lung function; well-developed, energetic lymphatic system; poorly-developed, flabby muscles; large energetic pancreas with excellent starch metabolism; weak respiration; normal secretions; large but erratic spleen; sluggish stomach; feeble, sometimes contracted tendons (during cold weather); ticklist, scratchy, catarrhal throat. Motor nerves are strong; sudden disturbances cause shaky nerves; nerve exhaustion is likely, as are nervousness and highly sensitive nerves.

Five Senses

The Nitropheric type has the keenest senses of taste and smell of the twenty types. His vision is often nearsighted, and there may be optical illusions. Audio function is very keen; olfactory sense is exceptional; taste perception is excellent; sense of touch is very good.

Metabolic Functions

Respiration is easily disturbed and oxygen often lacking; good but temperamental digestion rejects foods containing chemical additives or preservatives; elimination channels are sometimes sluggish; oxidation is extremely poor; sweat may be oily; nutrition is excellent; metabolism of starches is excessive; deficient of calcium. Sexual system is weak, generally passive; sexual appetite is not easily aroused, though the individual can be amorous and affectionate on occasion.

Mental Characteristics

The Nitropheric type has a calm, relaxed appearance; he is pensive, reliable, tactful, reserved, only subtly aggressive and commanding. Misfortune drives him into seclusion; grief is suppressed within; change is disliked; habits are fixed. He is studious, domestic and home-loving; a better listener than conversationalist; rarely quarrelsome; exclusive in associations; generally introverted. He prefers reading to outdoor activity or exercise. His faith in himself is great, although he may be plagued by fears, phobias, illusions. He may feel alienated from the world (when nitrogen is in excess); weep without apparent reason; fear evil, harm from others and travel. His wants, emotions and sentiments are more powerful than his reason, logic or will power; he is highly affected by unpleasant situations; eventual nerve collapse is possible. The mind is slow, lacking concentrative ability; thinking is arduous; faculties may be dull and unresponsive. Although will is weak, obstinacy and tenacity are powerful.

Brain Faculties

Strong Faculties. Vitativeness, bibativeness, alimentiveness, amativeness, secretiveness, destructiveness, parental love, acquisitiveness, conjugality, self-esteem, caution, continuity, conscientiousness, inhabitiveness, idealism.

Weak Faculties. Cerebellum (muscular brain), medulla, firmness, individuality, weight, calculation, benevolence, veneration, hope, locality, combativeness.

Brain Itself. Large brain, square-shaped; insufficient development of medulla, motor department and pons varolii; cerebellum slow in directing muscular movement; cerebellum small and slow in general.

Talent and Career

Nitropherics make successful office managers and supervisors; they attain their goals without direct confrontation. They are good at photography, journalism, mass communications, accounting, secretarial and legal occupations. Musical talent may lead to professional performance.

447

Biochemistry and Diet

Leading elements in the Nitropheric type include nitrogen, carbon, hydrogen, oxygen, of which hydrogen and nitrogen are most often excessive. Calcium, iron, iodine, nitrogen, potassium, oxygen, silicon, sulphur, sodium, fluorine may be lacking. Starch assimilation is high; protein metabolism is poor. The Nitropheric frequently craves cold foods, wine, fruit and vegetables, cereals, meat, acid foods; experiences strong hunger pangs without reason and heartburn from calcium foods; is fond of ice water; has a large appetite at night, poor in the morning; prefers sweets, starches and nitrogen-carrying foods. Beneficial foods for this type include those high in sulphur, phosphorus, iodine, chlorine, manganese, magnesium, silicon, potassium, sodium, iron; vegetable proteins, unrefined grains, warm foods. To be avoided are animal proteins, milk, water, fats, starches, milk, stimulants, sugars, chilled foods. Vitamin supplementation is not usually required. Fresh vegetables and juices are very beneficial. supplementation is not usually required. Fresh vegetables and juices are very beneficial.

Additional Requirements

Tepid water is best for bathing. A breezy, humid, balmy climate is beneficial; chilling, damp air is unfavorable. The best altitude is between 2000 and 5000 feet, with a liberal supply of ozone. Light exercise, particularly walking, is necessary; isometrics and stretching are helpful; a change of scenery may be of benefit. Sleep should not be excessive (Nitropherics are very heavy sleepers.); fresh air is needed in the sleeping room.

Common Ailments

Afflictions and diseases likely to manifest in the Nitropheric type include abscesses, involuntary muscle ailments, aphonia, apoplexy, asthenia, blisters, impoverished blood, blood fungi, blood poisoning, choking, coma vigil, contusions, dislocations, distension, enteralgia, excoriation, heart failure, lethargy, infections, megalopsia, necrosis, numbness, phlebitis, rheumatism (muscular), typhoid, tetanus of flexures. The mind is generally calm; body health is subnormal and constitutional strength is lacking. This type prefers the advice of natural healers to medical methods. Life expectancy is below average; Nitrophercs frequently do not reach old age.

Special Notes

Under the influence of nitrogen, this type is diplomatic, conservative, clannish, slow, deliberate. He is well-qualified for high posts requiring diplomacy, honesty and refinement.

The following fundamentals, according to Kenneth R. Pelletier, Ph.D., have a great deal to do with a person's state of health.
  1. How you think.
  2. How you deal with stress.
  3. How you eat.
  4. Your physical activities.
  5. Your environment.
  6. How you respond to economic and political issues.
  7. What you think about living a long and healthly life.

THE CARBOFERIC TYPE

Definition

The term "Carboferic" means carbon carrying.

Classification

Vital temperament. Combinations include (infrequently) Vital-Mental or Vital-Osseous types.

Leading Element

Carbon.

General Characteristics

The Carboferic type is generally restless and slow moving. In youth he may be stout, energetic, solidly built, attractive, even beautiful; but such strength is deceiving, for this is the weakest of the twenty types. When immobile Carboferics appear natural and graceful; when in motion, they appear awkward. Their first impression is favorable. As age advances, clumsiness, obesity and laziness often set in. The build is stout, chubby, short; equilibrium and composure are easily disturbed; fingers are used energetically when explaining something; vital force is low; appearance is more coarse than refined; gait is unsteady; voice is weak, sometimes squeaky, hoarse or pleasant, feminine. Although this type resembles the Nitropheric in some ways, the Carboferic is light-skinned and has other opposite characteristics. Ninety percent of Carboferics are female, ten percent male.

Head and Facial Features

Skin is milky-white and clear in youth but has a muddy cast during illness. Wrinkles are rare in this type, no matter the age. Face is fleshy, circular; neck is short and thick; forehead is low and hair plentiful. Facial expression is shy and credulous. Cheekbones are small; cheeks are convex, ample; chin may be double. Many Carboferics are blond; a few are brunette, but rarely are they as dark as the Nitropheric; hair is often long, abundant and lovely, though many begin to lose hair while still young. Mouth is usually open; lips are large and full. Face is short from mouth to eyes; it is broad or round and heavy in lower part; features are broad-circular or conic in shape. The face seldom wrinkles because responsibilities and worries are few.

Physical Exterior

Height: Medium.
Weight: Stout to obese (200 pounds or more).
Because carbon and carbohydrates build fleshy tissues, the Carboferic type is inclined to severe overweight; the greatest weight is carried in hips and thighs. Feeble bones and muscular system promote lack of physical vitality. The abdomen is massive, often bloated and puffy. Other external characteristics include small but sometimes swollen ankles; weak wrists; arms heavier near shoulders, narrowing toward hands; feeble small of back; plump, rounded, very heavy body; massive chest; tiny, sensitive feet, with much foot trouble; tiny, feeble, soft hands; large, often bloated hips; feeble, easily-quivering knees; short legs (except in Vital-Osseous); thick neck; voluptuous physique; massive, fleshy shoulders; large torso in contrast to appendages; waist set low on body.

Physical Interior

Assimilation is excellent (too good for elimination to keep up); sugars and starches are most easily absorbed; sugar metabolism is good. Arteries are inferior in development; veins are generally expanded; circulation is poor, erratic; hands and feet especially lack good circulation so become numb easily. Bones and joints are feeble, small, sore; muscles lack strength; tendons and ligaments are poorly developed, feeble. Sugars and starches often ferment and form acids in the body; glands are large and energetic; heart lacks strength; intestines are massive but overworked by excessive carbohydrates; kidneys and liver are large but overworked; respiratory capacity is poor due to medulla weakness, sodium deficiency and lack of artery tone; lymphatic system is large and vigorous; secretions are plentiful; spleen and lungs are overworked but well developed; throat is often swollen and sore. Nerves are sensitive and weak; nervousness and nervous collapse are common.

Five Senses

The senses are generally inferior, with the exception of the Carboferic's excellent sense of taste. Vision is often blurry, farsighted; sense of touch is dull; auditory and olfactory functions are generally poor.

Metabolic Functions

Fresh air is craved and breathing is inadequate under physical exertion; insufficient oxygen is inhaled to eliminate the gas generated. Digestion is exceptionally good, although digestion of proteins and tissue salts is below normal. Eliminative channels are not active enough to rid the body of carbon ferments and end-products generated in the body. Nutrition may be excessive; face perspires readily; pulse rate is feeble; sexual system is energetic but not strong.

Mental Characteristics

The Carboferic is charitable, good-hearted, receptive rather than aggressive, faithful, forgiving, complimentary, soft-spoken. Generally exclusive, he is extroverted with familiar associates. His intuition and sensitivity are well-developed; he has lofty ideals and philosophy, grand intentions, but is weak-willed and physically below par; his shortcomings cause him extreme depression and self-condemnation. He is deeply appreciative of kindness and compassionate toward others.

Judgment may be poor; imagination weak; mental processes slow. He is readily confused or fearful; and his ideas, thoughts, plans, beliefs and notions are clouded, unclear. He may feel sorrow over trivial things; his mind is sensitive although somewhat shallow. Strong minds can easily dominate the Carboferic, who lacks will power and strength.

Brain Faculties

Strong Faculties. Amativeness, bibativeness, alimentiveness, parental love, approbativeness, friendship, human nature, imitation, caution, spirituality, benevolence, comparison.

Weak Faculties. Medulla, cerebellum, combativeness, firmness, self-esteem, acquisitiveness, calculation, weight, conscientiousness, continuity, hope, causality.

Brain Itself. The brain becomes fatigued easily, even when reading; brain substance lacks tension and solidity. Internal nerve tremors or diarrhea may result from use of the brain. Diminutive, inefficient cerebellum causes indolence from deficiency of cerebellar energy. There is weak development of motor faculties (hence no combativeness); little or no self-esteem (hence humility); faulty memory.

Talent and Career

Carboferics make better followers than leaders; they need guidance from more enterprising individuals. They make successful fiction authors, photographers, retouchers; sedentary occupations such as dressmaking, packing, assembling are preferred. Areas in which they can comfort and minister to others are suitable; domestic settings are favored.

Biochemistry and Diet

Leading elements are carbon, hydrogen, oxygen. Calcium, fluorine, iodine, magnesium, iron, manganese, phosphorus, oxygen, silicon, potassium and sulphur are often deficient. Carbon and hydrogen are the only elements likely to be excessive. The appetite of the Carboferic is tremendous, with carbohydrates being the favorite food group. Overeating is likely because will power is lacking; starches, alcohol, sweets are favored to the detriment of health (Carboferic females are the greatest consumers of carbohydrates.).Fortunately, few vitamins are needed to supplement the diet, unless wrong diet has led to exhaustion, obesity or illness.

Suitable foods are those which contain high quantities of iodine, calcium phosphorus, potassium, silicon, manganese, magnesium, sodium, iron. Although needed, foods such as bitter greens, unsweetened dishes and tart foods are disliked. The best foods for this type include lean veal, fresh vegetables, bitter green salads, tart foods and tonics. If a strict diet is adhered to, individuals of this type can greatly increase their general health and well-being.

450

Additional Requirements

A cold, arid, hilly climate is most beneficial; much sunlight, high altitude, sandy and rocky soil are helpful. Sunbaths are suggested. Exercise should be strenuous, heavy, continuous; breathing exercises are vital. The mind needs to be developed in the directions of science, mathematics, technology, intellectual subjects.

Common Ailments

Maladies common to the Carboferic type include alcoholism, arterial degeneration, blood disease, boils, bruises, carboluria, carboemia, carbonic acid poisoning, fears and shyness, mental deficiency, overeating, glycosuria, hemigrania, myalgia, nephritis, paralysis, phosphaturia, prolapsus, rheumatism (nervous), sugar-induced acidity (saccharic acidosis), sexual disorders, sleepiness, spermatorrhea, sugar in the urine, throat afflictions, torpor, tympanitis. Ailments of the Carboferic are related to climate and seasons, to optical and auditory distortions. The health level is generally low, especially after menopause; mental health is also low. Life expectancy is average or short; old age and obesity may begin early.

Special Notes

Carboferic individuals are highly valued for their kindness and compassion; they make the best domestic companions of the twenty types.

THE HYDRIPHERIC TYPE

Definition

"Hydri" refers to water; "pheric" means carrying: "Hydripheric" thus means water-carrying.

Classification

The temperament is generally classified as Vital, though Vital, Osseous and Mental characteristics are combined.

Leading Element

Water (hydrogen).

General Characteristics

The Hydripheric constitution is a product of a powerfully active lymphatic system, excessive assimilation of hydrogen and a shortage of oxygen and solid elements. The body contains much heat, resulting in intake of moisture to cool it. The system is generally acidic because it contains so much hydrogen. The Hydripheric type often gives a false impression of health but in reality is quite fragile. The manner is remote, unattainable or disinterested, with a serious expression and little smiling; there is a constant wariness of strangers. The body is built on the principle of wideness—of hips, feet, torso, hands. The face is usually placid, sorrowful, loving, restful, kind. No magnetism is found within this type; others find them cold. The carriage is dignified; voice is kind, pleasant, soft unless angered. Movements are slow, deliberate, calm except when excited. Eighty percent of Hydripherics are female, twenty percent male.

Head and Facial Features

Eyes are large and calm, even soulful; face is cubic, padded with flesh. Cheekbones are moderately prominent; cheeks are rounded; chin is wide and pudgy, heavy. Complexion is generally blond or medium (darker in hot climates). The central portion of the face is curved inward; chin and eye regions are more convex. Face is masculine; lower face is large; healthy complexion is pinkish to ivory. Features are generally rounded; there may be bags under eyes; mouth, nose, eyes and ears are small. Hair falls easily, is light-colored, thin and fine.

Physical Exterior

Height: Ranges from short to tall.
Weight: Normal in youth, but water retention causes obesity in adult years. The Hydripheric has much difficulty losing weight because of excessive

water retention; water is also absorbed directly from the air in humid areas.

Torso and limbs are heavy or unwieldy; flesh lacks good tone; tissues are generally flabby; individuals appear to be waterlogged. Exterior characteristics include heavy lower abdomen; large arms; weak ankles; massive chest with loose flesh; small hands; wide, generally straight back; sloping shoulders; very large hips; weak knees because joints are weak; short legs, especially shin bone; large, heavy neck; rosy complexion; thin, soft skin; very full thighs; long, wide, ponderous torso; waistline low on torso; large waist. Body is generally large, fleshy, soft, weak and nervous.

Physical Interior

Arteries and veins of the Hydripheric type are weak and rupture readily; circulation is poor. Assimilation is good, especially of water. Muscles of the abdomen are weak; bones are rigid, awkward in movement, medium in length, slim, tender and lacking in strength; joints are weak; muscular system is feeble; eye muscles are jerky; tendons are feeble. Glands are active; heart is slightly weak; digestive system has troubles (enlargement of bowel, etc.); kidneys and lacteals are active; lungs are below average in activity; lymphatic system is very active, as is pancreas; secretions are adequate; venous system is sluggish due to many toxins. Nerves are softened by hydrogen, making the Hydripheric type liberal and gentle; nerve function is, however, more uneasy than it appears; nerves are highly sensitive. Fatty tissue is a result of lymphatic water retention; watery deposits build up around abdomen, hips, glands and under skin.

Five Senses

The five senses are variable in their development. Vision is usually poor; touch and hearing are keen; smell and taste are very acute. All physical senses are active.

Metabolic Functions

After midnight breathing becomes more difficult. Eliminative channels are very active. Metabolism is faulty because excessive water fills the tissues; nutritive system is active but solid nutrients are not assimilated; liquids are readily absorbed. Perspiration is more profuse under emotional stress, in bright sunlight and out of doors; stuffy and closed rooms do not stimulate perspiration to such a degree. Pulse rate is variable, more rapid in the morning and slower at night. The sexual system is not active; platonic love is of more interest than is sexual desire.

Mental Characteristics

The Hydripheric appears calm and serene and has a calming influence on others; his intuition is strongly developed; his is a quiet nature. He is infrequently talkative but interesting at those times; imagination is vivid. Harmony, serenity, relaxation, comfort are important. He desires pleasant associates. The earth's magnetism has a great influence on this type. Knowledge, belongings and friends are shared readily; he is unselfish and always willing to aid others. The exterior impression is of unemotionalism, passivity; deep emotions are unexpressed and feelings rarely surface.

Judgment regarding food, tonics and their relative purity is good; lack of sanitation is easily detected. Tears come easily to the female but are usually shed in secret; she may be exclusive, wary, observant, sensitive, shy and/or fearful. Trances and self-hypnosis come easily. Memory is good for past events but less good for recent happenings; dates, figures, details are not remembered; names are more easily recalled. The will is based on emotion and feeling, rather than on reason.

Brain Faculties

Strong Faculties. Amativeness, bibativeness, parental love, conjugality, comparison, human nature, alimentiveness, imitation, approval, inhabitiveness, language, caution, often destructiveness.

Weak Faculties. Combativeness, sublimity, acquisitiveness, eventuality, firmness, time, locality, suavity, benevolence, cerebellum, self-esteem, individuality, weight calculation.

Brain Itself. Sluggish intellect and will power faculties; strong emotional faculties, physical function faculties and base of brain. Diligent work, hard study, great will power, concentration on scientific subjects or mathematics, prompt action or deep reasoning are not qualities of the Hydripheric type. Cerebellum is too relaxed for sufficient nerve force; its development is weak; slow response of cerebellum and muscular system result. Amativeness is one of the strongest faculties of this type but love is platonic, loyal, lasting and often exclusive. The brain is under the influence of the overly active lymphatic system.

Talent and Career

Suitable occupations include those of family physicians, therapists, beverage manufacturers or tasters, nature cure physicians, home economists, fishermen; hobbies include music and music appreciation, art, sculpture, ceramics, handcrafts.

Biochemistry and Diet

Biochemical elements most often deficient are silicon, potassium, oxygen, calcium, sodium. Hydrogen, the leading element in the Hydripheric constitution, is often excessive. The appetite of the Hydripheric type is enormous and demanding, not easily controlled; this type often wakes up in the night and raids the refrigerator. He mistakenly craves the very substances which contribute to water retention: soft drinks, water, liquids and watery foods. A low liquid diet allows this type to remain reasonably slim and to maintain health.

Additional Requirements

Warm baths are beneficial; massage is not necessarily indicated. An arid, balmy, cloudy climate with a rich ozone belt and low altitude are recommended. A liquid diet is contraindicated; neither are large quantities of vitamins needed. Most suitable foods include those with liberal supplies of iodine, chlorine, calcium, phosphorus, nitrogen, potassium, silicon, dry foods, tonics, berries and juices.

Common Ailments

Disease tendencies of this type include asthma (watery), atrophy of tissues and membranes, bone decay, catalepsy, anemic convulsions, cysts, bloating, dropsy, hydric dyspnea, eczema, effusion, fevers, heart disease, enlarged heart, hemorrhages, infiltration, mesenteritis, hydric obesity, exhaustion and sudden collapse, nervous plethora, sores, spasms, dental caries, low temperature, moist tumors, venous stagnation.

Constitutional weaknesses are due to excessive hydration, overabsorption of moisture, lack of solid nutrients, gases and acids, circulatory anemia, oxygen deficiency, excessive body heat. Preventive measures include a salty diet to take up excess water (especially sodium foods); cold water; warm milk (especially goat milk); muscle-developing foods; frequent moderate exercise; large quantities of oxygen. This type appears much more healthy than he actually is; a state of general weakness pervades the body. Longevity is average; usually age does not exceed 75 years.

Special Note

Hydripherics are effective peacemakers and harmonizers.

THE PALLINOMIC TYPE

Definition

The term "Pallinomic" comes from two Greek words *Pallas* and *osmen*. *Pallas* is the Greek goddess of wisdom, crafts and the arts; *osmen*, from os, mouth, refers to an omen or significant warning fromth of a god.

Classification

Vital temperament. Harmonious type with Vital system predominant.

Leading Elements

Nearly balanced.

General Characteristics

Temperament is somber, melancholy, dark; appearance is not attractive. The Pallinomic type is a deep thinker, wise, serene, serious, courageous, stately, aristocratic, defensive or offensive; he has a corpulent or portly body which is well-proportioned but large with much flesh; his skin is dark, olive, swarthy; his manner is grave, reserved, modest, respectful, sedate, independent, disciplined, well-mannered, composed; his countenance is pensive, grave. The Pallinomic is not magnetic to others but has a strong vital force, good mentality; his walk is ponderous, heavy, slow, long-strided; his voice is deep or low, controlled, subdued, resonant, strong. Sixty percent of Pallinomics are female, forty percent male.

Head and Facial Features

The face is wide at the cheekbones; forehead is prominent. Cheekbones are large and noticeable, though cheeks are often concave. Complexion is dark and swarthy, ivory-rosy or whitish; severe and regular features alternate; hair is stiff, bristly, strong, wiry, coarse, usually brunette; lips are medium-sized, set; mouth is wide, masculine; skin lacks tone and has deep, rough wrinkles.

Physical Exterior

Height: Under six feet.
Weight: Usually between 145 and 200 pounds.
Torso is wide, a mixture of vital and muscular build. Abdomen is well-developed but not prominent. Other external features include well-developed, stiff ankles; normal-sized arms; broad back; fair chest development; broad shoulders; wide, flat, heavy feet; bony but soft hands; wide but not deep hips; large knee joints; long legs in relation to body; short and stocky neck; strong, portly, large-chested physique; normal-sized thighs; long torso with larger-than-average waist; balanced waistline, sometimes slightly high on torso.

Physical Interior

Internal features include well-developed abdomen; erratic digestive function; defective assimilation; sluggish circulation; blood lacking alkalinity; overworked, chaotic veins; massive, strong heart which is sporadic in activity; feeble, erratic glands; intestinal weakness; active but sometimes troublesome kidneys; overworked and weakened lacteals; weakened liver (from excessive toxins); good lung structure but shallow breathing; sluggish lymphatic system; sporadic pancreas; variable secretions; weak, erratic spleen; digestion of animal food superior to that of vegetable products; wide, average-length bones; normal joints; well-developed, efficient muscles; throat which must be protected from cold and moisture. Nerves are well-nourished, strong and smooth in function; their activity is slow and powerful; they are well-controlled, as are mental faculties.

Five Senses

The physical senses are not exceptional in the Pallinomic type. Vision is normal; sense of touch is fair; auditory ability is average but interpretation of vibrational pitch is keen; sense of smell is fair; taste ability is moderate.

Metabolic Functions

Breathing is good but could be deeper. Digestion is good. Elimination, especially through kidneys, is weak. Catabolism is superior to anabolism. Perspiration is not uniform. Sexual system is strong and efficient unless undermined by toxins and acids.

Mental Characteristics

The Pallinomic is very diligent, constructively critical and positive in attitude, sincere and stable, a better listener than conversationalist; his likes and aversions are pronounced; he is punctual, realistic, practical, frugal, solid; he may be intolerant of nomadic habits or radical ideas of others. His judgment is usually rational, practical; he is a good judge of morals, honesty, ethics, values, virtue, quality, form, rank, regulations, safety, debits and credits, discipline, punishment, politics, standards, uses, purposes. His will power is mighty, decided, unswerving, persistent. His mind is pensive, forcible, convincing, thoughtful.

Brain Faculties

Strong Faculties. Combativeness, continuity, caution, causality, acquisitiveness, firmness, destructiveness, inhabitiveness, secretiveness, conscientiousness, form, tune, constructiveness.
Weak Faculties. Language, vitativeness, self-esteem, hope, individuality, weight, eventuality; mirthfulness, veneration, comparison, bivativeness, often calculation.
Brain Itself. Exceptionally large brain; some weakness in medulla; normal cerebellum. Mind is serious, prudent, wise, honest, ethical, practical.

Talent and Career

The Pallinomic has a superb grasp of business and monetary values. In any vocation he is dependable, loyal, stable, thrifty. Pallinomics may be skilled engravers, craftsmen, designers, watchmakers, dental technicians, business managers and advisors, farmers, ranchers, sailors. They are creative and original.

Biochemistry and Diet

Leading biochemical elements in the Pallinomic type include carbon, potassium and (less strongly) calcium. Unless ill, no elements are lacking; during illness alkaline salts may be deficient. Carbon is sometimes excessive. The appetite of the Pallinomic is generally exceptionally vigorous, though there may be periods when appetite vanishes entirely. Abnormal cravings are unexplainable; craving for sweets causes flatus. Animal proteins are better digested than an exclusively vegetarian diet. Foods to avoid include canned and adulterated foods, acidic fruits and vegetables, refined starches, sweets, gravies, potatoes, fatty meats, fried foods, sugary drinks.

Suitable foods include veal, young fowl, alkaline fruits and vegetables, foods rich in potassium, dairy products, iron-rich foods, laxative foods and drinks, warm goat milk, lamb, fish, mint and other herbal teas, low carbohydrate foods. Vitamins are also recommended, especially with advancing age.

Additional Requirements

Warm baths and deep massage are suggested; sunbaths are also beneficial. Moderate exercise is helpful, as are sunshine, breezy weather, oxygen, high altitude, pure air.

Common Ailments

Common illnesses of the Pallinomic type include bladder disturbances, colic, cramps, emphysema, enteralgia, hematemesis, hemorrhaging, jaundice, depression, pleuritis, pneumonia (typhoid), rectitis, rheumatism, sour stomach, varicose veins. Health is fair and life expectancy is not long.

Special Notes

High technical skill enables the Pallinomic type to be successful professionally. Also helpful are his talents of thrift, diligence, persistence and good judgment.

THE LIPOPHERIC TYPE

Definition

"Lipo" refers to fats and "pheric" means carrying; the Lipopheric is therefore the fat-carrying type.

Classification

Vital, Vital-Osseous or Vital-Osseous-Mental temperament.

Leading Element

Fats.

General Characteristics

The Lipopheric type is chubby, stout or obese; merry, festive and fun-loving; even-tempered, congenial, spirited, animated, vigorous, expectant, familiar, reachable, hopeful. The body is built disproportionately, with too much flesh and an overly-large trunk, especially in the lower abdominal area, near shoulders, in upper chest, neck and cheeks. Complexion is generally light; countenance is happy, alive; vital force is great but stamina is lacking. Lipopherics appear poised but are not; they may become magnetic healers. Their voices are powerful, high-pitched, loud; their step is

455

generally light and lively. Fifty percent of Lipopherics are male, fifty percent female.

Head and Facial Features

Cheekbones of the Vital types are small (though Vital-Osseous are larger); cheeks are massive, often baggy and bloated. Face is convex, usually large, fleshy, conic-round, long, wide, flat, full. Complexion has a whitish-gray cast and may be greasy, muddy, coarse. Features are fat-padded and regular; eyes are large; lips are full but curvy; mouth is optimistic. Hair is straight, oily, coarse (sometimes fine), greasy, very thick, bushy and brittle; it may be dark, light brown or blond. Head is wide with low forehead; face does not wrinkle, except for occasional lines on forehead and hands.

Physical Exterior

Height: Varies from short to tall.
Weight: 200 pounds or more.
Entire body is heavy, thick, rounded, tapered from shoulders downward. External features include oversized abdomen, especially in lower bowel area, giving a paunchy appearance; feeble, small ankles; short arms with upper arms extremely heavy; elongated, rounded back; massive chest; small but fleshy feet; cool, soft, small, tapering hands; feeble knees; medium-sized hips but heavily-padded groin area; short legs; short neck, well-padded with flesh and fat; massive, rounded shoulders; heavy, fleshy thighs; large waist, larger with age; waistline set low on body. Physique is generally corpulent, fleshy, loose, flabby; skin is pale, white, rosy, creamy, gray-white or muddy-white, but always whitish; skin is smooth and cool and may feel greasy.

Physical Interior

Interior features include active stomach; good digestion; superb assimilation; weak arteries and veins; slowly-moving blood; subnormal oxidation; perfect fat metabolism; well-developed, energetic glands (except mammary); large heart weakened by obesity; peristaltic action hindered by fat in bowel; well-developed but overworked kidneys; excellent lacteals; massive but overworked liver; large and active lungs; outstanding lymphatic system; fair muscular development and activity; short, small bones; feeble joints; fair tendon efficiency; well-developed pancreas, respiratory system and secretion functions; normal throat development but throat susceptible to many ailments. Nerves are well-fed as is brain tissue (because lecithin is well supplied); joy facilitates efficient nerve activity.

Five Senses

Efficiency of the senses varies in the Lipopheric type. Vision is fair; touch is acute and may have magnetic healing power; auditory function is fair to keen or sometimes dull; olfactory sense is good, often acute but sometimes distorted by catarrh; taste is exceptionally good.

Metabolic Functions

Breathing is superb but air requirements are excessive; digestion is excellent, except when intake of fats, sugars and starches is excessive; eliminative channels are active unless diet is improper; metabolism of fats is excellent of proteins, not so good; nutrition is exceptional; oxidation is subnormal; perspiration is copious; pulse rate is variable, weak to normal; sexual system is powerfully developed and active but Lipopherics are not producers of large families because concepotion requires an alkaline medium.

Mental Characteristics

The Lipopheric is friendly, well-groomed, vivacious, emotional, unselfish, pleasant, outgoing, interested in world and local affairs, persuasive, open and familiar with associates; the personality is magnetic; much thought is given to pleasing others, especially for own gain; charm and friendliness are impressive. Judgment in management, catering, brewing, public service, manufacturing of beauty products, etc., is good; there is skill in caring for the sick and for children, for diagnosing disease and administering anesthesia.

The mind is optimistic, lively, agile, abstract, mysterious, occult, fun-loving, positive, playful. Mental inclinations are to pleasure, satisfaction, fun, service, accomplishment. Will power is feeble and sentimentality powerful. Memory is best for sports, games, pleasure, social events, food, style, fear, as well as for the mysterious, occult and supernatural. Mental deficiencies include lack of will power and concentration, lack of physical and moral courage, lack of conviction, lack of judgment of good and evil, lack of interest in scientific study, lack of executive ability.

Brain Faculties

Strong Faculties. Bibativeness, destructiveness, amativeness, friendship, benevolence, hope, mirthfulness, spirituality, language and faculties dealing with physical senses (especially taste).

Weak Faculties. Pons varolii, corpus callosum, motor areas of cerebellum, combativeness, self-esteem, continuity, weight, firmness, acquisitiveness, conscientiousness, veneration, secretiveness, constructiveness, causallty.

Brain Itself. Medium sized; cerebellar energy is low.

Talent and Career

Friendliness and sociability make this type suited for public service and public relations where one-to-one contact is important: as hostesses, greeters, sales personnel, hosts; entertaining in the home is more important than private and personal enjoyment of home life. Lipopherics are successful club work organizers. Many become psychics or mediums.

Biochemistry and Diet

Leading elements in the Lipopheric type are carbon, oxygen and hydrogen; fats and oils are dominant. Carbon and hydrogen are most often excessive; oxygen, silicon, calcium, iron and potassium are most often deficient. Carbohydrates, especially refined ones, and fats should be severely limited in the Lipopheric diet; fatty meats and oils or fried foods must be avoided. Good foods for this type include lamb, lean veal, fish, fresh fruits and juices, bitter salad greens, low carbohydrate vegetables, sauerkraut and juice, asparagus, steamed cabbage and milk, cheese, cucumbers, goat cheese, leaf lettuce, barley and rye (moderate quantities), strawberries, soups rich in potassium, calcium, sodium, iron, silicon. Few vitamins are needed in supplement.

Additional Requirements

Warm baths daily or warm showers and rubs with rough Turkish towels are suggested, along with vigorous skin brushing. A warm, breezy, fresh aired, cloudy climate is best; abundant ozone is helpful. Good forms of exercise include brisk walking, games and field sports, swimming in warm water, fishing, gymnastics, track, isometrics, sailing, skating, fencing—all actively and for extended periods. Little sleep is required.

Common Ailments

Illnesses common to the Lipopheric type include abscesses, acidosis, acoria, strengthless legs, anemia, chest oppression, congestion, constipation and indigestion (due to fats), dizziness, fatty degeneration, foot and joint disturbances, flatus, heartburn, hyper- and hypo-glycemia, injuries, liver ailments, catamenial disturbances, miscarriages, obesity, hemorrhoids, seborrhea, ulcers, torpidity, throat problems, sleeping sickness. Maladies are generally related to oppression, fatty degeneration of deposits, nutritional disturbances, heart or throat.

The Lipopheric type has a high natural capacity for health of both body and mind. Correct diet, climate, work, habits, friends, study, breathing exercises, home life and love life help maintain this health; above all, a fatty diet must be avoided. Weaknesses result from intemperate diet and sexual activity; from destructive habits and vanity; from shortage of necessary biochemical elements in childhood (silicon, calcium, potassium, oxygen, iron). Life expectancy is short; surgery is often fatal.

Special Notes

Like the Sillevitic, the Lipopheric type is magnetic and persuasive when dealing with other people.

Dong Quai, a popular food supplement in China for centuries, has been found to be high in B-12 and vitamin E—higher than comfrey and wheat germ.

THE PARGENIC TYPE

Definition

"Par" or "para" means side, aside, beside or incorrect, wrong; "genic" means producing or begetting; the Pargenic type therefore bears a taint of "wrong birth."

Classification

Vital temperament; Osseous-Vital or Vital-Osseous.

Leading Element

Fat.

General Characteristics

The Pargenic's general manner is unrefined, common, coarse; he has a sensuous nature, an aged appearance; he appears rough, unkempt, fat, ungraceful, fleshy, strong, clumsy; he is known as being unfortunate, uncouth, shabby, shameless, dangerous, cruel, vindictive, corrupt, insulting. He lacks poise and composure; his expression is threatening, primitive, vicious. When communicating he uses powerful, clumsy gestures; his mental processes are slow but powerful; his voice is nasal, emphatic, deep, gutteral, sarcastic; his walk is ponderous, clumsy, rigid, jarring, slow; his nerve force is slow but efficient. Sixty-five percent of Pargenics are female, the rest male.

Head and Facial Features

The face is heavy and fleshy, even bloated; features are irregular; expression is sulky, resentful or indifferent; eyes are distrustful, cautious, secretive; eyebrows are bristly, stiff, unmanageable; cheeks are heavy, puffy; complexion is ruddy with earthy cast or inflamed with bluish tint, or it may be pale, reddish and yellowish; hair is unmanageable, coarse, bristly, often greasy, oily, dirty; hair color is usually dark or brown; lower lip is thick, parched, ruddy or red-blue; upper lip is more normally sized and set; mouth is wide, pessimistic, unyielding; nose is large and wide; deep furrows and wrinkles give an aged appearance.

Physical Exterior

Height: Medium to tall (six feet).
Weight: Often heavy, overweight.
Torso is heavy and wide, causing limbs to appear disproportionate; body is rigid, inflexible. External features include massive lower abdomen; weak ankles; heavy, plump arms, especially at shoulders; massive, wide lower back, long from neck to tailbone; healthy-looking body; deep-barreled, broad, long chest; flat, wide, often odorous feet; rigid, unattractive fingers and hands; wide, fleshy hips; well-developed but not strong knee joints; malshaped, possibly crippled, legs; thick neck; broad, heavy shoulders in Osseous-Vital type, less so in Vital-Osseous; mottled, flaky, scaly, parched skin; large thighs; large waist, set low to middle.

Physical Interior

Internal features include slow but efficient abdominal functions; good water assimilation; exceptional protein assimilation; often excessive fat assimilation; moderate absorption of sweets; efficient arteries but impaired veins; poor, fatty, overly-rich or tainted blood; slow, sporadic circulation; rigid bones; large, powerful, but subnormally mobile joints; large, irregular uncoordinated muscles; fat deposits on lower abdomen, nape of neck, lateral chest, groin area, intestines; large but overworked glands; long, large, sluggish intestines (due to fat deposits); large but overworked kidneys, liver; energetic lacteals; well-developed lungs but shallow breathing; very efficient pancreas; excellent secretions; large, sluggish spleen; large, efficient stomach which fails only when overstrained; catarrhal, parched, sensitive throat. Nerves are powerful and well nourished, disrupted by miasms, heat and fatty acids; extreme nerve irritation may result in psychopathic or psychotic behavior, mania, alcoholism, seizures.

Five Senses

The physical senses are not well developed in the Pargenic type. Good vision is eventually lost; sense of touch is moderately active; auditory function is chaotic; senses of smell and taste are poor.

Metabolic Functions

Breathing is shallow, difficult, short, often through the mouth; digestion is superior, especially of fats and proteins; eliminative channels are defective; metabolism is exceptionally good; body is well nourished; perspiration is active; pulse rate is short, weak; passions are intense, sexual impulses excessive.

Mental Characteristics

Regular job routine and details are detested by the Pargenic type. Knowledge is absorbed slowly, but the mind has good retentive ability and force. Mental tendency is toward caution, wariness, gravity, soberness, wisdom, secretiveness; intentions of others are often mistrusted. Actions and speech are carefully considered beforehand; impulsive action is rare. Haughty pride is often evident; independence is highly valued.

Judgment is good in matters regarding animals, meat, poisons, foods, alcohol, combat, weather, law enforcement, evil. Memory for information in books is poor; there is inefficient recall of details, numbers, statistics, mathematics, history, systems. The mind runs to immorality, evasion, sports, sarcasm, gluttony, disobedience, dissipation, sulkiness, treachery; mind is slow, ponderous, unresponsive, possibly diabolical. Will is strong but stubborn, rebellious, insubordinate.

Brain Faculties

Strong Faculties. Amativeness, vitativeness, cerebellum, destructiveness, secretiveness, alimentativeness, bibativeness, combativeness, causality, acquisitiveness, at times constructiveness, infrequently spirituality and mirth.

Weak Faculties. Veneration, conjugality, self-esteem, hope, suavity, human nature, individuality, locality, continuity, imitation, eventuality, time, sometimes weight.

Brain Itself. The brain of the Pargenic type is influenced strongly by the miasms or taints inherent in the constitution, as well as by calcium and carbon. Amativeness and destructiveness are the principal dictators of the Pargenic mind.

Talent and Career

Suited for positions as labor leaders, businessmen, ranchers, livestock breeders, brewers, truckers, railroad managers, farmers, veterinarians, political figures, criminal lawyers. Commercial aptitude is high. Financial understanding and shrewd monetary judgment are qualities of this type; they may even be geniuses, great world benefactors.

Biochemistry and Diet

Leading biochemical elements are carbon and calcium. Fluorine is most often deficient; silicon, sodium, potassium, sulphur and chlorine are rapidly precipitated; fat is excessive. The Pargenic should avoid fatty foods such as butter, coconut cream, ham, lard, oils and oily nuts, fatty gravies and soups, shellfish, oily fish, refined starches and sweets, stimulants, spices, liquors, wines. Weight tends to get out of control and toxins invade the body; autointoxication is possible.

Suitable foods include foods high in formic acid, fluorine, chlorine, sulphur, potassium, silicon; mint and other herb teas; bone broths, lean veal, fish, lamb, fowl, game; vegetables such as watercress, mustard greens, leeks, garlic, sauerkraut and juice, dandelion greens. Vitamin supplementation usually necessary.

Vigorous outdoor exercise is indicated and a breezy climate may be beneficial; sunshine helps to expel carbon dioxide. Hot baths, packs and air baths are helpful; a high altitude near the ocean and with high ozone is recommended.

Common Ailments

Common diseases of the Pargenic type include asthma, bone ailments, biliousness; convulsive, congestive, catarrhal, eruptive, degenerative, sexual, hair, liver, lymphatic, mastoid, menstrual, nasal, ovarian, scrofular, phlegmatic, pustular, salivary, ulcerous, venous, visual complications; warts, tumefaction, paralysis, boils, blindness, bronchitis, enlarged liver, epilepsy, fatty degeneration, mania, skin eruptions, swellings, vaccinosis, impotence, gangrene, homicide or suicide. The health of the Pargenic is superb until illness strikes; illness may last for the duration of the lifetime; the mind is questionable and unstable.

The Pargenic has a pessimistic, melancholy attitude and bodily imbalance.

twenty-four

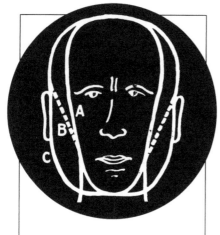

The mental types of man

Neurogenic, exesthesic, pathetic, nervimotive and atrophic

Sketch of the Mental Temperament Types

Five varied types comprise the mental temperament. The *Neurogenic* is the best "stereotype" of this temperament. Phosphorus is very active in the brain of the Neurogenic, giving him a prolific mentality and a responsive mind. Stoutness or obesity is unlikely because little bulk building material is utilized by this type. Well-developed muscles are impossible because muscle-building material is not well used. A large bone structure is not realized because not enough calcium is assimilated.

The *Exesthesic* is another mental type. The word exesthesic means one who expresses feeling. Sulphur, potassium and phosphorus are the dominant elements. Sulphur contributes to emotionalism; potassium works in the muscle structure to cushion bones evenly; phosphorus gives an alert mentality. The stature may be short or tall; the build is gracefully slender. The face is oval and the manner and countenance selective and remote. Women make up the majority of Exesthesic types.

The *Pathetic* type puts on weight easily because carbon and phosphorus are active. Still, these people have a mental nature. The height is usually short to medium. Hands and feet are small and well padded with flesh; joints are supple, limber and elastic to the touch.

The *Nervimotive* type is generally short-to-medium in height, slim and strong boned; face is long and narrow. This type gives the impression of slenderness but toughness or ruggedness at the same time; he is retentive and strong. The leading elements are sulphur, phosphorus and calcium. Sulphur lends qualities of depth and intensity; calcium contributes endurance and power; phosphorus gives keen mentality. The expression of the eyes is penetrating; the overall appearance is compact and efficient.

The *Atrophic* type is often six feet tall, the tallest of the mental temperaments, efficient assimilation of calcium for bone structure. Phosphorus is also active, making this type a competent mental worker. The body shape is angular; forehead is large and the cheeks often concave. This type is characterized by a sober expression and a businesslike attitude or intellectual bearing.

Neurogenics are well mannered and refined, tactful, mentally prolific.

The manner of the Exesthesic is refined, flawless in appearance and behavior.

The Pathetic type is the most amicable, kind hearted, genial of the twenty types.

The Nervi-Motive type is positive and optimistic, brave and extremely active, not easily controlled or intimidated.

Creative ability and intellect are particularly strong in the Atrophic type.

THE NEUROGENIC TYPE

Definition

"Neuro" refers to nerve(s) and "genic" means producing; hence, nerve producing.

Classification

Mental temperament. Mental Osseous.

Leading Elements

Phosphorus.

General Characteristics

The Neurogenic constitution is a result of low physical vitality; brain and nerve malnutrition; deficiency of calcium, carbon, nitrogen, silicon, sodium, magnesium and oxygen; excess of phosphorus, creating an acidic system. The body is fragile, small, out of proportion; vital and motive systems are poorly developed; the individual is easily injured, sensitive-to-rough treatment, lacking in stamina. Refinement and culture are evident in poise and composure; expression is sorrowful, aged, cultured, selective; countenance is changeable; body is active. The Neurogenic type is short, slim, tidy, dainty and has excellent taste; he is attentive to activity around him; his eyes are bright; when in good health, his expression is intelligent and alive. He is often nervous and restless, although his vital force is low; his nerve force is easily exhausted by trivial worries; his voice is gentle, soft, cultured, pleasant, high pitched; his step is lively, more gentle than forceful. He is finely tuned physically and intuitionally and is interested in the welfare of others; he is intellectual, orthodox in behavior. Seventy-five percent of Neurogenics are female; twenty-five percent are male.

Head and Facial Features

The forehead is the most prominent feature; head is widest in temple region; lower part of face is narrow or small. Cheekbones are small to medium sized; cheeks are concave, diminutive, short (showing low oxidation, poor nutrition). Most

Neurogenics are light complexioned, some medium and brunette; hair is usually fine textured, soft, thin; it falls easily and grays early; color ranges from light to black but is most often light brown. Features are sharp, angular, chiseled, aristocratic; eyes are large and soulful; mouth is small and feminine; lips are small, thin, sometimes shapely. A fine network of wrinkles covers the face, giving an aged appearance.

Physical Exterior

Height: Usually five feet or shorter.
Weight: Generally 100 pounds or less.
The body is delicate and fragile, too weak for work requiring physical exertion. External features include flat abdomen; bony ankles; slender, weak arms; narrow, concave-shaped, slender back; weak, delicate backbone; cold, moist skin with gray or waxy pigmentation (due to phosphorus excess), color ranging from pale gray to ashen to waxy-gray, texture soft and elastic and very sensitive; small, flat, narrow chest; long, narrow feet; small hips, bony knees; flexible, bony, slim fingers and hands; long, slim legs and neck; thin, square, sloping shoulders; slim thighs; masculine, slim, frail torso, sometimes short in comparison to legs; small waist set high on torso.

Physical Interior

Absorption is faulty and all vital functions are generally weak in the Neurogenic type. Interior features include weak veins and arteries; blood deficient in salts and fibrin, poorly circulated and unable to nourish the body properly; pliable bones, soft, small in joints, slender, fragile, sometimes tender and painful; glandular ailments or diseases; poor fat metabolism; brain and nerves poorly supplied with cholesterol; small, relatively weak heart, small, irregularly-functioning intestines; feeble tendons, ligaments and joints; small kidneys overworked by excessive phosphate metabolism; small, inconsistent liver; undersized lungs which function spasmodically; feeble, faulty lymphatic system; undersized pancreas which is susceptible to diabetic disturbances; erratic respiratory function; undersized, easily-disrupted spleen; small, inconsistent stomach; feeble muscular system; parched throat. Optic nerves lack strength, as do other nerves in the body; nervous system is erratic, morbid, ailing due to excessive phosphorus by-products; nerve force is dissipated by extreme criticism or roughness; nervous system is very finely, delicately organized and highly sensitive; nerves are overly active and brain oversized for the amount of nutrients actually assimilated; brain and nerve energy is deficient in the entire nervous system.

Five Senses

With the exception of vision, senses of the Neurogenic are exceptionally keen; vision is fair (due to weak optic nerves and brain centers); touch perception is excellent; hearing is acute, distinguishing; smell and taste (both for food and for culture) are keen.

Metabolic Functions

Breathing is shallow; eliminative channels are inefficient; elimination is often too rapid (especially through the bowel) and liver function is irregular. Metabolism is defective; brain and nerves are malnourished; oxidation is poor; perspiration may be deficient; pulse rate is irregular, nervous, brief; sexual function is feeble but excitable, lacking in strength; digestion is rapid or delayed.

Mental Characteristics

Neurogenics are well mannered and refined, tactful, mentally prolific; on the surface, they appear calm and remote; they are gifted speakers and writers, creative and original; occult, mystical or metaphysical subjects fascinate them. Judgment is superb in art, literature, music, poetry, fine architecture, interior decorating; color perception is excellent. The mind tends toward the occult. Memory is good for criticism, reprimands, disapproval because feelings are extremely sensitive, sympathetic, nervous, emotional. The will is weak.

Brain Faculties

Strong Faculties: Destructiveness, caution, approval, parental love, ideality, form, time, color, sublimity, tune, causality, mirth, spirituality, constructiveness.

Weak Faculties: Cerebellum (including muscular brain), pons varolii, medulla, amativeness, vitativeness, bibativeness, alimentiveness, combativeness, acquisitiveness, firmness, self esteem, weight, locality, continuity, hope secretiveness.

Brain Itself: Between 10 p.m. and 3 a.m., the brain of the Neurogenic is most active; it is sluggish in the morning. Excessive activity overheats the brain and exhausts the brain force; the brain is so active that vitality is rapidly precipitated. The cerebellum is diminutive, promoting a weak muscular system and lack of animal heat (producing great sensitivity to cold). Phosphorus has a powerful influence over the mind of this type, making the individual dreamy and unrealistic; he has powerfully developed faculties of sensitivity, sentimentality, idealism and refinement.

Talent and Career

The Neurogenic type is inclined toward such vocations as psychology, psychiatry, astrology and psychic research; his creative endeavors include art, creative writing, fashion designing, hairdressing, watch or jewelry making; he is amiable, often acting as peacemaker or diplomat because he can view all sides in a detached manner.

Biochemistry and Diet

Phosphorus is the leading biochemical element in the Neurogenic constitution and is the only element likely to become deficient. Frequently excessive elements are silicon, calcium, carbon, fluorine, iron, magnesium, free oxygen, organic elements and most blood salts. An abundance of phosphorus foods is needed by this type, along with vitamin and mineral supplementation. Suitable foods are nut butters, nut and seed oils, wheat germ and wheat germ oil, fish and seafoods, fowl and wild game (expecially dark meat), veal, fresh vegetables (plenty of greens), fruits, egg yolks, raw milk, herbal teas; foods rich in sulphur, phosphorus, iodine, iron, chlorine, potassium, magnesium, neurol, vitamins. For weight building, the most helpful foods are juicy meats, juicy fruits, carrots, ice cream, buttermilk, strawberries and raw cream, other juicy foods. The Neurogenic type has difficulty maintaining good health; compliance with dietary needs helps ensure health and lengthens the life expectancy.

Additional Requirements

Considerable sleep is needed by this type, as are rest and relaxation to reduce nerve pressure.

Sunbathing, air bathing, warm water, limited cold baths or showers, deep massage after bathing are beneficial. The most suitable altitudes range from 4,000 to 10,000 feet; plenty of ozone and a cold or cool climate with plenty of fresh air are recommended. Vigorous exercise in the outdoors is helpful, if not essential.

Common Ailments

Principal ailments of the Neurogenic type include anemia, asthma, brain deterioration, catalepsy, colic, dementia, emaciation, fatty degeneration, seizures, gas pressure, heart disease, hemorrhages, myasthenia, myelosclerosis, nervous prostration, neuralgia, neurasthenia, paralysis, pneumonia, mental impotence, pus generation, scrofula, sterility, insomnia, weak joints, jaundice, albuminuria; ailments are related to the nervous, vital and spasmodic functions.

Weaknesses in this type are generally attributable to lack of phosphorus in the bones and excess phosphorus in brain and nerves; overly-developed upper part of brain; lack of brain development at base; low oxidation; insufficient animal heat and magnetism; impracticality; low energy; shortage of blood and tissue salts; weak vital functions. Anemia results from blood deficiency, as required elements are not sufficiently extracted from foods. Vitality is lacking because of deficient oxidation in tissues and nerves. Many Neurogenics die in younger or middle years.

Special Notes

The Neurogenic type is the most highly evolved of the twenty types; he is in contact with both the physical and the spiritual worlds and finds it easy to interpret mystical and metaphysical symbolism and phenomena.

THE EXESTHESIC TYPE

Definition

"Ex" means out, "esthesic" or "esthetic" means feeling; hence the Exesthesic type throws out feeling.

Classification

Mental temperament. Mental-Muscular, Mental-Muscular-Vital, Mental-Vital-Muscular, Vital-Mental, Muscular.

Leading Elements

Sulphur; potassium, phosphorus.

General Characteristics

The extreme electrical activity generated by phosphorus, sulphur and iron in the body create the Exesthesic constitution; sulphur and phosphorus by-products result from intense emotions and an active nervous system. The physical stamina and power of this type are limited; the constitution is generally acidic; appearance is youthful, with pale complexion in the morning and rosier in the evening; the nature is highly refined, cultured, regal,

stately, poised. This type is one of the most attractive and well proportioned; the body is usually shapely and svelte, tall, slim and graceful. Emotions are held in check in public but may explode forcefully in private, especially when the individual is fatigued or irritated. The face is sober, kind, sensitive, indicative of good breeding. In general, the Exesthesic is vivacious, spirited, lively, attractive but not magnetic; conduct is proper, except in unexpected circumstances. The voice is high-pitched, often soprano. Ninety percent of Exesthesics are women, ten percent men.

Head and Facial Features

The face is oval with regular features; the forehead is prominent, the face widest in the temple area. Cheekbones are not prominent but are well-padded with flesh, having a rounded appearance. Features are regular and pleasing to the eye; mouth is small, lips thin or small, nose aristocratic but not large. Hair is usually wavy or fluffy, never oily, attractive with good growth; it is often red, auburn or blond (beautified by sulphur). Because of nervous activity, a fine network of wrinkles may develop by age 30.

Physical Exterior

Height: From about 5 feet to 5 feet 7 inches or taller.

Weight: Proportioned to small frame.

The body is slim and well-proportioned; size is medium to small; chest development is moderate to small; fingers are long, pliable, pale, thin; skin of hands is soft, thin, flexible, hot to the touch; flesh of hips is firm, sometimes with some fat; legs are long, slim, attractive; neck is long; shoulders slope gracefully; complexion is rosy but light; body skin is soft, fragile, smooth, satiny, with small pores; thighs are firm with some fat; waistline is small to medium (about 26 inches) and set high on the torso.

Physical Interior

Internal features include poor assimilation; small, fragile arteries and veins; poor circulation; varying body temperature; active glands; heart which is weaker on right side; some intestinal troubles; weak joints; long, pliable, small, fine bones; highly mobile muscles; average tendons and ligaments; weak kidneys; small, overworked liver; underdeveloped lacteals; small but active lungs; average lymphatic system; overworked eyes; average pancreas; small, feeble spleen; problems in throat and tonsils. Nerves are stressed, high strung; spells of nervous debility are likely; nerves become overheated and painful. The Exesthesic type does not become obese because he avoids fatty foods. His weakest areas are the digestive and sexual systems.

Five Senses

Sensitivity is great; eyesight is keen, touch sensation acute, auditory function superb; taste and smell are somewhat less sensitive, although appetite is finicky.

Metabolic Functions

Fumes and by-products generated in the body affect breathing unfavorably; elimination is faulty; metabolism is active; nutrition is generally good; oxidation is deficient; perspiration is minimal; pulse rate is variable, short; sexual system lacks vitality reserve and desire is inconsistent.

Mental Characteristics

The manner of the Exesthesic is refined, flawless in appearance and behavior. He is outgoing among associates but shy among strangers. The mind is excessively active (due to sulphur) and sensitivity is high. Judgment is good in matters of rhetoric, art, acting, literature, people, music, architecture, landscaping, metaphysics, philosophy, religion. Memory is good for faces, poor for details. As the name suggests, the Exesthesic is an aesthetic and appreciative of beauty, refinement or culture; much pride is taken in appearance, dress, social status.

Mental inclinations are toward sympathy, worry over trivial things, an emotional will, serious delusions, forgiveness, expression of feeling and emotion, irritability when nerve force is low. The mind is agile and responsive; reality is perceived at a glance; emotions cause lack of reason. Educated and wise Exesthesics are revered and appreciated.

Brain Faculties

Strong Faculties. Parental love, approval, caution, ideality, sublimity, language, tune, spirituality, comparison, conscientiousness, veneration.

Weak Faculties. Bibativeness, secretiveness, weight, continuity, self esteem, conjugality, calculation, acquisitiveness, conscientiousness, causality.

Brain Itself. Moderately large muscular brain is very active; cerebellum is often overheated and easily exhausted; mental response is quick. Nerve irritation should be avoided to prevent precipitation of lecithin from brain and nerves.

Talent and Career

Creative, artistic fields appeal to this type; Exesthesics are often found in the entertainment world. They seek a refined atmosphere in which to work and may be successful as singers, voice or speech coaches, fashion and beauty consultants, librarians, interior decorators, fashion designers, actors or actresses, language teachers or in other intellectual and/or cultural pursuits.

464

Biochemistry and Diet

The most active biochemical elements in the Exesthesic constitution are sulphur, phosphorus, potassium, magnesium, carbon. Most often deficient are magnesium, manganese, nitrogen. Sulphur raises the level of sensitivity; heats the liver, brain and nerves; increases skin activity; augments mental dissatisfaction. Sulphur fumes are detrimental; cooked sulphur foods generate gas; sulphur foods are craved. Indigestion results from eating an early breakfast and occurs about an hour after meals; digestion is almost perpetually disturbed.

A diet rich in phosphates, magnesium, manganese, potassium and iodine is necessary to counteract nerve depletion, exhaustion, insomnia. Good foods for this type include game and fowl, sea vegetation, fish and fish roe, fresh fruits and vegetables, fruit and vegetable juices. Foods to be avoided include sulphur vegetables (onions, cabbage, turnips, mustard greens, rutabagas), condiments, refined carbohydrates, desserts, pastries, fatty gravies, rare meats.

Additional Requirements

An altitude from 2000 to 5000 feet is most favorable; climate should be breezy, cool, dry, with plentiful ozone. Cool baths and showers are beneficial, as is deep massage. Walking and other outdoor exercise is suggested. Also useful are solitude, water, fresh and pure air, love, understanding, optimistic associates, travel and variety, freedom, much sleep, foods that feed the brain and nervous system, foods rich in magnesium, manganese, potassium, sodium.

Common Ailments

Maladies common to the Exesthesic type include acidity, aberration, cerebral congestion, chest oppression, cramps, sensation of crawling skin, delusions, eruptions, eye problems, fermentation, gastro-intestinal troubles, headache, hematuria, hemorrhages, hypersensitivity, hysteria, indigestion, low oxidation, miscarriages, nervous troubles, neuralgia, numbness, prolapsus, nervous exhaustion, menstrual complications, spleenitis, tumefaction, throat constriction, spasmodic rheumatism, weak ankles or back or knees. Further ailments include pains in eyes, neck, small of back; coughing, hot urine; fainting; mental ailments; sexual disorders; lack of nerve force.

Sources of inherent weaknesses include excess sulphur products; lack of oxygen and tissue salts, notably nerve elements such as phosphorus; extreme emotion and nervousness; ferments; small liver and sluggish portal system. The Exesthesic type is not long lived; his health is fair, but he is not hardy. He lives mostly in the realm of the mind. To maintain health, he must find happiness and peace and avoid excesses.

Special Notes

Frequent changes of scenery, vacations, interesting friends and hobbies are needed by the Exesthesic type. Associations and environment should be refined, cultured, pure.

Low blood sugar (hypoglycemia) can cause depression.

Asthma sufferers are almost always hypoglycemic, according to Larry Christiansen, Ph.D. Attacks come when blood sugar is low, never when it is high. There is a close relationship between brain function and blood sugar, which means that the most important effects of hypoglycemia may be in the area of mental health. Low blood sugar is estimated to affect about 40 million Americans.

465

THE PATHETIC TYPE

Definition

"Pathetic" is derived from the Greek term "*patheticus*," meaning full of feeling or pathos (emotion, suffering).

Classification

Mental and Vital temperaments combined; Mental-Vital or Vital-Mental.

Leading Elements

Phosphorus, carbon, hydrogen.

General Characteristics

The Pathetic constitution results from heredity; the predominance of carbon, hydrogen and phosphorus; shortage and faulty combination of biochemical elements. The general appearance of this type is healthy, well proportioned, tidy, professional, well dressed, youthful, stout but not obese, well mannered, friendly, polite, rosy complexioned, of medium height. Bones are small and muscles lack tone; countenance is pleasant, responsive; body is calm; vital energy is high though individual seems passive, well poised, subdued; voice is rich, well modulated, soft, sympathetic, understanding; walk is quiet, short strided. Ninety-five percent of Pathetics are female; only five percent are male.

Head and Facial Features

Face and features are rounded; prominent forehead indicates keen intellectual ability. Cheekbones are usually obscure; cheeks are rosy, fleshy; features are regular, finely molded; lips are well shaped, full; mouth is short. This type seldom develops wrinkles.

Physical Exterior

Height: Usually between 5 feet and 5 feet 5 inches.
Weight: Proportioned to small bone structure.
The body is frail in bone structure but well rounded (soft in women) and well proportioned.

External features include averaged-sized abdomen; feeble ankles; short, fleshy arms; attractive, well-formed back; weakness in small of back; long torso; waistline set low on body; well developed but not large chest; small, well-formed feet; long, symmetrical, tapered hands and fingers; medium-sized hips; small, weak knees; long, shapely, symmetrical legs; large thighs relative to lower legs; long, symmetrical neck; regal, aristocratic, artistic, professional-looking physique; soft, fine, sensitive, rosy, attractive skin.

Physical Interior

Internal features include good digestion; normal assimilation; feeble, sluggish arteries and veins; deficient, acidic blood; poor circulation; weak, sluggish heart; normal fat metabolism; energetic, normally-developed glands; large, energetic intestinal tract; strong, active kidneys; feeble joints and ligaments; average development and activity of lacteals; normal liver; underactive lungs; above-average lymphatic system; weak osseous system (motive); good muscular coordination but subnormal strength; normal pancreas and secretions; subnormal protein digestion; throat weakness and easily-impaired vocal chords. Nerves appear to be under control but are actually acutely sensitive and responsive; nerve activity is steady but easily disrupted; nerve shock and nervous collapse are possible.

Five Senses

Except for poor eyesight, the senses are highly developed. Hearing is acute, easily disturbed by noise, commotion, rattle; sense of smell is keenly developed; touch and taste are highly developed; eyesight is mediocre or fair.

Metabolic Functions

Breathing capacity is mediocre or fair; digestive ability is average or above average; eliminative channels are normal; anabolism is good, catabolism average; nutritive function is normal; oxidation is fair; pulse rate is often chaotic, soft, interrupted; sexual system functions below par and manifests weakness.

Mental Characteristics

Memory is best when related to child psychology, habits of animals, color in art or home decorating, human nature, service and comfort of others, social activity, amusements, plants, songs, music, poetry, styles of dress, acting, speech, conversation, commitments. The brain is slow and deliberate, even sluggish or uncentered; will is weak, lacking in leadership, execution, confrontation, resolution. Concentration is difficult; there is little self esteem, lack of courage and initiative, instability, lack of stamina, persistence, force, aversion to violence, punishments, altercations. The mind is too resigned, bendable, tenacious. There is a love of the aesthetic and an inclination to ask advice of palmists, fortune-tellers, astrologers, tarot readers.

The Pathetic type prefers the home and domestic duties; he is easy-going, placid, devoted, affectionate, self examining and self critical. Unfounded inferiority complexes are common. Ambition and capability often outweigh fortitude. These individuals are adaptable, attentive listeners, easily influenced by kindness, adverse to roughness and cold ambition, susceptible to environmental vibrations, hypersensitive, predisposed to worry, loyal and devoted to mates and duties.

Brain Faculties

Strong Faculties. Parental love, conjugality, friendship, tune, benevolence, agreeableness, alimentiveness, bibativeness, hope, ideality, language, amorousness, approval, form, color, human nature, caution, sublimity, spirituality, comparison.

Weak Faculties. Destructiveness, combativeness, firmness, self esteem, continuity, motoria in the brain.

Brain Itself. Mental functions are sluggish; cerebellum is small, especially the motor department, causing weak muscles, ligaments, tendons. Humane faculties are active, making the Pathetic very respectful, even reverent, loving and tolerant. Especially prominent faculties are agreeableness, benevolence, friendship, parental love, which are responsible for respectfulness.

Talent and Career

This type is not suited for great responsibility, high pressure or extremely hard work. They are successful as kindergarten teachers, librarians, writers of children's stories, pet store owners, toy designers, fashion designers, floor walkers, stenographers, secretaries, telephone operators. Their primary purpose is to serve and help others; their environment must be harmonious and serene.

Biochemistry and Diet

Leading biochemical elements in the Pathetic type are phosphorus, hydrogen and carbon. Nitrogen is occasionally excessive; calcium, iodine, iron, magnesium, manganese, nitrogen, potassium, silicon and sometimes fluorine are often deficient. This type has poor bone and muscle metabolism; a diet rich in calcium, potassium, iron, lecithin, manganese and iodine foods is essential. Suitable foods include raw goat milk and cheese, sea vegetation, fresh white fish, unpolished rice, wheat germ, game and fowl, fresh vegetables (including root vegetables), fresh fruits and berries. Foods high in protein should be limited; meat, fatty foods and stimulants should be avoided. Assimilation of biochemical elements is subnormal, but little vitamin supplementation is needed. Health and life expectancy can be enhanced if wise dietary habits are observed.

Additional Requirements

Eight to twelve hours of sleep are essential for the Pathetic constitution. Tepid baths are beneficial, followed by massage. Balmy, arid, warm climates are best, with altitudes from 2000 to 4000 feet. Exercise should be light or moderate, increasing gradually in duration; although it is essential, exercise should be wisely guided. Brain and nerve tonics may be beneficial, as is a diet high in lecithin, blood salts and tissue salts. Mental conditioning may help to steady and strengthen nerves.

Common Ailments

Conditions common to this type include anemia, anergia, muscular troubles, nervous ailments, ovarian and uterine disturbances, paresis, cardiac complications, fatigue, low energy, extreme and sad emotional disturbances, brain fatigue, dislocations, ruptures, headaches, difficulties sleeping, hemorrhages, neuroses, unrequited love, blood ailments, neuralgic disruptions. Because the health level is low and constitution somewhat weak, good health is difficult to maintain. Life expectancy is often below 60.

Special Notes

The Pathetic type is the most amicable, kind hearted, genial or the twenty types.

THE NERVI-MOTIVE TYPE

Definition

"Nervi" has to do with nerves; "motive" means movement, moving. The Nervi-Motive is a nerve and bone type combined; nerves are as active as are bones.

Classification

Motive temperament. Mental-Osseous or Osseous-Mental (less frequently).

Leading Elements

Phosphorus, sulphur and calcium.

General Characteristics

Emotional and volative (changeable) forces are most active in this type because phosphorus, calcium and sulphur are used extensively. The nerves, bones and bone energy,and brain are highly charged with heat; thus, the Nervi-Motive type is hot-tempered, intense, emotional, stubborn, hardworking, energetic, nervous, volatile, spiteful, hostile, revengeful, even cruel. Excessive work creates an acidic system. The general appearance is described as aged, wrinkled, slightly pale; face and head are small with angular features; body is slim or emaciated; manner is short and abrupt to others; expression is severe. Body appears disproportionate, small to medium in size, with short torso and long limbs. Countenance is grave, stern, forbidding; composure and poise are lacking; life force is average but nerve, bone and brain energy are strong, however spasmodic. The voice is squeaky, gutteral, rough when offended, whiny in children. Gait is irregular, jerky; head is often carried ahead of feet. Fifty percent of Nervi-Motives are men, fifty percent women.

Head and Facial Features

Face is usually long and narrow; expression is alert, tense. Cheekbones are high, cheeks concave. Hair is usually dry, rigid, unmanageable, dull; color ranges from light gray to light red and sandy. Head is broad and wedge-shaped, small or medium sized. Lips are thin, harshly set, small. Wrinkles are numerous.

Physical Exterior

Height: Usually 5 feet 7 inches or under.
Weight: Porportioned to slenderness and light or average bone structure.
The body is slender with strong bone structure; calcium contributes to its durability and strength. External features include concave abdomen; powerful ankles; bony, gnarled, strong, long arms; incurved back; short, flat torso and chest; bony feet; slim, bony, dry hands, square in shape, unrefined and large for body size; medium-sized hips, wide across but narrow on sides; strong, bony knees; ungainly, slim legs; long, heavy neck for body size; broad, square, slender shoulders, medium or small thighs. Physique is medium-sized to small, sometimes tall, slender, masculine, wide compared to thickness from front to back. Sunken appearance of abdomen, thighs and hips makes this type appear delicate but actually great strength exists. Skin is fair to ruddy, fine, freckled, sensitive.

Many similarities exist between the Nervi-Motive and the Neurogenic types. The major difference lies in the refinement of the Neurogenic, compared with the coarseness of the Nervi-Motive. The Neurogenic has impeccable manners, a pleasing voice, a kind countenance, fluid movements; the Nervi-Motive has rough manners, a harsh voice, a severe countenance, jerky movements.

Physical Interior

Internal features include mediocre, slow digestion; sluggish intestinal activity; weak assimilation; resilient, efficient but overworked veins and arteries; deficient blood; much arterial pressure from extreme emotions; bones are rigid, elongated, large for body size, dense, with active metabolism; excessive blood flow to head; fat not metabolized; diminutive glands; rapid, strong heart; large, efficient joints, powerful ligaments and tendons; overworked, average-sized kidneys; small, sparse lacteals; medium-sized liver; active, good-sized lungs; slow lymphatic system; average pancreas; efficient respiration; scanty secretions; sporadic spleen; strong throat. The nervous system is malnourished and chaotic in function; nerves are easily riled, excited; females particularly find temper and nerve control difficult. Optic nerves are moderately strong but overwork and nerve depletion cause vision problems.

Five Senses

Vision is inherently good, notwithstanding intense use of brain and nervous system; eye weakness comes through strain, overwork, strong emotions, lack of sleep, rash behavior. Touch perception is moderate; auditory faculty is acute; smell is very sensitive; taste varies from good to deficient.

Metabolic Functions

Breathing capacity is average; digestion is poor; elimination is sluggish; bone metabolism is excellent; other metabolism is good; oxidation is above average; muscle oxidation is often excessive; perspiration is profuse; pulse rate is fast, nervous, strong; sexual system is not strong and its power is variable.

Mental Characteristics

The Nervi-Motive type is positive and optimistic, brave and extremely active, not easily controlled or intimidated. Phosphorus in the brain lends mental attentiveness and quick menta reflexes. Sulphur contributes creativity, expressiveness, emotionalism, quick temper. The individual readily airs his opinions, enjoys debates or quarrels; he is generally a poor listener, has much faith in his own abilities, is obedient to laws, enthusiastic for new knowledge, creative, studious, organized, scrupulous, honest, security-oriented. Making money is his prime concern and money is highly esteemed. Judgment in matters of money, finance, commercialism, business is excellent.

Memory for offenses, money, income, valuation, lawsuits, taxes is outstanding. The mind is extremely energetic, enduring, though it may become exhausted by intense use. Will is very strong. Qualities include bravery, strength, endurance, diligence, promptness, combativeness, expediency, patience, determination, activity.

Brain Faculties

Strong Faculties. Combativeness, approval, acquisitiveness, form, ideality, constructiveness, conscientiousness.

Weak Faculties. Friendship, conjugality, self esteem, order, continuity, veneration, locality.

Brain Itself. Exceptionally active brain; restless nerves; spasmodic muscles; large cerebellum compared to cerebrum (giving tremendous stamina and energy, good nerve force). This type drains vital, motive and cerebral energy exceedingly rapidly. His behavior is erratic, impatient, extreme, intense, irascible, excitable, rushed, impulsive, revengeful, bitter or spiteful, passionate, hot-tempered. (A sulphur diet intensifies and stimulates these mental faculties and emotions; magnesium has the opposite, relaxing effect.)

Talent and Career

This type is best suited for independent undertakings; they prosper as insurance salesmen, property appraisers, auditors, investigators, tax collectors. They also make law-respecting judges, politicians, attorneys, stockbrokers. Discipline is one of their best traits.

Biochemistry and Diet

Leading elements in the Nervi-Motive type are calcium, phosphorus, sulphur; calcium, chlorine, sulphur and silicon are likely to be excessive; carbon, iodine, manganese, magnesium, sodium and nitrogen are most often deficient. The great quantities of sulphur used by this type are responsible for many of their fickle, contradictory, volatile characteristics. Appetite and cravings are capricious; there is little hunger in the morning; appetite needs to be well supervised. Suitable foods are those high in phosphorus and magnesium, berries, clabbered milk, cheese, fish, onions. A high alkaline diet is essential. Other good foods include mulberry juice, cooling (sodium) fruit juices, fowl and game, avocados, papayas, persimmons, fresh fruits, nut and seed butters, fresh vegetables and greens, unpolished rice, wheat germ, barley, herbal teas. If alkaline foods are consumed in proper quantities, the Nervi-Motive type is likely to maintain good health and to have a long life, because he is inherently strong.

Additional Requirements

Cold baths or showers are helpful in winter or summer; deep massage is also suggested. A low altitude and humid, warm climate is best; ozone is not needed in large quantities. Exercise should consist of relaxation exercises, riding, isometrics, driving; love sentiments should be developed; restful sleep is a requisite.

Common Ailments

Diseases likely to develop in the Nervi-Motive type include anacusia, angina pectoris, bleeding hemorrhoids, cerebral membrane disorders, coryza, neuralgia, cyanosis, enteralgia, exostosis, falling hair, fungi, ganglioma, hay fever, insomnia, migraine, neuratrophia, neuritis, obsession. ovarian and uterine complications, psoitis, rectitis, sciatica, swellings, toothache, uremia, phobias. Other disorders may be nervous, cerebral, hysterical, mental, alcoholic, digestive, pancreatic, venous, anemic, gastric, blood-related, urinary or inflammatory.

Inherent weaknesses are attributed to the small backhead, hot temper, malnourished nerves, talkativeness, overwork. Because stamina and will are strong in this type, health may be maintained or regained with plenty of rest and sleep, relaxation, recreation, laxative foods, brain and nerve foods, solitude, magnesium foods.

Special Notes

The basis of the Nervi-Motive constitution is the intensification of bones, nerves, brain and emotions due to highly active sulphur and phosphorus. This is the longest-lived of the twenty types.

Dr. Edward Feldman, a New York nutritionist, reports that fresh fruit and vegetable juices are excellent for detoxifying the body.

Cirrhosis, hardening and enlargement of the liver, is the most common liver disease and is usually caused by excessive use of alcohol over an extended period of time. In its early stages, it can be reversed by quitting alcohol consumption and using a diet with plenty of protein foods, vegetables and supplemental B vitamins.

THE ATROPHIC TYPE

Definition

"A" means not; "trophic" means nourished. The Atrophic type is not properly nourished.

Classification

Mental temperament. Mental-Osseous or Osseous-Mental type. Pathogenic constitution or individuals hereditarily inclined to disease and disharmony.

Leading Elements

Phosphorus and calcium.

General Characteristics

The medulla (chest brain) is inherently weak in the Atrophic type, curtailing efficiency of respiration, digestion, oxidation, assimilation. Malnutrition and lack of oxygen are likely, due to weak lung function. Toxins and impurities are not properly removed from the system. The four vital processes—oxidation, digestion, circulation, nutrition—are all below par in this type.

An Atrophic individual may wander in a daze for weeks; others consequently think him peculiar. His body odors are often fetid; water and bathing are distasteful to him because dampness intensifies his ailments; complaints of constant coldness are common. The Atrophic system tends toward acidity, partially because an unbalanced diet of meat, potatoes, gravy, fatty foods, pastries and desserts is favored. An Atrophic person is identified by his husky, empty or hollow voice. Seventy-five percent of Atrophics are female, twenty-five percent male.

Head and Facial Features

The face is long and narrow, with a large forehead. The face may often appear fatigued; eyes appear dull and lusterless. Features may be severe, irregular or angular, bony. Hair color ranges from light brown to black; hair is often oily, heavy, matted, odorous. The face has a fine network of wrinkles.

Physical Exterior

Height: Six feet or taller.
Weight: Underweight in proportion to height.

The body of the Atrophic is tall, slim, lanky; chest and abdomen appear sunken; limbs are long and slender. Other exterior characteristics include large, unpadded ankle bones; incurved back; generally long, slim bones; narrow chest capacity (weak lung function); cold, damp, tender, elongated, rough feet; long fingers with sizable knuckles; narrow, untapered hands; narrow hips; large, bony knees; long, skinny neck; slender, angular build; pale or clay-like skin, taking on color from excess carbonic acid in body; flush on cheeks just below eye bones; damp or clammy skin; well-developed thighs; slim, flat torso, especially above waist (little space for vital organs); waist set high on trunk; small, frail wrists.

Physical Interior

Internal features include poor digestion; sluggish bowel; deficient blood, deep red and lacking in healing power; flexible, long, slender, fragile bones; subnormal circulation; glands susceptible to illness; weak heart due to weak medulla; active, but not powerful, small intestine; average kidney strength; well-developed lacteals; heavy, sensitive joints; weak ligaments; feeble tendons; weak liver; average lymphatic efficiency; inflexible, flabby muscles; weak pancreas; lack of secretions; weak spleen; weakness in throat. Nervous system is active but erratic; there may be stabbing, smarting pains through the nerves; nerves are restless as morning approaches; optic nerves are generally feeble. Internal organs are usually weak in this type.

Five Senses

This type has unusual sense traits. Vision is usually far rather than nearsighted; sense of touch is very acute; poor hearing may result in partial deafness; snese of smell is faulty. Sense of taste is variable; fickle and finicky appetite causes individual to avoid eating many good foods such as salads and vegetables.

471

Metabolic Function

Breathing is difficult, defective, short, rapid; eliminative organs are sluggish, except for active perspiration; body metabolism is generally sluggish. Malnutrition of bones, blood, tissues and sexual system is likely; oxidation is low; pulse rate is weak, irregular, jerky. Calcium and phosphorus may become deficient because they are used in such large quantities. The sexual system is the strongest facet of the Atrophic type.

Mental Characteristics

The Atrophic individual has an intelligent, serious expression. He is an avid student; creative; serene and calm; very private; quick to offer advice; decisive; in constant quest of further knowledge; disciplined and self sacrificing; self confident; learned; wise beyond his years. He favors education and study over social functions. His abilities are well developed.

The mind is prolific though the body is relatively inactive; lack of physical vitality may keep this type from true creative genius. Atrophics are lovers of books, philosophy, literature, science, mathematics, mechanics and technology; in comparison, recreation, animals, plants and people are not enjoyed; study and seclusion are preferred to social and cultural activities. Habits and behavior tend to be fixed and predictable; if a change is undertaken, the new direction is followed diligently. In youth, vital energy may be squandered; the price must be paid in later years. There is physical strength but lack of vital energy.

This type has great faith in miracle cures, the future, laws of nature, God, ethics, outcomes. There is little faith in humanity, medicine, religion, government. The mind is highly active. Reasoning ability, common sense and abstract understanding are strong. Will is also strong and resolutions unshakable. The individual is slow to anger but unforgiving if maltreated; he may be critical, easily offended, stubborn.

Brain Faculties

Strong Faculties. Combativeness, firmness, inhabitiveness, language, form, size, weight, individuality, order, color, comparison, calculation, constructiveness, causality, benevolence, conscientiousness; may also be strong in ideality, caution, sublimity, approbativeness.

Weak Faculties. Alimentiveness, bibativeness, medulla, eventuality, imitation, time, destructiveness, friendship, conjugality, secretiveness, acquisitiveness.

Brain Itself. The brain is active and strongly influenced by phosphorus and calcium. Medulla is small, as is muscular center of cerebellum. Reasoning power is good; interest in metaphysical, logical, philosophical matters is strong.

Talent and Career

Suited for creative arts, scientific research, invention, photography, journalism, mass communications, advertising, public relations, secretarial jobs, landscaping, postal service. Indoor jobs must be balanced by outdoor activities, in order for health to be maintained.

Biochemistry and Diet

The Atrophic type is most often deficient in calcium, carbon, chlorine, fluorine, iron, magnesium, manganese, oxygen, phosphorus, potassium, silicon, sodium. Calcium is the only element likely to be excessive in the body. Malnutrition throughout life is a real possibility. Phosphorus and calcium, the leading elements, are precipitated and utilized too rapidly. Suitable foods are cod liver oil, sarsaparilla and other herbal teas, garlic, game, fowl, lamb, fish, veal liver and liver supplements, whole grains, raw goat milk and cheese, fresh vegetables, nut and seed butters, fruit juices, all fresh fruits in season, honey.

Additional Requirements

Refrigerated air and dampness must be avoided. Moderate outdoor activity and exercise are essential. A breezy, arid, fresh-aired climate with rich ozone is recommended. A diet high in essential vitamins is necessary. Health of this type may always be subnormal; nevertheless, success in work is feasible because of quaillties of diligence, studiousness, self confidence.

Common Ailments

Maladies likely to develop in the Atrophic type include bone tumors, dental caries, conjunctivitis, spinal curvature, bone decay, yellow and green discharges, dislocations, earaches, lymphatic enlargement, gastric inflammation, lung hemorrhage, malnutrition, night sweats, Pott's disease, pus generation, pustular eruption, rheumatism in bones, rickets, tuberculosis. Inherent weaknesses are attributed to malnutrition; poor oxidation; deficiency of fluorine, chlorine, calcium, phosphates; weakly-developed circulatory system; overstudy; pus formation. Diseases are principally attributed to malnutrition, deficiency of oils in the system, shortage of calcium, lack of other tissue salts, shortage of oxygen. The Atrophic type is inclined to develop tuberculosis.

Special Notes

Creative ability and intellect are particularly strong in this type.

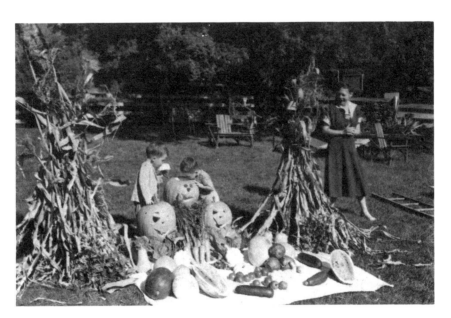

A Halloween celebration at the Ranch.

I personally believe that temperaments, foods, types, culture, climate, altitude, environment, inheritance, living habits and sunshine all go together to make the man.

—Dr. Bernard Jensen

twenty-five

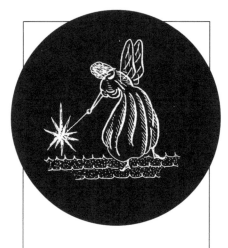

Fundamental laws of health

I believe the greatest means of preventing disease is good health. We must take our minds off disease. We can look at it and not be afraid of it, but we need not dwell on it. The fear of death may be strong, but the instinct to life is still stronger. For our health's sake, we are going to live the ideals that we can, wherever we go in life. We have been given life to enjoy, to master, to direct. If we can wink an eye or lift a finger, we can make a change for the better. The change we make depends entirely on our knowledge and how close to God and Nature we stand. We must return to God and Nature; this is a return to our true self. I am speaking of ideals here; some we may never attain, but we must reach for the stars, otherwise, what will we get? For health to come in, we must reach for it.

Disease is a lack of ideals. Old age is a lack of ideals. Sickness is a lack of ideals; so let's talk ideals. I don't like to say, "I'm only human"; we all give this excuse when we're not really happy with our lives. Each day I wake up with the idea that I'm going to make this a better day. I'm going to live the spirit more, serve more, be better in the sight of God. Whatever I do, I want to have the approval of God. I believe we will all be taken care of when we live this way.

Lift Others

If you really want to stay in balance, go out and lift others. The more you lift other people, the more you will do for yourself. We live on what we pour out. The only thing we have is what we give.

Good thinking is the beginning of good health. Good thinking leads to a body that is in chemical balance. When I speak of health from a physical standpoint, the dust of the earth standpoint, I recognize this as only one part of the balance that brings health. There must be beauty, loveliness and godliness throughout our life. This is why we must reach for the spiritual in our life if we would have the physical. We are grounded but we belong to heaven, too.

We must return to God and Nature; this is a return to our true self.

Good thinking is the beginning of good health; it leads to a body that is in chemical balance.

Thinking can exhaust the chemical reserves we have stored in our organs.

It is a lovely healing thought to know that God considers our bodies "good."

Nature does the curing; all she needs is an opportunity.

Yes, We Are A Sculpture

We are a sculpture and a sculptor. We have come to earth to refine. How we are made, how we are put together, how we look when we are feeling well and what we do to change that—all this is done with Mother Earth. What we do with our minds is done with the divine principle within us.

The Chemistry of Man, we realize, may be based on the dust of the earth, but before the physical was the spiritual. We have a spiritual "chemistry" as well as a physical chemistry.

Here is a summary of the fundamental laws of health, axioms and principles for proper nutrition and good health.

1. The chemical elements that build our body must be in biochemical, life-producing form. They must come to us as food, magnetically, electrically alive, grown from the dust of the earth.

2. Healthy plant life requires all the chemical elements in the proper, balanced order.

3. The animal that lives on plant life molds to the food it eats.

4. Man has the ability to transmute, develop, transcend. This is the cycle of life we go through. The grasshopper eats the plant; the chicken eats the grasshopper; the preacher eats the chicken. Whether we eat meat or not, our food must still come from growing material.

5. Each of the chemical elements has a story to tell. Each has attributes and functions, and serves man in a specific way that can be studied and used to our advantage.

6. Our body is a storehouse for the chemical elements. Each organ tends to use one specific chemical element more than others, according to the law of balance and proportion.

7. With a knowledge of the workings of the chemical elements within the body, we can look at a person and tell immediately when he lacks certain chemical elements. When we burn out the specific chemical reserves held in our organs, we produce symptoms which indicate these deficiencies.

8. Whenever we are sick, we are short of at least one chemical element. We must pay back what we "owe" the body. When we take in these chemical elements, health returns.

9. Every symptom is a sign of a chemical shortage in the body. When you feel sick or even look sick, you are lacking in one or more chemical elements.

10. When regaining health, you don't take "two tablespoons" of some remedy and get immediately well; however, you're on the way to getting well the minute you begin filling the body with the missing chemical elements.

11. Because "two tablespoons" are good for you, that doesn't mean "four tablespoons" are even better. Nature builds one drop at a time. You take two tablespoons every day for six months; that's how you get well.

12. As long as you are moving and active, the body will take up the chemical elements from food provided, just as parsley will take iron and calcium from the soil to make its leaf structure.

13. We are like a plant. We can get well, but we must have the right nutrients and other conditions to grow and thrive. We have to take care of our environment, and take care of ourselves "within"—inspirationally—so we have the incentive to really live.

14. When we are lacking any element at all, we are lacking more than one element. There is no one who has ever lacked just one element. We don't have a food that contains only one element, such as a carrot entirely of calcium or sprouts totally made of silicon.

15. Foods build specific systems within us because they contain chemical elements high in the minerals supporting that system; i.e., when the mental energies are depleted, we go to foods that support our nervous system and brain.

16. When we have depleted our body or work at a job requiring a great deal of nerve energy, we have to back up this depletion with foods that will rebuild accordingly.

17. Vegetarian foods have a vibratory rate that must be balanced with an appropriate peaceful and low-key lifestyle. If you want to become a good vegetarian, your mental and spiritual attitude must match the diet.

18. The same foods that feed the glandular system, feed the nervous system. A good deal of the natural healing art is based on treating a system rather than a symptom. Falling hair, disappearing eyebrows, skin trouble, the jitters—all come from the nervous system and they go away when we feed the system properly.

19. "Disease preys on an undernourished plant." We can't kill all the germs we encounter in life, but we can pay attention to our nutrition.

As soon as we change our "soil," germ life responds to us differently. If you want to be free of germ life, you must be clean inside.

20. None of the diseases will come upon you if you live the laws that have been given you to live by. The spiritual laws of the universe are just as inviolable as physical and natural laws.

21. Different types of people need certain chemical elements to fit their type of life. Since we are different types, we should each know the chemicals in which we are likely to become deficient in our particular job and lifestyle. Our food pattern should be in harmony with this knowledge.

Lifestyle and Nutrition

We can burn out the vitamins, oils, proteins and chemical elements in our body through our character, job and emotions faster than we can build them up. This is the mental side of the chemical story. We must learn to live a balanced life that does not burn the building materials out of our body faster than we can replace them. Sometimes we have to change our environment or change ourselves in order to get into alignment with our higher potentials.

Our thinking can exhaust the chemical reserves we have stored in our organs. We become depleted and we must change our way before we can change the way the chemicals are drawn out of the body.

The wife of a well-known lotion manufacturer spent time in the hospital every time her husband went off without telling her where he was going. She would break out in a terrible rash because of her emotional upset. She finally got a divorce. That was the only way she could find to solve the rash problem.

Our Temple Needs Care

If we just left our body to the forces of nature without any care, it would be like leaving a house unattended. It deteriorates and breaks down. If we don't paint, re-roof, repair and rebuild this house we live in, it becomes a shack. When it becomes a shack, we're not living the beautiful ideal we're meant to live. When we do

not care for this body, it's really not the temple of the living God.

One day my little five-year-old girl came running into the room. "Who's beautiful in here?" I asked. Her face lit up and she exclaimed, "Me!" That's the way we should all feel. We have to get this beautiful idea going for us. When we feel beautiful, it's really not something we have to talk about. People will know.

Poor Mental Thinking

There are people who really go through life not knowing that through their own negative mental thinking they are destroying themselves and adversely influencing others around them. We don't benefit from others who make a habit of talking about states of sickness or other negative ideas, and it's difficult to be around negative people. That's why we have to master our own feelings. For some of us, exterior influences from others can be more than our nervous system can handle.

Many people say they are only "human." They give an excuse and then stand behind it. It's not enough for us to stand behind, "I'm only human." Instead, we must stand behind the divine principle. The divine principle made us perfectly; when God made this body, he said, it was good. It is a lovely healing thought to know that God considers our bodies "good."

Built in God's Image

Did you ever stop and think how much more your body can do than what it actually does? The Good Book says that man is built in the image of God and that there are no impossibilities on this earth. Some of us are limited in what we are doing, because we limit ourselves. We have to get to the place where we realize how much more we are capable of. We have an opportunity to improve our health. That's easy. Nature does the curing; all she needs is an opportunity. God made our bodies to be self-healing.

"The real voyage of discovery consists not in seeking new lands but in seeing with new eyes." —Marcel Proust

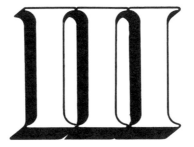

A vital course on foods

Although I traveled and studied with V. G. Rocine over a period of years, I cannot distinctly recall the occasion of our first meeting. What I do recall is what a striking man he was, what authority he exercised over his material. I was awed by the depth and extent of what Rocine knew about food—and the implications of food chemistry in terms of its effects on the body and temperament.

V. G. Rocine knew several languages, including classical Greek, and he had studied the writings of everyone who had written with originality and insight about nitrition, psychology and spiritual wisdom. He was convinced that there was much more to nutrition and body chemistry than simply physiological effects and processes, so as a young man, he launched into his own investigations concerning how these fields were interrelated.

Genius does not consist in rearranging the furniture of other men's ideas, but in drawing upon the best they offer and striking out in bold new directions. A great part of Rocine's genius and originality came from seeking answers from a source he often recommended to others—the Great Within. Applying the homeopathic principles to foods was

important, but not necessarily original. What was original in Rocine's work was the discovery that body chemistry and human psychology are related, that the spiritual and mental aspects of life depend, in the type and degree of their expression, on the cleanliness, character and chemical balance of the body. He also found that the spiritual and mental life affected body chemistry, so that a reflex relationship exists both ways.

If all body functions are controlled by brain centers, as Rocine believed, then any malfunction in the body is accompanied, preceded or followed by malfunction in the corresponding brain center— either repression or overstimulation. Since all brain centers are interrelated, this means all of them will be affected, and every cell of the body, every thought and emotion of the mind, every aspect of personality will be altered to some degree. Rocine also believed that this was a two-way street.

Not only could the body affect the mind, but the mind could affect the body as well.

In other words, Rocine had developed the concepts of wholistic health and psychosomatic disease before these terms found their way into the literature and popular thinking of our time.

To a great extent, Rocine believed that sensory, intellectual and spiritual experiences are as necessary to feed the mind, soul and spirit as food is necessary for the health of the body. Poor food habits that result in nutrient deficiencies in the brain could lead to mental dis-ease and mild to bizarre misbehavior. So could long-term exposure to an environment stripped of beauty, meaning and hope. Rocine understood that poor nutrition was often at the root of undeveloped or underdeveloped gifts and talents, the source of which was to be found in brain centers. In other words, he believed that the right foods, the right experiences and the right teachings were necessary to awaken the brain centers and to allow each human being to develop his or her full potential on this planet.

The fact that human development is so often blocked gives rise, in Rocine's view, to deviant forms of human behavior such as criminality, cruelty, sexual deviation, alcoholism, drug addition and other similar behaviors. The solution to these problems, he believed, was at hand in the form of scientific nutrition, a correct understanding of the various temperament types, climatology, spiritual wisdom and other subject areas. There was only one problem. Of all the thousands of students he had taught, Rocine once wrote to me, most were only "nibblers." The student must want to learn these days or very little of any consequence can happen.

It has seemed to me that V. G. Rocine was one of those rare geniuses who was so far ahead of his time that few of his contemporaries really understood his teachings. These days people seem to be more receptive to new concepts about health and life. Perhaps the people of our time would have understood and accepted V. G. Rocine and his work.

We find that some of Rocine's work is "dated," and although I have edited some of this out, I have also left much of it in so the reader could see how Rocine thought about things. Keep in mind that Rocine, like everyone else on this planet, is human and capable of error. Nevertheless, the main thrust of his work is still so practical and far-reaching that those who have eyes to see will reap much benefit from it.

The reader will notice that chapters on the elements carbon, hydrogen and oxygen are not included in Rocine's Course on Foods. That is not, we assume, accidental. These three elements are in all food groups—protein, carbohydrates and fats—as Rocine knew. So, he did not discuss them.

I am grateful to Dr. Rocine not only on account of my own work, but on behalf of thousands of patients who have reaped the benefits of the seeds this great man planted in my life.

This Course on Foods was developed from Dr. Jensen's notes taken in Dr. V. G. Rocine's classes.

Bernard Jensen, DC

ACID AND ALKALINE BASIC FOODS

The word "basic" is derived from the Greek "basis," meaning foundation. In a chemical sense, the word relates to the properties of acidity and alkalinity. Thus when a metal ion is with a hydroxyl ion, we have a base, and when a hydrogen ion is with a negative ion such as chloride or sulphate and so forth, we have an acid. The term "alkali" means the same as soda ash, and alkali metals such as sodium and potassium make strong bases. When these bases engage with acids, there is a sort of chemical "warfare" between them, and we find a chemical salt left on the battlefield when the struggle is over. A base will turn red litmus paper blue, while an acid will turn blue litmus paper red. Acids and bases are chemical opposites, so to speak. Alkaline chemicals are important for saponification, whether in the stomach or in a soap factory. Yet, we must realilze that the human body is not the same as the chemist's laboratory; the former is more complex, with acids, bases, enzymes, heat, fermentation and so forth, with the emotions capable of shifting the chemical environment at any time. Foods that are basic in the laboratory may not be in the stomach, nor will they respond the same in the digestive tracts of different people. That which neutralizes acidity in one stomach may not do so in another.

The most alkaline food element is sodium. Next comes magnesium. Food potassium is alkaline to the muscles and urinary system. Calcium is alkaline to the bones, magnesium to the nerves. Manganese is alkaline to the brain, and iron to the blood. Sodium is alkaline to the alimentary tract. The alkaline principle in foods can cure most diseases without doctors or pills.

CHEMISTRY OF FOOD CHART

This food map, from European research, may vary from U.S. food analyses because of soil differences. The food can be no different from the soil in which it is grown.

Name of Food	Water	Protein	Fat	Carbohydrates	Ash	Potassium	Sodium	Calcium	Magnesium	Iron	Phosphorus	Sulphur	Silicon	Chlorine	Manganese	Fluorine	Iodine	Acid Forming or Basic	Contains	Kind of Acid
Acorns	4.0	8.2	37.2	47.8	2.8	16.4	0.2	1.8	1.4	0.4	4.7	1.2	0.06	0.5	0.06	-	-	Hyperacid	Tannin	Tannic acid
Almond nuts	4.9	21.3	53.9	16.7	3.1	21.2	0.9	3.6	4.0	0.3	11.3	1.0	0.90	0.1	0.03	-	-	Hypobasic	Amygdalin	Fatty acids
Apples, dried	28.1	1.0	2.6	67.3	1.0	33.9	35.9	4.2	1.0	1.4	13.6	3.7	4.20	-	-	-	-	Hypobasic	-	Oxalic, malic, etc.
Apples, fresh	84.6	0.4	0.5	14.2	0.3	36.9	24.9	4.1	8.4	1.1	13.6	6.1	4.20	0.6	-	-	-	Hypobasic	-	Malic, oxalic, etc.
Apricots	85.1	1.1	-	13.2	0.6	19.8	4.0	1.2	1.6	0.2	4.8	1.0	2.00	-	-	-	-	Hypobasic	-	Malic, several
Artichokes	79.6	2.5	0.3	16.4	1.2	26.4	6.4	1.3	1.8	2.3	8.1	2.0	6.10	2.3	-	-	0.01	Basic	Scolymin	Solvent acid
Asparagus	94.0	1.6	0.3	3.0	1.0	21.1	15.3	9.4	3.8	3.0	17.1	5.4	10.00	5.3	-	-	0.20	Hyperbasic	Asparagin	Antacid
Avocado	70.3	2.3	20.0	6.2	1.1	12.3	9.0	2.3	2.4	0.6	8.7	5.0	0.90	6.9	-	Trace	Trace	Basic	-	Fatty acids
Bacon	31.8	15.0	45.2	-	7.9	4.0	35.6	0.2	1.0	0.3	7.1	2.1	-	15.6	-	-	-	Hypoacid	-	Fatty, etc.
Banana	75.2	1.3	0.8	21.6	1.1	18.0	6.3	0.8	2.6	0.05	3.1	1.4	0.90	2.8	-	-	-	Hypobasic	Volatile oil	Starch acid
Barberries	84.1	1.6	0.9	12.9	0.4	20.1	1.4	6.8	9.3	0.9	8.1	1.3	0.06	1.6	-	-	-	Hypobasic	Berberin	Antacid; antitoxic
Barley	12.0	10.0	2.6	72.8	2.6	24.1	6.4	2.4	8.2	0.3	35.5	0.9	21.60	0.4	-	Trace	Trace	Hyperacid	Avenin	Starch, etc.
Barley, pearl	11.6	8.3	1.2	77.9	1.0	12.6	0.4	0.2	3.9	0.1	16.0	1.0	-	0.3	-	-	-	Hyperacid	-	Amylic
Bass	76.7	20.0	1.9	-	1.3	20.2	6.3	3.6	3.4	0.04	24.4	3.9	-	28.1	-	0.2	0.05	Acid	-	Flesh acids
Beans, garbanzo	7.3	26.0	1.6	60.8	4.3	19.6	1.0	1.6	17.7	0.09	31.8	1.4	0.10	0.9	-	-	-	Hyperacid	-	Fatty
Beans, kidney	80.6	9.0	0.3	9.2	0.9	24.7	1.8	3.0	1.8	0.03	6.4	6.4	-	1.8	-	-	0.30	Hyperacid	Asparagin	Amylic, oxalic
Beans, kidney, dry	14.0	23.6	3.3	54.7	4.4	21.0	0.8	3.0	4.1	0.05	17.6	2.9	0.40	0.4	Trace	Trace	0.10	Hyperacid	Asparagin	Oxalic, starch
Beans, lima, fresh	68.5	7.0	0.7	21.9	1.9	34.1	6.2	2.6	4.4	0.1	7.2	3.3	0.05	0.4	-	-	0.01	Hyperacid	Toxin	Amylic
Beans, lima, dry	11.6	20.9	1.1	61.6	4.8	29.8	5.9	2.6	4.5	0.9	6.9	3.1	0.03	0.4	-	-	0.01	Hypobasic	Toxin	Starch
Beans, string	88.7	2.1	0.3	7.6	1.2	36.4	4.5	5.6	6.2	0.06	6.6	11.5	0.05	2.2	-	-	-	Hypobasic	Toxin	Tannic, etc.
Beef	71.6	20.2	6.6	-	1.6	16.3	3.3	0.09	1.4	0.1	8.4	3.2	Trace	2.7	-	-	-	Basic	-	Flesh
Beechnuts	4.1	22.1	58.4	11.3	4.1	7.6	3.2	7.3	6.0	0.4	13.6	1.3	1.5	1.0	-	-	-	Hyperacid	Toxin	Fatty
Beef, dry	51.0	31.1	7.4	0.3	10.1	16.4	31.4	0.08	1.4	0.1	8.5	3.3	0.01	16.1	-	-	-	Hypobasic	Flesh toxins	Flesh acids
Beer	87.9	Alcohol 3%		0.3	0.3	33.6	8.9	2.7	6.2	0.5	31.3	3.4	9.30	2.9	-	-	-	Hyperbasic	Alcohol	Many
Beets	83.1	2.1	2.0	11.8	0.9							Not reported				-	-	Hyperbasic	Betaine	Citric, Tartaric
Beets, sugar	87.0	0.6	-	11.3	1.0	46.1	9.8	4.2	3.0	0.2	8.3	0.4	2.30	3.0	reported	-	-	Hyperbasic	Betaine	Citric, Tartaric
Beets, red	87.5	1.6	0.1	9.7	1.1	44.0	10.3	6.2	3.1	0.3	9.4	-	-	-	-	-	-	Hyperbasic	Betaine	Solvent
Beets, white	86.1	2.0	0.8	8.9	1.6	54.0	15.9	4.1	4.5	0.8	8.4	3.1	2.40	6.4	-	-	-	Hyperbasic	Betaine	Solvent
Bilberries	84.2	1.6	0.1	13.1	0.9	20.0	1.2	6.1	5.0	1.0	7.4	1.0	0.50	1.4	-	-	-	Basic	-	Quinic, malic
Biscuit, shredded	9.5	12.3	1.9	74.1	1.5	31.2	3.1	2.6	11.3	1.3	26.2	0.4	1.80	0.3	-	-	-	Hypoacid	Toxin	Starch
Blackberries	87.7	0.9	0.5	9.7	1.0	20.0	0.9	7.6	4.7	0.9	7.2	0.9	0.03	1.7	-	-	-	Hyperbasic	Berberin	Tannic, tartaric
Blackberries, wild	84.8	1.1	1.0	11.9	1.2	21.0	1.1	8.0	5.0	1.2	7.6	1.0	0.45	1.7	-	-	-	Hyperbasic	Berberin	Tannic, malic
Blackfish	78.9	18.0	1.6	-	1.4	19.4	9.6	3.4	2.6	0.4	24.5	3.7	0.02	7.3	-	-	-	Acid	-	Flesh
Blood	68.7	30.2	-	-	1.0	13.8	5.9	0.5	0.3	5.0	3.5	0.3	Trace	5.7	-	-	-	Hyperbasic	-	Mild
Blueberries	87.8	0.8	1.5	8.9	1.0	58.2	5.1	8.0	6.1	1.1	17.4	3.1	0.90	-	-	-	-	Hyperbasic	-	Citric, malic

Chemistry of Food Chart (Cont'd.)

Name of Food	Water	Protein	Fat	Carbohydrates	Ash	Potassium	Sodium	Calcium	Magnesium	Iron	Phosphorus	Sulphur	Silicon	Chlorine	Manganese	Fluorine	Iodine	Acid Forming or Basic	Contains	Kind of Acid
Blueberry juice	87.4	0.3	1.4	10.1	0.7	32.1	5.1	3.9	4.4	0.3	12.0	2.0	0.09	-	-	-	-	Basic	-	Malic, tartaric
Bluefish	78.6	18.4	1.6	-	1.4	12.0	4.3	1.0	3.0	0.09	39.4	1.4	-	0.1	-	Not reported	-	Hyperacid	Toxin	Flesh
Bone	-	-	-	-	-	-	-	24.0	8.0	10.0	34.5	0.4	0.07	12.0	Not reported	-	-	Acid	-	Phosphorus
Brain	80.6	8.5	9.3	-	-	19.5	-	0.4	0.7	0.1	27.3	1.2	1.5	4.3	-	-	-	Hyperacid	-	Phosphorus, fatty
Brazil nut	5.3	17.0	66.8	7.0	1.1	8.0	6.8	8.0	6.0	0.3	13.3	0.8	-	1.6	-	-	Trace	Acid	Toxin	Fatty
Pumpernickel	42.2	12.2	0.7	43.3	3.9	32.3	2.3	1.6	8.4	0.4	24.5	0.3	0.2	6.8	0.03	-	-	Basic	-	Amylic
Rye bread	49.8	11.2	1.3	36.4	1.3	25.0	6.4	0.3	2.0	0.08	18.7	2.9	-	12.9	-	-	-	Hypobasic	Mild toxin	Amylic
Ry-Krisp	8.1	18.0	3.6	70.1	1.2	5.6	11.0	1.0	1.2	0.4	5.8	Trace	-	1.9	-	-	-	Hypobasic	Mild toxin	Starch
Bread, white	34.4	8.7	1.3	54.2	1.9	11.7	2.7	1.4	1.4	0.2	2.0	0.6	0.4	Table	-	-	-	Hyperacid	Mild toxin	Starch
Bread, whole wheat	32.4	8.1	0.4	57.9	1.2	7.1	9.4	0.6	1.9	0.9	11.0	-	3.2	2.1	-	-	-	Acid	Toxin	Starch
Broccoli	90.9	2.4	0.2	5.5	1.0	41.4	1.5	6.1	3.9	0.3	19.1	12.1	0.5	3.1	-	-	0.7	Basic	-	Brassidic
Buckwheat	14.5	12.1	3.1	67.3	0.8	27.2	6.0	1.3	3.4	0.03	19.1	1.2	-	2.6	-	-	Trace	Hyperacid	Grain toxin	Several starch
Butter, cow	11.0	1.1	84.4	-	2.8	11.1	1.8	0.8	0.1	0.1	0.09	5.8	-	14.0	-	-	Contains dope	Hypobasic	-	9: Capric, butyric, etc.
Buttermilk, cow	91.6	3.4	0.1	3.4	3.4	14.0	12.6	13.0	2.4	0.08	19.0	2.1	0.06	5.0	salt	-	-	Basic	-	Lactic, etc.
Buttermilk, goat	-	3.6	0.2	3.5	1.0	14.6	10.1	13.2	2.6	0.4	20.2	2.4	Trace	4.2	-	-	-	Hyperacid	-	Milk acid
Butternuts	4.4	27.9	61.3	3.5	1.2	16.3	11.2	1.4	2.1	0.2	17.3	0.01	0.6	-	-	0.08	-	Hyperbasic	Sovariol	Fatty
Cabbage	92.7	1.3	1.1	3.8	2.9	35.9	0.6	18.0	5.2	1.4	12.0	10.3	5.6	6.0	0.01	-	-	Hyperbasic	Brassin	Brassidic
Cabbage, red	90.4	2.1	0.2	6.3	1.1	44.5	11.9	16.2	2.9	0.2	4.2	10.1	4.5	9.8	-	-	Some	Basic	Brassin	Brassidic, etc.
Cabbage, savoy	88.2	3.4	0.8	6.1	0.8	24.8	10.0	16.5	8.6	0.9	19.0	6.0	5.9	6.0	-	-	0.2	Hyperbasic	Brassin	Brassidic, etc.
Caraway	20.9	28.6	26.3	16.1	1.4	18.6	10.9	11.9	6.4	1.1	15.9	4.0	-	3.4	-	-	0.2	Basic	Caruin	Phosphorus
Cardamom	9.7	19.6	25.9	36.2	8.1	35.2	5.1	10.9	6.4	2.3	21.8	3.7	5.9	2.2	0.2	-	0.02	Acid	Ether	Tannic, etc.
Cardoons	80.0	3.1	0.2	15.5	8.6	26.0	5.3	2.1	2.6	2.9	8.6	2.7	2.0	2.3	-	-	-	Basic	-	Solvent
Carrots	89.0	1.2	0.5	8.2	1.2	53.7	13.4	7.3	2.8	2.8	9.8	High	1.0	-	-	-	-	Hyperbasic	Scolymin	Antacid, malic
Carrots, white	87.1	1.5	0.9	9.4	1.1	30.9	1.4	7.8	3.1	2.0	8.5	1.9	3.9	Not reported	Not reported	-	0.6	Hyperbasic	Carrotin	Malic, formic
Casaba	91.0	0.7	-	7.6	1.2	19.0	14.2	2.3	1.6	0.8	4.3	12.0	3.2	3.2	-	-	0.1	Basic	Carrotin	Starch
Cauliflower	93.1	2.1	0.8	3.1	0.6	46.7	4.7	5.8	3.7	0.7	17.4	4.2	0.03	0.8	-	-	-	Hyperbasic	-	Brassidic
Celery	94.8	1.3	0.2	2.5	0.9	29.0	5.7	10.1	4.8	1.0	14.6	1.2	0.3	4.4	-	-	-	Basic	Brassin	Tannic, antacid
Chayote	95.7	0.6	0.1	3.3	0.3	32.2	26.0	7.2	5.4	1.1	14.1	0.3	-	6.2	-	-	-	Hyperbasic	Apiol	Several
Cheese, cow, cot.	67.8	23.4	1.8	4.9	2.2	16.1	12.6	16.0	1.5	1.8	14.9	0.6	-	7.0	-	-	-	Neutral	-	Lactic
Cheese, goat, cot.	62.7	23.4	1.8	6.0	6.1	14.2	4.2	15.1	1.6	1.4	16.0	0.1	0.3	9.1	-	-	-	Basic	-	Hircic, milk
Cheese, cow, brown	17.6	21.0	22.0	5.0	34.0	4.9	4.3	4.1	3.8	0.2	6.4	1.5	-	45.0	-	0.06	-	Basic	-	Mild
Cheese, goat, brown	19.1	18.4	12.1	6.1	44.3	5.4	36.5	3.0	5.2	0.4	4.1	0.4	-	41.7	-	-	-	Hyperbasic	-	Mild
Cheese, Roquefort	37.4	23.0	28.3	2.1	9.1	16.1	34.2	15.0	1.5	0.9	16.0	5.8	3.0	9.1	-	0.05	-	Neutral	-	Hircic, milk
Cheese, Swiss	32.9	28.8	29.6	1.8	6.8	18.8	18.6	26.9	0.2	6.0	20.4	1.8	3.2	7.2	-	-	-	Hypobasic	-	Lactic, antacid
Cherries, wild	80.1	0.1	1.8	17.0	1.0	57.7	6.8	4.2	5.5	0.09	15.1	1.6	4.2	0.5	-	-	-	Hyperbasic	-	Malic, oxalic
Cherry juice, wild	86.8	2.1	0.9	9.0	1.2	77.5	1.0	4.7	1.8	-	4.5	14.1	0.4	3.4	-	-	-	Basic	-	Fruit
Cherries, light	78.9	1.6	0.9	16.7	1.9	18.8	0.8	2.6	1.4	3.3	5.0	3.0	-	6.9	-	-	-	Hyperbasic	-	Sugar
Chervil	86.7	4.9	0.4	6.1	2.0	41.9	0.2	3.8	2.4	0.6	21.6	0.1	2.4	0.1	-	0.02	-	Hyperacid	Anthriscin	Several
Chestnuts	5.9	10.7	7.0	74.2	0.3	31.4	0.3	1.0	1.9	0.8	5.5	4.0	-	2.1	-	-	0.04	Hyperacid	Nut toxin	Amylic, tonic
Chicken	75.6	20.8	2.5	-	1.1	14.6	3.3	0.2	1.6	0.2	8.6	2.7	-	2.7	-	-	-	Hypoacid	-	Lactic, meat
Chicory	78.8	0.8	0.2	18.3	0.7	13.2	5.0	2.4	1.6	0.9	4.3	1.6	-	-	-	-	-	Hypoacid	Tannin	Oxalic, tannic
Chinese cabbage	91.4	1.7	0.5	3.9	2.6	18.8	35.4	12.2	9.0	1.9	10.0	-	2.4	7.3	-	-	0.2	Hyperbasic	Brassin	Brassidic

Chemistry of Food Chart (Cont'd.)

Name of Food	Water	Protein	Fat	Carbohydrates	Ash	Potassium	Sodium	Calcium	Magnesium	Iron	Phosphorus	Sulphur	Silicon	Chlorine	Manganese	Fluorine	Iodine	Acid Forming or Basic	Contains	Kind of Acid
Chives	82.0	5.8	0.5	10.0	1.0	28.0	2.3	11.3	2.9	0.8	8.1	6.7	-	2.3	-	-	-	Hyperbasic	Alliol	Several
Chocolate	6.9	12.9	48.6	30.9	1.3	17.1	0.6	1.1	3.1	0.04	15.2	1.0	-	0.9	-	-	0.08	Hyperacid	Theobromin	Tannic, linoleic
Cider	-	-	-	-	3.2	53.7	1.2	2.7	2.0	0.4	12.6	-	0.9	9.4	0.5	-	-	Acid	Alcohol	Acetic, malic
Collards	84.7	4.9	0.8	7.1	1.5	14.3	21.1	19.7	7.3	4.0	11.1	1.2	5.0	0.5	-	-	0.2	Hyperbasic	Brassin	Brassidic, oxalic
Cocoa	4.6	21.6	28.9	37.7	7.2	27.6	0.6	4.7	19.7	0.2	39.2	4.2	0.4	3.4	-	-	-	Hyperacid	Theobromin	5: oleic, oxalic, etc.
Coconuts	14.4	6.5	50.0	27.1	2.0	41.8	8.4	4.3	9.4	-	17.0	5.1	0.5	1.2	-	-	-	Hyperacid	Myristin	Many: Capric, oleic
Coffee	1.1	51.0	31.1	11.7	4.9	59.8	0.5	7.2	10.7	0.9	12.9	4.4	0.9	1.1	-	-	-	Hyperacid	Caffeine	Tannic, etc.
Corn flour	12.9	7.6	1.8	77.2	0.6	2.4	0.1	0.1	1.0	0.05	4.0	3.7	0.5	Not	-	-	-	Hyperacid	-	Amylic
Corn on the cob	75.4	3.1	1.1	19.2	0.7	8.5	3.2	0.5	2.6	0.07	8.3	0.9	1.3	0.09	-	-	-	Neutral	-	Amylic
Corn, yellow	14.0	12.2	3.3	67.4	2.8	33.9	7.7	3.1	18.0	0.5	30.3	-	-	1.9	-	-	-	Hyperacid	-	Amylic
Crab	75.3	17.1	2.1	1.6	3.9	16.1	12.3	Undetermined	Undetermined	Undetermined	23.0	High	-	2.2	reported	reported	1.8	Basic	Flesh toxin	Flesh acids
Cranberries	87.6	0.5	-	10.6	0.2	10.2	0.1	9.6	0.6	0.05	2.0	15.3	0.02	6.6	-	-	-	Hyperacid	-	Many
Cream, cow	73.6	2.6	18.6	4.6	0.6	5.0	1.6	3.1	0.9	0.09	3.6	0.4	0.1	0.2	-	-	-	Hyperacid	-	8: fatty
Cream, goat	73.4	2.8	19.1	4.5	0.6	7.0	2.1	3.1	0.6	0.2	5.0	0.7	-	0.4	-	0.02	-	Hyperacid	-	9: hircic, etc.
Cucumbers	96.0	1.0	0.6	1.8	0.6	41.2	10.0	7.3	4.1	1.4	15.0	6.9	7.4	0.4	-	-	-	Hyperbasic	Cucumin	Oxalic, etc.
Currants, black	77.4	1.6	-	20.0	1.0	14.0	2.0	0.9	1.3	0.03	13.6	13.0	0.03	2.0	-	-	-	Hypobasic	Ribin	Citric, oxalic, malic
Currants, red	85.1	1.6	-	12.3	1.0	12.1	0.01	1.6	1.0	0.04	12.2	18.1	-	2.7	-	-	-	Acid	-	Malic, oxalic
Currants, white	83.2	0.4	-	16.1	0.4	17.0	0.2	0.4	0.5	0.06	11.5	24.4	0.03	4.1	-	-	-	Acid	Ribin	Several
Currants, Zante	15.5	4.9	5.0	66.0	8.6	32.1	4.1	1.8	2.0	0.2	12.6	3.5	-	2.8	-	-	-	Hyperbasic	-	5: fruit
Custard apple	72.1	2.6	-	9.1	1.2	18.4	-	0.8	0.3	-	2.4	1.7	-	1.2	-	-	-	Hyperbasic	-	3: fruit, malic
Dandelion	82.0	2.6	1.1	9.3	5.0	32.0	10.1	20.0	9.8	1.2	11.0	3.0	8.0	10.9	-	-	-	Hyperbasic	Leontodin	Several vegetable
Dates, dry	15.0	2.1	3.0	78.0	1.4	10.1	1.0	1.4	1.5	0.02	1.6	1.1	0.04	2.0	-	-	-	Acid	-	Amylic
Dewberries	80.1	1.0	1.2	16.8	0.9	14.1	12.0	3.9	4.6	0.3	4.3	0.6	-	6.8	-	-	-	Basic	Berberin	5: citric, malic
Dill	84.0	4.0	0.8	8.6	2.6	21.2	3.0	19.0	6.0	1.0	18.6	14.0	2.6	8.9	-	-	-	Hyperbasic	Anethol	Several
Duck	67.8	19.6	8.8	2.1	1.7	14.5	3.3	0.3	1.6	0.04	7.4	3.6	0.01	20.8	-	-	-	Hypobasic	Flesh toxins	Lactic, meat
Eggplant	92.8	1.3	0.3	5.0	0.6	41.0	5.1	3.4	4.6	0.3	8.6	4.6	0.02	1.9	-	0.02	-	Hyperbasic	-	Mild plant
Eggs, boiled	71.7	12.5	12.1	-	3.5	17.4	22.9	10.9	1.1	0.4	34.6	0.4	1.9	7.3	-	-	-	Hyperbasic	-	Several
Egg white	82.7	12.4	0.2	-	0.6	31.3	31.6	2.8	2.8	0.5	4.4	2.1	2.0	0.3	-	-	-	Hyperbasic	-	Antacid
Egg yolk	49.6	15.9	32.0	-	2.9	9.3	5.9	13.0	2.1	1.6	63.4	Trace	0.4	0.5	-	0.01	-	Acid	-	Phosphoric, etc.
Endive	82.0	1.1	2.1	8.0	2.1	35.1	3.4	10.4	3.6	1.4	12.3	14.0	0.09	Not	-	-	-	Hyperbasic	Bitters	Tannic, etc.
Figs, black	79.1	1.5	0.7	18.8	0.6	55.8	-	2.4	5.6	-	12.4	3.9	0.02	33.1	-	-	-	Hyperbasic	-	Amylic, oxalic
Filberts, dry	3.9	15.6	64.6	12.9	3.0	7.2	0.3	3.7	2.2	0.5	8.0	4.7	0.7	0.4	-	-	-	Hyperacid	Nut toxin	Oily
Flour, white, low	13.1	12.3	1.2	71.0	2.1	36.3	-	5.7	6.4	-	49.3	0.2	0.8	0.5	reported	reported	-	Hyperacid	-	Starch
Gizzard	71.0	24.9	1.8	-	2.3	8.1	44.0	1.0	5.0	0.04	7.1	1.9	-	Not	-	-	-	Hyperbasic	Ingluvin	Antacid
Gooseberries	89.6	0.6	-	9.1	0.6	12.0	11.9	3.2	4.0	1.3	6.0	1.2	0.1	0.9	-	-	-	Hyperbasic	Ribin	Malic, citric, etc.
Grapefruit	90.9	0.6	-	8.0	0.5	13.3	-	2.3	2.6	0.4	4.1	4.3	0.9	0.1	-	-	0.01	Hypobasic	-	Citric, formic, etc.
Grapes	77.4	1.3	1.6	19.2	0.5	50.9	-	5.0	3.0	0.04	21.2	3.4	-	3.4	reported	reported	0.05	Hypobasic	Arsenic	Tartaric, etc.
Grapes, wild	78.9	2.0	1.3	17.0	0.7	56.0	0.9	5.4	2.6	0.9	18.6	3.1	0.8	2.3	-	-	0.02	Hyperbasic	Almerin	Tartaric, etc.
Grapes, green	78.1	1.0	1.2	19.1	0.5	44.1	1.0	4.3	2.9	0.4	14.0	6.4	0.1	-	-	-	-	Hyperbasic	Iodine	Tartaric, etc.
Green turtle	90.0	3.8	0.6	4.1	0.6	39.0	9.1	1.0	0.9	0.8	12.8	3.4	0.9	-	-	-	5.8	Hyperacid	-	Several
Grouse	64.0	19.0	16.0	-	1.0	15.1	4.1	0.3	1.4	0.09	11.6	1.8	Some	-	-	-	-	Hypoacid	-	Meat
Ham, smoked	53.6	20.1	18.2	-	8.0	16.4	11.8	3.2	1.3	0.1	18.9	3.6	0.4	13.4	-	-	-	Hypobasic	-	Boric, saltpetre, etc.
Haddock, smoked	73.0	22.6	0.3	-	4.1	35.1	10.3	5.1	3.2	0.08	26.4	2.9	0.04	12.4	-	-	0.7	Hypobasic	-	Meat
Halibut, smoked	51.2	18.6	14.9	-	15.3	29.2	13.1	2.3	3.6	0.04	24.2	3.2	0.01	15.6	-	-	1.0	Hyperbasic	-	Fish acids
Hazelnut	5.4	16.5	64.0	11.7	2.4	19.9	0.8	3.8	2.0	0.4	18.3	2.1	0.6	0.3	-	-	-	Hyperacid	-	Oily
Herring, fresh	69.5	19.2	9.5	-	1.8	17.0	3.4	3.4	2.2	0.02	22.0	2.3	-	4.6	-	-	1.8	Acid	-	Fatty
Herring, smoked	35.1	37.8	16.3	-	10.8	17.8	9.9	3.4	2.3	0.02	22.0	9.1	0.01	11.6	-	-	1.5	Hypobasic	-	Meat acids
Hickory nut	4.1	15.0	67.4	11.3	2.2	30.1	1.8	3.7	7.3	0.03	21.6	-	0.4	0.03	-	-	-	Hyperacid	-	Fatty
Honey, alfalfa	19.6	0.4	-	79.7	0.2	0.08	0.1	1.1	0.09	0.1	0.21	0.02	-	0.02	0.01	-	-	Hyperacid	-	Formic, fatty

Chemistry of Food Chart (Cont'd.)

Name of Food	Water	Protein	Fat	Carbohydrates	Ash	Potassium	Sodium	Calcium	Magnesium	Iron	Phosphorus	Sulphur	Silicon	Chlorine	Manganese	Fluorine	Iodine	Acid Forming or Basic	Contains	Kind of Acid
Honey, eucalyptus	18.4	0.8	-	80.0	0.8	0.2	0.2	1.1	0.1	0.1	0.2	0.01	-	0.03	-	-	-	Hyperacid	Eucalyptol	Honey acids
Horseradish	86.6	1.3	0.2	10.3	1.6	21.8	3.6	5.8	1.9	1.3	10.6	35.8	9.8	9.3	-	-	-	Hyperacid	Thiosinamin	Sulphuric, etc.
Huckleberry	86.1	1.8	0.7	13.9	0.4	27.8	4.1	3.8	2.9	0.6	9.3	1.6	2.0	0.06	-	-	-	Hyperbasic	-	Citric, malic, etc.
Juniper berry	69.1	9.8	0.9	14.1	6.1	55.1	4.5	4.0	4.9	2.1	16.0	1.8	2.0	2.8	-	0.02	0.2	Hypobasic	Juniperin	Mild acid
Kale	93.1	2.1	0.1	3.1	1.6	31.8	6.4	19.4	8.1	1.4	17.6	10.4	0.08	4.3	-	-	-	Hyperacid	Brassin	Brassidic, oxalic
Kohlrabi	91.0	2.4	0.1	5.1	1.4	30.2	11.3	12.2	7.5	2.7	12.9	11.6	3.3	7.5	-	-	-	Basic	Brassin	6: brassidic, etc.
Lamb	66.9	20.1	12.0	-	1.0	31.0	4.2	0.9	2.1	0.1	23.0	2.1	0.6	12.1	-	-	-	Hypobasic	-	Meat acids
Leeks	92.1	1.3	0.6	4.9	1.1	23.3	10.0	11.6	3.2	4.8	19.2	13.7	5.0	6.0	-	-	0.1	Hypobasic	Allyl	Onion acids
Lemons	89.4	1.8	0.1	8.2	0.5	48.3	0.8	29.9	4.4	0.2	11.1	2.8	0.3	0.2	-	-	-	Hyperbasic	Essence	Citric, formic, etc.
Lentils	12.9	26.8	1.6	55.1	3.6	35.0	5.2	3.1	1.6	0.6	19.2	2.0	0.9	2.0	-	-	-	Hyperacid	Toxin	Starch, etc.
Lettuce, common	92.5	3.7	0.7	2.6	0.5	46.6	3.3	5.1	0.8	9.4	5.3	High	-	Not	reported	-	-	Hyperbasic	Asparagin	Lactucic, etc.
Lettuce, head	94.9	1.4	0.3	2.2	1.0	27.9	13.5	10.6	4.2	2.4	16.6	6.9	4.6	3.8	-	-	0.01	Hyperbasic	Lactucerol	Lactucic, etc.
Lettuce, lamb's	93.0	2.9	0.4	2.7	1.0	29.0	12.8	8.4	6.5	2.1	12.0	5.8	4.9	3.6	-	0.02	0.09	Hyperbasic	Asparagin	Lactucic, etc.
Lettuce, sea	90.8	2.1	0.7	5.1	1.3	30.0	13.5	12.1	5.0	2.6	13.2	5.0	4.0	3.4	-	-	0.20	Hyperbasic	Asparagin	Lactucic, etc.
Limes	95.6	2.2	-	0.8	1.4	31.1	-	6.3	1.9	1.4	6.9	2.8	0.03	3.0	-	-	-	Basic	-	Citric, formic, etc.
Liver	71.5	20.0	3.7	3.2	1.5	13.9	7.9	2.0	0.1	0.04	27.3	0.5	0.1	1.3	-	-	-	Hypoacid	-	Several
Lobster	79.5	16.5	1.3	0.4	2.2	28.0	11.1	2.1	1.6	0.3	32.0	12.6	-	1.9	-	-	1.70	Acid	-	Meat
Lung	79.8	15.2	3.6	-	1.9	1.2	24.7	1.8	3.0	0.08	46.1	1.3	0.4	6.4	-	-	-	Hyperacid	-	Fatty
Loquats	86.7	7.0	0.3	4.3	1.1	12.3	4.4	1.6	2.0	-	1.4	1.2	0.02	3.9	-	-	-	Hyperbasic	-	Malic, citric, etc.
Mandarine	88.3	0.7	0.4	10.0	0.6	18.0	-	2.6	2.9	-	12.6	1.6	-	1.4	-	0.02	-	Basic	-	Citric, malic, etc.
Mangoes	87.4	0.6	0.4	9.9	0.5	17.9	-	2.6	1.7	-	9.7	1.6	-	1.4	-	-	-	Basic	-	Tartaric, malic, etc.
Maple syrup	27.6	-	-	71.6	0.5	2.7	0.1	1.4	0.5	0.06	0.3	0.09	0.03	0.1	-	-	-	Hyperbasic	-	Sugar acids
Marjoram	74.6	14.1	0.2	7.0	3.4	28.7	4.6	12.6	4.0	1.9	14.1	11.56	16.2	6.4	0.03	-	-	Basic	Origanin	Plant acid
Meat, game	58.6	18.6	21.0	-	1.6	16.1	3.4	1.6	1.6	0.01	8.3	3.4	Trace	1.7	-	-	-	Hypoacid	-	Many: uric, lactic
Meat, goat	51.2	24.4	23.1	-	1.3	17.8	4.9	1.6	1.9	0.6	19.3	2.3	0.02	3.6	-	0.02	-	Hyperbasic	-	Meat
Milk, cow	87.1	3.2	4.0	5.0	0.7	26.6	12.5	24.8	0.9	0.05	21.2	0.7	0.02	10.3	-	0.06	-	Basic	-	Lactic
Milk, goat	84.8	4.3	4.9	5.1	0.8	28.6	14.6	13.8	2.6	0.7	22.0	0.8	0.3	13.6	-	0.01	-	Basic	-	Lactic, hircic
Milk, mother's	87.8	2.1	3.0	6.4	0.5	11.8	3.2	13.0	2.0	0.09	16.8	0.8	0.09	9.9	-	-	-	Basic	-	7: fatty
Milk, skimmed	90.2	3.5	0.4	5.1	0.8	24.4	8.8	23.9	0.9	0.04	20.4	0.7	0.01	10.0	-	-	-	Acid	-	Milk, preservatives
Millet	11.8	10.6	3.9	71.5	2.0	19.0	0.8	1.0	3.2	0.4	19.6	0.3	1.9	1.9	-	-	-	Hypobasic	Panacin	Starch acid
Mirabelles	84.8	0.7	-	14.0	0.4	11.6	1.7	1.0	1.3	0.2	3.9	1.0	-	-	-	-	-	Hyperbasic	-	Mild fruit
Molasses	26.0	1.9	-	69.3	2.8	21.1	0.3	3.1	1.1	0.01	6.7	1.9	-	0.1	-	0.02	-	Hyperbasic	Preservatives	Sugar, preservatives
Mulberries	83.6	0.6	0.04	15.2	0.6	10.1	3.6	3.8	2.9	0.5	8.3	1.2	0.6	5.9	-	-	-	Hypobasic	-	Moraxytic, tartaric
Muscle	75.5	18.7	3.7	1.0	1.1	18.2	2.8	0.5	1.9	3.0	23.0	1.0	0.3	2.7	-	0.06	-	Hypoacid	Often choline	7: uric, lactic, etc.
Mushrooms	73.3	4.4	1.1	18.6	2.0	48.1	2.0	0.9	2.6	1.4	16.8	2.9	0.7	0.9	-	0.01	0.20	Hypoacid	Choline	Sugar, etc.
Muskmelon	82.1	7.0	-	9.6	0.6	9.4	1.2	0.9	0.9	0.9	2.7	0.9	-	0.7	-	-	-	Neutral	Betaine	Neutral
Mussels	83.4	8.9	1.4	4.2	2.1	11.1	16.3	2.5	3.0	0.7	18.0	11.1	1.9	9.0	-	-	0.40	Hypobasic	Fixed oil	Meat, germ
Mustard						18.3	0.2	9.3	6.5	1.0	15.0	48.2	-	0.1	Sand, etc.	-	-	Hyperbasic	Thiol	Sulphur, etc.
Nasturtium	92.1	2.0	0.1	1.0	4.3	38.6	6.0	14.0	6.1	1.0	14.0	11.8	1.1	4.4	-	-	-	Hyperacid	-	Sulphur, etc.
Nectarines	80.1	7.0	0.04	11.1	0.6	17.4	4.9	6.0	4.9	0.1	9.4	2.2	0.9	0.3	-	-	-	Hypobasic	-	4: fruit
Nettles	92.5	2.2	Some	1.2	4.1	30.4	16.0	12.1	8.0	3.0	11.1	18.1	3.0	0.9	-	-	-	Hyperbasic	Tannin	Tannic, formic, etc.
Plumcot	81.2	1.0	1.1	16.8	2.0	18.1	1.9	1.5	1.8	0.6	3.9	1.0	0.7	0.1	-	-	-	Neutral	-	5: Tartaric, malic
Plums	78.3	1.1	0.1	20.0	0.5	17.1	0.2	3.1	11.9	0.9	4.3	1.8	0.7	0.7	-	-	-	Hypobasic	Prunin	Several
Plums, Blue Damson	80.4	1.0	0.1	18.0	0.5	19.1	1.1	2.9	10.4	0.7	4.1	1.6	0.6	0.9	-	-	-	Hypobasic	-	Laxative acids
Pomegranate	80.1	1.6	0.2	17.1	1.0	14.6	16.3	2.3	9.9	0.1	3.2	0.2	0.04	0.4	-	-	-	Hyperbasic	Pelletierin	Many: citric
Popcorn	4.4	11.0	5.1	78.1	1.4	12.1	0.2	0.6	2.9	0.01	16.4	0.8	0.4	0.3	-	-	-	Acid	-	Starch
Pork	64.7	18.5	15.6	-	1.2	10.0	6.4	0.1	1.3	0.01	8.0	2.2	0.2	1.8	-	-	-	Hyperacid	-	Fatty
Potato, baked	78.1	2.2	0.1	18.4	1.1	60.4	2.6	2.6	4.9	1.2	17.3	6.5	2.1	3.1	-	-	0.01	Acid	-	Starch
Potato, sweet, raw	55.2	1.5	0.6	22.0	0.9	34.0	2.2	2.4	2.6	0.4	13.1	4.6	1.2	3.0	-	-	0.01	Hyperacid	Solanin	Starch

482

Chemistry of Food Chart (Cont'd.)

Name of Food	Water	Protein	Fat	Carbohydrates	Ash	Potassium	Sodium	Calcium	Magnesium	Iron	Phosphorus	Sulphur	Silicon	Chlorine	Manganese	Fluorine	Iodine	Acid Forming or Basic	Contains	Kind of Acid
Prunes, American	79.6	0.9	-	18.9	0.6	63.8	Some	4.7	5.5	-	14.1	2.7	-	Not	reported	-	-	Hypobasic	Prunin	Malic, oxalic, etc.
Prunes, German	84.9	2.4	0.8	11.2	0.7	59.2	0.5	10.0	5.5	3.2	15.5	3.7	2.4	0.4	-	-	-	Hyperbasic	Prunin	Sugar acids
Pumpkins	92.8	1.2	0.2	5.0	0.8	16.9	16.1	5.7	2.8	1.8	23.0	1.7	5.1	1.9	-	-	-	Neutral	-	Plant acids
Quail	63.7	19.1	16.0	0.2	1.0	17.0	3.4	0.4	1.5	0.02	9.0	4.7	0.02	6.3	-	0.02	-	Hypobasic	-	Meat acid mild
Quince	70.0	0.5	0.4	14.6	1.4	20.0	10.6	9.5	5.1	1.03	10.9	1.9	3.3	4.0	-	-	0.01	Acid	-	Malic, etc.
Radish, black	90.7	2.0	0.1	6.1	1.0	30.6	6.4	11.0	5.1	3.0	13.9	16.1	0.9	4.8	-	-	-	Hypoacid	-	Many
Radish, red	94.3	1.2	0.2	3.7	0.7	38.1	7.2	11.9	6.0	3.2	19.0	17.1	1.1	2.0	-	-	-	Hypoacid	-	Plant acids
Raisins	14.7	2.5	3.7	75.4	3.7	52.8	2.9	5.1	3.1	0.6	21.6	4.4	0.1	1.9	-	-	-	Hypobasic	-	Tartaric, malic
Raspberries, black	84.1	2.2	1.4	12.6	0.7	14.6	6.0	2.8	2.0	0.1	3.8	4.8	0.09	2.9	-	-	-	Hyperbasic	-	Tannic, tartaric, etc.
Raspberries, red	86.6	1.9	0.9	10.0	0.6	16.9	1.9	3.0	1.6	0.07	4.6	12.0	0.04	2.9	-	-	-	Acid	-	Malic, tannic, etc.
Raspberries, white	87.0	1.7	0.9	9.8	0.6	16.8	1.9	3.0	1.6	0.04	4.5	11.8	-	4.2	-	-	-	Acid	-	Tannic, malic, etc.
Rhubarb	94.6	0.5	0.6	3.6	0.7	44.0	8.4	10.9	2.9	1.8	16.7	2.0	2.6	0.9	-	-	0.1	Hyperacid	-	Oxalic, etc.
Rice bran	13.9	11.1	7.8	62.1	4.6	6.0	-	1.3	9.2	4.0	22.8	0.1	8.8	0.8	-	-	0.1	Hyperacid	-	Starch
Rice flour	11.8	8.1	0.4	78.6	0.4	26.1	12.7	4.9	9.8	1.16	35.8	0.4	6.4	0.7	-	-	0.1	Hyperacid	-	Starch
Rice, processed	14.0	11.3	0.7	82.9	0.5	20.8	13.9	4.4	9.6	0.8	40.2	0.2	6.1	1.0	-	-	Some	Hyperacid	-	Starch
Rice, polished	12.5	8.0	0.4	78.8	0.3	5.9	10.2	4.0	8.4	0.4	42.6	0.1	6.5	1.9	-	-	Trace	Hyperacid	-	Amylic
Rice, wild	11.8	8.2	0.4	79.2	0.5	20.1	12.7	4.9	9.1	1.2	37.8	0.4	0.9	4.3	-	-	0.2	Hyperacid	-	Amylic
Roe	92.5	1.5	0.4	4.2	5.0	10.4	6.1	14.1	2.1	1.8	55.4	0.3	2.1	1.1	-	-	0.04	Acid	Asparagin	Fatty mainly
Romaine	88.9	1.3	0.2	8.5	1.4	27.9	25.0	12.0	6.1	1.4	14.1	5.0	1.1	0.6	-	-	-	Hyperacid	Asparagin	Mild plant
Rutabaga	10.9	17.4	3.7	69.1	1.1	43.6	10.2	9.4	8.8	1.4	11.7	5.2	0.4	0.5	-	-	-	Hypoacid	Brassin	Brassidic, etc.
Rye bran	13.0	6.9	1.1	78.3	3.0	15.7	0.8	2.0	2.8	0.5	26.7	6.0	2.9	0.6	-	-	-	Hyperacid	Secalin	Starch acids
Rye flour	11.4	13.6	2.0	71.5	0.7	13.0	0.2	1.9	2.3	1.0	16.6	0.6	2.4	0.5	-	-	-	Hyperacid	-	Amylic
Rye meal	12.1	9.1	0.1	78.1	1.5	29.4	17.0	5.9	12.0	6.1	24.0	0.5	0.2	7.0	-	-	-	Hypobasic	-	Cereal
Rye, Minn.	65.6	20.0	13.0	-	0.5	27.6	4.6	5.6	11.7	5.2	40.8	2.7	24.0	0.4	0.01	Trace	-	Hyperbasic	Secalin	Amylic
Salmon, silver	7.8	16.9	7.0	64.5	1.4	13.1	5.0	4.0	3.8	0.3	19.6	4.0	0.9	10.1	Some	Trace	1.5	Acid	-	Meat
Oats, rolled	7.3	16.0	7.2	67.0	3.8	6.0	1.1	1.4	2.0	0.1	7.6	5.4	0.2	0.9	-	-	-	Hypoacid	-	Starch
Oats, steel cut	86.8	2.0	0.5	10.0	2.0	13.6	3.0	2.9	5.2	0.2	18.2	4.9	0.2	0.7	-	-	0.01	Hypoacid	Avenin	Starch, etc.
Okra	9.5	6.3	Some	6.0	0.7	9.0	12.6	20.0	2.8	-	8.4	1.8	9.1	0.4	-	-	-	Hyperbasic	-	Mild acid
Oleomargarine	9.5	1.3	83.6	-	4.8	0.5	8.1	7.7	-	-	0.4	-	0.3	10.9	-	-	-	Hyperacid	Cholesterol	Fatty
Olives, dry	30.7	5.3	52.0	9.6	2.4	61.6	6.3	3.7	2.0	0.2	4.9	0.6	0.08	0.9	-	-	-	Hyperbasic	Cholesterol	Arachidic, oleic
Olives, ripe	64.5	1.8	26.0	4.4	3.3	19.0	2.6	6.4	1.0	0.2	0.9	0.5	0.09	10.0	-	-	0.2	Hyperbasic	Volatile oil	Arachidic, oleic
Onions, white	83.1	4.6	9.0	10.3	1.1	30.2	1.6	22.6	3.0	2.3	12.6	4.0	9.1	1.6	-	-	-	Hyperacid	-	Onion acids
Oranges, Florida	81.5	1.2	0.2	16.3	0.6	48.9	1.0	10.1	5.3	0.4	12.8	2.7	0.3	0.4	-	-	-	Basic	-	Formic, citric
Oranges, California	81.5	0.9	0.2	17.0	0.4	39.8	0.8	4.0	3.6	0.2	9.8	0.3	0.08	0.2	-	-	-	Basic	-	Citric, formic
Oysters	83.2	6.3	1.9	6.0	2.6	16.9	21.2	1.5	3.0	0.05	34.0	6.0	-	16.1	-	-	1.3	Hypoacid	-	Mild
Papaya	87.9	0.5	Some	11.0	0.5	9.1	9.6	19.0	4.6	0.3	5.0	2.0	0.09	4.0	-	-	-	Neutral	Caricin	5: Malic
Parsley	86.6	3.7	0.7	7.0	2.0	41.0	2.2	6.0	3.1	0.9	7.1	6.0	0.04	2.3	-	-	-	Basic	Apiol	Tannic, malic, etc.
Parsnips	82.5	1.8	0.7	13.4	1.6	42.2	0.4	4.6	3.1	0.3	12.8	7.2	9.4	1.0	-	-	-	Hypobasic	Fruit ether	Starch, etc.
Peaches, Hale	89.1	0.9	0.1	9.4	0.5	31.0	3.2	1.0	1.8	0.4	7.0	2.4	0.1	0.8	-	-	-	Hyperacid	Toxin	Malic, etc.
Peanuts	9.6	25.1	40.8	22.4	2.1	12.0	0.2	1.8	2.3	0.2	12.0	0.9	6.0	0.3	-	-	-	Hyperacid	-	5: Arachidic
Pears, Bartlett	83.8	0.8	0.7	14.2	0.5	11.0	6.0	1.4	1.9	0.08	5.3	0.5	0.02	0.3	-	-	0.1	Neutral	-	Mild fruit
Peas, sweet green	81.1	3.6	0.5	14.1	0.7	16.0	1.2	1.4	2.7	0.4	16.1	3.9	0.08	1.2	-	-	0.08	Hypobasic	-	Mild
Peas, Scotch, dry	2.8	9.5	71.0	14.5	2.0	7.2	1.1	1.3	3.3	0.8	3.4	3.4	0.1	1.9	Some	-	-	Hyperacid	Asparagin	Many: Oxalic
Pecans	2.7	9.7	70.8	14.6	2.0	7.1	0.4	3.1	1.9	0.8	6.8	6.8	0.04	2.6	-	-	-	Hyperacid	Toxin	Fatty acids
Persimmons	65.8	0.7	0.7	31.6	1.0	19.0	3.0	4.2	1.9	0.1	6.0	1.0	9.4	0.2	-	-	-	Hypobasic	-	Gum, fruit
Pike	80.0	18.0	1.0	-	1.0	15.1	13.0	3.4	2.3	0.01	24.0	0.5	6.0	1.9	-	-	-	Hyperbasic	-	Meat acid
Pineapple	88.9	0.5	0.3	10.0	0.4	13.0	8.2	3.0	2.6	0.5	4.2	2.9	0.02	2.6	-	-	01	Hyperacid	Toxin	Many: Citric, malic
Pinons	3.6	15.0	61.5	17.0	2.9	16.8	0.8	3.4	2.6	0.5	14.1	0.1	0.08	0.2	-	-	0.3	Hyperacid	Nut toxin	Terpene, several
Pistachio	4.2	22.3	54.0	16.3	3.2	Unreported	-	-	3.6	-	14.1	-	0.1	Not	reported	-	-	Hypobasic	Verin	Oily

483

Chemistry of Food Chart (Cont'd.)

Name of Food	Water	Protein	Fat	Carbohydrates	Ash	Potassium	Sodium	Calcium	Magnesium	Iron	Phosphorus	Sulphur	Silicon	Chlorine	Manganese	Fluorine	Iodine	Acid Forming or Basic	Contains	Kind of Acid
Salmon, smoked	44.2	35.6	10.1	-	10.1	41.0	15.1	4.1	3.8	0.3	19.5	2.0	-	10.0	-	-	1.4	Basic	-	Fish acids
Salsify, black	80.0	1.4	0.5	17.0	1.1	46.0	7.8	5.1	3.4	6.4	14.0	5.9	0.1	1.5	-	-	-	Hyperbasic	-	Oxalic, tannic, etc.
Seacrab	76.0	18.2	1.8	1.1	2.9	18.9	High	6.0	-	-	36.1	1.4	-	Not reported	-	-	-	Hypobasic	Pagurin	Flesh acids
Shallot	64.6	5.9	0.1	27.9	1.4	26.1	12.0	6.0	3.2	2.0	11.6	1.4	0.09	0.08	Not reported	-	-	Neutral	Allyl sulphol	Active
Shrimp	70.8	25.4	1.0	0.2	2.6	Others not given	-	-	-	-	-	-	-	-	-	-	5.9	Hyperacid	Iodine	Several
Smelt	78.0	18.0	2.0	-	2.0	26.4	12.8	6.0	3.2	0.4	31.6	1.0	-	3.9	Not reported	-	-	Hypoacid	-	Flesh acids, mainly
Sole	79.2	17.1	2.1	-	1.6	15.0	1.0	4.2	2.4	0.2	22.5	0.6	-	1.8	-	-	0.2	Hypoacid	-	Flesh acid
Sorghum	14.8	9.1	3.6	69.8	2.1	6.0	0.9	0.3	4.9	0.4	9.8	0.2	-	0.2	-	-	-	Hyperacid	-	Amylic, etc.
Sorrel	92.6	1.9	0.4	4.0	1.1	34.0	1.0	9.1	8.9	2.9	17.4	10.4	-	9.1	-	-	0.1	Hyperbasic	-	Oxalic, etc.
Spinach	91.8	2.3	0.4	3.3	2.2	39.9	9.4	2.6	2.2	6.0	2.2	12.4	8.0	11.0	-	-	-	Hyperbasic	-	Oxalic, etc.
Spleen	75.5	17.1	4.2	1.0	1.6	6.1	28.3	4.8	0.3	4.6	17.3	1.0	0.1	0.3	-	-	-	Hyperbasic	-	-
Squash	87.0	1.6	1.1	9.6	0.7	21.3	16.8	4.3	3.1	0.3	22.0	1.0	2.1	0.2	-	-	-	Basic	-	Mild plant
Strawberries	90.0	0.7	0.4	8.1	0.8	13.4	19.6	8.7	1.6	3.8	5.1	1.9	7.0	1.0	-	-	0.1	Often basic	Euonymin	5: Malic, citric
Sugar beets	81.6	1.2	0.2	16.0	1.0	42.9	11.0	6.2	3.0	0.03	9.0	-	0.01	1.3	-	-	0.1	Hyperbasic	Betaine	Solvent, sugar
Sugar beet leaves	88.1	2.2	Trace	9.1	0.6	31.4	12.3	17.2	9.4	0.9	3.6	2.0	-	0.09	-	-	-	Hyperbasic	-	Plant acids
Sugar, brown	-	-	-	95.0	Lacking in other elements	Ash elements unreported	-	-	-	-	-	-	Same as granulated sugar	Same as granulated sugar	Not reported	-	-	Hyperacid	-	Sugar acids
Sweetbreads	69.0	19.2	9.5	-	2.1	-	-	-	-	-	-	-	-	-	-	-	-	Basic	-	Antacid
Swiss chard	85.5	3.1	Trace	10.0	1.4	26.8	23.0	12.2	6.8	1.9	14.3	7.7	6.0	1.0	-	-	-	Hyperbasic	-	Many, oxalic
Tamarinds	67.5	1.0	-	31.0	0.5	37.0	1.0	0.9	9.4	0.08	20.0	16.1	7.6	1.4	-	-	-	Hyperacid	Essence	Many, malic, citric
Tangerines	87.6	0.8	Trace	11.0	0.5	46.7	1.0	21.0	5.0	0.3	13.1	5.3	0.3	0.4	-	-	-	Basic	-	Formic, citric, etc.
Tea, Japan	10.6	21.0	Unreported	11.0	6.1	37.5	1.4	9.4	8.0	1.8	12.3	4.2	11.3	1.5	2.1	-	-	Hyperacid	Thein	Tannic, boheic
Thyme	88.2	3.8	3.2	1.9	2.9	30.0	4.6	12.5	4.2	1.2	21.6	11.1	6.6	5.9	-	-	-	Neutral	Thymol	Several
Tomatoes, red	90.3	1.2	1.3	6.5	0.7	39.9	9.4	2.6	2.2	0.9	2.2	5.1	1.6	7.0	-	-	0.02	Hyperbasic	-	5: Citric, malic
Tomatoes, Burbank	90.1	1.3	1.3	6.5	0.8	36.4	12.3	2.7	2.3	0.8	2.0	1.8	1.0	6.0	-	-	0.09	Hyperbasic	-	Many
Trout	77.6	18.6	2.4	-	1.4	16.2	8.3	1.5	2.0	0.04	26.0	2.0	1.0	3.0	-	-	0.08	Hypoacid	-	Fish acids
Turbot	69.7	14.7	14.40	-	1.3	18.9	6.0	1.9	14.0	0.3	29.8	1.8	0.9	4.0	-	-	0.09	Neutral	-	Flesh acids
Turkey	51.6	28.0	19.1	-	1.2	20.1	4.0	0.4	2.0	0.08	18.6	4.0	0.03	2.9	-	-	-	Hypoacid	-	Meat acids
Turnip, white	89.6	1.3	0.2	8.1	0.8	43.0	8.3	8.8	2.7	-	11.4	12.0	1.6	5.0	-	-	-	Hypoacid	-	Amylic
Turnip leaves	83.1	5.2	0.1	10.3	1.3	41.0	7.0	11.9	5.1	0.7	13.2	10.0	1.8	6.5	-	-	-	Hyperbasic	-	Plant acid
Turnip, Russian	87.1	1.2	0.9	7.9	0.7	43.4	9.8	10.6	3.7	0.8	12.7	11.2	1.8	5.0	-	-	-	Hypobasic	-	Starch
Veal joint jelly	70.4	7.6	0.7	18.6	2.7	16.6	10.9	19.2	6.8	0.8	29.8	2.1	2.4	10.6	-	-	-	Hyperbasic	-	Gelatin acids
Vegetable marrow	86.0	1.8	1.6	9.9	0.7	20.4	14.0	4.5	3.2	0.4	20.9	1.0	2.1	0.9	-	-	-	Hypoacid	-	Mild plant
Walnut, black	2.7	27.6	56.3	11.4	1.9	12.7	0.1	5.6	16.6	1.6	57.8	1.3	0.7	0.7	0.3	-	-	Hyperacid	Toxin	Fatty
Walnut, English	2.5	19.0	65.0	11.1	1.6	36.1	0.3	1.2	3.0	0.3	41.9	0.7	0.9	0.1	-	-	-	Hyperacid	Toxin	Oily
Water chestnut	42.6	4.6	1.3	49.6	1.9	14.0	0.09	1.2	2.15	0.04	11.8	0.9	0.02	0.9	-	-	-	Hypoacid	-	Oily acids
Watercress	93.8	2.0	0.1	2.3	1.8	21.6	4.1	16.0	6.2	0.4	7.17	29.4	0.03	4.6	-	-	0.2	Often acid	-	Many
Watermelon	92.1	0.5	0.2	6.9	0.3	21.6	7.7	5.0	3.4	1.8	7.6	1.1	1.6	2.0	-	-	-	Hyperbasic	-	Negative
Wheat bran	12.4	16.6	3.5	62.1	4.9	15.1	2.3	8.6	9.4	0.3	27.8	0.2	0.5	1.1	-	-	-	Hyperacid	Often toxin	Starch
Wheat, Oregon	13.6	12.4	1.7	70.5	1.8	29.7	3.0	7.1	13.2	0.2	42.1	0.1	1.0	0.2	-	-	-	Hyperacid	Often toxin	Starch
Wheat, Canadian	15.4	12.2	1.5	69.5	0.6	24.0	6.5	10.5	13.2	0.5	44.1	1.9	2.2	0.01	-	-	Some	Hyperacid	Often toxin	Starch
Whey, cow	93.8	0.6	0.1	5.1	0.4	21.8	9.8	13.6	0.3	0.4	12.0	1.9	-	11.2	-	-	-	Hypobasic	Zinc oxide	Milk acids
Whey, goat	92.5	0.8	0.1	6.2	0.5	23.7	10.0	11.0	0.5	2.3	10.6	2.7	0.2	13.9	-	0.06	-	Basic	-	Milk acids
Whitefish	68.8	22.9	6.6	1.6	1.6	13.0	4.7	2.3	0.1	0.09	30.6	0.3	3.0	4.6	-	-	0.3	Hypobasic	-	Fish acids
Whiting	69.0	20.9	6.5	2.0	2.0	32.3	7.7	4.5	9.3	0.03	50.1	1.3	1.6	-	-	-	-	Hypobasic	-	Oily acids
White flour	12.0	14.0	1.9	71.3	0.9	13.6	1.1	1.1	0.9	3.9	6.9	1.9	Salt	1.3	-	-	-	Hyperacid	-	Starch acid
Wild strawberry	89.2	1.3	0.7	7.9	0.9	62.8	0.9	10.0	1.8	3.6	4.7	1.7	7.9	0.9	-	-	-	Often basic	-	5: Malic, citric
Wild cherry	86.6	6.4	0.8	4.1	2.1	30.2	1.8	4.6	5.6	0.02	32.4	0.1	4.3	-	-	-	-	Often basic	Euonymin	5: Malic, tartaric
White crackers	6.8	11.9	5.0	74.7	1.6	32.4	0.9	2.6	6.1	0.5	5.6	0.6	Salt	1.3	-	-	-	Hyperacid	-	Starch acids
Yeast	65.1	11.7	0.4	21.0	1.8	32.4	0.1	5.5	6.1	0.5	5.6	0.6	1.3	-	-	-	-	Acid	Fungi	Fermentative
Zapote	74.7	1.9	0.5	21.7	0.6	9.2	8.1	1.7	1.1	0.04	2.4	-	-	0.9	-	-	-	Hypobasic	Pagurin	5 acids

Notes within the bottom rows: "High in phosphates and chlorides" and "Also tender protein."

WHAT THE CHEMICALS DO IN THE BODY: VITAL LESSONS IN THE CHEMICAL STORY

FOODS AND CHEMICALS
SODIUM

No previous lesson has been as important as this one lesson on sodium. It is a lesson for people who suffer from acidity of the stomach, gas generation and gout. Such patients should eat sodium foods in abundance.

The ordinary common table salt is a combination of sodium and chlorine, in almost equal proportion. Salt is inorganic sodium and chlorine. For that reason, it is not so valuable as that sodium which we find in organized foods. Sodium which we buy in drugstores is not so valuable as that which we find in organic foods. The human being is organic or organized. Sodium which we get from plants and vegetables is organized sodium.

When we take out from foods some certain salt, we are likely to alter the chemicals in those foods. When extracted from food, that certain chemical salt extracted, may even become a poison. Potash by itself is a poison, whether it comes from food or from the drugstore. This is also the case with phosphorus. You thereby overtax your system, and your functions must work that much harder, in order to throw off those inorganic salts or poisons introduced, either through drugs, or through so-called tissue remedies or otherwise.

When we are sick, we should eat such foods that contain the salts needed. We obtain sodium salt from spinach, strawberries and carrots. If we put sugar and cream on the berries, we are not wise, for the sodium that the berries contain, will be overcome by the sugar, cream or whatever else we may put into the food. We should eat the food the way the Almighty is manufacturing it for us. The sodium which we need is often used up by the cream or by the sugar, as the case may be. It mixes with the cream in the stomach and the power of the sodium salt is almost lost.

We should eat strawberries without cream and sugar. If we would do this, the sodium salts, which the Almighty has put into the food, would do us more good. You should eat the foods as they are; and when you are in need of much sodium, you should eat those foods that are very rich in sodium salts.

When you cook spinach and you pour the juice into the sink, you get spinach minus the salt. The salts you need, you pour into the sink.

The Almighty did not make sugar. The sugar you use on the table you have manufactured yourself—the Almighty had nothing to do with it. When He made wheat, He did not intend you to eat it in the form of white flour and doughnuts. If He intended you to eat doughnuts and coffee, He would have made doughnuts and coffee for you, and would have had them in the Garden of Eden.

The sodium we get from plants is organic sodium. French vichy water is organic. Sodium is a Latin word. Natrium is the Greek word for the same thing.

Chemicals that are alkaline are most valuable for the sick man. Every food that is acid or makes the system more acid, is bad for the sick man. Every food that generates gas in the alimentary tract is bad for the sick man. Coffee may have a good taste and is as inviting as the wine in the glass, but it makes the stomach acid. Tea generates acid and gas, and yet there are many people who drink 12 cups of tea a day. Then they wonder why they suffer from nervousness and gas in the stomach. Some of them drink so much tea that they become hysterical. There is no nutrition in tea. Why should you drink it or why should you drink coffee?

Sodium combines with chlorine. Chlorine is an important element. Chlorine is the laundryman of the body. It carries impurities out of the body. It is associated with sodium to make the cells clean and pure. It kills germs that are always associated with foods that are rich in sodium. Sodium makes the cells alkaline. If you take sodium- and chlorine-containing foods or drinks in abundance, your cells are purified, then you get very thirsty and you want pure water in abundance; you should then drink distilled water and fruit juice.

There is a strong affinity between sodium, chlorine and oxygen. Foods that are rich in sodium are often rich in chlorine and oxygen also. Oxygen foods are often rich in chlorine, also in sodium, in potassium or in potassium oxide. Sodium neutralizes acid. It is used in soap manufacture. Sodium and chlorine in soap take off the dirt. The same kind of soap manufacture is going on in the body and the same kind of cell-cleansing processes.

Saponification is a physiological function. If you take sodium and potassium out of the body, saponification stops. If you then eat fat of any kind, your stomach becomes acid. Sodium and potassium are the two elements necessary for soap making. If those two elements are low, you cannot take care of the fat. Hence also you grow lean; and the more fatty food you eat, the more lean you grow. If you are lean, you grow leaner on a starchy and fatty diet; and if you are fleshy, you grow fleshier. You well up with water and fatty substances; you become food drunk, and you cannot get all of those fermented substances out of your body.

Do you think that you can starve all such fatty substances out of yourself? No, no! If you suffer from obesity, that fat stays in your body even if you starve yourself to death. Even after you are dead, you have those same fatty linings in the stomach; and if you are a lean man and you eat fatty foods at such a time, you cannot take care of the fat. Supply yourself, at such a time, with sodium and potassium foods in abundance for a long, long time and you will find that lastly your system will take care of fatty foods. At such a time, do not forget the necessity of fresh air. If you do this, you can put on flesh; you can convert oil and fat into good tissue. As a general thing, people at large do not understand the human machine, nor the foods that go into the human machine. Even doctors are not acquainted with the human body nor with the chemistry of the body nor with the chemistry of foods, we are sorry to say. They do not teach this in medical colleges.

Sodium neutralizes acid. Gout is caused by nothing but acid. Neuritis is caused by acid. Celery juice will cure neuritis when it is caused by acid around the nerves. It is the acid that makes the nerves ache. The nerves would never ache if there were no acid in the system around the nerves. When you neutralize the acid around the nerves, the pain stops.

If you eat sodium foods, do not drink a great deal of water afterwards, for if you do, you wash the sodium out of your system. Hot water will convert sodium into sodium carbonate. If you drink cold water after eating sodium foods, it will have a decomposing effect upon the stomach. The man who tries this diet should not introduce water into his system. Eat sodium foods so that sodium may act upon other foods and so that it may neutralize the secretions and make the secretions alkaline, as well as the tissues. When you are acid, eat nothing but celery one whole day, and eat nothing but oranges and good rye bread the next day, then eat celery the third day and then chew something, for instance, raw bran and swallow the saliva and spit out the bran. Keep this up until you make your stomach more alkaline and then see how you feel. By making the stomach more alkaline, you can overcome indigestion. The reason that the eating of bran cures indigestion is because it constantly increases the saliva in the salivary glands which secrete the most alkaline secretions in the body. If you manufacture great quantities of these salivary secretions and swallow them, it will neutralize the acid in the stomach and thus overcome indigestion. Indigestion is always caused by acidity in the stomach or at least perhaps 90 cases out of 100. The eating of bran is no good for any other purpose except for making the saliva flow more readily. You could chew almost anything just so you get the saliva to flow freely. Do not chew gum, however, as you abstract and swallow the gum compounds and they are not good for the stomach.

Water decomposes in the stomach. Water drinking leads to diabetes, dropsey or acidity in the course of time. Decomposed water is subject to the formation of acidity and fermentation. The tissues are full of decomposed water. You cannot cure diabetes or dropsy by drawing out the water from the system. When the tissues lack sodium, potash and chlorine, the water in the tissues decomposes. This decomposed water, going to the kidneys, decomposes the kidneys also. If you suffer from dropsy, go to the hills and fall back upon foods that are rich in sodium, chlorine and potash—especially chlorine.

The lower types of people have more sodium in their system. They are seldom sick. The more highly organized man or woman does not have enough sodium and yet he or she needs more sodium than one of a lower type. Highly-organized people have too much phosphorus in the system. They are always burning up the phosphorus in the brain, and thus throw too much work upon the liver and other eliminative organs. At last, when the liver cannot function sufficiently or efficiently, the tissues become acid; the entire alimentary tract also becomes acid. Highly intellectual people suffer mostly from acidity.

We have been told that gout is caused by high living, but we find gout among the lower types of laborers also who live on the cheapest kind of food. We find gout among highly organized people. The Osseous or bony and Desmogenic people are the most intellectual and they are the ones who suffer from gout.

The more sodium the tissues take up, the more alkaline and stronger they become. Desmogenic people are the strongest people we have; they are strong because they have a great deal of sodium in their tissues, tendons, ligaments, joints. Almost all of the sodium foods eaten by Desmogenic people goes into the tissues, so that the spleen, the alimentary tract and the secretions, as well as the blood, are all robbed of sodium. Thus they suffer from sodium starvation; although their tissues are full of sodium. Desmogenic ladies are also powerful, in the majority of cases, unless they are sick from the lack of sodium and other important salts.

The synovial membrane secretes sodium. If there is a lack of sodium in the joints, the joints crack. Creaking joints show that there is too much calcium, and that there is a lack of sodium in the joints. There is a low supply of sodium. Creaking or cracking in the joints is a calcium-excess symptom.

You can digest albumin well if you have plenty of sodium and chlorine. When you eat the white of an egg, and you put plenty of salt on it, you can digest it better. Nervous people should never eat the white of an egg nor other foods that are rich in albumin. Tired nerves cannot handle albumin. A man who is pulling heavy loads, like a mule, should eat albumin or the white of an egg, but he should always put plenty of salt on it.

If you eat too much calcium in the form of foods and there is not enough sodium in the system, you are likely to suffer from rheumatism and stiffness everywhere.

If you bleed easily, there is not enough of fibrin in the system. It means that you are not able to handle fibrin nor manufacture fibrin because there is a lack of some salts.

A man who suffers from albuminuria, lacks chlorine and sodium. Breathing is difficult without sodium. There is more sodium salt in the ear and in the big toe than elsewhere and there is also more calcium in the ear and in the big toe; because of the great quantity of calcium those parts usually are subject to calcium deposits. Hence also gout starts in the big toe and sometimes also in the ear. An excess of calcium in the system results in boils of a special kind. If you suffer from gout, fall back upon a correct diet. Drink distilled water in abundance and fall back upon a low calcium diet.

Lack of sodium salt results in catarrh. If you suffer from catarrh, you need foods that are rich in sodium such as celery, spinach, lettuce, etc. Doctors usually say that the appendix is of no use indicating that the Almighty did not understand His business when He made the appendix. Doctors cut out the appendix; and yet, the appendix is a germ killer. It secretes a certain secretion that contains germicidal properties; this secretion kills a great many germs that happen to be in the colon. This is the function of the appendix and that is a very important function. The appendix cannot secrete this secretion if it is cut out. Then bacterial gases and toxins fill the colon and the entire alimentary tract.

The thyroid gland keeps poison from passing up into the brain. When the thyroid gland cannot do its work autotoxins pass up into the brain. This has a bad effect upon the brain function. When the Almighty made the appendix, the thyroid gland and a great many other glands, He knew His business, whether the doctors know this or not.

The saliva is rich in sodium. That secretion should pass into the food every time we eat. When the saliva does not pass into the food, some parts of the food are not so well digested. Hot applications, applied to the stomach, create action in the stomach and the bowels so that the excreta may pass out of the bowels and so that bowel gases may be dissipated.

Hydrochloric acid does not burn in the upper stomach. Such acid would be at the bottom of the stomach. The burning in the upper part of the stomach, which people suffer from who suffer from indigestion, is not caused by hydrochloric acid. A man who suffers from indigestion and burning in the stomach usually always lacks hydrochloric acid. Lack of sodium is another cause of constipation and also other salts. If there is a lack of sodium in the system, the brain cannot perform its function so efficiently.

If you injure the feelings or the purse or the interests of a Desmogenic man, he will always remember it. You may be good to him 99 times, but if you are bad to him or mean to him only once, he will remember that one bad deed forever. The Desmogenic man is often a stormy man. He has his ugly spells; he wants to quarrel and fight in between.

Gout is a disease that proves conclusively that there is not enough sodium to keep calcium in solution.

A sodium patient feels well one day and the next day he is sick. He feels that all of the time something wrong is going to happen. He is sleepy during the day and at night his brain is very active. His brain is very active after 12 o'clock at night. Then he plans and feels as though he can accomplish great things, but during the day he is always sleepy, always tired, always drowsy.

Lack of sodium results in palpitation, gas in the stomach, liver trouble, slow digestion, lack of the gastric juice and lack of the saliva. A sodium-hungry patient is hard to please. A wife cannot get very much love out of a husband when that husband suffers from sodium starvation. If your husband is ugly, because of lack of sodium, give him plenty of celery at every meal.

So sure as the sodium supply runs low, so sure you will suffer from weak eyesight. It is better to eat celery for weak eyesight than to go to an oculist. When the sodium supply is low, the memory is poor.

In 99 people out of 100 there is a lack of sodium rather than an excess.

A heavy potash diet requires from 40 to 60 times more sodium. If you live on an exclusive vegetable diet or on greens that are full of potash, more sodium is needed than you can supply. When potash passes out of the system, it precipitates from 52 to 65 ounces of sodium to every ounce of potassium. If you have an excess of potassium salts, you can overcome the effects of excess of potassium salts by introducing foods that are rich in chlorine. All people should increase the sodium supply in the body by eating foods that are rich in sodium.

A hot climate uses up sodium salts in the body, and a very cold climate also uses up sodium salts. A love state enables a man to take up more sodium salts. Under favorable emotions, sodium is more rapidly assimilated or utilized; but under unfavorable emotions or passions, the sodium salts are precipitated and appear in the urine. A loving state of mind is favorable to health. Temper, excitement, jealousy and ugly melancholy passions, always have an unfavorable effect upon the chemistry of the body or upon health.

The sick man requires sodium salts or a sodium diet. People between the ages of 7 and 21 do not require very much sodium for at that time, the body is usually alkaline. When sodium runs low, it means malnutrition and this malnutrition even terminates in tuberculosis.

Sodium excess is usually excess of sodium in the tissues not in the secretions. There is never an excess of sodium in the blood and secretions; but there may be an excess of sodium in the tissues, in the joints, as for instance, in the Desmogenic man. Let a chemist analyze a Desmogenic man and give us a report of the analysis.

The gossiper is usually lean, broad-headed, sharp-nosed and has drawn lips. Such a lady knows what is taking place in the neighborhood. She thinks every man is a rascal and that every woman is a flirt. The gossiper is the "Devil's neighborhood directory."

When sodium is lacking, the nerves are on fire, judgment is unreliable, concentration is poor and there is a greater tendency to sunstroke or heatstroke.

The sodium man is different from the calcium man. The calcium man is persistent; his diseases are persistent; his love, his anger, studies, are all persistent.

When you require newer and newer spectacles, you are in the greatest need of sodium-containing foods such as celery, strawberries, raspberries and others.

The Desmogenic man is a real sodium man. He has sodium in his tissues, but not enough in the blood nor in the secretions nor other fluids.

If a Desmogenic man gets interested in some special thing, it is difficult to get him to stop. If he is interested in a certain science he never stops until he has mastered the science in every detail. Try to stop him and you increase his interest and determination to go on. If he falls in love, he cannot stop, he must go on. Try to force him, and he will soon stop. We can never force a Desmogenic man, nor a Desmogenic woman.

When a man suffers from flu, you should analyze his urine. When he suffers from pneumonia, you should also examine the urine. If you do, you will find that the blood salts are precipitated from the body; in times of flu and pneumonia you should supply the blood salts and forget almost everything else. Supply sodium salt or supply blood salt and you will cure flu, unless the disease has progressed to such an extent that the flu germ has taken full possession of the body, in which case the man will die. When all of the chemical food salts are supplied in the body there can be no symptoms, no ailments, no peculiarities to bother you and others. You are simply healthy. Indigestion is caused by a lack of hydrochloric acid or it may also be caused by inflation of the stomach, inflated by gas. Foods containing sugar, starch or fat are converted into gas when the stomach is acid. Gas in the bowel produces sleeplessness. When you cannot sleep at night, it is because of gas generation in the bowel or because of acid formation. Do you think it is wise to go to a doctor and have him give you morphine at a time when you cannot sleep, when this sleeplessness is caused by gas or acidity? One-sided headache comes from the bowels.

A certain eruption on your chest or on your backs, arms or neck is caused by lack of sodium in the body. The best way to improve your complexion is not by going to a beauty specialist but by eating plenty of celery when the skin is murky from lack of sodium.

When there is a lack of sodium in the system, there is anxiety around the heart. A person must stop to rest while walking, because his heart bothers him. When the tissues feel bruised or seem bruised without any seeming reason, there is lack of sodium. When the urine sinks in specific gravity there is a lack of sodium. Urine is nothing but tissue water passing away from the system. You can tell by the urine what is going on in your tissues.

If you increase the sodium supply in your system, you increase saliva. If you increase salive, you increase the flow of the gastric juice and by increasing the flow of the gastric juice you increase digestion. When there is a lack of sodium and you go to a doctor, he is likely to think there is perhaps a tumor in your stomach or that you suffer from cancer or that you have an ulcer. In fact, he is very likely to think anything. If he doctors you, he cannot cure your disease. Sodium, chlorine, magnesium and potash are the food chemicals that enable your stomach to carry on its functions. When these elements are lacking you suffer from constipation and autointoxication, gastritis and many other ailments. A burning pain in the upper part of your stomach is an indication that there is a lack of sodium.

A minister of the gospel should be a dietician. It is not easy to pray when you suffer from indigestion. It is not easy to be a good Christian when there is acid and poison in the stomach and bowel. A minister should tell his congregation what to eat. We imagine that the prayer of a Dyspeptic does not go very high, perhaps no higher than the ceiling.

Your stomach is a laboratory. If you put fermentable food into your stomach the food ferments. If you put acid food into your stomach, your stomach will become acid. When you suffer from congestion in the bowel or when you are consiptated, you should remember that foods rich in magnesium, sodium, chlorine and potash will help. Drink salty water at such a time, it will help.

Chlorine is another salt that the Almighty put into the system to improve the metabolism of starch, fat, sugar, albumin and protein.

If you wish to convert fat into heat, you should eat potash-containing foods, sodium-containing foods and silicon-containing foods; those salts are necessary for the purpose of converting the fat into heat units. If there is not enough oxygen, sodium, chlorine, potassium, iron and silicon, all of which are tissue salts, you cannot convert fat into heat units nor can you convert sugar into heat units. You cannot convert fat into calories without breaking down some of those salts.

People are more nervous in hot, sultry weather, because of lack of sodium. Heat or sultry weather, precipitates the salts. People are in danger of heart trouble during July and August, when the heart is weak. You are in danger of heart failure yourself, even when your heart is strong, during July and August, if there is a lack of sodium salt in your system. During the Fall and Spring, and in the evening, there is a great deal more carbonic oxide in the air. At that time, the fever of the consumptive increases and keeps increasing until about 12 o'clock at night. Then the fever passes away, perspiration starts and he suffers from exhaustion and night sweats.

The Almighty never intended that we should drink ordinary water, full of germs and minerals. He made vegetables and greens which contain from 50% up to 98% or more of water. In greens and vegetables, we get organized water. That is the kind of water needed in the human organism. The sodium supply is lowered by drinking ordinary water or in fact any kind of water. Water-drinking washes the sodium salts out of the system. People are drinking too much. They are drinking coffee, ice cold water, chocolate and all sorts of drinks not good for the stomach nor for the health in general.

The harder you study, the more sodium you need. Have you noticed that your perspiration is salty?

Temper and excitement uses up sodium salt. The more high temperature, the more you burn up or destroy sodium salt. At last you will suffer from indigestion because of your temper. It is much better to cultivate affection than to cultivate temper. If you cultivate love, you will cure your indigestion; but if you cultivate temper, you fill your system with toxins and impurities.

A mother needs calcium, sodium, iron and silicon in abundance because the baby is taking up all of those salts and a great many others. Morning sickness is an indication of a lack of sodium. Supply sodium in abundance and morning sickness disappears. Gizzard contains an abundance of sodium. The coming mother should eat gizzartds, drink gizzard extracts and eat plenty of celery. This will cure morning sickness. Menstruation is impossible when there is an absolute lack of sodium and iron salts.

Fluorine, sodium and chlorine are the three salts that the spleen needs. The spleen is the most bloody organ in the body. The spleen has a good deal to do with the circulatory system and the vital organs. The spleen is also the dumping ground for the red blood corpuscles as we have been told by physiologists.

When there is a lack of sodium, the canal walls become more and more covered with calcium salts. To get the calcium out of the walls of the stomach or out of the canal walls, out of the arterial walls, it becomes necessary to eat sodium foods in abundance. The very best way to cure arteriosclerosis is before you get it, merely by eating foods that are rich in sodium.

There are two functions of sodium going on in your body—tissue sodium and free sodium. Tissue sodium is found in the tissues. Free sodium is used by the functions.

Sodium, potash, chlorine and fluorine are needed when germs are prolific.

Milk is full of calcium salts. When there is an excess of calcium salts in the blood or in the tissues, boils are prolific.

FOOD ANALYSIS EXPLAINED

CARROTS are one of the very best foods we can eat. They may be eaten raw or cooked. If we cook them, we cook out most of the sodium salts and if we pour the juice into the sink, we pour the salts into the sink also. If you cook carrots, do not use very much water, then drink the water; or steam the carrots. Carrot juice is excellent for the kidneys, liver, digestion and the bowel. Carrot juice makes the stomach walls alkaline.

CELERY. You may think that celery is of no special value, but it is of the greatest value to the nerves and brain. It supplies sodium to the tissues, organs and secretions. Celery is important because it is rich in sodium. It has a neutralizing effect upon the tissues and nerves.

When you suffer from gas generation, press out celery juice and drink it in abundance. Eat celery for one whole day, two days, three days or a week if it is necessary. If you are not then well, eat celery another week, and do this until you feel better.

LENTILS are rich in potash, but they do not contain much silicon or sulphur. Eat lentils together with food containing silicon and sulphur when you suffer from dropsy. A salty, dry diet will save you, but drugs will not—and operations will not.

ALMOND NUTS are said to be the "king of nuts." They are rich in nearly all the elements needed by the body but they are low in silicon and chlorine. This is the reason that you should salt the nuts. They are rich in phosphorus and are therefore good for brain workers. Do not eat almond nuts by themselves; eat them with other foods. The skin outside the nut should be taken off, as it contains certain toxins which are not good for your system. When you bake almond nuts, they are improved, providing you use plenty of common salt. Bake the salt into them. Do not eat bitter almond nuts, for they contain a small percent of Prussic acid, which is a very energetic poison.

PISTACHIO NUTS. They are high in sodium and contain also fluorine in a small quantity. Those nuts are valuable in times of indigestion caused by a low sodium supply.

OKRA is rich in sodium and chlorine. Eat okra in conjunction with other foods. No other food is so rich in sodium and in chlorine.

SPINACH. This is one of the best foods we can eat. When constipated because of lack of potassium salts in the alimentary tract, eat spinach and more spinach and still more spinach. Stasis is that kind of constipation which is caused by lack of potassium. It is cured by eating plenty of raw spinach, cooked about 3 minutes in its own steam. When you eat spinach, be sure to wash it in running water and cut into fairly small pieces. Sprinkle it with distilled water and cook it in its own steam for 3 minutes. Spinach contains all the salts needed by your system. It is especially rich in potassium salts. Spinach also contains iron salts.

STRAWBERRIES should be fresh. They must not be decayed nor unripe. If a strawberry has a white end, do not eat it. Do not eat hot-house strawberries. Do not pour cream on strawberries and do not put any sugar on them. Eat them as the Almighty made them. Strawberries are excellent for gout. Canned strawberries contain too much sugar. The manufacturers spoil strawberries by canning them in sugar.

SWEET APPLES are good, if eaten raw. If you bake apples, do not use much sugar. Always use sweet apples not sour. Sour apples are too high in malic acid.

ASPARAGUS is good for indigestion. It contains sodium, also sulphur. Of course, sulphur is not very good for indigestion but the sodium salts are. If you have an acid stomach, the sulphur contained in asparagus, is turned into gas.

BEETS are rich in sodium and also sugar.

COCOANUT contains an acid called myristic acid. The kind of fat that cocoanut contains has a remarkable reconstructive effect upon the chest in ladies. Cocoanut contains no iron but it is rich in chlorine. Cocoanut is excellent for the nerves and for the brain and lung substance. For some reason not known, cocoanut, in connection with breathing exercises, will build up a very large chest in ladies, the same as cream and buttermilk will enlarge the lower bowel and the hips.

CUCUMBERS are rich in sulphur. They are very cooling and therefore an excellent food during July and August when it is hot and sultry.

EGG YOLK is lecithin. It is rich in the vitamins. It contains nerve salts, brain salts, fluorine, protein, fat, iron, sulphur, calcium, phosphorus and a certain digestive principle called diastase. The white of the egg should not be eaten except by the man who does hard, physical work. The brain worker needs the yolk not the albumen. Egg albumen is poison to the nerves; a nervous person should not eat egg white.

FIGS are rich in all the salts. They are especially rich in calcium, sugar and worms. People who eat figs may be sure they are also eating worms, but fig worms will hurt no one except for the taste or sight of the worms. Figs are excellent for constipation.

FISH are rich in calcium, chlorine, sodium, potash, phosphorus but fish contain no iron, sulphur or silicon. We should eat foods containing those elements lacking in fish. Fish is good food for the brain worker because of the fat, phosphorus, chlorine and sodium it contains.

LOBSTER is full of phosphorus. Whiting and smelt are high phosphorus-containing fish.

GOOSEBERRIES are rich in potash, phosphorus and calcium.

COW'S MILK is good for calves but not for human babies. There is too much calcium in cow's milk for babies. No food is richer in calcium. It is also rich in potash and chlorine to some extent.

GOAT'S MILK contains the blood salts. Goat's milk and cheese are good for people who are weak in the medulla or in whom the circulation is defective. It is rich in fluorine. Outside of goat's milk, goat's cheese and pistachio nuts, it is not easy to get foods that contain fluorine.

STEEL-CUT OATMEAL contains a greater quantity of silicon than any other food. We find also potash and phosphorus in steel-cut oatmeal; also avenin, which is one of the most strengthening and stimulating principles for the sexual system.

PRUNES are good for people who suffer from constipation. If there is a lack of bile in the system, eat prunes and drink prune juice. But do not drink more than your body can assimilate. Remember that you have your limitations.

RADISHES are full of sulphur. When you eat radishes, be sure there is no acid in your stomach; for if there is acid, you will suffer from gas generation. The sulphur in the radishes will be converted into gas and this will pass into your red blood corpuscles.

RUTABAGAS are excellent for the tissues and brain. They are also rich in sulphur, but not high in sulphur. If your stomach is acid or if you already have too much gas, rutabagas are not a good food.

TURNIPS are fine for the tissues and the brain. If your stomach is acid, you cannot tolerate them due to the high percentage of sulphur contained in turnips. This sulphur will be converted into gas and will make you ill.

QUESTIONS AND ANSWERS

1. Are radishes difficult to digest? Answer: A medical doctor said that radishes are one of the hardest foods to digest and they cause acute indigestion. Radishes are not difficult to digest but they contain considerable sulphur. If your stomach is already acid, the sulphur is converted into gas and this is the gas that would produce acute indigestion. It is not the radishes but the sulphur in the radishes that produces indigestion. The sulphur in cabbage also produces gas. All sorts of sulphur foods produce gas when there is acid in your stomach but not otherwise. Radishes digest in about 38 minutes; they digest easily but they generate sulphur gas.

2. Why does a person get cramps in his legs at night? Will sodium cure it? Answer: Cramps in the legs are caused by low tissue oxidation, acid in the tissues and lack of the blood salts in the blood. Sodium food will not cure it but it will help.

3. What are the symptoms of albuminuria? Answer: Albumin in the urine.

4. Are there any special gizzards from the fowls that you recommend or do you refer to chicken gizzards only? Answer: All sorts of gizzards are rich in sodium. Any gizzard is valuable.

5. Some of the sodium foods listed require cooking. How about the sodium above 130 deg Fahrenheit? Answer: Yes, some sodium foods require cooking. We should cook in such a way that we may preserve the salts. Carrots should be steamed, if not eaten raw. When we cook food in a very high heat, foods are not so valuable.

6. If the central nervous system of an insane person is affected, would sodium foods cure him? Answer: No.

7. Are there any food compounds in the body besides sweets and water that destroy sodium salts? Answer: Yes.

8. How should gizzards be used? Whole or just the outer skin or the meat? Answer: The inner part. It is not the skin that is valuable but the inner part.

9. Is there any sodium in egg plant? Answer: Yes, but there is so much acid in egg plant that it will make our stomachs more acid.

10. Should celery be eaten alone at a meal? What foods should be eaten with celery? Answer: Celery may be eaten in any way you choose. Any foods may be eaten with celery, the same as you may eat any kind of food with spinach or carrots. And why? Because such foods are rich in sodium salts. You should always eat some kind of sodium-containing food at your meals. The more starch, fat or sugar you eat, the more you should eat of sodium-containing foods.

11. If sodium decomposes water, is it well to drink celery broth made from the coarse parts and leaves? Answer: Sodium decomposes water, but celery is organized sodium and does not decompose water in the stomach. It helps to organize water instead of decomposing it. When we eat celery or any kind of sodium food, we should not drink water.

12. Do celery seeds contain much sodium? Answer: Yes. They are rich in sodium, also in potash and sulphur.

13. Which is the best way to obtain celery juice? Is there any way to keep it for any length of time? Answer: You should never try to keep it for any length of time but use it right away. The best way is to use a press.

14. Does the body need more sodium than any other salt? Answer: No. The body needs more chlorine than any other salt.

15. Does the continued use of drinking salt water have a tendency to harden the arteries? Answer: If there is a lack of sodium salt in the system it will.

16. Can a man lack hydrochloric acid and still have acidity in the stomach? Answer: Lack of hydrochloric acid would result in acidity. It should be remembered also that there are many different kinds of acids in the body. One kind of acid is caused by phosphorus products; another kind of acid is the result of carbon products; and still another kind of acid is a result of sulphur products. There are many kinds of acidity.

17. What chemical salts do the stomach lack when beans are hard to digest? Answer: Sodium and chlorine salts.

18. What is the cause of bilious headache? Answer: Lack of sodium, chlorine and magnesium.

19. If sodium is precipitated in times of great heat, how will hot celery water effect inflammatory rheumatism? Answer: Precipitation of sodium salts by external heat or by excess heat in the blood or by inflammation in the stomach or by inflammation in a joint, are very different processes of precipitating sodium in the system than the application of celery water on an affected rheumatic part. If you apply hot celery water applications to a rheumatic part, you are simply reducing the inflammation, that is all. Inflammatory rheumatism, however, is not caused by precipitation of sodium salts so much as it is caused by a certain germ. Inflammatory rheumatism calls for dry heat.

20. What can be done for excessive sodium in tissues? How can it be equally distributed to blood, fluids and secretions? Answer: If the tissues take up too much sodium, it requires time and patience to overcome this tendency.

22. What difference does it make if sodium salts are in solution in the stomach by the drinking of water at meals? Answer: If there is much water in the stomach, the sodium and chlorine will mix with the water and pass out of the system through the kidneys.

FOODS AND CHEMICALS
CALCIUM

Calcium is the same as lime but not exactly. Lime is calcium-oxide, while calcium is an element. That is one reason why we should not drink water from a hydrant, well, river, for the simple reason that all such waters, without exception, are rich in calcium. Calcium which is inorganic, cannot be taken up by the human system. It will collect in the various structures of the body and produce many ailments and diseases.

In Calciferic people, oxidation is always low. In people of the phosphoro-calcium type (Atrophic), oxidation is exceedingly low; in other words, there is a great affinity between people of the Califeric constitution and the Carboferic, Sillevitic and Exesthesic. Calcium usually associates itself with sulphur, silicon and carbon.

We study plants and soils, but we forget man. Why is that? People of the Atrophic constitution, Carboferic constitution, Pathetic constitution, Hydripheric construction always suffer from calcium deficiency. They seem healthy. They are fat, yet they have no strength, or power because they do not get enough calcium. Calcium is the fertilizing agent; it is the tiller of the soil. It is also the tiller of the human soil in the human organization. The various soils are compelled to give up their vitality under the influence of calcium.

Mothers who are of the Calciferic constitution bear from five to fourteen children or more. Calciferic mothers give rise to strong children. Carboferic mothers give rise to weak children. You look at a Carboferic girl and you think she is very beautiful. You marry her. Then you find she has no strength. You have to prepare your own breakfast, sweep the house and do everything yourself. When it is a question of reproduction, you get a baby that is a weakling. You work all your life to raise that baby. You bury your wife when she is about 45 years old and also your children.

The Carboferic often has a sour odor. If she sleeps in a room, the room itself may have a sour odor. It is because there is not enough calcium in her system. Every person who has calcium in abundance is clean, on the inside, although he may be dirty on the outside. The calcium man does not need to clean and brush because the calcium takes care of that. Calcium is a deodorizer. It throws out impurity. If there is plenty of calcium in the system, there is greater vitality, there is stronger sexuality, there is greater cleanliness.

We learn that hens lay better and more eggs when they are fed cracked oyster shells and food rich in calcium. The farmer has found this out, but the human farmer has not found it out, neither has the doctor, nurse or cook. If we want to give rise to gifted children, we should eat foods rich in calcium during the period of gestation, because then the mother is laying the foundation for the life of her baby. That is the time that calcium salts are being used up. If that mother-to-be is not sufficiently supplied with calcium, she is in danger of disease after she is through with gestation. Most milks are rich in calcium. There is 24% of calcium in cow's milk and in mare's milk more than 24% of the salts contained because the colt and calf must build bones, horns, hooves. Therefore, cow's milk is not the best food for the human baby. The baby does not build such big bones; the baby does not build horns, hooves or a heavy hide. The baby that cannot get mother's milk is to be pitied.

You can never get a product as good for the baby as mother's milk. It contains only 4% of fine sugar. Some infant foods contain a great deal of cheap sugar; therefore, they will do your baby more harm than good. We should pass up science when we get so scientific that we kill the baby with our science and "scientific" food.

The rain water is at work in the rocks manufacturing calcium. We do not know that it is calcium that makes the bones of man. We do not know that it is phosphorus that is in the brain. We do not stop to think that those inventions, arts, geniuses we admire, those excellent books on science and philosophy, are nothing else than stone talking to us.

The bones that we have are originally nothing but stone. They come from stone and go back to stone. We are nothing but living soil. A man with a great deal of calcium in his organization is a man of endurance. It takes him about 2 weeks to get angry, but once angry, it may take him, perhaps, 50 years to get over it. A calcium man never forgets. When a calcium man gets angry, you are dealing with a loaded man. A weak person, one of the Pathetic type or a Carboferic type, gets angry in a second but there is nothing to it. A man is loaded when he has considerable calcium in his organization. Look at those policemen and those criminals who empty pistols at each other and neither one falls. If a calcium man points a pistol at you, you are a deadman.

Many Russians are calcium men. Napoleon said that you would have to shoot a Russian and then push him down. Calcium people are slow, patient, steady, heavy. It is nothing but calcium that makes them so.

If people do not have enough calcium in them, their ankles are weak. Calcium and fluorine hold the bones together. When a child is slow in walking, it is because there is not enough calcium in its system. That child needs a sensible doctor, cook and mother to give the right foods to that child so he may gain in strength. If boys or girls do not have enough calcium in their systems, they are feebleminded. Put them on calcium-containing foods. Keep them on a calcium diet for a long time and they will not be feebleminded any more.

If there is an insufficiency of calcium in the bones when they are being formed, when the solid structures are being formed, when vitality is needed in abundance, the child will be feebleminded. It cannot be helped until a heavy calcium diet is supplied.

A person interested in humanity should study every detail of diet. It is well to be a doctor, but we should be something else. It is all right to be a scientist, but we should depend more upon the Almighty and upon nature. We should use the science of the Almighty. He has given us our reason to use.

You have noticed sometimes that a person bleeds easily, more or less, of nose, chest, bowel, because of the lack of calcium. A man who bled easily went to a specialist and took serum injections for one year which cost $500. He bled just as easily as ever all because there was not enough calcium in his system.

If you want to learn concentration, do not waste your money on a concentration course, but fall back on a calcium diet. After you take a calcium diet, you will not need a concentration course. These are facts we are just finding out.

If you cut yourself and you do not have enough calcium in your system, the wound will not heal. Then you should fall back on a calcium diet. Some people suffer from hemorrhages of the lungs, stomach; they need a heavy calcium diet.

Calcium gives greater power to the heart. Judgment and motion of a calcium man are slow. He is a bit awkward, but he is sure. When he strikes, he strikes hard. Of course, a quick man can get out of the way before the calcium man can hit him.

If there is a lack of calcium, there is little vitalization. The calcium man has the most perfect offspring, if he has the right kind of a wife. If she is Calciferic or Isogenic, she will have gifted children. The most gifted children in the world come from Isogenic mothers.

If you were running an insurance company, you would make money by taking in only Calciferic and Isogenic people and refusing all others. That is something the insurance companies should do. They also should teach people how to take care of themselves. Then that insurance company would make more money.

If there were no calcium in the system, there would be danger of oxalic acid symptoms. There are many people who suffer from acid symptoms. When the tissues can find no more calcium, when the secretions can find no more calcium—the whole man will suffer. When the calcium salts are extracted from the body or when the body has been robbed of calcium, decomposition sets in.

What do you think of yourself as a mother when you buy the cheapest kind of candy and give it to your child at the time they are building bones? What kind of teeth will that child have when it is grown? Can you expect a child to build a good set of teeth on candy? The sugar we are giving children will use up the calcium. There is a very strong affinity between sugar and calcium. You can put teeth into a sugar solution and it will never affect them at all because the teeth have a coat of fluorine on them to protect them. But if you eat sugar, it goes down into the stomach and takes up the calcium, and your blood is robbed of the calcium, and your teeth do not get the calcium salts needed. The child becomes lastly a fermentation factory if the mother feeds it candy. That child will have poor bones and at last will walk on crutches, if at all. The thing to do is to take the crutches away from him; he must exercise; he must do something; he must be put on a calcium diet and kept on it. If you continually feed your boy or girl candy, sweets and starches, you may be sure that child will walk on crutches. When a person is building bone, calcium is needed for bone building.

To give the body one and one-half grams of calcium salts needed each day, a person would have to eat eight loaves of white bread daily; if you expected to get your calcium salts from white bread. Therefore you are compelled to fall back on some food that is rich in calcium. As white bread does not fall back on some other foods that are rich in calcium, in order to supply enough of calcium salts for bone and tissue. It would be better to give our white bread to our pigs. White bread will fatten pigs, but our child cannot find enough bone-building material in white bread and similar food products.

You must give your child foods containing fluorine because fluorine is a co-worker with calcium. Fluorine is a sort of a bone cement and helps to keep the bones together. If it were not for fluorine, the bones would fall apart like wall plaster.

All people have stomachs, brains, tissues, joints, blood, all people think more or less. All people require a certain degree of endurance. All people must concentrate their mind to a certain extent at least. If there is a lack of calcium in the body, the brain is too soft; and if there is not enough calcium in the system, the brain cannot use itself in concentrating processes. If you make a chisel of mush, you cannot cut through a stone wall with that chisel. If you make a chisel of hard steel, you can cut through any kind of a stone wall. So it is also with the brain. If there is a lack of calcium salts in the body, the body, including the brain, is too soft. Hence, also the brain has no power of mental concentration. And what good would it do to take lessons in concentration? Would it not be better to eat foods that are rich in calcium? If you want to improve your power of mental concentration, you should fall back upon a very heavy calcium diet and you should take heavy, persistent physical exercise.

The calcium man does not need a concentration course. He is so powerful in the processes of mental concentration that he would even concentrate himself into the asylum with his thoughts of invention.

People who are soft in tissue or Carboferic people, do not have enough power of mental concentration. Carbon people are very poor mathematicians, but calcium people are always better mathematicians. Where there is an abundance of calcium, there is greater power of mental concentration. All people who are low in calcium cannot concentrate their minds.

When we know all such facts, we smile at "concentration courses."

If you suffer from calculi, you should eat foods that are rich in sodium salts. A poultice of bran and milk will draw impurities out of a sore. A poultice made of milk and bran contains calcium or calcium salts; and, such a poultice put on a sore or a swelling containing ferments and impurity or sick blood, will draw the impurity, soreness, heat and inflammation out of that swelling or out of that sore.

A very powerful electric light applied to a sore, will kill a greater number of germ species; hence, also, a strong electric light applied to a sore or to a swelling where pus formation is taking place, will kill a great number of germs and thus help to heal up the sore.

We often talk scientifically but we neglect common sense. We should never neglect or forget what the Almighty has given us, viz. reason and common sense.

Milk is a fine food product. It is rich in calcium and also in a great many other salts. Sometimes you may suffer from a swelling in the knee or a sore; remember at such times that a milk cloth kept on that sore place as hot as you can stand it very often will cure that swelling and draw out the impurity in that sore. Even gangrene may be prevented to a certain extent, at least, by hot milk applications. Put on a bran and milk poultice for several days and you will be surprised how that poultice will help to heal up a sore or draw out the swelling. It is the calcium in the milk or bran that cures.

A man who has plenty of calcium in his system is never nervous. Other temperaments, lacking calcium, are always nervous. Women, as a rule, are lacking in the calcium element, as well as other salts; they are forever complaining about nervousness.

Diseases are chronic in Calciferic people. When a Calciferic man begins to fail, he reaches a climax. He goes down rapidly. It is difficult to cure his disease and medical men call his disease chronic.

It takes a Calciferic man a long, long time to gather knowledge or to learn or to memorize; but that which he does learn, he can use forever. He does many times more with his knowledge than any other man.

After we are about 35 years of age, we should cut down our calcium diet, especially if we are Calciferic people.

If there is a lack of albumin, fibrin and calcium salts and you cut yourself, the cut keeps bleeding. But when there is calcium salt, albumin and fibrin in abundance in your system, the sore heals quickly. Fibrin forms in the cut and the calcium salts will promote coagulation of blood in that sore and will soon heal it.

Nervous people are defective in calcium. If we pay no attention to diet, we cannot cure.

A Calciferic man believes nothing but science and facts. When a man has calcium in excess in his system, he becomes a skeptic and often a materialist. The more calcium a man has in his bones and blood and the smaller his back head, the more developed his brain at firmness and at combativeness. The more scientific the man becomes, the more courage he has. You cannot scare such a man. The more calcium a man has in his bones, the more of a critic he is.

Habits always grow and become permanent in a calcium man. The older he grows, the more set he becomes in the bone and the more stern he becomes. His wife can do nothing with him. If a calcium man becomes a clerk when he is young, he remains a clerk and dies a clerk. If he becomes an inventor, he knows of nothing but invention; he hears nothing but invention; he thinks of nothing but invention and he dies an inventor. If he goes to heaven, he will likely continue with his inventions and if he goes to hell he will in all probability, invent things there.

If you want to become a first-class salesman, I would advise you to fall back on a calcium diet and to develop the faculty of conviction, viz. combativeness. I would also advise you to inhale fresh oxygen in abundance and thereby develop your chest and your conviction power. This would be better than to take a salesmanship course. It is well to take such a course, but you should also remember the value of a calcium diet and the necessity of developing the faculty of conviction. If a salesman cannot convince he will not make many sales.

Mothers usually suffer from displacement after gestation because they have lost too much calcium and other salts in order to build bones and solid structures in the baby. Such mothers need a calcium diet after delilvery and also after lactation. When there is a lack of calcium salts, the breath is short; there is very little power in the lungs; respiration is laborious, as may be seen in the consumptive. It is difficult, at such a time, to take enough air and hold it long enough.

Colleges do not say much about the material that should be taken into the human machine. If we want to learn all about diet, we must leave the university and the medical college and also all other colleges for such colleges teach simply about proteins, carbohydrates, hydrocarbons and about a few "oses," such as hectoses, lactoses, etc. and "ides," as for instance, saccharides, bisaccharides, etc.

Calcium is the strongest element in the human body. By eating great quantities of sugar or sugary foods, we always reduce calcium in the body. Lime salts associate themselves with the sugar and are eliminated. If we live in the sentiments largely and eat sugary foods in abundance, that stops bone building to a certain degree. If we live in the will faculties and do very heavy persistent work, we build bone to a greater degree. Heavy exercises develop bone. The less we work as we are growing up, the less strength we will have in the bones and the smaller the bones.

A girl of a Vital temperament, who sits still all the time, who sleeps much and who reads novels, is likely to become so weak in bone structure that she could almost be said to be boneless. Look at the man who is carrying heavy planks and you will find that he has very heavy bones. Heavy, persistent work builds bones, heavy bones and compact bones.

The consumptive requires calcium, not because he lacks it, but because the calcium element is being deposited in tubercles in the lungs. Those tubercles are hardened calcium. When calcium is locked up in tubercles in the lungs, there will be an insufficiency of calcium. The consumptive may have plenty of lime salts in his system, but when the lime salts are locked up in tubercles, the blood is being robbed of its calcium and so are also the bones. Hence, the consumptive suffers from calcium hunger, although he has calcium in excess.

Calcium salt is one of those salts which is being consumed by the mother during gestation and lactation. Those are the two periods requiring calcium salts in abundance. Calcium is in great demand during this time. A mother who is carrying a child that is hungry for calcium at that very time will after the time of delivery, feel almost like an empty shell. Think of a doctor who is giving this mother suffering from calcium hunger, drugs instead of calcium foods. Later on, when she gets sick, perhaps from tumors, he performs an operation and calls this "science." All mothers who are giving rise to offspring, are in the greatest need of calcium salts during gestation and lactation. The milk function is almost impossible, unless there is a plentiful supply of calcium salts in the system at this very time.

Perhaps a mother may neglect the eating of such foods and drinking of such drinks that contain calcium salts, simply because she depends upon her appetite and eats according to her appetite instead of eating according to science. The less calcium we have in our system, the less we want. The less calcium a mother has in her system. the more calcium has been broken down in her body during gestation, the less appetite she will have for calcium. At last, when a dietician begins to supply that mother with the calcium salts or ordering such foods containing calcium salts in abundance, she may become sick; because when the system has been robbed of calcium salts for a long time—and they are suddenly supplied—they create a revolution in the system and the mother is likely to think that the food does not agree with her. That which we need may be the very thing we do not want. It may be the very food article that goes against us and that our appetite does not call for. The man who drinks whiskey has an appetite for whiskey, and he thinks that whiskey is the very thing he needs.

If there is too much calcium in the system, bones, joints, arterial walls, canal walls—here, there and everywhere in the body, too much calcium in the blood, too much everywhere in the body—it is likely to result in some sort of calcic hardening. Too much calcium in the blood results in epilepsy, especially when there is an insufficiency of sodium and chlorine.

Lower the calcium supply for 5, 6 or 8 months, and that man becomes sick. Try this, viz., a calcium-free diet on another man and he becomes sick. Try it on a third man and he becomes sick. They all suffer from the same thing. When we say this and know this through experimentation and observation, we know positively that we are on the right road. If we can make those sick men well by placing them on a high calcium diet, we know that we are doing the right thing. Unless we find such facts through dieting (all our knowledge is based on such facts), we are not scientific dieticians. Formerly I paid people to let me practice diet on them. Put a man on a one-sided diet or on a diet that does not supply a certain needed salt in the system and that same man soon becomes ill.

It is well to remember also in connection with experimentation through diet on human beings that we must not go too far, for if we do, the chances are that the body refuses to take up that same needed chemical food salt. If the body has been robbed of a certain chemical food salt for a long time, until actual starvation for that same food salt takes place, the body may never assimilate that chemical food salt again, then the man would die.

At that time, when we are most healthy, we should build up and not wait until we are sick. As a general rule, when we begin to build up, it is too late.

A man who lacks calcium has many peculiar symptoms. He is full of fear; something hangs over him; he thinks something terrible will happen; he is gloomy; he stays around the house and refuses to do anything.

When there is too much calcium in the system, it results in calcic diseases or in hardening, calcic acid formation, formation of calcic by-products and calcic deposits.

At about the age of 55, a man usually suffers from brain shrinkage. When that brain shrinkage is rapid, there will be a vacuum between the brain membranes and the skull. This causes a very peculiar sensation. If such a man lies down suddenly, he feels dizzy; he feels as if he is going down. There is danger of insanity. The brain rolls in the cranium because of this shrinkage and this may produce feeblemindedness or some form of insanity. A man, at this age, in whom the brain is shrinking, should take a long time to lie down. He should lie down gradually, a little at a time; and in the morning, he should get up slowly. Such a man must not bend down suddenly nor lie down suddenly nor arise suddenly.

A cataract is caused by excess of calcium in the diet. Calcium, chlorine and sodium are the three elements that keep the blood in condition. If there is too much calcium, there is danger of thrombosis. This may also happen when there is not enough calcium. Sodium keeps calcium in solution. Fluorine keeps calcium at work in the bones. Without sodium and fluorine, it would not be very easy to build bones nor would it be easy to keep calcium in working condition in the body, blood and in the bones.

When people grow old, they become stiff. Calciferic people, or bony people, are the most long-lived people that we have, yet they often suffer from calcic ailments or hardening.

Gout is taken from the word "gutta," which means drop. Doctors formerly thought that patients had a certain "drop" which traveled here, there and everywhere, something similar to mercury and they called this kind of ailment gout. That gutta or gout is caused by acid. This acid is everywhere. This is why it seems to the gout patient that the pain jumps, for the pain is first here, then there, then somewhere else. That stiffness in the bones, tendons, joints, is hardening, caused by calcium deposits. If a man eats calcium food all of the time, there will eventually be an excess of calcium and he will suffer from calcic ailments. You cannot cure a man like this by giving him drugs. You cannot cure him by punching his back, nor by giving him osteopathic treatments. There is only one way of curing him and that is by placing him on a calcium-free diet; also by giving him a high eliminative diet with plenty of foods that are rich in sodium, to keep the calcium in solution.

Calciferic people are the greatest constructors or builders that we have. They are the best engineers; they are the greatest mathematicians we have. They are highly scientific. They are for nothing but studies. Calcium people are interested in geology, and in all sorts of agricultural problems. The Calciferic man contradicts the minister. He is from Missouri. He tells the minister "Show me your God and I will believe in Him; show me where heaven is and I will believe in your heaven.

Every tubercular patient feels better in the morning. He feels worse as soon as the sun passes the Meridian. Then he grows worse until about 12 o'clock at night. After midnight, he breaks into perspiration; this is called night sweat. Then there is a change in temperature. The carbonic acid in the atmosphere is a change in temperature. The carbonic acid in the atmosphere is partly dissipated and there is more oxygen in the atmosphere. The oxygen increases more and more until the sun rises in the east; and it keeps increasing until about 12 o'clock noon. During all this time the carbonic acid in the atmosphere is decreasing. At this time, the tubercular patient seems better. We should put the tubercular patient in an airship and send him up into the air afternoons or after 12 Noon, and when night comes, so he may obtain Ozone in abundance. Then you could cure your tubercular patient quicker. He can never be cured, however, if you put him inside four walls in a sanitarium where there is no air, and give him one pint of cream and twelve raw eggs a day. This would surely kill him; and would not this be enough to kill anyone?

A calcium hunger patient cannot digest food. His appetite is stronger than his digestion. He overeats at every meal. The more he eats, the leaner he gets and the more his consumption increases. A tuberculosis patient should be placed on a dry diet. He should, however, not go according to his appetite. Appetite knows nothing about science. Appetite knows nothing about assimilation and digestion. Most Calciferic men are fond of whiskey, which is also the case with most Oxypheric men. The tubercular patient is weak in the sex brain, yet he is sensual and excitable because of inflammation of the sex brain.

Some people wonder how we can tell when a certain diet is necessary. This is very easy. Every food element, when it is lacking, has its own peculiar symptoms. Iron-hunger has its anemia; calcium-hunger has its tuberculosis and its catarrh and earache. Calcium excess has its symptoms in the form of poor hearing, poor eyesight, stiff joints, gout, chronic rheumatism, arteriosclerosis, irritability and so on. When we are acquainted with the symptoms peculiar to a certain chemical food element or the lack of the same, we know when that chemical food element is lacking or when it is excessive. Certain symptoms precede certain coming diseases; certain symptoms and diseases call for a certain diet. When a man suffers from anemia, we know that he needs iron for his blood. When a man suffers from cerebral neurasthenia, we know his brain is starved, and that he is in great need of a diet that is rich in phosphorus.

FOOD ANALYSIS EXPLAINED

CRANBERRIES generate hippuric acid in the system. When a person eats cranberries, there is always hippuric acid in the urine. Calcium is abundant in cranberries; but they do not contain salts except in small quantities.

CABBAGE is a very high calcium food. It is rich in vegetable calcium. There is a difference between vegetable calcium and animal calcium. The calcium which we find in milk is animal calcium. Some people can handle animal calcium better than they can vegetable calcium, which is the case with the Calciferic patient. Cabbage should be eaten raw or it may be eaten cooked if it is sauerkraut. Chinese cabbage is rich in calcium; it is also rich in sulphur. Some people can handle Chinese cabbage in its raw form. Those who eat it raw always get the vitamins. If you cook cabbage, you get only a dead food. Anything cooked is dead. Anything cooked, baked, fried, boiled does not contain any of the vitamins. Cabbage juice is a fine tonic if rightly prepared. If it is not, it is not a good food.

MILK. Cow's milk is high in calcium. Mare's milk is even higher in calcium. Cows and mares secrete milk very rich in calcium for their offspring are in need of calcium for heavy bones, solid structures, hooves, hair and hide. But mare's and cow's milk are not good for human babies. Babies do not build such items as hooves or hides.

KUMISS is high in calcium unless it is made from goat's milk or sheep's milk. There is much more calcium in cow's milk than goat or sheep milk.

LEMONS. When you buy lemons, always buy those that feel soft. This holds good in regard to oranges and limes. Never buy those that feel hard or have a thick skin. Citrus with thin skins are more juicy and they were ripe when picked. Thick-skinned oranges contain an acid that does not belong in the orange. Thin-skinned oranges contain more citric acid.

ONIONS contain calcium in abundance, also sulphur. It is the sulphur and oxygen acid that goes into the tissues everywhere when you eat onions. It is the sulphur in the onions that give you that odor. Do you remember what a girl sang, viz. "I am to remember the kiss you gave me, pet, you had been eating onions and I can smell them yet." If you eat onions you will have an onion odor for two or three days that will reach out perhaps five, ten feet away from you.

RHUBARB is a high calcium food. It contains also oxalic acid. There is no food so stimulating to the brain as rhubarb. If you have citric acid in the body and uric acid, you are in no danger; but if there is an excess of uric acid and you then eat some foods such as rhubarb, containing oxalate of lime, the two will unite and form a quadriuratic deposit, which will cause inflammation and you will suffer perhaps from chronic rheumatism; or perhaps from gout or arthritis. Arthritis is that kind of gout that lives in the joints. It is a diet disease. Rhubarb is injurious to a man who has that kind of acid in his system or who suffers from gout or chronic rheumatism.

SAUERKRAUT is a very good food—if prepared rightly or as the Germans prepare it. But if you prepare it with considerable vinegar or prepare it in some way that is not favorable, it is not good food. Remember that vinegar is acetic acid and this is bad for the liver.

SPINACH is a very fine food unless it is grown on hot beds. Spinach is high in chemical food salts. If you drink hard water for a long time you may be sure that the calcium in the water will collect around the kidneys and on the walls of the arteries, in the bones and in the walls of canals. Lastly, you will suffer from rheumatism and will become stiff and unyieldy. Your hinges will become rusty. Never drink ordinary water. It is not necessary for the Almighty has made foods that contain enough water even up to nearly 100%. He never told us to drink ordinary water. The Almighty distills the water for us through the vegetable kingdom and through rain. We should do the same.

LIMA BEANS are very high in salts, also calcium salts.

EGG YOLK is rich in the vitamins, if you do not boil it or fry it. You need not think the white of the egg is rich in vitamins, because it is not. If you cook the egg, you kill the life in the egg. A boiled egg is dead food. There is no life value in a boiled egg. There is no food of such high value to the brain and nerves as raw egg yolk. Raw egg yolk is full of life. If you boil eggs and set a hen on them, do you think you can get chicks? Certainly not.

GOOSEBERRIES are excellent. They contain potassium acid of high value for gonorrhea. The potassium acid in gooseberries and in red or black currants is simply fine for Medeic impurity. The pulp of the grapes does not have any vitamins. You find the vitamins in the seeds. Any food that reproduces itself or that germinates in the soil has the vitamins. It is the vitamins that are the life principles in foods, seeds, berries and plants.

GRAPES are said to be excellent for the complexion because they contain a small percent of arsenic; also because they contain grape sugar and tartaric acid. They should be used sparingly, nevertheless.

LENTILS. You can never get a better food than lentils. If you knew the value of lentils you would plant them and eat them to a greater extent. They give you all the protein your system needs and more. You could work like a mule on lentils. They contain more protein than beef. They are more easily digested; they have more of the organometallic salts with the exception of two of those salts. They are low in calcium.

LETTUCE is a fine food, if clean. Lettuce should be eaten with other foods.

HUMAN MILK is low in organometallic salts.

DRIED PEAS are high in salts and low in calcium. They are fine for a man who is stiff in the spine.

YELLOW PEAS are much better than any other kind of peas. You can cook these in steam at a temperature of about 125 deg Fahrenheit. You can work like a horse on such food. If you want to grow strong muscles, eat plenty of peas.

PRUNES are of value, not for all people, but for some.

WALNUTS are high in fat but low in calcium. Walnuts are an excellent food after the age of about 51 years when a man begins to stiffen up in the hinges. Lentils, peas and walnuts are high protein foods.

CHEESE. Goat's cheese is low in calcium but high in the blood and heart salts. It is a fine food for the old gentleman, the grandfather. This is true in regard to sheep's cheese. Such cheese does not fill the system with calcium. Goat's cheese contains blood salts in almost equal proportion. There is no food that contains the blood salts and the heart salts so equally as goat's cheese or milk. In goat's cheese and milk, we find fluorine that valuable element so essential in times of tuberculosis. There we find the salts that are needed in the blood and tissues; we find more of the salts in a more equal proportion than in any other food. That is why goat's milk and cheese are such valuable foods.

CUCUMBERS are valuable when sores do not heal; where there is proud flesh; when there is a tendency to congestion; when it is hot and sultry.

RADISHES are rich in sulphur-containing food but not in calcium.

Vitamins found in impure water, viz., germs, are the very kind of vitamins we do not want. They would send us into eternity.

When we study the percent of the salts, we mean the percent of the salts found in the various foods. For instance, when we say that wheat contains 2% of mineral matter, we mean that it contains 2% of mineral matter as compared to the wheat itself. But when we say that wheat contains 31% of potash, we do not mean that it contains 31% as compared to the wheat itself, but compared to the 2% of mineral matter found in the wheat. Or in other words, wheat contains 31% of potash of the salts found in wheat. We are talking about the percent of the salts and not the percent of wheat. Wheat bran is usually recommended for constipation, but wheat bran is not a cure for constipation, in very many patients. There may be an occasional patient who is benefitted by a wheat bran diet, but most become constipated by eating it. Wheat bran will not cure constipation in the Calciferic patient; it would increase the constipation. Bran is not a laxative food to the calcium patient. It is a good food for some people but not for the Calciferic. If you eat the bran raw, you get the vitamins but not otherwise.

All citrus fruits are high in calcium. Some people are sensitive to calcium as for instance, Desmogenic, Myogenic, Pathetic and Neurogenic people. Some patients get sick from milk because it is too rich in calcium. If we do not know types of patients as doctors we will doctor the people into their graves. One man is cured on a certain diet, another patient is killed on the same diet.

The main element in the Calciferic man is calcium. The Calciferic man is a sort of a calcium factory. He craves for foods that are rich in calcium. The Calciferic man thrives on a milk diet, because milk is rich in calcium. If you give a Myogenic patient calcium or milk, he becomes sick. The Myogenic man is a vegetable man; he likes greens, vegetables and nuts, but a milk diet will make him sick. The Neurogenic man or patient is a sort of a brain or nerve factory. There is a vast difference between man and man. People differ in chemical elements and in characteristics and therefore also they differ in dietetic needs. One man thrives on a fruit diet; another thrives on a milk diet. One requires a nut diet and another requires an eliminative diet. One needs a brain diet, and so on.

When we improve upon a certain diet, we are likely to recommend that diet to everyone. This is wrong. Just because a certain food cured one is no sign that the same food will cure another. We never stop to think that one person is different from another; that a certain disease in one person has one cause and the same disease in another may have another cause. We never stop to consider that one person has a different body chemistry from another.

The citric acid and the formic acid found in limes are beneficial for the nerves. There is nothing better than cucumbers for congestion of the blood. If the sexual system is too energetic, there is nothing better than the juice of limes and cold baths. If you want to break down fat, there is nothing better for this purpose than hot sour lemonade made without sweetner.

If your vitality is running low, do not drink pasteurized milk and do not give it to your baby. We are told that ordinary cow's milk is rich in germs. That is true. One teaspoonful of milk contains more than 40 million germs in many instances. It is not the germs we need, especially dangerous germs. It all depends on what kind of germs they are. It is not the germs in the milk at the time of milking that we need be afraid of, so much as it is the germs that have been added to the milk by the dirty milkman and his dirty cans and his dirty methods. Moreover, there is no food that grows germs so fast as milk.

When a prominent man recommends a certain food article, we are ready to recommend that food article also without knowing anything about it. When we pasteurize milk, we kill the vitamins, and we alter the chemistry of the milk. It would be much better to instruct the milkman to wash his cans, wash the cow, watch out for the germs flying around in the atmosphere and to have a first-class chemist inspect the milk cans; this would be much better than to pasteurize the milk.

In times of chronic rheumatism, we should fall back upon foods that are rich in citric acid and formic acid and in times of great nervousness or brain trouble, we are in the greatest need of such fruits or foods that are rich in formic acid. High-tempered people need fruits that are rich in formic acid. Sensualists need foods that are rich in formic acid. If you are excitable and you are subject to the growth of tumors you are in the greatest need of foods that are rich in formic acid.

QUESTIONS AND ANSWERS

1. Would calcium and fluorine foods help sober a drunkard? Answer: No. They would increase his drinking tendencies. A heavy calcium diet will increase drunkenness.

2. What is the best substitute for mother's milk for the unfortunate baby? Answer: Goat's milk.

3. What is the aura and is it more pronounced in some constitutions than in others? If so, which ones? Answer: It is an electrical condition or a magnetic substance in the human organization very closely associated with life, as I understand it. If you put your finger in front of the light, you will find that your finger is translucent. It is the life principle or the aura that makes it translucent. When the aura is gone from your finger, your finger is dead. When the aura has left your body, your body is dead. The aura is the soul in man; the soul that lives in the body is the aura. The soul in some people is larger than in other people. People who have a large soul are called magnetic; people who have a small soul are called unmagnetic. If you increase the aura or if you develop the soul itself, you will increase your own personalilty. People who have very strong back heads are interested in humanity; they have a larger aura or a larger soul. They are interested in humanity. Christ is a remarkable example of that kind of a man. Tolstoi is another example of a large-souled man. The aura is not exactly electricity in the body. Electricity has no aura, but a Christian, who has a large soul, always has a large aura. A Medium claims to see the aura in the dark; a Medium comes in contact with your aura and is able to tell what is in your mind. The Medium believes he is guided by a spirit or Indian guide, but he is not. They get the information from you or from some other human soul. Spirituality is of such a nature that it is symbolic. If you dream a symbolic dream, it will come true.

4. Will calcium make a Carboferic person stronger after he has attained his growth? Answer: Yes. It will make him strong if he will only work and make effort at the same time. A Carboferic man does not want to work, nor make effort in which event a calcium diet would not make him any stronger.

5. Would Calciferic and Desmogenic people be happy together? Answer: This would not be a

favorable matrimonial combination. They are not affinities whether they could live well together or not.

6. Do Calciferic people make good classical dancers if they move slowly? Answer: No. They would dance like oxen or in an awkward way. There is strength in a Calciferic girl but you would not like to dance with her; she would step on your corns.

7. Does cow's milk supply the calcium needed at the rate of a pint a day, for the adult? Answer: Yes, unless you are a constitution that cannot tolerate milk; in which case, you must get your calcium from the vegetable kingdom.

8. Is lack of calcium associated with rheumatism in a young person? Answer: No. It would not result in rheumatism but in acidity, and that acid could result in rheumatism.

9. What is calcium lactate? Answer: It is sort of a milk of lime.

10. When a Myogenic or a Desmogenic suffers from muscular rheumatism, what diet is the best? Answer: If a Myogenic suffers from muscular rheumatism, it is because of the condition of his blood. In the Desmogenic, it is caused by acid and lack of oxygen.

11. Kindly explain how hypertrophy of the heart and tricuspid regurgitation are brought back to normal condition when valves are pathologic. Answer: Take the water out of the system and fall back on calcium, potassium and chlorine food salts. Give a dry diet. It is necessary to manufacture fibrin also.

12. What is the cause of some people being born left handed and can they become right handed? Answer: The reason why some people are born left handed is because the right side of the cerebellum is the stronger. If you are right handed, the left side of the cerebellum is stronger. If a child is born left handed, it is better not to interfere.

13. Is Ozena or Atrophic catarrh caused by lack of silicon and will a silicon diet cure it? Answer: Not altogether; but it will help.

14. If a Myogenic man does brainwork only, is it not necessary for him to take regular exercises or become interested in athletics? Answer: The Myogenic should spend at least 6 hours out of doors every day and be in action; otherwise, he will get sick. He cannot sit indoors and remain healthy. The Isogenic man can sit at a desk 18 hours a day, where there is little fresh air, and work, work, work, day in and day out for 50 years, and feel great, as for instance, Edison. But not so with the Myogenic. He must be in action and outdoors every day.

15. What is the cause of a cystic tumor and what cures it? Answer: It is a watery tumor. Wherever there is dead tissue, water will form. It is cured by work, massage and a chlorine diet.

16. Are some types more subject to epilepsy than others? If so, what types? Can epilepsy be cured by diet? Answer: Yes. Some type are more subject to epilepsy than others. The Oxypheric, Calciferic, sometimes the Exesthesic. Yes, it can be cured by diet, when it is caused by diet.

17. Is not the fertilization of soil with manure instead of with chemical fertilizers or pulverized rock or coal ashes, the cause of germs on vegetables? Answer: Whenever fertilizing is done with animal manure there is great danger of germs. Chemical fertilizers are better.

18. What does a prominent zigzag vein on the temple mean? Answer: It means that hardening of the arteries is at work.

19. What are the leading faculties of the mechanical engineer? Answer: He is a mechanical engineer by reason of his temperament. The Calciferic type is the most scientific and successful mechanical engineer. But that does not mean that others are not good mechanical engineers also.

20. Can a person overcome an excessive development of the parietal region of the brain? Answer: Yes. He can overcome fear. He should develop courage; feel that he can do anything; fight anything; not be afraid to meet the devil himself. When a man feels strong, there is no fear in him and we cannot scare him.

21. Is a meat juice diet less dangerous than a vegetable diet? Answer: We should never live exclusively on a meat juice diet. That would not be a diet. It may be a tonic in time of sickness but meat juice would not constitute a diet.

22. How can we find out what constitution we are in order to know what our diet should be? Answer: Take a good look at yourselves. Study yourselves and take a first-class inventory of yourselves before a mirror; then determine your own characteristics, mentally and physically.

23. What affect has prayer on the brain? And why should we pray? Answer: We should pray,

not because God needs it, we should pray, not because other people need it, we should pray because it does US good. We should pray to bring blood to the areas of the brain that make us highly religious, so that we do not become un-Christlike, desperadoes, undesirable people. We should pray to develop ourselves.

24. What causes an Oxypheric to experience periods of exhilaration and periods of despair? Answer: Oxygen. The more oxygen there is the more fire there is. At last the fire goes out. This is the climax.

25. If there is no prenatal influence, can a literary genius spring from illiterate parents? Answer: Yes, indeed. We have noticed this hundreds of times. Very often a great literary genius gives rise to an ordinary child. Geniuses very often spring from ordinary parents; and the most highly educated parents very often give rise to simple-minded children.

FOODS AND CHEMICALS
SILICON

Silicon is contained in the outside of oats. People who use their brains a great deal use up the phosphorus element. If they do not eat foods that are high in silicon, eventually the system becomes acid. Phosphorus products lead to acidity. The starch in potatoes is a very different starch than the starch in oats. A diabetic can tolerate the starch in oats, but the starch in sugar, potatoes or rice passes through the kidneys.

Oats is a valuable food. You may think that wheat is the king of cereals, but barley is a much better food for man, and oats are still better, provided the outside of the oats has not been milled away. The miller takes almost all the outside and gives us only the inside. All chemicals needed in the human system are found in oats. The outside of the oats contains silicon to the extent of 39% of the salts. Meat and vegetables do not contain as much silicon as oats. Avena sativa contains avenin, and has a remarkable tonic effect upon the entire sexual system.

When goat experts want to increase the milk production, they give goats oats. Barley is next to oats as a silicon food. Agriculturists know more about the value of foods than doctors. Medical men do not know as much about goat milk as the experts. Avenin is valuable in times of neurasthenia. If you want to cure the brain, weak nerves and a weak heart, eat oats. There is no better tonic for the sex brain nor for the cerebellum. Eat oats in connection with goat's milk, spinach and carrots and you supply the blood salts in abundance.

A certain amount of silicon is used by the various functions. It is called free silicon consumption. The silicon that is used in the tissues, in the secretions and in carrying on the functions of life, is called free silicon. We must absolutely supply the silicon that is needed. Some is needed every day. It is impossible to build good nails, solid tissue, a good skin or to grow beautiful hair without silicon. Fall back on a silicon diet and take care of your hair roots, if you want good hair. You will be surprised how glossy your hair becomes in a very short time. Women of the silicon type have the longest and the most beautiful hair of all.

When a grandfather becomes weak and sick, we ought to give him various oatmeal dishes, so he can regain his former strength. Also give him raw egg yolk. We can keep well and strong and live a long time unless the digestive system gives out. When it goes, we cannot digest food. When a man cannot digest food nor assimilate it, he is beyond repair. So long as food can be digested, utilized and waste matter eliminated, we can build up again, and make a new man out of an old one. We can make blood, build a new stomach and a new set of bones in seven years. So long as food can be digested and utilized, that long it is possible to build and rebuild.

The alkaline food salts are sodium, magnesium, potassium, silicon. Those are the food elements that we must absolutely fall back upon.

Magnesium is the most essential for the nerves and brain. Silicon acts upon all sorts of solid tissue, which must be made strong; also upon the skin and hair. Silicon makes the more solid tissues alkaline. Potassium makes the muscles and vital organs more alkaline. Magnesium acts upon phosphorus products. Sodium keeps calcium in solution and acts upon the blood and digestive juices. After the tissues become acid, we get sick and no doctor can cure us. You may go to a hospital and be operated on, but when you come out you are as acid as when you went in. If you do not fall back on sodium, silicon, potassium and magnesium, the Almighty's remedies, which He puts into foods to make the tissues alkaline, it is impossible to get well. So long as the tissues are alkaline, we can keep well. Those alkaline properties are the Almighty's remedies. He is a better specialist than any specialist in our hospitals. I believe the Almighty understands His business. He puts those elements into the human organization to keep it alkaline. Silicon should never be forgotten. Silicon is found in barley and oats, but barley is acid producing. Oatmeal food is more beneficial to the human organization.

The sheep is a silicon animal. The goat is too. The goat always likes high places. People with considerable silicon in their organization always like high places. Goats and other silicon animals are fond of silicon-containing feed, grasses, leaves and grains. You can put any kind of food in front of goats, but if you put oats in front of them, they devour the oats first.

There is nothing better for impotence than oatmeal, raw egg yolk, iron, phosphorus and sleep. Any one suffering from sexual weakness will become more invigorated by such a diet. If a wife would fall back on an oatmeal diet, she would be more able to retain her husband's affection.

Neurosis is a nerve habit, as for instance, the "writer's cramp." In such an ailment, silicon, sulphur and neurolin are used up in the nerves. Neurosis is in the nerves. In times of nervous debility, fall back on oatmeal. Eat oatmeal muffins. They are essential in an alkaline diet. So long as the tissues are acid, so long as there is acidity in the secretions, so long as the sexual system is acid, that long we will be weak and sickly.

Silicon has a remarkable effect upon the intellect or that part that thinks and observes. Take out that part of the brain and we are as helpless as babies yet we may have as strong a will as we ever had. Then we are human beings without intellect. We are next to animals. The monkey has no brain in front of the fissure of Rolando; it has no tophead. A man has a different head from the monkey. A man has a large tophead. He also has an intellect which a monkey never did have and never will have.

Love acts as an invigorating tonic and is of the greatest value in sickness. A love life often cures some people. It is not generally known that formic acid is of value to the brain and to the performance of the functions in some of the tissues. When there is a lack of formic acid, there will be a lack of the necessary salts and then there is a greater tendency to insanity. The insane people in hospitals are people in whom those important salts are lacking.

If a man does not have any silicon, he lacks "sand," or courage. Silicon increases courage. Silicon people are never afraid. A silicon man would fight a half dozen other men. It gives a man as stated before "sand."

Vaccination serum is harmful to the tissues. That serum breaks down important salts. Oatmeal diet is important in times of such infection. Silicon, in connection with potassium, prevents paralysis. When the cerebellum contracts to such an extent that it cannot obtain blood, the patient is paralyzed. Sometimes you may suffer from sewer gas poison; then you should fall back on a silicon diet. Silicon has a beneficial effect upon the various tissues of the body.

If you show the children where there is a sandpile, they will run to it and play from morning to night. If a child suffers from eczema, give him a silicon diet and let him play in a sandpile when the sun is shining down on him.

Silicon is beneficial for the nerves, the canal walls, alimentary tract, lungs and the entire system. If children are not supplied with silicon, they suffer from catarrh. Catarrh develops in membraneous tissue or in canal walls. If we supply silicon in abundance, we become more alkaline; we feel as if we could do anything. A silicon man is here, there and everywhere. He is like a goat. He likes to be high in the air. The goat likes to get up among the highest rocks. Silicon people are elastic and prone to exaggerate. They see everything through magnifying glasses (imagination). It is nothing else than hyperbolism. They exaggerate. Alkaline people are imaginative. They are busy all the time. When they are not talking, they are singing. Silicon people are just like goats in disposition. You find silicon people mostly among the Swiss. The Swiss girls have the most beautiful hair in the world.

I have never seen a silicon type talk long on any one subject. There are two elements that make us feel important: One is silicon, the other is phosphorus. If there is an excess of phosphorus a man feels like a king. He walks with a stately bearing. The only difference between silicon people and phosphorus people is that silicon people talk, while phosphorus people stand and look. The silicon man talks all the time, looking this way and that. He talks on a thousand different subjects. He acts like a goat.

The silicon man is sociable, just like the goat. If you buy a goat, be sure you buy two. If you do not buy two, you will lose the one you buy. That is the way with goats. The silicon man is the same. He can never be by himself. A silicon man does not need very much sleep. He may retire at one and sleep until four. Some Desmogenic people do not require very much sleep. Silicon people never live to be very old. They become so excessively active that they simply wear themselves out. They are like electrical motors. Full of activity. They think anything they go into will succeed. They are moved by a child-like hyperbolism.

There is a similarity between silicon hunger and tuberculosis. Both affect the patients to such an extent that they become anxious about themselves. They cannot forget themselves for one minute of the time. They tell you all about themselves. They talk about their symptoms, diseases, diet and wants. They are not interested in the scheme of the world. They just want to talk about their own selves and their own ailments.

Silicon hunger patients think they are going to die. They cannot bear noise. When they are tired, they cannot get hold of their thoughts; they cannot form ideas; they cannot recall subjects. They feel as if they are losing their minds. They may have everything they could wish for, but they think they have nothing to live for.

When a doctor gets hold of a silicon patient, he is likely to send him to an asylum for the insane. If you are a doctor you should build your sanitarium in the hills, where the goats thrive, in a high altiltude, a sandy soil.

Silicon patients perspire on the head and face. If you tell them to look at some certain thing and keep looking at it, they look, then look away; they get restless and uneasy. They have very little control. It seems as if the brain itself is loose. They suffer from catarrh in the lungs, throat, stomach; catarrh somewhere. They are spitting and coughing. They should eat foods that are rich in the organic elements and should cut out starch, fat and sugar from their diet. There are not very many foods that are rich in silicon.

When you are using your intellect, you are also using your cerebellum, because you can never talk or reason without using cerebellar energy; it is the function of silicon to supply cerebellar energy. If you feel exhausted or overworked, fall back on silicon. It does not feed your brain, nor your nerves, but it stimulates them. That is the way silicon acts. It tones up the cerebellum and the motor nerves. When there is a normal amount of silicon in the system, the brain and nerves are stronger. Increase the silicon and the nerves become strong. But if you do not work, you cannot assimilate silicon. Silicon requires action. When we labor, we take up a greater amount of silicon. But if we sit around, ride in automobiles, never walk, we do not take up silicon and we grow weaker.

To increase silicon in the body, leave fats, starches and sugars alone. Eat plenty of oats and oatmeal and you will grow stronger as you increase the silicon in your body. People in Southern California where there is sandy soil, high altitude, dry climate, have engaged in the goat industry. Everything there favors silicon metabolism, both in goats and in people. People in a cold climate are disagreeable as in Colorado and Montana. But in California, it is dry, the altitude is high, sandy soil and the functions of the people are more alkaline and the dispositions more genial.

When silicon is in excess and when it is lacking, it affects the nervous system. A silicon hunger patient complains that his teeth are aching. Pathophobia is a disease which causes him to think that other diseases are creeping upon him and he thinks that he can never get cured. Alkaline diseases and alkaline gout, so far as I know, we can never touch with diet. When the cerebellum is exhausted, you suffer from a neurasthenia called psychentonia; you cannot memorize, you cannot see nor hear as you should.

When the alkaline elements are too excessive, it results in suffering in the solid structures of the body. Too much silicic acid causes suppuration in the bones and in the membranes. The silicon constitution is subject to excessive energy which is also the case with the Desmogenic and the Nervi-Motive, but the Desmogenic never suffers from the same kind of ailments as the Sillevitic.

If the frontal sinuses become catarrhal, you suffer from a catarrh because there should be a free outlet through the frontal sinuses. There is a sieve-like bone at the root of the nose, leading up into the brain; if this is filled with catarrhal mucus, your thinking, memory, concentration and health are unfavorably affected.

The nose has another function besides that of inhaling air for the lungs and that is the function of communication with the brain. If there is a stoppage in the nose, the perspiration of the brain is retarded, resulting in brain heat, coryza, stupidity and lack of energy in the brain's function. The perspiration cannot pass down into the nose. If the frontal sinus is closed up, there will be a multiplicity of ailments. When there is a lack of silicon, these nasal canals become catarrhal and filled with mucus, resulting in sickness. Our memory and faculty of understanding as well as other mental faculties, are inefficient. A certain amount of evaporatiove moisture passes from the brain through the nose every hour. If the nasal canals and the othmoid bone are congested, the brain avenues of elimination are closed, resulting in colds, catarrh, disturbances of the brain, headache and other ailments.

A great many people drink mineral water. We have heard from many sources that mineral waters are health, in various diseases. The climate at all mineral springs is usually beneficial and the altitude favorable. When a man or woman goes away from his own neighborhood or his own city that same man or woman is different in the new surroundings. If you take away the mineral water, there would be the same results, yet we are told it is the mineral water that does the work. Very often,

when the patient returns from the mineral spring, he is just as sick as before. In the majority of cases, those mineral waters do very little good. Mineral waters contain inorganic salts that do harm.

We should always remember that the human body is organic. And we should remember that everything we put into the body should be organic also. If we can find mineral springs in which the minerals that the water contains are organic, those salts would be beneficial to the human body. All substances, foods or liquids that go into the human body should be organic. If we drink mineral waters for any length of time, we will soon suffer from some kind of ailment. Hardening processes will take place in the body. The kidneys may have so much work to do that they may give out.

The kidneys make take up those inorganic salts. The kidneys cannot do the work and there will be kidney disease. We should never drink mineral water. If we can find a mineral water that contains organic salts, we may drink it, but not until them.

So long as a doctor does not know what kind of salts the body needs, and so long as he does not know which food salts are beneficial for certain symptoms, he is not a desirable doctor. If you ask physicians why they recommend some special mineral water, they may say because it contains iron or carbonic acid or bicarbonate of sodium. If you ask whether it makes any difference whether you take inorganic or organic mineral water, they will tell you that it is one and the same thing. Doctors should be very careful in regard to that which goes into the human machine—that which we eat and drink "Why should we drink mineral water anyway?"

We can find the necessary elements in food. If we need silicon, we find that in oats and barley. If we need calcium, we find it in milk and cheese. If we need chlorine, we find it in sauerkraut. We find sulphur in all sorts of cabbages. We find arsenic in grapes. Why should we go to mineral springs for these elements, when we can find them in foods?

If we need a higher altitude, we can go to the hills. We should remember that different temperaments require different altitudes. One doctor sent an Exesthesic lady to Pike's Peak. Long before she arrived there, blood came out of her nose and mouth. You cannot cure anyone with poison, and poison is what they study in most medical colleges. Studying poison will never enable us to cure man of his diseases.

The medical colleges should teach us the value of climate and altitude; the chemistry of the human body, foods, peculiar tendencies, diseases and functions of the body. If we were taught those facts in medical colleges, we could cure people and people would not talk against doctors, as they do now.

Because doctors cannot cure their patients, they send them to mineral springs to be cured. When patients go there and get well, it is because of the high altitude and favorable environments and not on account of the waters. When there are unfavorable conditions at home, it has a bad affect on health.

Perhaps it is the work the patient is doing that makes him sick. If he is a bookkeeper and sits all day, the mathematical centers in the brain become weak because he overworks those centers of his brain. Too much blood is brought to the mathematical centers and they become weak. The blood congests. When the vital centers become congested, there is trouble with the stomach. When the vital areas become congested, there is lack of nerve force. No energy is transmitted. The mechanism is weakened. We need all the knowledge we can get in order to cure people. We need electricity and all the "ologies" combined and still more. We need knowledge of diet and still more. We never can know too much when it is a question of health.

We cannot cure a man who is filled with impurities by putting poison into him. We must eliminate those impurities.

Silicon is needed when a patient thinks that something or someone is after him. A man who suffers from silicon hunger is in the same kind of condition as an electrical motor that has run itself out. Now he sleeps so you cannot wake him; then he cannot sleep. When he tries to talk to you, he tires quickly. He thinks there is some disease at work in his system.

I believe that if we would supply oatmeal, egg yolk, neurolin and marjoram tea in abundance to men they would never commit self abuse. Put such patients on a heavy diet of the above, give them cold applications on the central section of the body, sudden cold applications and plenty of massage; tell them to go on top of a high building and go through all sorts of massage; let the sun shine on the nude body, let them fall in love and they will soon be cured.

Weak kidneys require a silicon diet. The function of silicon is to keep parts in a first-class alkaline condition. A silicon hunger patient complains of being cold on the left side. Put a St. Vitus dance patient on a heavy oatmeal diet; keep him away from school; put him in a room all by himself and keep that room dark; let him sleep much; pay no attention to him; do not talk about him because when he hears it his ailments will grow worse. Chorea is a silicon symptom. We call it a disease, but it is nothing but a symptom the result of a wrong diet.

You cannot massage silicon into a patient, but give him a silicon diet together with the treatment. A silicon patient always staggers to the right side, never to the left.

Silicon is needed when the canals of the body close up (stenosis). When a patient tells you that his arm is upstairs and his foot is in the down, he suffers from silicon hunger. Silicon is needed when a patient craves stimulants.

When we know the symptoms and ailments peculiar to silicon hunger, we know the cure.

The cerebellum, in times of pregnancy, works like a factory. That is also the case in a silicon hunger patient. There is a peculiar cerebellar pulsation in the pregnant mother; also in the silicon man.

A man who does not have silicon in abundance in his system and becomes a father, does not transmit himself properly. That is one cause of defective offspring. We should give to our children the best we can. It is better to give children health and character than it is to give them a million dollars.

Supply silicon for the teeth in growing children.

The word "phosphorus" means to carry light; "phos" means light; "phor" means to carry. Carry light or intelligence. It is the element of intelligence. The silicon element works in membranes, bones, ligaments, skin, teeth and solid tissue. Phosphorus works in the brain. If there is no phosphorus, there is no cerebration.

If your patient suffers from headache, put hot applications on his head. If his headache stops it is a sign that he lacks sililcon. Massage will not cure that kind of headache.

One peculiarity of patients is that if anything is wrong with any part of the body, they always carry the hand to that part, unconsciously. You may be sure that is where the trouble is. If it is his head, face, sexual system, he carries his hand there. An insane man carries his hand to his head. He tries to think. His eyes are wide open, as if something is wrong. Coming insanity has this symptom also.

When you see a little boy on whom, all at once, there is a heavy perspiration on head and face, you know that silicon is lacking in that boy. When you have studied hard and have been deeply interested in your studies, at last the brain gives out and you do not care to think or study any longer. Your enthusiasm disappears. You lose interest in your studies. When you know those symptoms, you know there is a lack of silicon and lecithin.

A silicon hunger patient feels that he is going insane. He is sure of it and you can't make him believe otherwise. Suppose you want to experiment; you take your patient and give him foods high in silicon and no other foods and keep that patient on that diet and watch him. Ask him all sorts of questions. The constitution that lacks silicon is the one to experiment with. You must not take a silicon type. If I wanted to experiment, I would take a man who already suffers from excessive silicon consumption and therefore silicon hunger. Simply stuff him with silicon foods. Then write down those peculiar symptoms which he never had before. When you experiment that way, you will learn things you never knew before. It is certainly interesting. The more you understand types of people, the more interesting those experiments become.

Remember that silicon is found in the outside or in the peelings which are usually thrown away. When we peel the outside, we cut away all those important elements that the Almighty put there for us. When we get sick, we think we can get well and healthy by patronizing drugstores. When the housewife peels away all the important elements and feeds her family only the inside, she cooks them into the hospital.

All foods that enter the human machine should be organic, because we are organic, so everything must be organized. We should go to the vegetable and animal kingdoms for everything we need in the way of minerals.

Do not let anyone lead you to think that vitamins are found in the juices of foods. The juices are fine; but they do not contain the vitamins. Everything that produces life contains the vitamins. If you eat the raw seeds, the principles that germinate and grow you get the vitamins. If you boil the seeds, you kill the vitamins. If you eat boiled food, you eat dead food. If you eat boiled foods, you do not get all of the salts. If you do not eat the seeds raw, then you do not get the vitamins. The vitamins are always in the seeds. You get the vitamins in egg yolk if you eat it raw.

FOOD ANALYSIS EXPLAINED

BARLEY (unpearled) is one of the best silicon foods. Never eat pearl barley, because almost all of the salts have been taken out. Get the whole barley and buy a mill and mill it yourself.

Some barley preparations are hard to digest. If there is a tendency to fermentation in the system, you should not eat barley. Then eat oatmeal. If you are somewhat fleshy do not eat barley. Eat oatmeal; it will make you lean. Barley will make you fat. If you must put on flesh and if your kidneys are strong, eat barley and you will gain flesh.

If a patient has sores in his mouth, put him on a heavy barley diet. Give him barley drinks. If you are lean, a barley diet makes you fleshy. If you are fleshy, you can reduce on an oatmeal diet.

OATMEAL. If you are a Desmogenic type, you are active in the brain. Then you would gain on an oatmeal diet. Oatmeal is the highest silicon food there is. Silicon is on the outside of the grain not on the inside. Be sure the oatmeal you eat contains silicon.

RICE is very low in salts and low in silicon. It is inferior to oatmeal.

ASPARAGUS. The best asparagus is found in California. There is no corrosive acid in asparagus. It contains silicon to a certain extent.

BEECHNUTS contain nearly 3% silicon.

CABBAGE is an interesting food. Sauerkraut is better than cabbage, as it contains more chlorine. Sauerkraut is excellent for the nervous system. It has a cooling effect upon the brain. The Ocypheric has too much heat in the blood, nerves and brain. The Oxypheric is an active talker and uses his brain. When the brain is on fire, the liver and nerves are also on fire. This is excess of oxygen. The brain and nerves are burning up. They need sauerkraut and mulberry juice in abundance; also perspiration to get rid of some of the heat. They must turn that heat in the liver and the blood into steam or perspiration. Put them to sleep, and give them plenty of sauerkraut or any food that reduces heat.

CUCUMBERS. If you eat too many cucumbers, you may suffer from neuritis. But cucumbers are good, cooling food.

FIGS are high in salts and sugar. You find plenty of worms in figs. You find worms either on the outside or the inside or both. If you eat figs, you will eat worms, but that does not make any difference. The fig worms can never hurt you. We should eat figs because they are rich in those salts. But if we eat too many figs and cannot take care of the sugar, we may have trouble. That extra sugar may be converted into gas.

HORSERADISH is a stimulating food. It stimulates the brain, blood and tissues. We should not prepare horseradish in vinegar. It is better to grate it and prepare it in a more natural way. It does not contain much silicon. If you have a taint in your system and want to drive it out, horseradish will drive that impurity to the surface of the skin and may produce eczema as a result. If you suffer from eczema you are healthy or you need vegetable salts. Horseradish drives impurities to the surface of the skin.

LETTUCE contains silicon in addition to other salts and is a good food.

MILK. Pasteurized milk is not a good food. Pasteurization kills the vitamins. It is a bad practice. Instruct the milkman to wash his hands and clean his pails and have the cow washed so that everything is clean before he milks. If a germ gets into the milk, there will be millions of germs, because germs multiply tremendously in milk. There is very little silicon in cow's milk but there is more silicon in goat's milk. Goat's milk is closest to mother's milk. It is high in chlorine and lactic acid. That is the reason that goat's milk passes through the alimentary tract in a little baby, while mother's milk may constipate the little bowels of the baby. Evaporated goat's milk is a very fine product. The real goat's milk comes from the Toggenburg goat.

SPINACH is low in silicon.

STRAWBERRIES are high in silicon and contain many salts. They are also rich in sodium.

FOODS AND CHEMICALS
<u>IODINE</u>

NATURE AND CHARACTERISTICS

Under the influence of iodine, the brain becomes more active. Iodine affects the function of the brain more favorably because it helps to neutralize all toxins that may possibly pass up into the brain. The thyroid gland in the throat secretes Iodothyrin. If the thyroid secretion is not thrown upon the blood, all of the toxins that may be in the blood, as it passes into the brain, will affect the brain. The thyroid gland guards the brain. It guards against all of the toxins that otherwise would pass up into the brain and cause disease, insanity, decay of the brain, softening of the brain and many other ailments of a mental nature.

Iodine and the thyroid gland with its secretion are there to guard the brain. If a child is not sufficiently supplied with iodine food and with thyroid secretion, the child becomes feeble-minded, and cannot study successfully in school. The child goes about with wide open eyes under lip hanging down and mucus running out of the mouth.

Iodine is an element about which nothing was known 30 years ago. We did not know then that there is iodine in the human system. We found that out about 1890. Also, we know now that there are sixteen different chemical elements at work in the human organization. Previous to 1890, we wrote and talked about fifteen chemical elements. But after we learned about iodine, we began to write about sixteen elements. There may, possibly, be another chemical element but we rather doubt it, because every secretion in the human body has been analyzed.

Physiologists, doctors and chemists have found out a great deal more about iodine and its influence upon the human organization than they ever knew in regard to any other chemical element. Potassium-iodine is being used in times of tertiary syphilis. When there is not sufficient iodine in the system, a person is exceedingly sensitive to venereal miasms or diseases. Iodine has its effect upon syphilis and other sexual diseases so much so that when a patient suffers from venereal disease, foods that contain iodine are of the highest value.

If there is a lack of iodine and silicon, the lining of the lungs of the throat, bronchial tubes and a great many others are likely to suffer. In times of chronic consumption of the throat, foods that contain iodine and silicon are very important. After the disease has gone too far, we cannot cure it with an iodine and silicon diet because the system may not assimilate iodine and silicon any more.

Whenever you suffer from catarrh or bronchitis, eat foods rich in iodine and silicon and breathe oxygen in abundance. It is well to take treatments in connection also.

People of the Hydripheric constitution are usually well supplied with iodine. It is because they are so well supplied with iodine that their lymphatic glands are so active. If you wish to reduce, eat foods rich in iodine. That is one of the functions of iodine. When it is supplied to excess, it will reduce obesity.

Iodine does not supply the brain with vitality but it is invaluable to the normal brain in prevention of toxins. The secretions will destroy toxins that would otherwise pass up into the brain and injure brain function. If the thyroid gland could not secrete that important thyroid secretion which is essential for the brain and its function, the person would be in danger of brain trouble.

The person who suffers from catarrh lacks iodine and many other salts. There are many kinds of catarrh, but anyone who suffers from catarrh suffers from lack of oxygen or lack of some one of the salts and iodine.

The gland becomes overworked when there is a lack of iodine. There is an enlargement of the gland. Sometimes that enlargement may affect the eyesight, sexual system, lumbar center in the spinal cord or perhaps some other organ. Iodine also has a great deal to do with oxidation. Everyone who suffers from catarrh suffers from low oxidation or lack of oxygen.

If some kind of metal enters the system it will pass to some certain part of the body. If it is not organized metal and an excess of that metal is taken up, the function may become transmuted and disease follows.

Medical men are injecting goat glands. This is only a fad. Sacks of pus under the teeth are there not because of rheumatism but because a person is acid in the tissues. The stomach and secretions are acid. A doctor who understands diet would not tell you to go to a dentist and have your teeth taken out. He would give you a diet to neutralize the acid. Otherwise you may become acid everywhere. Your joints will become acid. You will suffer from gout, rheumatism and other ailments. The doctor should treat that patient with electricity and a basic diet and he will render the secretions more alkaline.

The function of iodine has been studied by doctors everywhere. They are more acquainted with the function of iodine than they are with the function of any other element. I have read several articles written from Japan, Sweden, Germany, Austria and other countries on iodine and its function.

If you suffer from intestinal trouble, stomach trouble, gas generation or acid stomach it is because of a high albuminous diet. If you do not have enough iodine, your stomach is acid; if there are already toxins in your system, egg white or any albuminous food may become toxic. That is why if a person suffers from chronic indigestion or acidosis, acid formation or tubercular ailment, we should not give him egg white.

Do not give a patient egg white in any form when he is sick or weak. All sorts of fats, starches, meats and egg white are dangerous foods. They cause sickness when you live on such foods and neglect iodine.

FUNCTIONS OF IODINE IN THE HUMAN ORGANIZATION

We dig our graves with our teeth. We eat ourselves into our graves. If we knew how to eat, drink, live, work, develop, I believe, perhaps, we could live to be as old as Methusalah. Scientists tell us that bones last 2 to 3 thousand years. They tell us the muscles would live indefinitely; that we build a new heart every 30 days. I see no reason why we cannot go on and live. But we must know how to eat and drink.

When there is a lack of nitrogen and phosphorus or when there is an alarming increase of nitrogen and phosphorus, it results in death. Iodine has much to do with the prevention of death.

When we speak of demineralized food articles, we refer to foods from which some chemical elements have been removed. White flour is a demineralized food product. The principal minerals have been taken out; the minerals are in the bran that is given to the horses. We give that demineralized white flour to children. The bran should be left in the flour; then we would get all the salts the Almighty put there for the normal functions of the body.

When the thyroid gland finds no mineral for functioning, it gets sick. Then comes the surgeon with his knife. He cuts out this gland and that gland. All at once tumors may form. Perhaps the whole intestines may be nothing but a mass of tumors.

The thyroid gland should be well supplied with the thyroid secretion. When children cannot get enough of the thyroid secretion, they become simple minded. It is a crime to try to force mathematics into a child's brain when that brain lacks the thyroid secretion. Give the child iodine foods and you will not have to try to force mathematics into him; he will study it all right himself and enjoy it too.

The thyroid gland does not function in a child before he is two, three or possibly five years old or even up to 12. Never give a child meat or the white of eggs until he is from 3 to 12 years of age, because the thyroid gland function cannot destroy albuminous or protein toxins in the blood of the child. That is the reason the Almighty supplies the little child a milk diet. The Almighty created cow's milk, goat's milk and mother's milk so the child can get milk in early life.

Never give babies food rich in sugar. Mother's milk contains only 4-5% sugar.

Keep protein out of a child's system until the thyroid gland functions. If you suffer from catarrh, avoid albuminous foods. That is the time you need a milk diet.

The brain cannot take up oxygen very quickly. Oxidation in the brain is exceedingly slow. The more phosphorus you have, the slower oxidation is in the brain. That is why we need more iodine in our food when we have a large brain. That is why it is dangerous for us to use our brains when the thyroid gland is weak.

Iodine spurs the brain into action. Under the influence of iodine, a man is able to expand the lungs more, take in more air and hold it longer. When there is a lack of iodine in the system, the range of respiration is decreased and the pulse runs up above 95 beats per minute.

Iodine increases oxidation in the system. Iodine is creative or has a creative effect. It is not the iodine in itself, it is the affect of iodine upon calcium secretion, metabolism and oxidation that increases oxygen in the system. Anything that increases oxygen will also increase the creative power in the system. You know, if you suffer from anemia, you need iron, potassium chloride, vitamins and iodine in abundance. It is very important that you be placed where the altitude is high and the air is breezy in order to make the proper use of all these foods. Formerly medical men recommended iron for anemia, but at last, they found that iron did not cure anemia because it was the drugstore iron. That is why the iron did not cure. They omitted potassium-chloride, iron, iodine and a high altitude. Anemia is likely to affect ladies of all constitutions especially if the domestic life is not favorable.

Iodine increases oxidation in the brain; hence, it has a constructive effect.

We should supply iodine to growing children. That is one period of life when iodine seems more important than at any other time. Between the ages of 14 and 18 years, iodine should be well supplied—while vigorous growth is going on. Iodine has a great deal to do with puberty. If iodine is then lacking in the system that period comes much later, or may not come at all. If iodine is well supplied at the time of puberty, blood is made abundantly and the person becomes more vigorous. Therefore

512

supply an iodine diet to growing children; then oxidation becomes more perfect. The sexual functions and the brain become more complete.

Do not go to the goat or rabbit for blood. Aim to manufacture your own serum. The Almighty never told us to go to the sheep or rabbit for serum. There is life in blood. The life in a certain individual changes the chemistry of the blood. If you take the blood from one person and inject it into another person, you may kill that person. If somebody offers, when needed, look him over very carefully and be sure the blood is pure; but, best of all, manufacture your own blood and iodine.

Iodine has its period, calcium has its period. To build good teeth start in at the age of 7 or sooner. So it is with other elements. Every element has its own period; its own organs; its own functions; and its own faculty.

CONSTITUTIONS IN WHICH IODINE IS INHERENTLY EXCESSIVE

Iodine is excessive in no constitution unless we supply it to excess. No people eat abundantly foods rich in iodine. They do not know what foods contain iodine.

Every man should develop his own functions. Nature's work is very slow. It takes nature 20 years to build a man out of a baby. During that time, nature's work goes on more efficiently than at any other period.

SYMPTOMS WHEN IODINE IS EXCESSIVE

There are some nerves in the system that are not functioning equally with the brain. The patient goes from one extreme to another. He is first pessimistic then optimistic. At one time his nerves are drawing him in one direction at another time in another direction.

He cannot tolerate anything sharp. If you take up a knife and show him the point, he gets uneasy and restless. He cannot tolerate a scraping sound on glass. It works on his nerves. He does not want to see an animal with bristles.

You know phosphorus is of such a nature that it forms certain habits. If a phosphorus man or woman begins to think of a certain disease, maybe hydrophobia he thinks about it and at last he gets it. He reads of the symptoms of it and

at last imagines he has it himself and pretty soon he does. Perhaps he will die of it. The brain becomes neurotic. There are many phosphorus people who suffer from neurotic nerves, even from psychotic ailments.

If you tell a phosphorus man that he is being killed and another man meets him and tells him the same thing; then another man tells him he is being killed; at last, the phosphorus man thinks he is being killed and he will die.

Some scientists experimented on a criminal condemned to death. They told him they were going to bleed him to death. They blindfolded him and brought a tub of water. Just at the time when one man dropped water into the tub, drop by drop, the surgeon put a sharp knife to one of the arteries of the criminal. He was not cut at all, but he thought that drop of water was his own blood. He heard the doctors talking about how pale he was getting. Before the night was over, he was dead. But you could not do that with a Calciferic or Isogenic man; only with a man who suffers from lack of phosphorus and iodine.

We talk about powerful imagination. That is what we can do with imagination. We can do that with certain people but not with others. If it is a Neurogenic man, we can kill him with all sorts of stories. We can make him sick; we can tell him his liver is diseased and he believes it. It is his nerves working unfavorably on those organs. It is a case of neurotic nerves when a man suffers from iodine hunger. He becomes neurotic. It is a morbid disease.

When you talk about disease, he feels that he has that disease. When you talk about a cat living in his stomach he believes he has a cat living in his stomach. That is imagination. People like that are psychotic or neurotic.

HELPFUL HINTS

If you want to experiment in regard to iodine diseases, always pick a Pathetic or Sentimental type, one who cries easily, interested in humanity, a little weak in the heart. Put her on a strong iodine diet and see how quickly she responds to iodine foods. There are some who do not respond to iodine at all or very little, as for instance, the Calciferic man or woman are not very sensitive to iodine foods. In fact, the Calciferic is not sensitive to anything because calcium resists. The Calciferic has that same combativeness and firmness that causes him to throw off anything that comes to him. If you tell him something in regard to himself, he contradicts it. When we deal with a calcium man, we must deal with him in the way of suggestion. We must say it in such a way as if to insinuate that he believes it. Tell him that, "If I understand you rightly, I think you are in sympathy with so and so." The same with a Calciferic girl. If she has fallen in love with some man then you have just simply to force her to marry him and she leaves him alone. The more we try to force a man like that, the more he resists. You cannot force a Calciferic man into heaven with a club.

If there is an excess of iodine, the eyes go to sleep. The eyelids fall down and cannot lift. It is difficult to lift the upper eyelid. That is the iodine patient. If you listen to the heart mechanism in an iodine patient, you find tremor in the heart; also in the nerves. The iodine patient and the tobacco patient have the same kind of a heart or heart beat.

The iodine or phosphorus patient would never pass an insurance examination. It is not a "screw" loose in the brain but brain decay. The brain is deteriorating. In other words, iodine is degenerating.

He is uneasy and restless if there is a deficiency of iodine. He is first here then over there. Now he is in the waste basket, then he is up on the desk. You know the iodine patient can never sit still. If he sits down, he is doing something with his fingers. All sorts of peculiar motions like a jumping jack. You can see little children like that. There is not enough iodine in the system and too much oxygen. You know oxygen is full of motion. The iodine is being used up too rapidly. You try to make him behave himself. That is lack of iodine. A doctor will give him bromin when what he needs is iodine foods.

Amyloid means starch generation. He becomes starch drunk. Then he grows heavy. The flesh is hanging over everywhere. That is starch poison.

The anatomy of the body is very peculiar. There sits the thyroid gland in the throat. The Almighty placed it right there where the blood is going up into the brain to increase oxidation in the brain. The brain is burning up with phosphorus. oxidation is slow between phosphorus and oxygen. Iodine increases oxidation. In other words, it sets the brain going. It puts fire to the brain.

It increases heat and oxidation in the brain. It arouses the brain cells, increases memory, intellectuality and personality. In iodine starvation, the brain is sick. It is diseased. It cannot think or reason. The pupil is a dull student. If you use the intellect too much, you use up the iodine in the thyroid gland or the iodine secretion. Then you must fall back upon a strong iodine diet.

FOOD ANALYSIS EXPLAINED

SMOKED SALMON. The amount of iodine found in smoked salmon and certain other salts also found in smoked salmon, make it a very good food. That is, smoked salmon, not canned; not the fresh salmon either—just smoked salmon.

SHRIMP. I would not recommend shrimp because it contains a poison in the first place, and it will generate a great deal of gas since it is rich in sulphur.

You find a small trace of iodine in oatmeal and whole wheat, but it is very little. Iodine is not found in Irish moss to any great extent, only 0.003%, yet that is the richest iodine food.

Iodine is found in these foods only in the smallest quantities. If there is any trouble with the thyroid gland or any trouble with the brain, various nerves and linings, in the system, then we must fall back on a heavy iodine diet.

The best iodine foods are: cod liver oil, green turtle, smoked salmon and Irish moss. Feed backward boys and girls who cannot understand anything at school green turtle, smoked salmon and Irish moss.

QUESTIONS AND ANSWERS

1. What can be done for a young girl who is showing signs of a goiter? Answer: Place her on a heavy iodine diet and the goiter will disappear in the course of a year or two. Give her also plenty of fresh air and a constructive diet.

2. What about numbness when a person sleeps and then wakes up due to numbness in hands, arms or legs? Answer: Numbness is not a good indication, whether it be numbness in the daytime or numbness at night. There should be none. If there is it shows that some of the motor nerves or one of the motor centers is weak and

this means that it is necessary to recuperate and nourish the cerebellum and the motor nerves or the motor centers.

3. Will honey reduce vitality the same as sugar? Answer: Honey will neither reduce vitality nor increase it. Honey is nothing else than one kind of sugar.

4. Will honey develop all backhead faculties in the same manner that it develops the sexual system? Answer: Honey does not develop the backhead faculties and neither does it develop the sexual system. Eucalyptus honey contains a certain principle that is called Eycalyptol and this acts as a tonic or stimulant to the sexual system. This is the reason why we recommend eucalpytus honey in times of sexual weakness. Honey supplies a certain sweet and also certain salts needed by the muscles—and if this sweet is needed, honey helps development.

5. The Carboferic people suffer from sugar fermentation. People with weak alimentiveness suffer because they cannot utilize sugar. Do they both suffer from sugar fermentation? Answer: Yes, if they eat foods that are rich in sugar. If a man is weak in alimentiveness, he cannot utilize very much sugar. Hence, also he must exclude sugar from his diet; i.e., he should not use any more sugar than he can utilize for if he does, he will surely suffer from gas and sugar fermentation.

6. If coffee is taken away from a person all at once after many years of constant use, does it not cause a great reaction in the body? Answer: Yes, it results in headache, weakness and general disturbances, but those are for the better.

7. What is the cause of tartar on the teeth and how can it be removed and the teeth made white again? Answer: The tartar is the result of mineral salts that do not belong in the body or else the eating of foods that do not contain the vegetable salts which have a soluble effect upon mineral salts. Tartar on the teeth can only be removed by the dentist. The acid which strawberries and raspberries contain, acts upon the tartar of the teeth; if this juice is held in the mouth for some time, especially by leaning forward with the head so that the juice may come into contact with the tartar on the teeth. However, the juice or the acid in strawberries and raspberries would not remove the tartar altogether.

8. What causes cold spots above the knees? Answer: When there are any cold spots on the body, you may be sure that the red corpuscles of the blood have been broken down and that acid is at work on the nerve structures at that very spot. Eat vitamins and a strong iron diet and also foods rich in iodine.

9. What is the cause of lines in the face? Answer: Lack of vegetable salts. Those lines can be removed by breathing plenty of fresh air, by retiring at 8 o'clock in the evening and introducing foods that are rich in vegetable salts.

10. Which are the salts that keep the cerebellum in perfect condition? Answer: Potassium chloride.

FOODS AND CHEMICALS

<u>IRON</u>

Hemoglobinogenesis is a word that means blood production or the manufacture of hemoglobin. "Hemo" means blood; "globe" means ball; and "genesis" means production. The manufacture of hemoglobin stands in close relation to oxidation. If there is a lack of hemoglobin, there is usually also low oxidation in the blood.

When a man falls in love, there is a greater production of the red corpuscles. The red corpuscles are manufactured in greater abundance during a happy state of mind. A happy state of mind stimulates the sexual system. When a man marries, he should be at his best, which holds good in regard to the lady also. Abundance of iron in the blood and abundance of red corpuscles result in better offspring. A man who is sexually weak should marry for developmental purposes but should not become the father of offspring before he is strong.

The hemoglobin of the red corpuscles of the blood contain iron. Iron is necessary when it is a question of health. Many people take drugstore iron. Some businessmen have heard that iron is good for the blood so they manufacture a certain kind of iron and advertise it heavily. We should remember that the human organization is organic and cannot assimilate iron in drug form or in an inorganic form. We should remember that nature must manufacture the iron which is to be taken up by the body. Without iron, we could not live very long.

When there is a great deal of carbon and sulphur in the iron, it is not so good. The railroads do not allow the construction of locomotives from that kind of iron which contains too much carbon and sulphur for that kind of iron would fall to pieces. Locomotives could not stand the strain if they were made of that kind of iron.

There is an affinity between oxygen and iron in the blood. They rush into each other's "arms."

If we had sense enough to eat foods that are rich in iron, we would have plenty of iron in our blood.

If you take drug iron for a long time, that iron will eventually be eliminated by your kidneys and in doing so, will break down your kidney cells, decompose the walls of the kidneys and you will die from dropsy, albuminuria or some other kidney disease. Leave such iron alone.

Metallic iron will disturb the iron that you have already in the blood. If the spinal marrow becomes weak or weakened by heat, germs, gas or some other condition, eventually the red corpuscles will not be manufactured in the bone marrow. Lastly that same person will suffer from anemia, which may also run into diabetes and dropsy. When there is a lack of iron, some kind of dropsy is usually the result. The red corpuscles must eventually go to the liver. There the iron undergoes a certain process and becomes duly qualified to enter into the hemoglobin of the red corpuscles of the blood and enter the vim of tissue life.

If you take drug iron, you may improve temporarily but you will improve at the expense of your own life. People used to take arsenic for a beautiful complexion. They had a bright eye and a beautiful complexion for a time, but all at once the arsenic did its work and the complexion or the beauty disappeared and they looked old and homely and died before their time. This is also true in regard to drugstore iron.

Green grapes will improve the complexion but if you eat green grapes to excess, your blood will be too rich in sugar and your liver will become enlarged.

Whenever you have too much iron in your system, you have a tired feeling somewhere in the forehead, eyes or elsewhere. You have that same sensation when you suffer from iron starvation. Iron is stimulating. It gives energy to functions. When a man grows weak, has no power, no strength, it is perhaps because there is a lack of iron in his blood, and he cannot oxidize his blood. When you cannot oxidize the blood nor your tissues, you grow weak day by day.

When there is a lack of iron there is often a lack of potassium also. When you have plenty of iron in your blood, your nerves are stimulated and you are usually better nourished. If you marry when you have plenty of iron in your blood or when you have red corpuscles in abundance and all the hemoglobin in the red corpuscles are charged with iron and you become a father or a mother, you have greater power of transmission to send energy into every little cell, resulting in strong and healthy offspring, as well as gifted. Is it not better to know this or is it not better to know how you can get iron and oxygen into your system than it is to have a thousand volumes of eugenics on your shelves? Without iron and oxygen, you cannot transmit yourself to your child. Your child becomes Atrophic—a weakling; perhaps that child fills the consumptive's grave before reaching the age of 21 years.

When you have iron in your blood and potassium in your tissues and oxygen to act upon your functions throughout, you are more fascinating, more beautiful, more useful. You have more energy, more magnetism, greater transmissive power. You know what you are doing; you know your duties; and you fulfill those duties.

When there is a lack of phosphorus, the patient suffers from neurasthenia; the patient is so weak that he can hardly hold his jaws together.

If you want to become more efficient, more successful, if you want to love to the fullest capacity, if you want to attract attention and become popular among the opposite sex, eat foods rich in iron. Do not take drug iron; fall back on that kind of food which is rich in the iron element. Eat wild blackberries from the iron belt in Michigan or from the iron belt in Oregon.

If you have a weak stomach, you cannot digest bran nor take the iron out of the bran. Some foods do not give up their iron readily. It requires a very strong stomach to take iron out of bran, but it does not require a strong stomach to take the iron out of wild blackberries from the hills in Michigan or Oregon.

Before going up stairs, carrying a heavy object, running fast, always fill your lungs full with oxygen. If you get out of breath easily, you do not have enough oxygen in your blood; you suffer from oxygen hunger quickly. This means that you do not have iron in the hemoglobin; it means that the red corpuscles cannot carry enough oxygen for your system. It means that the hemoglobin cannot take up very much oxygen. It is not a question of how many red corpuscles you have in your blood, so much as it is a question: How readily those red corpuscles are charged with iron and oxygen. If they are healthy, vigorous and if they have plenty of iron in their interior, they carry oxygen to lungs and tissues in abundance. Lack of air is lack of hemoglobin or it is lack of iron. This results in asthma. A man needs plenty of oxygen in order to run fast. The faster you run, the more it is necessary to hold your lungs out and fill them with air. The more aggressive you want to be, the more you want to argue, the more positive you want to be the more it is necessary to charge your lungs with fresh air. It is through iron that oxygen comes into your blood.

When oxygen is at work in the tissues, there is plenty of energy, life and heat in the tissues. When there is heat generated in the muscles, you feel warm even when it is cold. Then you feel energetic. You can fill your lungs with air and you feel that life is a pleasure.

The Almighty wants us to have iron and oxygen in abundance and therefore energy and life, especially when it is a question of transmission of life. You may write and read volumes on birth culture, but it would not do you very much good unless you have iron and oxygen—energy and a strong sexuality. You cannot give birth to vigorous and gifted offspring merely by reading works on eugenics and birth culture.

Iron is used up, to a great extent, in the liver and the spleen and in other parts of the body. There is considerable iron in the red marrow of the bone. If the marrow is red, it indicates energy in the marrow cells. If there is a lack of iron in the liver, blood or spleen, there is a deficiency of oxygen. Whenever there is a deficiency of iron in some parts of the body, there is also a deficiency of oxygen.

You find iron and oxygen at work vigorously in the Myogenic and Oxypheric constitutions; never iron to excess in any other constitution. The Atrophic constitution is low in iron and therefore also low in tissue oxidation and in the oxidation of the blood. In Pathetic people, oxidation is low; in Desmogenics, oxidation is often low; in Carboferic people oxidation is almost always low, especially after they reach the age of about 35. Some people suffer from iron hunger and from oxygen hunger after 35 years and sometimes often before.

Plethoric temperament means that there is an excess of iron and certain other salts as well as of oxygen. When oxygen is too dense, it results in Plethora. When there is an excess of iron, a man may become a sensualist. There is an increase of nerve power. Excess iron attracts oxygen, perhaps even to excess. When oxygen is in excess, the man is under a heavy oxygen pressure. If a woman lacks iron, she cries readily. She craves love and sympathy almost all the time. She is like a baby.

Furnish iron to the tissues and phosphorus to the brain in abundance and you can do mental work efficiently without fatigue. When there is a lack of phosphorus, we are weak in brain function and also physically. When there is a lack of iron for any length of time in a young girl or woman, she lastly becomes hysterical. Starve the body too long and it cannot take up iron. The tongue becomes thick, when there is a lack of iron.

If you eat sulphur foods to excess that sulphur which is not taken up by the system is converted into gas and passes into the red corpuscles and fills up the hemoglobin so that the hemoglobin cannot carry oxygen normally. Then the iron in the hemoglobin will do you no good. People who suffer from sulphur gas, suffer also from low oxidation and yet there may be nothing wrong with their blood so far as the blood count is concerned.

Animals always become more tubercular towards Spring and Fall, when there is a tendency to tuberculosis, simply because animals—during Winter and Spring—cannot obtain the right kind of food. The feed that the animals get during the Winter does not contain iodine in sufficient quantities. This is the reason that oxidation is low in animals during Winter. It should be remembered that iodine has a great deal to do with oxidation. Whenever a girl suffers from low oxidation, she is likely to suffer from goiter. She suffers from goiter because there is a lack of iodine in the thyroid gland. To cure goiter of this kind, it is necessary to eat foods that are rich in iodine and practice breathing exercises in abundance.

We always obtain more oxygen when the air is attenuated, where the altitude is high. If we live in a dense atmosphere and low altitude, we lack oxygen.

The Calciferic and Desmogenic need iron and potassium foods in abundance.

When you use your brain vigorously all the way from 10 to 20 times as much blood goes to the brain. If you become very excited, the blood flows to the brain tremendously and the red corpuscles die in great numbers. At last, the brain becomes hyperemic or overcharged with blood. How do you think this will affect your health for a day or more?

A disturbance of specific gravity in the blood, either one way or another, affects the function of sleep, even the function of the brain.

Oxypheric people usually have the blood salts in abundance. They are full of energy. If you are a businessman and you want a partner for the purpose of promoting your business, you must hire an Oxypheric man. Such a man is a great talker and can always get people interested. He can inspire confidence and enthusiasm.

When a man grows old, the red corpuscles die in great numbers and he cannot manufacture red corpuscles fast enough. The iron in his blood is below par; he becomes weak and feeble. The hemoglobin cannot carry enough oxygen to his various functions and there will be an insufficiency of oxygen in his system. As he grows still older, his strength fails, because oxidation fails—then he must die.

To influence people, we must have an abundance of red blood corpuscles and plenty of oxygen in the system and also the essential vegetable salts by means of which the functions carry on the complexity of life. We must have iron in abundance in the hemoglobin of the blood.

If a man is not vigorous, he does not eat right and he has undesirable habits. A young man has more executive power and power of organization than an old man because of an abundance of iron, oxygen and potassium, which he has in his system. The business house always wants young men in its service. After a man is 55, 60 or 65 years of age, business firms do not care for him, because he is not vigoroius enough.

A business house does not always know how to keep its men vigorous. If you want more work out of a machine, you must feed the machine right and take care of it. This is exactly what businessmen forget. They never think of placing their employees where they can act according to their talent nor do they ever teach their employees how to eat and live. If employers would teach their employees how to eat and live, they could increase the efficiency of their employees and obtain perhaps twice as much work out of them. It is not easy to get work out of a tired mule, neither is it easy to get work out of a dyspeptic, nor speed out of a consumptive, nor patience out of a nervous sickly lady.

Everything that weakens the red corpuscles of the blood, weakens also the oxygen-carrying capacity of the red corpuscles. Anything that weakens the iron in the hemoglobin of the blood leads to inefficiency in the oxygen function. If there is too much blood, too much iron and too many blood salts, the result is plethora—resulting in inefficiency again.

People who have a normal quantity of iron and oxygen are never depressed. When there is an excess of iron in the blood or when there is an insufficiency of iron in the blood, in both cases there is mental depression. The man who lacks oxygen feels that everything is against him. The man who has iron and oxygen in excess also feels that everything is against him. When you are going to make a transaction you must have a face that makes your customers feel that you are a success. You should be optimistic and enthusiastic. If you are a pessimist, people do not want your goods.

We must remember that the body requires organic iron; the system needs food iron not drugstore iron.

We have been told that is used over and over again in the body. This is relatively true. But iron is eliminated from the body and after the iron shall have been eliminated from the body, it is not in the body any longer. The menstrual function uses iron at each period to carry out the function. That iron which is broken down and precipitated is lost and not in the body any longer. When there is a lack of iron in the blood, the menstrual function is inefficient; blood clots form and menstruation is painful. The iron that is used in the muscles is broken down and eliminated. Therefore also that iron which is eliminated or precipitated, cannot be used over and over again. We need a new supply.

The more iron a man has in his system, up to a normal amount, the greater capacity that same man has in his various functions. A woman does not have as many red corpuscles to the count as a man. Neither does a woman have the same oxygen-carrying capacity as a man. A woman uses iron in carrying out the feminine functions. It is impossible for a mother to grow a baby without using up her own iron. It is impossible for a mother to menstruate without using up the iron in her body. Even the iron that the mother has goes to the baby and if she does not know enough to eat foods that are rich in iron so she may replenish her own blood with iron, she will suffer from iron hunger and therefore also from oxygen hunger.

If iron is not supplied, she lastly suffers from tumors, weakness, disturbances and female ailments that no drug doctor or osteopath can cure. When she is placed on the operation table, not a word is said about iron food. Then the white-robed, skillful surgeon operates but he himself does not know that that lady suffers from tumors because of a lack of iron in her blood. If you let her eat wild blackberries in abundance or drink the juice from wild blackberries, she would gradually improve and no more tumors would form for the surgeon to cut out; her complexion would improve and she would no longer be hysterical.

A lack of iron leads to the divorce court. A mother cannot be a good mother without iron; and a wife cannot be a good wife without iron, according to the scheme of the Almighty.

Sometimes we think that we catch cold. The fact is that we do not catch cold neither do we catch hot. We are perhaps inhaling germs or breaking down too many red corpuscles. Perhaps we have been doing too much brain work. Maybe there is a congestion somewhere in the system or not enough iron or oxygen in the body. Very few people know that there is a close communication between the brain and the nose. If this communication is disturbed, i.e., the nose stopped up, frontal sinus full of mucus—how do you think you would feel? Do you not think you would suffer from headache and catarrh and do you not think that the red corpuscles would die in great numbers in that very place? Do you not think that there would be pus formation taking place in the nasal membrane and frontal sinus? Do you not think that your brain would perspire and suffer from the effect of such nasal congestion?

These girls who have plenty of iron and oxygen in their blood, never need to go to a beauty parlor. Oxygen and iron are the Almighty's complexion specialists and beauty restorers.

If the duodenum is unable to take up the iron, the iron is not taken up. The duodenum is the iron absorber; it is hungry for iron.

Bran contains iron, but it requires a very strong stomach to digest and assimilate the food salts contained in bran. It is better to drink blackberry juice when you need iron. Drink blackberry juice and go out into the open air, up into the hills and breathe fresh air in abundance and you will improve.

How much iron do you think you get in white bread, biscuits made of white flour, pancakes made of white flour, doughnuts cooked in grease, coffee, tea, bacon and other similar foods? How much iron do you think there is in cake, pie, candy, vegetable drinks and other dishes of civilized cookery? We are wonderfully civilized, are we not? If you eat that kind of food do you wonder that you must have a good cry occasionally, or that you suffer from floating kidneys, prolapsus uteri, globus hysterious or menstrual pain?

If you suffer from floating kidney, you can fasten the kidney with wild blackberry juice. If you suffer from sleeplessness between 2 and 5 o'clock in the morning, you perhaps have sown avena fatua.

The word "vitamins" means life source. The vitamins are found in the seeds of foods. If you cook an apple, you kill the vitamins. Vitamins cannot stand any more cooking than you can stand. If you jump into a boiling pot for about an hour, how much life would there be left in you? Raw meat juice contains vitamins, but cooked meat juice or cooked meat contains no vitamins. Young meat contains more vitamins than old meat. Always get your meat from young animals if possible and eat foods fresh from the garden. You should live close to nature in order to get the vitamins.

FOOD ANALYSIS EXPLAINED

RYE BREAD. All people should eat rye bread if they suffer from calcium excess. There is an excess of calcium in whole wheat bread. If you are old and stiff you had better not eat whole wheat bread any longer nor should you drink milk or eat cheese or cabbage. If you suffer from hardening of the arteries, eat rye bread and drink plenty of distilled water but leave whole wheat bread alone.

BEEF. You do not find the vitamins in fried beef but you find the vitamins in the juice pressed out of raw meat. The best beef is tough beef, because it contains the salts simply because it has been exercised.

BLACKBERRIES. You find iron salts in blackberries. You can never get any other food so rich in iron as wild blackberries. Cultivated blackberries, however, never contain as much iron as wild blackberries.

HEAD LETTUCE. We find iron and sodium in lettuce. We find more iron in head lettuce than in leaf lettuce. There is more iron in a large dish of blackberries than in four gallons of cow's milk. The baby or fetus does not need an iron diet. The growing child does not need an iron diet. This is the reason the Almighty arranged it so the baby or child should get an iron-free diet because they already have iron in abundance.

ASPARAGUS does not contain very much iron.

BLACK CURRANTS contain a small percentage of iron. Currants are valuable because they contain potassium so important for the elimination of certain impurities from the body.

BARTLETT PEARS are low in salts and contain a small percentage of iron. They are rich in sugar. A sugar diet does not cause decay of teeth but sugar drinks the calcium and thus robs the teeth and bones of calcium.

SPINACH contains all the salts needed by the system; the vitamins are found principally in the seeds of spinach.

EGG YOLK contains the vitamins in abundance; the white, however, does not.

SHREDDED WHEAT BISCUITS. This is a fine food for anyone suffering from dropsy. Do not drink water if you suffer from dropsy. You need a dry diet one rich in chlorine.

STRAWBERRIES are good for rheumatism, if they are ripe. They contain iron and also the vitamins together with a great many other important salts needed by the body. When you eat strawberries do not use sugar or cream. If the Almighty had intended you to have sugar and cream on strawberries, He would have provided them.

DRIED FIGS are low in the salts and do not contain much iron. Figs, however, are laxative. They are also full of worms.

CONCORD GRAPES contain a certain percentage of grape sugar, also a small percentage of iron. They are low in the salts. If you eat grapes to excess, you will suffer from enlargement of the liver, because of the grape sugar. Remember that the liver must store up the excess sugar you eat. If you eat too much you will overtax your liver and soon it will go on strike—then you will be in bed or on an operation table.

GREEN GRAPES are good for the complexion because they contain arsenic. Your complexion will, at last, become as murky as the skin on a toad and you yourself will get sick and will die before time. Green grapes are excellent for syphilis because they contain organized arsenic.

LENTILS are high in organic salts. If you suffer from low oxidation, dropsy, neurasthenia, eat lentils. They are rich in potassium and exceedingly high in organic salts.

You must cook lentils otherwise you cannot eat them. They should be soaked overnight and cooked on a very slow fire for about two and one-half hours. When you eat them, you should not eat them to excess for they are so rich in protein you cannot digest and assimilate more than about three teaspoonsful.

QUESTIONS AND ANSWERS

1. How can wild blackberry juice be prepared in order to save the vitamins for a young child? Answer: Remember the vitamins are not in the juice but in the seeds. Eat blackberries in season; save the juice for Winter. This is the best to do.

2. Do you recommend eating salt or salty foods when the appetite is lacking? Answer: If there is a lack of appetite, there is not necessarily a lack of chlorine. Appetite may be lacking for many reasons. So long as there is no appetite, there is no gastric juice and the stomach cannot digest food. Eat only when you are hungry.

3. How can you keep blackberry juice from fermenting? Answer: Only by killing the germs in canning fruit. If there is a single germ in the fruit after it is canned, the juice will ferment. You should boil the juice and bottle up the juice when it is boiling. If you do everything rightly you need no sugar for canning.

4. Could a baby drink diluted fruit juice? Answer: A baby does not need diluted fruit juices containing iron. A baby usually has the red corpuscles in excess and also iron in excess or comparatively so. That is why the Almighty gives the baby milk. A baby needs an iron-free diet.

5. Can a complete loss of voice be caused by lack of iron and sodium? Answer: Yes. If iron and sodium are entirely exhausted in a Nitropheric lady, she is in danger of losing her voice temporarily, perhaps even permanently.

6. Has the lack of iron anything to do with varicose veins? Answer: Yes, but wrong eating and overeating have more to do with it.

7. If blackberries are not obtainable, will spinach juice supply enough of iron? Answer: No. You should drink the spinach juice eat the spinach as well, but whatever you do, do not pour out the spinach juice into the sink.

8. Can blackberry juice be obtained from canned blackberries such as purchased in grocery stores? Answer: The blackberries that are purchased in stores are mainly blackberry syrup. The best thing you can do is to take the berries out of this syrup and boil them in distilled water and take the juice out by this method.

9. How is the condition of mental perspiration determined? Is it theoretical or an established fact that the brain sweats? If so, does the heart and other organs sweat also? Answer: We said brain perspiration not mental perspiration. Brain moisture passes from the brain to the nose. You blow your nose but you do not know where that mucus comes from. The brain is a thinking organ. In thinking, certain moisture exudes from the brain and passes through the ethmoid bone, down into the nose. This is what the nose is for. If that moisture cannot find its way through the ethmoid bone you may suffer from catarrh and headache. When you suffer from headache, you know that it is a fact whether it has been established or not. If you experiment chemically, as a scientist, you soon find that phosphorus perspires and sulphur perspires also.

10. Can a Carboferic or Oxypheric lady suffer from lack of iron? Answer: Yes. An Oxypheric lady could suffer from iron hunger in 2 or 3 minutes merely by accidentally having an artery cut.

11. What diet is the best for a patient suffering from high blood pressure, running from 150 to 190? Answer: Determine the cause of the high blood pressure first, then remove the cause, then supply the diet needed.

12. Can we supply iron salts to the blood of an old man and thus chase old age away? Answer: When we grow old, we die fast. There is a lack of blood salts and a lack of oxygen; a hundred and one wrinkles appear and we look old. When we supply iron salts in abundance and the system takes them up, we increase the oxygen supply and impurities are eliminated from the body; the nutritive function is increased; youth is restored and the person looks younger than before.

13. Can you dry blackberries and thus keep them a year? Or are they dead food then? Answer: If you dry blackberries, the water passes up into the air. Thus you have all the salts and vitamins left. They are not dead food.

14. Can you supply the blood with the iron if you live in Chicago? Answer: Yes we can always obtain iron food in Chicago the same as anywhere else, but it is more difficult to get fresh air for the Chicago air contains all the way from 15% up to 27% gases, impurities, dust and fumes.

15. Is raw spinach juice rich in iron? Answer: The juice is not so rich in iron as the spinach. The iron is usually mostly in the leaves.

16. If the cheeks are faded and withered at forty, can iron iron out the wrinkles? Answer: You can eat in such a way that you appear young again at forty.

17. When the abdominal organs fall forward, almost to the knees, is this caused by iron hunger? Answer: Partly. In such a case, most of the salts are lacking and all of the muscles in the vital organs are extremely weak. The cerebellum then is also weak.

18. Is olive oil good when iron is lacking and constipation is chronic? What will cure this? Would you advise enemas? Answer: Olive oil is of no special value in such a case. It is much better to eat laxative foods. Enemas widen the colon in the majority of instances and only the water comes out. You cannot do very much with the hard excreta. The best thing to do is to eat rightly; breathe fresh air in abundance and spend much of the time outdoors. Also take horseback riding exercises when you suffer from constipation.

19. What shall we do if we cannot get blackberries in the winter? How can we supply iron? Answer: Eat those foods that you find under the heading of Iron Food.

20. Is blackberry juice that has been heated as good as fresh? Answer: No, but it contains iron nevertheless.

21. Does the system take up iron from spinach as readily as from raw egg yolk? Answer: Yes.

22. Should blackberry juice be given in times of ulceration of the stomach and in typhoid? Answer: It is better not to give anything in times of ulceration. Heal up the ulceration first and if you give any kind of food be sure that it is such foods that do not require digestion as for instance raw egg yolk with milk or raw egg yolk with orange juice. In times of typhoid fever, the walls of the stomach and intestines are almost rotten. You must not give a typhoid patient foods that require digestion.

23. Do loganberries contain iron? Answer: They are low in iron.

24. What causes hiccough? Answer: The diaphragm goes upward and is held with a tension, this causes hiccough. Lack of oxygen causes it. Breathe deeply and hold your breath long enough to stop the spasm.

25. What is the difference between ordinary sodium, sodium chloride and sodium carbonate? Answer: Sodium chloride is the table salt. Sodium carbonate is sal-soda. Sodium carbonate is used extensively in the arts. It is of great importance to all consumers of soap and glass, and glass and soap manufacturers. It is also important in the tissues.

26. Why are the skins of apples difficult for some people to digest? Answer: Because the apple skins contain the salts. Apples should be baked and they are more easily digested. Apples, however, contain malic acid which is not favorable to a weak stomach.

27. Are baked salmon, trout and halibut too high in protein for the Exesthesic lady? Answer: Salmon and halibut may be good for a laborer, but not for an Exesthesic lady; trout is better for her if it is baked but trout is not the cleanest food we can find.

28. Would a proper diet cure retroversion of the uterus? Answer: Yes in connection with other treatments.

29. Does a Neurogenic man need sodium? Answer: He needs magnesium rather than sodium. A man who has a great deal of phosphorus in his system and in whom phosphorus consumption is great should eat foods that contain magnesium and phosphorus.

30. Please give a diet suitable for a tubercular patient. Answer: We could hardly give a general diet for tubercular patients. As a general rule, such foods as egg yolk shakes, good rye bread, goat's milk, raw meat juice, blackberry juice tonics, oatmeal muffins, berries rich in vegetable salts and iron in connection with other foods are very good. A consumptive should have a regular diet system.

31. What salts are needed at a time of disappointment in love? When a man is languid and indifferent who was formerly happy? Answer: Anyone who is disappointed from whatever cause, is breaking down the sodium and filling the system with phosphoric products and fatigue poison, He needs oxygen in abundance. Send that man to the hills and let him forget his troubles and the girl; it will do him good.

32. How much iron is there in the blood of a full-grown man? Answer: Just about enough to make a tenpenny nail.

33. Should a Myogenic man drink buttermilk in abundance? Answer: No. His bowels would soon enlarge and he would suffer from rheumatism.

34. Does ice cream have any food value? Answer: Yes, but it does not give us very much strength.

35. What food value is there in milk chocolate with nuts? Answer: This is nothing but candy and nuts. The nuts are good but the candy is simply candy—no more.

36. Can fluorine be introduced into the system in youth and do good after the age of about 20? Answer: Yes indeed. If fluorine shall have once done its work in the bones and teeth, the teeth and bones may last perhaps 5 or 10 thousand years or longer. I have seen a skull that contained teeth and geologists claimed that that skull was 120,000 years old. Between the ages of 7 and 20, the teeth are forming. This is the time that we need a fluorine diet. Our parents, however, were not instructed in regard to the value of fluorine during the teeth building and bone building periods.

37. Is Cuba or the Adirondacks good for iron? Answer: You perhaps mean if iron foods come from the Adirondack Mountains. Do wild blackberries grow there? If so, I would say yes. Iron is found in the soil in Cuba and everywhere else, although there may be a difference in the supply of iron in the soil.

38. When sulphur is lacking in the system and sulphur foods produce gas and liver trouble, how then can sulphur be introduced into the body? Answer: Eat such sulphur-containing foods that the system can tolerate as for instance raw egg yolk, sauerkraut, figs. We should also remember never to overeat sulphur foods at such a time.

39. Can we eat raw sweet corn? If not, how long should it be boiled? Answer: We should not eat raw sweet corn for we cannot handle that kind of starch. If we must eat corn, we should boil it.

40. Do you compare the buttermilk made in this country with the kind made in Bulgaria which is from sheep's milk or goat's milk and prepared from the fresh milk not boiled? Answer: We do not compare buttermilk with buttermilk. The question is why should we eat buttermilk that is made with a germ and which is mainly a mass of germs?

41. Would albumin, injected into the blood, produce poison, the same as rattlesnake poison? Answer: No, I think not, although I have never tried it. It is true that albumin, as found in the white of egg, is identical to the poison found in the rattlesnake viewed from a chemical standpoint.

42. Does the cerebellum contract when sodium is needed, as well as when iron is needed? Does a person jerk from lack of sodium the same as he does from lack of iron? Are not the symptoms of lack of iron similar to iron excess? Answer: Yes. The cerebellum contracts also when potash is needed; it contracts when any of these salts are needed. Each and every salt has its own peculiar influence on the cerebellum. If you compare iron-hunger symptoms with sodium-hunger symptoms and if you compare iron-hunger symptoms with iron-excess symptoms or sodium-hunger symptoms with sodium-excess symptoms, you will find that they are widely different. Some may be similar but they are not identical.

43. What is iron carbonate? Answer: It is sort of a spar found in spathic and clay-iron stone often containing some manganese. It is manganese that is fitted for the manufacture of certain kinds of steel, hence it has been called a steel ore.

44. Could enough blackberries be put into chewing gum to make such iron chewing gum that would supply the system with iron? Answer: Would it not be better to eat iron-containing foods, just as the Almighty made them than to stick the iron into gum? When will we learn common sense?

45. What should stenographers do to regain red cheeks when they are compelled to sit still and

work 8 hours a day? Answer: Let them eat iron-containing foods and go into the hills for oxygen. This is better than to eat doughnuts and coffee and paint the cheeks.

46. How is the iron metal administered as a tonic? Answer: It is administered in the form of a fine powder as citrate of iron and also in other forms of drugs. We should remember, however, that that kind of iron tonic is not the best for the blood.

47. Should a child 4 years old be given iron pills? Answer: No. It is much better to give a child wild blackberries, blackberry juice or spinach, raw egg yolk, etc., the same as the Almighty made the foods.

48. Does celery cabbage contain sodium and iron? Answer: It is rich in sodium, but not iron.

49. Will breathing exercises, combined with iron food, increase oxygen? Answer: To increase oxygen, go out into the hills and then eat foods rich in iron and potassium.

50. Can the Desmogenic man become normal in iron and oxygen? Answer: Yes.

51. Does old age and study rob the blood of iron so much that the iron cannot be supplied? Answer: If we study too much or if we become too scientific we must suffer for it.

52. What cures rheumatism? Answer: It depends on what kind of rheumatism. It may be caused by acidity; it may be caused by phosphorus salts, excess of calcium, lack of sodium or germ life. When the cause is known, we can apply a remedy, but not before.

53. How can a sweaty scalp be cured? Answer: When there is too great activity in the hair glands and roots and too much carbon in the system of a baby or child that child is likely to suffer from a sweaty scalp. Cut down the carbon foods or cut down the food in general and this ailment disappears.

54. Do people who suffer from arthritis need iron? If not, what do they need in the way of diet? Answer: They need sodium and oxygen in abundance.

55. How fast are the red corpuscles manufactured? Answer: It is difficult to tell. They are manufactured rapidly after eating foods rich in iron. They are manufactured rapidly when in a high altitude. They are manufactured more rapidly during love states as may be determined in the laboratory and as we

have seen ourselves demonstrated again and again. They are also manufactured rapidly by a great many other means and methods.

56. How long does it take to build up the blood in anemic people? Answer: This depends on the constitution or the type of patient. We can supply enough iron to the body in 24 hours but whether the system can assimilate enough iron is another question. We can lead a horse to water but we cannot force the horse to drink.

57. Are the elements in Roquefort cheese easily taken up by any constitution? Answer: Yes. Why? Because those salts are organic and easily digested and utilized, especially if the Roquefort is made with goat's milk. It is, however, made of sheep's milk.

58. Should celery root be eaten raw or cooked? Answer: Raw is the best.

59. Would you recommend a patient who suffers from hyperacidity to eat sodium foods in preference to chlorine or should he have a combination of both? Answer: Hyperacidity means excess acid. When there is an excess of acid it should be neutralized, should it not? How can we neutralize acid? We can neutralize acid by another acid as for instance, citric acid, formic acid; also by supplying foods that are rich in potash, sodium, magnesium or some other alkaline salt.

60. Why is the brain constructed on a dual plan, divided into two hemispheres, the right and the left? Answer: I am not so sure but I think that one part of us is feminine and the other is masculine. I do believe that if a man were not constructed on this principle it would be impossible to give rise to more than one kind of offspring. There would be either no men or no women. There is another reason: When one side is useless the other side can be used. When one lung is gone, we can still breathe with the other lung. When one ear cannot hear, the other can. When one eye cannot see, the other can. When one hemisphere cannot think the other can. Man is dual but we really do not know why.

61. Are fruit juices, raw egg yolks, steel-cut oatmeal and graham toast with milk, sufficient for a baby one year old? Answer: This would be a strong diet for a child only a year old. It would not be a suitable diet. It would be a very good diet for a Calciferic child, but it would be a wrong diet for a Neurogenic child.

62. What causes fibroid tumors? Answer: Lack of alkaline salts.

63. How can a Desmogenic man make sodium act upon the blood, the secretions and the functions instead of on the tissues? Answer: By supplying it to excess. That is about the only thing that a Desmogenic man can do, unless he wishes to study developmental methods and form habits for developmental purposes.

64. If the appendix is removed is there a greater tendency to colitis? Answer: There is a greater tendency to germ life. A man who has undergone an operation for appendicitis, will never live so long nor ever enjoy as perfect health as he would otherwise have done, if he had kept himself in condition by means of a scientific diet. Operations do no one any good. We should live in such a way that we do not need to undergo operations.

65. How can sodium be introduced into the fluids as well as into the tissues? Answer: Only by supplying too much sodium. Sodium is not contained in foods to excess.

66. Will honey spoil sodium in strawberries? Answer: Why should you put honey on strawberries? Are they not sweet enough without it? If the strawberries are very sour, you should not eat them.

67. Should a Neurogenic patient eat sodium-containing foods to the exclusion of fats such as butter, cream, fat meats, etc.? Answer: A Neurogenic patient is in the greatest need of sodium, but he should also introduce certain fats. Not such fats that come from the cow, but fats that come from other sources. He needs oleic fat, cocoanut fat.

68. Does a lack of sodium in the blood produce nervous diseases? Answer: Yes.

FOODS AND CHEMICALS

POTASSIUM

Potassium is used by soap manufacturers. The human body is also a soap factory. The function which physiologists speak about, called "saponification," which means soap-making, is a physical or physiological process going on in the human organization. When there is a lack of potassium salts in the body, fats are not converted into the proper compound. Then, fatty food elements are converted into fatty acids and gases. This may result in a certain form of rheumatism.

The organic food elements are not well taken care of when there is a lack of potassium in the body. Then the organic food elements are converted into acids so that lastly the entire body becomes acid and the secretions become sour. Because of these body acids, some foods will be converted into gas, resulting in ailments and diseases. If you do not have enough potassium salts in the body, you better leave fat alone. Sodium and potassium salts are absolutely imperative in order to take care of fat.

Potassium salts are needed also for sugar metabolism.

There is one brain center that is essential in order to take care of fatty products, viz., the sex brain. If this brain area has been weakened, it is almost impossible to take care of the fatty elements. Then fats and oils cannot be utilized by the system; then the spinal marrow, bone marrow, the brain, lung substance, joints and a great many other parts and secretions of the body will suffer, simply because the fatty elements cannot be utilized.

A certain substance called Neurolin is needed in the brain and nerves. When the sex brain is weak or has been weakened, Neurolin cannot be assimilated nor utilized by the nerves or brain. When the brain is not supplied with this important fatty substance, the brain becomes stiff and the brain neurons become unyieldy. Memorization is then impossible or at least difficult. A man will experience a peculiar sensation when sodium and potassium are lacking in the system and when the faculty amativeness is weak. When Ueurolin is lacking the membranes of the brain cannot function so efficiently.

The arachnoid membrane of the spinal cord and of the brain is a membrane that is concerned in the secretion of a fatty, oily element or substance for the brain and for the spinal cord. If there is a lack of potassium in the system, this important oily substance is not secreted for the spinal cord, nor the brain; nor is it secreted for the generative organs.

Never permit anyone to hypnotize you. You will never be the same person again. If you find anyone trying to hypnotize you, send him to "Siberia" immediately—in your imagination anyway.

Potassium and sodium have considerable to do with the generative function; with the utilization of fat for the generative system as well as for the nerves, brain, joints and for the sex brain; also for the spinal cord and other parts of the body requiring this very oily element of which we are speaking. When there is a lack of those elements, there will be a lack of the fatty element or at least it will not be properly utilized. This results in disease.

When we speak of the fatty elements needed in the body, we do not refer to the fatty element that is deposited under the chin or on the lower part of the abdomen or the fatty element which is deposited immediately under the skin. That kind of fat which is deposited in such parts of the body will never do you nor anyone else any good. It is superfluous fat; it will only do you harm.

When nature stores up fat in the blood, liver, under the chin, on the neck or anywhere, the fatty element is not being utilized properly. The fatty elements should be utilized in the bone marrow, nerves, lung substance, brain, generative substance; or in fact any and everywhere where it is needed. Even the muscles should carry a certain degree of fat.

When the potassium and sodium elements are lacking in the system, the function of saponification is not so good and then fatty foods do not agree. At such times we should also know what kind of fat will be most easily utilized. Butter fat, for instance, is never well utilized by the body for it is a different kind of fat than the body requires. Cocoanut fat is much better; even the fat from the "contemptible and dirty" hog seems to be nearer to the human body than is butter fat.

If there is a lack of potassium in the soil, the crops will suffer, so will the trees, nuts, plants, fruit and everything that grows in the soil. The crops will be backward; germs will thrive on the leaves of the plants. Potassium is important in taking care of the plants and preventing germs from thriving on leaves and fruit.

If we do not have enough potassium in our tissues, germs will take hold on the tissues. Certain salts protect our tissues as, for instance, potassium, fluorine, chlorine. Fluorine protects the bone; potassium protects the tissues and chlorine protects the alimentary tract. Fluorine also protects the lungs. When the system is charged with fluorine, it is impossible for consumption germs to take hold of the lungs. The fluorine element will send the consumption germs into eternity.

Potassium works in muscular tissue, sugar and fat. The muscles are vegetative in growth, as the hair. If it were not for the potassium element, germs would take hold of the roots of the hair and beard, resulting in their loss.

The scientific agriculturist recommends potassium for the soil to help the crop, trees, plants, nuts, fruits and also to protect them from certain species of germs.

The Myogenic man is red faced because he has the potassium element at work in his tissues. Because he has more potassium in his tissues, his tissues attract more oxygen. This is why he is red faced. He has more red blood and better functioning in the tissues. All people who have considerable oxygen in their tissues and their blood are red faced. They have a healthy color in their cheeks, magnetic eyes and an elastic walk.

If there is an insufficiency of the potassium element, tissue becomes sour. If you eat fat, butter, cream and all sorts of fatty products or fat meats, the tissues become acid and you suffer from gas generation and acid formation.

It may be very scientific to know how many red corpuscles there are in a cubic centimeter of blood. It may be interesting to know how great the blood pressure is. It may also be interesting to have an X-ray taken of our interior—but after all, when a doctor knows all of these facts and when you know all these facts yourself, what then? Can you then cure your disease or do you know after such scientific tests what you need? Does your doctor know? Can he cure you after he knows all the facts? If you need potassium, and you supply your system with the needed potassium foods, you will get cured whether you are in a sanitarium or a scientific laboratory, mansion or in the hills among the pines where the trees grow tall and where you do not know whether you have corpuscles in the blood or not.

When your tissues are acid, your system needs a greater supply of potassium. If you at such a time when you are sickwant to take a scientific count of your blood, do it. If you want your blood pressure determined, determine it. If you want your urine analyzed, analyze it; but whatever you do, do not forget that you need a high potassium diet. You can be as scientific as Darwin but do not be so scientific that you forget common sense.

Potassium is an alkaline element needed, not only by plants and animals but also by human tissues and secretions. If you are using up the potassium element in the muscles excessively and you do not supply enough of the potassium element, the tissues will soon become acid.

There are always germs wherever there is a lack of potassium, chlorine, fluorine and magnesium. So soon as there is acid in the stomach, bowels and tissues, there will be trouble. Acid and gas in the stomach and bowels results in constipation and autointoxication.

When there is an excess of the fibrin element in the blood, there is wonderful healing power in the blood. If there is a tiny hole or cut anywhere, it is soon healed up. If there is a hole in one heart ventricle or the valves of the heart resulting in regurgitation of the blood, and you manufacture fibrin in abundance, this leakage will soon disappear under a high fibrin and potassium diet. You can heal that leakage by diet but not by drugs. Nature can heal up a hole almost anywhere in the body; nature can cure you. The curative power is in the blood. Drugs may occasionally be necessary, providing they are not poisonous, but we should never forget diet. This does not mean that we do not need a doctor, chiropractor or osteopath. We need them all but their practice should be wide enough to include diet or that which goes into the human machine.

Hematogenesis is blood production. If there is an insufficiency of potassium, iron, sodium and chlorine, the right kind of blood is not manufactured. Internal oxidation is oxidation of the muscles. The muscles hold and utilize oxygen. Free oxygen is active in the muscles. We get animal heat through oxidation in the muscles. You do not get heat from fat. You may be told in your studies that fat is so many units of heat or so many calories. It is not so much a question of how much fat you have in your system, as it is a question, how are you able to utilize and convert that fat into units of heat? When we need bodily heat ,we must get it from the muscles not the fat. Seventy-five percent of the body heat comes from the muscles.

If you do not have enough oxygen in your tissues, you feel cold. Your arms, fingers, toes are cold perhaps all the time. Internal oxidation is at the foundation of thermogenesis or heat production. There is greater vibratory action in the cells when potassium is in the system. Under the influence of potassium, the cells receive greater power of life and action. During periods of potassium hunger, the tissues are cold and the handshake is dead; you feel as if you had hold of a dead fish. If such a man goes out to make sales what kind of a salesman do you think he will be? He has no energy. He cannot impress his customers. Even if he knew all about salesmanship he still could not make a sale. He cannot impress his customers. Courses in salesmanship never tell you anything about the necessity of a potassium diet. If a man lacks life, energy, ambition, power of conviction, personal magnetism, he cannot make a sale. A man can increase his self efficiency and efficiency as a salesman by the right kind of a diet.

Neuricity is the generation of nerve energy. When there is an abundance of potassium and high muscular oxidation, a man has more energy. He can sleep better. But when potassium is lacking there is unequal heat production in the body; one part may be hot and the other cold; one hand may be cold on one side and hot on the other. Lack of equalization of heat in the body is lack of potassium. If you want to make more fibrin for your blood, you must fall back on a high potassium diet.

The man who suffers from need of potassium is always in danger of falling. The power of balance is never good. When potassium salts are broken down in different parts of the body, this potassium precipitation must pass to and through the kidneys. The food ferments in the stomach and in the intestines when there is not enough potassium present in the system.

Butyric means butter. Butyric fat is not a good fat for the body.

Skatol and indol are protein poisons. If you are older than 27 years of age you better cut down your protein supply. You should look to other foods or eat other foods not containing so much protein. When we are protein drunk, we have the devil in us.

We should know what we are eating and drinking. If we do not cut out our protein foods, we will be compelled to go to the doctor. His pills will not cure us, however, before we cut down the protein diet. He can do us very little good as long as we keep up eating protein in excess.

When there is not enough potassium chloride in the tissues and blood, sickness sets in. Under the influence of potassium, the brain is able to function more vigorously. But when potassium is lacking, memory suffers from rheumatism and energy walks on crutches.

When potassium is lacking, sugar cannot be utilized in the muscles well. Hence, the sugar is stored in the liver until you suffer from enlargement of the liver. The liver may pass the sugar over to the kidneys and decomposition in the kidneys sets in and you suffer from dropsy or albuminuria or some other kidney disease.

Potassium and chlorine are important elements in the muscles. When the sugar goes through the kidneys, it causes fermentation. The kidneys are decomposed, resulting in diabetes. This is a tissue disease, although you think it is a kidney disease. This disease may start 5 or perhaps 10 years before you know there is any sugar in the urine. When you find there is sugar there it is sometimes too late. We should prevent this disease 5 years before it starts. We need preventive doctors. A doctor is too late when a man has one foot in the grave.

Neuritis is acid in the nerves or acid disturbing the nerves. Cramps are caused by acid. Neuralgia is nothing but acidity acting upon the nerves. Nerves will never ache unless there is acid which is producing the pain. When you suffer from neuralgia, there is acid in your system. When you suffer from sleeplessness, there is gas in your bowels, whether you know it or not. At such a time there is a lack of potassium or some other alkaline food element.

When there is acid or gas in your bowels it is not easy to sleep and when you do sleep it is a morphine-like stupor.

Animals sometimes eat grass to such an extent that they become bloated. Grass is very rich in potassium but does not contain chlorine to a sufficient extent. Let an animal eat grass until there is an excess of potassium in the system or in the alimentary tract and that animal will die from bloating unless ordinary common salty water is given that animal in abundance.

When potassium has been lacking for a long time and it is supplied, the patient may become sick. He thinks he does not need that kind of food because it makes him sick. He takes this for a sign that he must not eat it.

The eyesight is almost wonderful in people who have the potassium element in excess. They can see in the dark as clearly as a cat.

Deficiency of the potassium element in the body produces certain positive symptoms and perhaps also diseases. How do we know this? If you are a scientific man and want to find out for your self, cut out from your general dietary all such foods that are rich in the potassium element or cut out all such foods that are rich in the potassium element from the diet and watch for the results in 2 to 6 months. You will know not only the characteristics but also the symptoms, ailments, etc., which are peculiar to potassium-hunger. Remember you must know human constitutions.

There is a state of low tissue oxidation as a general symptom when the potassium element is lacking. This means that the tissues cannot function perfectly. Tissue water is formed. This decomposed tissue water decomposes the kidneys and lastly, the kidneys cannot function. All at once, you suffer from swollen ankles, which is a sure sign of low tissue oxidation. When we lower the potassium supply, the cerebellum cannot function efficiently. Hence, the patient feels like falling. Mental work and physical movements become difficult.

Periodic headache is a symptom that appears regularly, perhaps at 2 o'clock each day or perhaps in the evening. One peculiarity of potassium is periodicity. Plants, animals and people who lack the potassium element present periodic ailments or symptoms. When there is a lack of tissue oxidation, the muscles waste away, almost dissolve and are converted into water.

This is called dropsy. There is an inward fever but not an outward one. Something seems to be burning on the inside but not on the outside.

The skin itches and the patient scratches everywhere. The potassium patient complains of sensitive corns. There is a shrinkage in the cells of the cerebellum when there is a lack of potassium. Self abuse is often caused by a lack of potassium. A scar on the body itches more with a potassium lack.

When there is a lack of potassium, peristalsis is defective. This may result in acidity in the stomach. Even the muscles become acid and soon the whole system becomes acid. This results in many different diseases. That which you call disease is nothing else than the result of acidity in the system. So long as the system is alkaline there will be no disease; but as soon as the system becomes acid, gas is generated and finds its way to the nerves and even into the neurilemma of the nerves, between the nerve walls and the nerve substance itself, giving rise to what is called neuritis. These little gas wavelets find their way into the brain to disturb brain function. There is no such thing as an aching nerve as long as that nerve is alkaline. The Almighty has given us important foods containing salts of potassium, sodium, silicon and magnesium. The Almighty knew that without these alkaline elements, we would become acid and diseased.

Potassium is found in different greens, vegetables and cereals. Potassium is usually found on the outside but it is also functioning in the cells or the inner sanctuary of the tissues. The manufacturers put cereals through a mill and the potassium, silicon, phosphorus and other important organo-metallic salts are milled off. We get only the starch. The miller mills away— mother boils away—cook peels and pares away—that which we need so much. They may not mean to do it, but they are nevertheless. Thus those important foods that should contain the potassium element are eaten minus the potassium.

Lastly, stomach tissues and secretions become acid. Then the mother pays for her ignorance when her husband becomes a dyspeptic, a drunkard. She cooks him into an early grave, perhaps without knowing it. We should eat food the way the Almighty made it.

We have no business to mill away, peel away, boil away any part of food.

Potassium acts upon the intestines, motor nerves and makes them function more efficiently. The motor nerves are under the influence of the brain but if there is no potassium in the system to act upon the nerves, nerve action becomes spasmodic.

If we eat foods that are rich in fat, starch, sugar or gelatin, we cannot digest them nor assimilate them as we should. If we eat such foods which lack potassium it may produce autointoxication. This is especially true in regard to albumin. A lack of the potassium element in the system results in defective fat metabolism. Acid is a poison to the nerves.

The potassium-hungry person feels as if there is a grain of sand under his eyelid. He has a stitching pain in the left ear, never in the right. His mouth, throat and even stomach are full of pus and ropy mucus. He complains of pain in the lower back head. He turns from side to side and cannot sleep. He is restless, uneasy. A lady suffering from potassium hunger rushes home as fast as she can so she can take off her shoes, corset and other apparel touching her tender delicate skin. Her tissues are sore, tender, sensitive.

Displacement of the uterus is caused by a lack of potassium. A surgeon may cut in the muscles and sew in and around them—the patient may improve to a certain extent—but the muscles are too lax. The best thing a surgeon can do is leave the Almighty's workmanship alone, except in an emergency. An operation will do harm to people. Osteopaths do not care for operations. They may not be wise in all directions but they are willing to leave the Almighty's work alone.

Allopathic doctors are scientific men and are trying every possible way to cure people as for instance by electricity, baths, diet, climate, altitude. A doctor who recommends operations for the purpose of making money is not a real doctor. He is a mercenary. We have many such doctors, I am sorry to say. The doctor who says, "Eat what is placed before you and ask no questions," is no doctor.

The potassium hungry person likes his food sour and drinks great quantities of cold water, because his system is feverish. His liver is overheated and his spleen is in a state of fever.

He is fond of pickles. Hence we know that he lacks potassium.

Nausea from excitement is a positive symptom of potassium hunger. If you notice one single potassium-hunger symptom in your patient, you may know that he has perhaps a hundred or several hundred potassium symptoms.

When we are excited, we break down potassium salts. When we are jealous, we break down potassium. When we hate people, we also break down the potassium. The more we break down, the more acid we become and the more high-tempered we become also. It becomes more difficult for us to control our temper. Mental control, prayer and religion have their roots in the stomach. Ministers should know something about the chemistry of foods, how to eat and drink. They should understand the chemistry of the body.

Acidity acts unfavorably upon the nerves and cells. When there is an excess of acidity in the tissues, around nerves and perhaps in the brain, a man feels, acts and talks as though he is more devil than man. The time will come when ministers of the Gospel will be required to take a course in modern dietetics, according to the creative plan of the Almighty and thus explain to sinners how to eat, drink and cultivate good habits.

The more work we do the more potassium we break down. In a cold climate, we are able to increase the potassium supply in the body to a greater extent than during the hot summer months. Myogenic people usually have potassium in abundance. This is why he is unusually healthy. The vigorous man can undergo many hardships and yet keep up his health.

In times of emergency, the weak man collapses but the strong man goes on as if nothing has happened. He is sometimes like an elephant. A rabbit could not withstand great hardship nor could a rabbit stop the momentum of anything. It takes an elephant a long time to start but when he gets going he can sweep a thousand greyhounds out of the way.

An excess of potassium makes a man feel as if he is half drunk, as if he doesn't have full control of his muscles. A lack of potassium has the same approximate symptom. Give a musician a potassium diet in excess for a week and observe his mistakes in playing his musical instrument. His finger technique is partly lost and his music is not so good. This holds true when potassium is lacking. A lady in whom potassium is lacking in the tissues and secretions holds her finger on one key too long and another key isn't held long enough. This affects the harmony of the music.

All at once a man feels bloated, for no seeming reason when there is an excess of potassium. The motor cells are affected by a heavy potassium diet or by heavy potassium drugs. The potassium patient may imagine that he is flying away from the devil or that someone is after him, perhaps a police officer. He may dream he is trying to fly away from the devil, perhaps in some deep forest and that lastly, the devil gets hold of his feet and is pulling him into the dark forest. He may feel he is losing his mind. He fears the asylum. Such symptoms most medical men, osteopaths, homeopaths and others never pay any attention to or they call it nonsense or imagination but their patient is not cured.

Under a normal potassium diet, people can live more harmoniously together, but under the influence of a heavy starch diet, love takes wings and flies away. Excess acid in the stomach leads to the divorce court, to the insane asylum or to the operation table.

The potassium patient wants sympathy but if you sympathize with him he gets angry. The potassium-excess patient suffers from excessive alkalinity; the potassium-hungry patient suffers from the opposite, viz., acidity. There is a deficiency in the circulatory current of the blood and a weakness in the circulation center of the brain in the potassium-hungry patient.

The potassium-hungry patient suffers from albuminuria; the albumin is precipitated and appears in the urine.

When we speak of the potassium man, we have reference to the man of the Myogenic constitution. The Myogenic man is usually healthy or should be healthy.

The words "calisthenics" means "beautiful strength." Calisthenics is feminine gynmastics. The Myogenic man prefers to study in nature's university. The Myogenic man likes to see how things are done. He wants to see things move. He is interested in traffic action; he does not care to see anything stationary. When a Myogenic man has his steam up he wants lazy drones out of the way. The Myogenic man is a potassium man and believes in work, action and motion. Potassium is an element of energy and action, the same as oxygen.

FOOD ANALYSIS EXPLAINED

CHERVIL is a high potassium food and contains vitamins in the seed.

CHICKORY is a high potassium food.

BITTER GREENS. Potassium is one of the most bitter elements there is. It is bitter even when it is associated with sugar. All sorts of bitter foods, bitter greens, bitter vegetables, bitter nuts always carry potassium.

LENTILS are excellent. They should be cooked slowly after first being washed in running water so that any impurity may be washed off. Cook in distilled water about 2-1/2 hours. Lentils are very nutritious and better than meat for laborers. The person who sits a lot, doing only light work, should eat only about 2 teaspoonsful of lentils.

ALMONDS. The skin of almonds should not be eaten. Almonds should be grated and salted. You should never eat almonds by themselves, nor on an empty stomach, for this may produce stomach trouble.

CHESTNUTS are high in potassium. We should never eat chestnuts when chlorine and sodium are lacking. We should eat these nuts together with other foods.

SUNDRIED OLIVES. Never eat any other kind of olives. Green olives or ripe olives may poison you.

SCOTCH DRIED PEAS. This is another potassium food. Here you find potassium in connection with nitrates. In almonds you have potassium in connection with starch. In figs, you have potassium in connection with glucose. In one food, potassium may be associated with sugar; in another, it is associated with acid; in another, it is associated with fat and still another, with starch and another may be associated with nitrates. Then again, it may be associated with albumin.

One patient may need potassium with sugar, another may need potassium in connection with albumin, in still another, almond nuts or the starch in almond nuts may be needed in connection with potassium salts; in still another patient, the potassium associated with fatty substances may be the very thing he needs. Cook Scotch peas slowly and always in distilled water. Be sure to wash the peas first. Do not cook so that the steam comes out into the air because you are losing some of the important food odors. Do not eat green peas or Scotch peas or yellow peas or lentils to excess. Remember they are very high in nutrition.

BLUEBERRIES are of great value to certain constitutions. They are good for the muscles.

COCOANUT is a fine food for the nerves, bone marrow, lung substance and the brain.

ENDIVE is high in potassium. Cut it into small pieces and eat it raw.

LETTUCE is a sleep producer. It contains soporific properties. It cures sleeplessness in some cases.

OATMEAL. Steel-cut oatmeal contains silicon. Silicon is found mainly in the outside of the grain. Potassium is found in abundance in oats. Thirty-nine percent of the salts found in oats is silicon. It is of the greatest value to the sexual system, viz., the salt and other principles found in oatmeal. Oatmeal contains a principle called avenin, which stimulates the sexual system and the brain. A man who is weak sexually, who has abused himself, who wants to gain in manly strength, should take a heavy oatmeal diet. Cook oatmeal 24 hours in a fireless cooker and make also oatmeal muffins, oatmeal bread and other oatmeal dishes, and eat it in abundance—but not more than you can assimilate.

PARSLEY is an excellent food for one who suffers from sexual weakness. It contains a camphor of the greatest value to the sex brain. It is also stimulating to the nerves.

POTATOES should be baked and eaten with the skin. You find potassium salts in the skin. Take potato peelings and put parsley, endive and other potassium greens together and make a broth; drink this and you will obtain more potassium than any other method.

GERMAN PRUNES contain twice as much potassium as American prunes. They contain all the salts needed in the body. Before the war, German prunes sold for 75 cents a pound. American prunes are low in the salts but high in potassium. Prunes contain important laxative principles, viz., potassium, phosphorus, magnesium and sodium.

SPINACH should be cooked for 3 minutes in its own steam, poured on toast and eaten with broiled ham. This makes a fine meal. We should not pour the spinach juice into the sink.

BRAN. Some people think wheat bran is good for constipation but it is not. If you chew bran slowly and swallow the juice you draw out the salts in the bran. This would help constipation because it sweetens the stomach, but it will not cure constipation.

CARROTS are excellent as a food. You can eat them raw, grate, crush, grind or boil them.

CARROT WATER. Drink it by itself. It is better to drink than coffee and healthier.

GOOSEBERRIES are low in salts but high in potassium.

MEAT JUICE, RAW is high in chlorine but low in potassium. It has a stimulating effect upon the muscular tissues.

PEACHES are low in the salts but high in potassium. If you eat peaches the proper way they sweeten the stomach.

ROMAINE is a vegetable rich in distilled water. It is high in potassium.

All vegetables contain the vitamins in the seeds. It is not so easy to kill vitamins in figs. Figs should be eaten raw. They are excellent. They contain sugar that is associated with the organometallic salts for figs are rich in ash. We should wash figs before we eat them for germs are likely to cling to figs. Worms always grow in figs because they are rich in sugar and because they are rich in vitamins. You cannot taste the potassium in figs because it is associated with sugar.

We are eating ourselves into our graves without knowing it. After the age of about 45, we are in danger of eating too much. Lentils are rich in potassium. If we suffer from potassium hunger, we should eat lentils. If you lack potassium or if your system is not able to utilize potassium foods, drink dandelion wine as this would increase the potassium-assimilating capacity in your system so you may take up potassium to a greater extent. You can make dandelion wine yourself.

Potassium is one of the most virulent poisons available. If the stomach is empty and there is a lack of chlorine and sodium in the system, the potassium in nuts or olives may poison you.

We have possibly 60 or 70 different kinds of bitter teas. Potassium is the principal element in all of them. All sorts of bitter teas carry potassium. It is the potassium bitters found in those teas that is valuable.

BONESET TEA acts upon the liver.

BURDOCK TEA acts upon the muscles.

CHAMOMILE TEA acts upon the sexual system and is very valuable in times of defective menstruation or times of leucorrhea. No other tea equals chamomile tea for defective menstruation.

CATNIP TEA is excellent for gas in the stomach.

DANDELION TEA acts upon the liver and blood.

DANDELION WINE increases the potassium-assimilating capacity in the system, enabling the system to take up potassium from foods.

ELDERBERRY JUICE is important for the motherhood function. In fact, no juice is so valuable as elderberry juice to this function.

FLAXSEED TEA is good for coughs, bronchitis and consumption.

HOPS TEA is an excellent one for the Medeic constitution. The Medeic impurities may be sent out of the system by drinking Hops tea. This is also true in regard to sassafras tea. Germs, vermin, insects dislike the odor of sassafras. The gonorrheal germ feels uncomfortable under the influence of hops or sassafras teas.

LAUREL LEAVES is a mild, bitter tonic containing tannin and a trace of hydroanic acid; it acts upon the cerebellum.

MARJORAM TEA contains a remarkable principle which has a very beneficial effect on sexual excitement. It acts favorably upon the sex brain, sex glands and sexual system of a man who suffers from satyriasis or from self abuse or from some other ailment of the sexual system. Marjoram tea is highly favorable for excessive tension in sexual glands, nerves or cells.

MINT OR PEPPERMINT TEA is excellent for gas in the stomach. Everyone should have these teas on hand. You should raise such herbs in your garden and preserve the same for winter. Such herbs you buy are never as good as those you pick and dry yourself. The teas you buy often have lost their strength.

SAGE TEA is good for colds. We can stimulate the circulatory system, sexual system with strong sage tea.

SARSAPARILLA TEA acts on the liver. There is no tea or food that acts directly upon the blood. It is only by passing through the liver that it can purify the blood. Anything that acts upon the liver acts also upon the bloodstream indirectly but never directly.

SASSAFRAS TEA contains and spreads an odor that germs, fleas, bedbugs, chicken lice, etc. cannot stand. It is even disagreeable to ants. It helps to send Medeic and gonorrheal impurities out of the system. Germs do not thrive under the influence of sassafras.

SAVORY TEA (Satureia hortensis) acts upon the uterus, a tonic; a carminative; i.e., it is a soothing tea; relieves gas pains.

SENNA TEA acts upon the liver and bowels.

THYME TEA contains thymol, an antiseptic and stimulant.

WINTERGREEN TEA acts upon the liver.

WORMWOOD TEA acts upon the heart. It is also a stomach tonic, but will weaken the stomach and lastly, destroy sex capacity.

AILMENTS ON WHICH TEAS RICH IN POTASSIUM HAVE A CURATIVE EFFECT

BLOOD: Boneset tea, Sarsaparilla tea, Senna tea, Wintergreen tea.

BRONCHITIS: Flaxseed tea.

CEREBELLUM: Laurel leaves tea, Thyme tea.

CIRCULATORY SYSTEM: Sage tea.

COLDS: Sage tea.

COLIC: Peppermint tea, Catnip tea.

CONSTIPATION: Senna tea.

COUGH: Sage tea.

HEADACHE: Peppermint, Catnip teas; if headache is caused by flatus. Chamomile tea, roasted Corncob tea; if headache is caused by contraction of the uterus.

HEART: Wormwood tea.

INFLUENZA: Hops and Sage teas.

LIVER: Boneset tea, Dandelion tea, Senna tea, Sarsaparilla tea, Wintergreen tea.

MUSCLES: Burdock tea.

NERVES: Savory tea.

SEXUAL SYSTEM: Ailments and self abuse—Marjoram tea; Weakened condition—Chamomile and Sage teas.

SEXUAL (females): Leucorrhea—Chamomile tea; Menstruation—Chamomile tea; Motherhood functions—Chamomile tea; Uterus—Savory tea.

SLEEPLESSNESS (caused by gas): Peppermint tea or mint tea.

STOMACH (Acid, Gas, Fermentation, Flatus): Catnip, Savory, Peppermint, Mint teas.

TAINT (Medeic): Hops tea, Sassafras tea.

TUBERCULOSIS: Flaxseed tea.

QUESTIONS AND ANSWERS

1. Can a child get enough potassium from spinach juice? Answer: I would advise other foods for potassium rather than spinach juice. Potassium is in the leaves to a greater extent than it is in the juice.

2. Would a fall resulting in a broken knee cap, which the doctors diagnose as tuberculosis of the joint, be contagious? Answer: No, tuberculosis is not contagious unless the sputum containing the germs dries up and floats about in the air so that a person will inhale the germ.

3. How long does it require calcium food to be taken up by the system after eating? Answer: It is difficult to tell how long it takes. Calcium stays some time in the alimentary tract and even after it is assimilated by the blood, it stays there for a time before it is deposited in the tissues. How long, no one knows. It may take perhaps anywhere from 3 days to 2 weeks. The sugar would go into the tissues, alimentary tract and the liver and absorb the calcium out of those tissues and also out of the blood.

4. How is potassium obtained from the birch tree? Does fire destroy it? How is potassium best applied to plants? Answer: No, fire cannot destroy potassium. We obtain it from the birch tree by burning it. Organic potassium is better for plants than inorganic. Wood ash is better for plants than the potassium that comes from rocks or heavy soils.

5. What is the best method of curing a severe cold in the throat and lungs in an Exesthesic lady? Answer: Retire and drink hot bitter teas. Do not eat anything. Sleep as much as possible. Put hot applications on the stomach and bowels.

6. Does a baby need potash when the face is very red and rough? Answer: That is no indication of lack of potassium. Potassium hunger has very different symptoms.

7. Please tell how to eat cocoanut to get chlorine; How much per day? Is the milk as good as the solid? Should the skin be removed? Answer: Eat cocoanut at meals. Grate or grind it up. Take about 3 tablespoons. The milk is not as good as the solid. You can eat the inner skin, it contains more potassium.

8. Can amativeness be developed and virtue retained? Answer: Yes. It has nothing to do with virtue either one way or the other. A man may be strong in amativeness and be as virtuous as an angel. He may be weak in amativeness and be a sensualist. Amativeness is not lust. The best way to develop amativeness is to admire the people of the opposite sex and leave them alone, by cultivating platonic love and the higher Christian virtues.

9. What is the cause of running of tears from eyes when not in emotion? What indicates aching veins? Answer: It is nothing but weak sexuality. Of course this is not the only thing that produces running tears, but it is one of those conditions that produce it. Aching veins indicate that the blood is too sluggish in the veins and that the liver is torpid.

10. What causes the lips to dry and blister during cold and windy weather, and what helps to take the soreness away? Answer: The fatty substance and moisture are drawn out from the lips by cold and windy weather. Supply sufficient moisture and the right kind of fat to the lips and keep yourself warm or stay out of the cold and wind.

11. What is the cause of Erysipelas? Answer: It is caused by a germ; it is a contagious disease.

12. If the regurgitation is in the aortic valve, should the patient lie on the right side? Answer: Yes. He should lie on the right side and slightly on the back.

13. Is filtered rain water the best to drink? Answer: Yes. Filtered rain water is an excellent drink. It is distilled water. Filter it in a clean barrel, put a layer of charcoal then a layer of washed white sand then another layer of charcoal and a little layer of fine sand. Make layer upon layer until the barrel is full. Then let the water filter through slowly. You will have clean distilled water.

14. What type of patients are bothered mostly by chapped hands? What is the cause of chapped hands? Answer: Calcium types. Exesthesic men and women are bothered very much. Chapped hands are an indication of a lack of the fatty element in the skin. Not all Calciferic people suffer from chapped hands nor a great many Exesthesic. Chapped hands are a result of the dryness in the tissues; lack of animal heat in the skin; lack of skin food or silicon. Of course, no one would suffer from chapped hands unless he is out in the wind, cold, frost and dryness. Some suffer from chapped hands because germ life inhabits the skin or because germs are at work at the surface of the skin, producing skin disease of some kind.

15. How can we determine whether it is excess or a deficiency of some certain chemical element from which a patient suffers? Answer: We can always determine this by the difference in symptoms. It may be true that symptoms may be similar but they are never identical. If a patient suffers from excess, there are symptoms that appear from excess of a certain chemical element which never appear in times of deficiency.

16. Is potassium needed in a mental breakdown from excessive mental strain? Answer: Yes. A potassium diet is needed in cerebellar and muscular prostration.

17. How long does the average patient have to subsist upon a specific diet before results may be obtained? Answer: This depends upon how soon the constitution responds to the element. The longer you go without supplying the elements needed, the longer it takes for your system to assimilate it. If a constitution has been robbed of sodium for a very long time, we begin to supply it and that person may become sick simply because his constitution cannot accommodate itself to the sodium element. It may take a month or six months, possibly even longer before the body assimilates that lost food element in normal quantities.

18. How much ash is found in persimmons? Answer: 0.96% or nearly 1%.

19. Which is the best part of the carrot—the inside or the part near the surface? Does the carrot contain any potassium? Answer: The potassium salts are distributed through the whole carrot, nearly equally, but most potassium salts are found in the peelings, nevertheless. Carrots contain nearly 1% of organometallic salts and of those organometallic salts, it contains 36.90% of potash; 21.20% sodium; 11.30% calcium; 4.40% magnesium; 21.00% iron; 12.80% phosphorus; 0.45% sulphur; 2.49% silicon; 4.60% chlorine; a trace of manganese and fluorine.

20. Do breathing exercises after meals interfere with digestion or do they benefit it? Likewise bowel exercises? Answer: Vigorous exercises are not beneficial after meals. If you take any kind of exercise after meals, let it be walking and breathing exercises. If you do vigorous physicul exercise after meals, it will interfere with digestion by drawing the blood to other parts of the body.

21. Is it possible to reduce a goiter of two years standing in a man of 65 years? What diet and applications are best for it? Answer: He is too old unless he is vigorous in vitality and youthful in appearance. An iodine diet is good for him. He could not perhaps extract the salts from supplied food.

22. Should a potassium and sodium diet always go together to avoid exhaustion of sodium when a potash diet is given? Answer: As a general rule, except when potassium has been exhausted for some cause. A potassium diet always requires a heavy sodium and chlorine diet. It is well to remember also that sodium and chlorine are elements that are used every hour of the day in every man, woman and child.

23. Is potassium especially indicated in albuminuria? Answer: No, but chlorine is.

24. Do you mean that excess potassium has the same symptoms as a lack of potassium? Answer: Yes. The symptoms are similar but not identical. There are great differences in symptoms between potassium hunger and potassium excess, as you would learn if you were to place potassium-excess symptoms and hunger symptoms in contrast.

25. What would you do in a case where potassium is lacking? Also chlorine and sodium? You say that chlorine and sodium foods should be omitted. Answer: In times of potassium hunger, the chances are that sodium and chlorine are in excess or at least one of those elements. In that case, we should cut out that element which is in excess. If both are in excess, it would be better to supply potassium only. Of course, you will understand that it would be almost impossible to cut out sodium and chlorine entirely for all foods contain them to a certain extent, although some foods are comparatively lacking in these elements.

26. Give your opinion on wearing corsets, belts, supporters or anything that obstructs circulation. Answer: Tightness or pressure on the stomach, neck or any part of the body interferes with the circulation of blood in those parts. We should never produce pressure on the skin, circulatory vessels, organs throughout the entire body. Any pressure upon any part of the body produces ailments of some kind in the course of time.

27. How much sassafras tea and how many currants should one drink and eat daily to get the Medeic taint out of the system and how long should one take them? Answer: A Medeic taint is simply a taint. It would perhaps require from 60 days to 1 year or longer to eliminate a Medeic taint from the system.

28. What can we advise for high blood pressure? Answer: That depends on the cause. There are many causes of high blood pressure. The main thing to do is remove the cause first. There may perhaps be from 10 to 20 causes or more. High blood pressure is a general symptom and does not mean much until we know what is causing it. It may mean anything or nothing. Some types of people have normally high blood pressure readings.

29. Is one likely to get too much potassium in foods? Answer: Yes, it is possible. If we eat high potassium foods at every meal, day after day, month after month, year after year, in the course of time, there will be an excessive supply in the body. If there is potassium excess there would be a sodium and chlorine hunger also. Potassium always lowers the supply of sodium and chlorine.

30. Is not potassium excess found in people who have been drugged with potassium drugs? Answer: It is possible to develop potassium-excess symptoms and poisoning merely by drinking drugs high in potassium. If you take potassium-carrying drugs for a very long time, you will become a wreck and no one can ever cure you.

FOODS AND CHEMICALS
<u>CHLORINE</u>

Chlorine is one of the sixteen elements found in man. It is a great germicide. It cleanses and washes the cells land sends germs and impurities out of the body. Germs are at work in the body by the millions. We are fighting germs, all of the time, and they are killing us. This is called disease. There are thousands of different kinds of germs. This is the reason that fluorine, chlorine and magnesium have been organized into the human body to help throw off poisons, germs and disease. Fluorine kills many kinds of germs, including the consumption germ. Chlorine kills hundreds of different kinds of germs. When there is gas generation, poisons, fever, fatty acid in the stomach, a teaspoonful of ordinary table salt, taken in distilled water, sometimes is very beneficial. Chlorine cleanses the cells until they are purified. It does this by a sort of suction or pressure. Chlorine does the same kind of work in the human body that the laundryman and soap do to clothes. Chlorine kills germs in the system, passes them through the alimentary tract, out of the body. One teaspoonful of ordinary common salt in a little water sends germs flying to the earth and space.

If you feel bloated, uncomfortable, cannot sleep because of gas passing into the nerves and brain, all because of impurities and toxins at work in tissues and nerves, a teaspoonful of ordinary common salt in distilled water and a hot application on your bowels, taken as hot as you can stand it for about an hour at time after you retire, will put you to sleep in perhaps 90 cases out of 100. Germs, impurities, decomposed tissue water are sent out of your system.

The human system is a sort of a battlefield. Talk about Hindenburg's army—you ought to see the army of germs at work in your interior to conquer you. There is a greater battle going on in the body than was carried on between Germany and the Allies. Millions of little germs are at work in the body. Chlorine, sulphur, fluorine, magnesium are your artillery and powder. Chlorine is a powerful germicidal agent. Ordinary common salt is nothing else than chlorine and sodium.

If there is an excess of chlorine in the system, you are relieved by inhaling ammonia. Sometimes in a Medeic constitution and in the Marasmic constitution, chlorine consumption may be too great. Those people have a suffocating cough and can hardly get air enough. This is a chlorine symptom. Chlorine combines with phosphorus. If you are a mental temperament or of a Pathetic constitution or Nervo-Motive or Exesthesic, and there is a lack of chlorine in your system, you suffer from a certain kind of neurasthenia and this neurasthenia no doctor can cure before you eat rightly.

The brain itself is of such a nature that it must have chlorine. If there is an insufficiency of chlorine in the body, you will have trouble with the nerves and brain. Chlorine has an indirect influence upon the brain. Phosphorus and sulphur have a direct influence on the brain but chlorione has an indirect influence. Lack of chlorine results in poor brain and nerve metabolism. Under the influence of a chlorine diet, the nerves grow stronger and the brain is supplied with the nourishment needed.

Chlorine takes up water like a sponge. It takes up 50 times as much water as its own quantity. If you eat foods rich in chlorine, you are driving sick water out of your system. If you suffer from impurities and you drink chlorine-containing drinks or eat chlorine-containing

536

foods, the decomposed liquid that you have in your system is abstracted from the brain, nerves, muscles, vital organs and must pass out of your body. You lose weight. Thus in times of hydric obesity, there is nothing better than a dry and high chlorine diet. You can reduce almost a pound a day on such a diet. If you get thirsty when you drink salty drinks and you then drink hot lemonade, you can reduce that much more, providing you put no sugar into the lemonade. When you suffer from hydric obesity, you should eat foods that are below 30% water, low in starch, sugar, fat, and rich in chlorine.

When there is an excess of water in the system, there is a lack of chlorine. Much water drinking washes the chlorine and sodium out of your body. When there is an excess of chlorine, you are lean. A Chinese is usually a chlorine man; he is also a lean man. You seldom see a fat Chinese. The Chinese are mostly a Marasmic constitution.

Nervous prostration, caused by a lack of chlorine, requires a high chlorine diet. When there is an excess of water in the system, you require a salty, dry diet.

A man who is Marasmic in constitution, should be given a diet rich in magnesium to counteract the excess of chlorine in case he wants to put on flesh. Give such a man the white of egg, either raw or boiled. The more albumin you put into his diet, the more work you give the chlorine he has in his system to do. Chlorine works in albumin. When a patient suffers from albuminuria, give him chlorine foods in abundance.

The Irish people, as a rule, are witty because they have chlorine in excess and because they are wide-headed. When a man has a wide head, a small back head, a low top head and chlorine consumption is great, that man is witty and sarcastic. A man who has Hydrogen or water to excess in his body, is not witty. Did you ever see a witty Hydripheric or Carboferic person? A chlorine person is always witty, always full of arguments and sarcasm. Very often, such a person has running eyes, or eyes called sour eyes. Sometimes the eyelids hang down like bags. He looks sour and angry, and people keep away from him.

Sometimes the stomach and liver become an alcohol factory, even in the Christian. At such a time, a rich chlorine diet is needed. If you feel bloated, uncomfortable, full of gas, take a teaspoonful of ordinary common salt in distilled water and you will soon be relieved. This starts the peristaltic movements in your stomach and intestines. Then it is necessary to eat small meals. When you suffer from gas in the stomach, bloating, indigestion, you must not eat heavy meals. Old people and people who suffer from dyspepsia, do not need very much food, as they cannot digest it nor assimilate it. When a man is over 55 years of age, he does not need very much food but he needs an eliminative diet.

When there is sulphur gas at work in the interior, it is not easy to be agreeable, romantic, poetic. A salty diet is very beneficial at such a time. The function of chlorine is to send impurities and germs out of the system and to draw off decomposed water. Chlorine takes the bacterial impurities out of the system and relieves the nerves and brain cells.

It is difficult to pray properly when there is autotoxin and acid in the stomach. It is difficult to talk about joy, peace, heaven, reformation and conversion. So long as there is impurity in the interior, around the nerves and in the brain, the Holy Spirit will not be influenced very much to live in such an atmosphere.

Metabolism is upbuilding and tearing down processes in the body. These two processes are at work in daytime and nighttime. We are being torn down every minute of the day; we are being built up every minute of the day also. When we are being torn down faster than we are being built up, we grow lean; when we are being built up faster than we are being torn down, we grow fleshy. In some people, that apparent fleshiness is nothing but gas. In others it is water; in others it may be nothing but phlegm; and in still others, it may be nothing but fat or fatty growths. When we grow old, it is better to be lean than fleshy. If a man is fleshy as he advances in years, he is likely to die early.

Chlorine and potassium are the two elements by means of which the peristaltic action takes place, under the influence of psychical impulse. When there is a lack of chlorine and potassium in the intestines, we suffer from constipation. Everything is comparatively still and we suffer from stasis. You cannot start that peristaltic action in the stomach by colon irrigation. You must supply the chlorine and potassium elements. A colon injection may weaken the bowels in the course of time and may even injure the bowels. It is better to fall back on a high potassium diet. Remember the elements chlorine, potassium, silicon, magnesium and fluorine when you suffer from constipation and catarrh.

Internal baths or colon irrigations, are likely to weaken the muscles in the canal walls of the colon. These muscle fibers may become paralyzed by inflation to such an extent that you may suffer from intestinal paralysis or from a colon ailment that can never be cured. If you must take a colon irrigation, use plenty of salt water and let the water run in as slowly as it is possible. The water should pass along the intestinal walls and does pass along the intestinal wall in times of colon irrigation. If it does pass along the intestinal wall, it does not effect the hardened excreta. The excreta is there just the same after you are through with your colon irrigation. Is it not much better to eat foods rich in chlorine, silicon, potassium and magnesium? This is the normal way. Then you will strengthen the colon and the muscles in the walls of the alimentary tract.

If there is a lack of chlorine in the muscles, we cannot work so efficiently. Go to church and pray but study diet and your own needs as you pray and read your Bible. Use your own brain and common sense. If there is a lack of hydrochloric acid in your stomach, how can you digest your food? You simply suffer from indigestion, not because you have too much chlorine, but because you do not have enough.

Germs cannot thrive in the presence of chlorine. You use ordinary salt to preserve meat; use common salt to preserve your own intestines. You can keep meat for a year or longer by putting plenty of salt on it. This is a good lesson in regard to your stomach. When there are many germs anywhere, put a little chlorine on them, and they will feel very uncomfortable.

It is not wise to use an exclusive vegetable diet. We should remember that there are 16 chemical elements needed in the body. In an entire vegetable diet, you cannot get enough chlorine. There are also other elements you cannot get very much of. If you live on nothing but greens, you get potassium in excess. Potash will take chlorine and sodium out of your system so that lastly, you will suffer from many ailments. Vegetables, fruit and cereals are lacking in chlorine.

Rheumatism is often caused by lack of chlorine, sodium, fluorine, manganese and magnesium. You may obtain a temporary relief from a masseur when you suffer from rheumatism, but it will return and you will never be cured until you eat right.

Chlorine has a powerful pressing effect on the cells. It presses the cells together so that they become compact. The chlorine man is a compact man; he is strong. Dempsey was a chlorine man; Carpentier was a chlorine man.

We should eat plenty of chlorine foods so we may eliminate impurities and kill germs or they will otherwise kill us.

All animals that have an excess of chlorine are hypnotic. A chlorine man is a great talker, for a time, then he is as mute as a grave. If you speak to him, he may answer you in a disagreeable manner. Chinese sit in different parts of the same room or car, and never say a word to each other.

A dog uses up a great deal of chlorine. The dog is slavish in his devotion toward his master. The chlorine man is similar to a dog in this respect. A dog sleeps with one eye open and the other eye closed; he can hear with one ear. This is also the case with the chlorine man. He is an excellent watchman. If you want a first-class watchman, hire a chlorine man. Such a man is usually wide headed. The more wide headed the more chlorine he utilizes for the metabolic functions. Such a man or animal suffers from liver ailments in the course of time. They are lean and a woman is also lean. She knows everything that goes on in the neighborhood; she is talking about everybody; she is a sort of neighborhood directory. The chlorine man has a wonderful memory for evil. That is also the nature of the dog. If you injure a man like that he never forgets it and never forgives it. If you injure a dog, he never forgets or forgives either. When a man is wide-headed and chlorine consumption is excessive, this man is always a sensationalist, if he is a journalist. His mind runs to yellow journalism.

If you fall in love with such a man, he loves you one minute and throws you out a window the next. When chlorine consumption is excessive, there is a greenish tint to the eye; there is also jealousy, temper, cruelty in his disposition. If he has a green eye, there is something ugly in his very soul—something black in his blood. He may marry a lady and leave her within only a few days, to find another affinity.

Injure a chlorine man and he may come back in five or ten years to fight.

The faculties of observation are never active in a chlorine man, whether they are large in the brain or not. The imaginative faculties are always more active in a chlorine man. At times, such a man does not know just where he is, nor what is taking place around him. He is in a sort of hypnotic dream occasionally. He can, however, watch evil deeds and evil people. He sees everything that is bad and imagines bad things also. A chlorine man likes stimulants and has a leaning toward morphine habits and drinking. Chlorine people are always in a rush.

When there is a lack of chlorine in the spleen, there is tension in the spleen. The spleen cannot function well before it is well supplied with chlorine. If you tell such a patient to hold out his tongue, his tongue seems to stick in his mouth and is so large it fills his entire mouth. If you tell a phosphorus patient to hold out his tongue, he sticks it out all the way and it is long, slender and small.

When you lack chlorine, you suffer from pyorrhea. Then your doctor may tell you to go to the dentist and have your teeth plucked out. The osteopath gives you treatments for spinal lesion. When chlorine is lacking, the functions are disturbed. A chlorine patient may suffer from toothache while out in the cold.

You cannot perspire without using up chlorine. When you cannot perspire you lack chlorine, sodium and sulphur.

The more you work, the more you take chlorine out of your system. When a man works hard and perspires, chlorine is passing out of his body very rapidly, through the skin, also through the urine. When you use your brain very much, you use up chlorine, phosphorus and sulphur, as may be demonstrated in the laboratory, for such elements always appear in the urine. In times of heavy brain work, this is especially true in regard to phosphorus. At such a time, you must supply those elements by eating such foods that contain those elements. You must know what you are eating. Foods that are good for you now may not be good for you a year from now.

If you suffer from autointoxication, you are in the greatest need for chlorine, potassium, magnesium and fluorine.

The Calciferic and Isogenic should eat foods rich in sodium, to prevent calcic hardening.

When people lack chlorine, they crave sympathy. This is especially true in regard to women. If you give them sympathy at such a time, they become fussy and may probably refuse the sympathy, yet they crave it.

When we speak of disease tendencies in chlorine people, we have reference to chlorine-excess symptoms and diseases. When chlorine is being consumed excessively, it results in chlorine starvation in the body, especially in the blood and secretions. There are certain compound elements needed by the tissues of the heart, i.e., sodium chloride, potassium chloride and calcium phosphate. They are the heart salts or tissue salts.

If you add iron, you have all the important blood salts and tissue salts needed by the tissues. When any of these compounds are lacking, there will be heart disease or a tendency to palpitation or a tendency to contraction in the heart nerves or in the heart muscles.

When I was in a laboratory once, we took a rabbit's heart that had not beat for 4 hours and put it into a solution made of those very heart salts and the heart beat for 72 hours before it stopped completely. This proved to us that the heart and its function depends upon chemical food salts. Those food salts must be supplied at all times, otherwise the heart action is not so energetic nor so regular.

If you suffer from heart disease, it may be due possibly to a lack of those tissue salts. Do you think it would be wise for you to drug yourself with digitalis at such a time? Do you not think that you would die? But if you supply those foods that contain sodium chloride, potassium chloride and calcium phosphate in proper combination, you would overcome your heart disease. Your heart cannot stop so long as they are supplied. That is one way of keeping your heart going, viz., by chemical means. Even after you are dead, it is possible to start your heart by keeping it in a solution made of those salts in the proper combination.

Iron, lack or excess, has its eruptions as potassium, chlorine, sodium and certain poisons as, for instance, the Medeic man with his poisons. Eruptions are different kin kind. In the chlorine patient, the mouth is almost dark red from eruptions when there is an absolute lack of chlorine in the tissues, blood or secretions. He has his eruption on the arms, chest, neck and on the mouth.

Chlorine patients breathe all the way from 16 to 38 respirations a minute. I do not know whether I would call that normal, because I have found that the stronger a man, the more air he takes into his system and the slower his respirations. Some men take 8, 5, even 3 respirations of air a minute. I have found that very strong men take only 3 respirations a minute. The chlorine patient takes from 16 to 32, being quick and weak. When the chlorine patient inhales air, it seems to him and to others also, as if his lungs are too small. It seems that the linings of the lungs do not permit expansion hence the breathing of the chlorine patient "catches."

We hear a great deal about proteins and we are told that they give us strength. They are called the albuminoids. When protein is digested in the human system, it is called proteid. Foods contain protein but after protein is digested and properly prepared in the body, it is called proteid in physiology. If you lack the chlorine element or if there is an excess of chlorine, it is important that your diet supplies chlorine according to your needs. If chlorine consumption is excessive so you suffer from chlorine hunger, you should have a low protein diet which contains about 1-1/2% protein. Use a vegetable-protein diet. Animal protein is more difficult to digest and handle. Meat or beef protein is difficult to digest. When chlorine consumption is too great you suffer from weakness of some kind and principally because you cannot digest, utilize and assimilate the protein element.

When protein metabolism is low, you should go on a low protein diet. You should introduce chlorine-containing food to a greater extent. You know when you have eaten too much protein because you feel heavy, dull and stupid after eating. When you feel weak and you do not know what to do, when you have no ambition, you may be sure that protein

metabolism is low. Again, when you have trouble with your stomach, when you cannot digest your food, you suffer from low protein metabolism. The stomach must digest food material for the muscles and when the stomach cannot digest protein, the muscles suffer. Hence, also, low protein digestion results in muscular prostration.

Excitable people run so low in chlorine that the throat contracts to such an extent that the voice gets beyond control. The slightest excitement in the Nervi-Motive people, affects the voice. You cannot sing well when there is a lack of chlorine. See that you have plenty of chlorine in your system before you take a course in voice culture. You should remember that chlorine increases the strength of the voice.

A function of chlorine is to work in albumin. If there is a lack of chlorine, it results in albuminuria. When we speak of chlorine people, we have reference to that constitution in which chlorine consumption is excessive. A chlorine patient is usually interested in sanitary work. Anything dirty often appeals to him. He may not be clean himself in the sense of dress, but he is clean in habit. He likes to cut in a cadaver; he usually makes a good surgeon. If you have strong ideality, you will never be much interested in surgery. If you are of an Exesthesic constitution or if you are of a Nervi-Motive constitution, you will not be interested in surgery. If you are of a Nitropheric constitution, you will not be interested in surgery nor should you take up surgery—instead become a homeopath, osteopath or an idealistic doctor, i.e., one who merely gives advice.

Heavy work in the sunshine uses up the chlorine element in your body. In a hot, warm country where there is a great deal of iron in the soil, heat is oppressive and the chlorine element is broken down in connection with the sodium element. A vegetable diet breaks down chlorine, also sodium. If you live exclusively on a vegetable diet, you will get so much sulphur into your body that lastly you are likely to spread an odor about you like a cabbage patch. Cabbage is a sulphur plant; onions are sulphur plants and radishes are sulphur plants.

In times of pneumonia, chlorine is precipitated and appears in the urine. This is also true in times of flu. You can never build strong joints without a heavy chlorine diet nor without sodium. You need these elements for the building of joints. It is chlorine principally that builds joints.

If absolute starvation of chlorine prevails in your system, you are likely to die of albuminuria. When you suffer from this, go to a doctor who believes in diet, a doctor who knows the value of chlorine, one who knows which foods contain chlorine. Old material must be taken out of the tissues and new material supplied.

If there is a lack of sodium chloride and potassium chloride, the old material cannot be taken out of the body and new material cannot be supplied, simply because old material is in the way. This results in tissue congestion. You may go to a masseur and he may stir up or loosen up the dead stuff in your tissues for the time being and you may feel well for about an hour or more then you feel as bad as ever. When there is a lack of chlorine, dead material is not well eliminated. Chlorine is, so to speak, the laundryman in the body. It helps remove dead materials from the body.

If there is an insufficiency of sodium chloride in the system or in the blood, the red corpuscles cannot maintain their shape nor can they travel forward so actively as they otherwise would. They cannot move forward with the same power. They do not have sufficient kinetic energy. They cannot carry as much oxygen as is necessary. That is the reason the Almighty put those important food salts into the body so that the body may be supplied with oxygen and with all those powers that are so essential for perfect self-efficiency, in all the functions, habits, studies and otherwise. This is also the reason why we should study all the chemical elements, both as we find them in the body and in food. We should study the Almighty's laws of life and introduce them into our everyday action, thought and studies. We should make an attempt to study the scheme of life in its relation to food, diet and efficiency.

Study the living man not the dead man. After a man is dead, he is dead. Then there is no life, no functioning; the blood and secretions are not the same. We should know also that when we wish to cure a living man, we should study a living man and not a cadaver. We should find out what is needed in the normal man; how

much chlorine is needed and where it is needed and why it is needed.

Chlorine is found almost everywhere in the body. It is found in the tissues to the extent of one and three-quarter pounds. Chlorine is needed for memorizing, for the nerves, bones, tissues, for the sexual function, the generative function, the bile, in order to carry out the bile function. It is needed in the joints above all things. Bones cannot be built without chlorine. If you become passionate, you are burning up chlorine, also iron. If you want perfect children, it is more important to have chlorine-containing foods than it is to study eugenics written by great authorities. You will have better offspring if you have all the normal food salts needed in your body. When you cry, you use up chlorine. Tears are always salty; your perspiration is also salty. Chlorine is needed almost everywhere in the body.

It doesn't matter so much how much water there is in a certain food, how much protein, how much fat, how much carbohydrate; it is exceedingly important to know how much of the various organometallic salts you are supplying in your everyday diet. When the chemist has analyzed or perhaps burned up everything there is in a certain food, only ash is left. It is the ash that is more important to study. If you wish to cure a sick man, it is the ash that cures. In speaking of all these salts, it should be remembered that they always appear as Oxides, as sodium oxide, etc. We should know in which foods we can find those salts. We should know what those salts are needed for, how they may be supplied, especially to a sick man.

We should study the ash contents of food. The Almighty put these ash contents into the foods and into the body because He knew they are needed in the scheme of life. Burn up the drugs in your drugstore, especially the poisonous drugs, if you please, but study the scheme of the Almighty.

Christian Science may be an excellent doctrine, but it cannot cure you when you are sick from a lack of certain salts. When the Christian Scientist lacks these important tissue salts, blood salts, nerve salts, he also is sick however much he prays; however holy he may be or however much he may deny disease and death. Even Mrs. Eddy is dead with all her wise teachings. It is perfectly true that her teachings are noble, great, good; but it is also true that she neglected the study of that material which goes into man and which builds a more perfect body, cleaner blood and a more purified soul. If we follow the scheme of the Almighty, we can keep ourselves well, strong and vigorous when we are old. We can live longer and die nobler.

Sometimes it seems that sickness is a sin. So long as we need asylums for the insane and those are full of insane people, doctors have not done their duty. So long as we need hospitals, doctors have not done their duty. So long as we have jails and criminals, ministers have not done their duty. If you eat right, think right, live right and study the scheme of the Almighty, there is no need for jails, hospitals, sanitariums nor asylums. Then there is also less need of undertakers and gravediggers.

When we are studying the ash of carrots, for instance, we say carrots contain 8% silicon. That means the carrot contains in the ash content 8% of silicon. Suppose we find about 1.74% of ash in goat's milk and we find that of these salts found in the milk 31% is chlorine; it simply means that 31% of the ash is chlorine. Ox blood, of its 0.85% of ash, we find about 35% of chlorine. We learn from such chemical analyses that goat's milk contains a higher percentage of chlorine than ox blood. The comparative percentage of goat's milk and goat's cheese is a great deal higher than the comparative percentage of ox blood.

The vitamins are found in abundance in fresh goat's milk but in boiled goat's milk you do not find the vitamins for the boiling kills them. The vitamins are always in the seeds of food. Anything that grows as for instance, a chicken, spinach, carrots or whatever it may be that grows, grows because it contains the vitamins.

Vitamins are in germs. So long as you are feeding your patient boiled food, fried food, you are not giving him vitamins. You are feeding him dead food and therefore you cannot cure him. The vitamins constitute the living principle in food. There are no vitamins in spinach. The vitamins are in the seed of the spinach. In goat's milk you find vitamins in abundance. You find the vitamins in blood but boil the blood and it contains no vitamins. If you boil a dozen eggs and you set a hen on those eggs how many chicks do you think you will get? This ought to be a good lesson for those who are talking learnedly about vitamins. The vitamins are always in the germ.

No food contains so much salt as whey cheese made from goat's milk whey or even from goat's milk. It is better to eat goat's milk fresh. If you cannot get goat's milk fresh, you can get goat's milk containing the blood salts in the form of evaporated goat's milk. Evaporated goat's milk contains the blood salts and the heart salts. This is also true in regard to goat's cheese. It is true in regard to goat's milk whey cheese. Goat's milk is nearer to human milk.

FOOD ANALYSIS EXPLAINED

SWISS CHEESE made of goat's milk is high in ash content. Goat's milk is higher in ash content than other milk. It is more valuable when it is a question of blood and tissue salts. Goat's milk is one of the best foods you can purchase when it is a question of blood salts and tissue salts. This is also true in regard to goat's milk cheese and goat's milk whey cheese.

The consumptive should live in the hills of California on a goat's milk diet. Any milk that is heated or boiled does not contain the vitamins nor the fluorine. If you heat cow's milk, you drive out the fluorine. As soon as the heat temperature rises above 130 degrees Fahrenheit, the fluorine element evaporates or it is slowly dissipated. If milk is heated slowly, you can heat it as high as 172 degrees before fluorine dissipates. Fluorine is an element that cannot stand high and sudden heat. Pasteurized milk, we are told, contains less germs; but it contais less of the vitamins also. If you pasteurize milk, you have dead milk. Moreover, pasteurization of milk disturbs the salts in the milk. I am not sure if it would not be as well to drink the milk as it comes from the cow, germs and all, as to drink pasteurized. If you drink fresh milk from the cow you get the vitamins and you can fight the germs because you will have more vitality. Some germs cannot be killed by a temperature of 172 degrees Fahrenheit and if you boil goat's milk you get the milk minus fluorine. You cannot build good, solid tissue without fluorine, calcium, chlorine and other salts.

SALT. Ordinary table salt, contains 40% of sodium and 60% chlorine. If inorganic salt should pass into your blood, it would, possibly, result in hardening of the arterial walls. It is, however, not easy to introduce ordinary common salt into your arteries and veins for the lacteals refuse that which is inorganic. The lacteals have selective and rejective power and refuse rock salt. If there is a great deal of gas generation going on in your stomach, after eating fatty foods, there is nothing better than a drink made of distilled water and about a teaspoonful of ordinary common salt. If you suffer from heartburn, drink ordinary common salt and distilled water.

OX BLOOD, CALF BLOOD, CHICKEN BLOOD could easily be assimilated, if introduced in your diet. The blood is the cleanest part of all secretions, which is also true in regard to milk. Milk and blood are the cleanest and purest products we can get. The germs we are told about and that you see in milk do not come from the interior of the cow but from the outside, from the atmosphere in the stable, from the dirty milkmen and from dirty bottles. When a germ gets into warm milk, it grows rapidly. We should not drink milk by itself.

SAUERKRAUT is a very good food. I have seen patients who could not digest nor tolerate any other kind of food. The German people have a superior way of making sauerkraut. Sauerkraut contains organic and inorganic chlorine.

HAM should be broiled but it does not require a great deal of it.

COCOANUT is one of the best foods we can get. We should, however, not eat canned cocoanut for it is much better to get the fresh. Cocoanut contains myristic acid, which is a fatty substance of great value to nerves and brain. If you are nervous, eat cocoanut. If you are small chested, eat cocoanut. Cocoanut builds up your chest if you breathe fresh air in abundance. There is no food so valuable to the nerves and to the lungs, but do not patronize manufacturers who are not giving you a natural product. I would advise you to patronize nature as much as possible. Canned foods are never so good as foods that come directly from nature. It may be that some canned foods are good during the winter season. We cannot get fresh foods during the winter.

When you suffer from cerebral neurasthenia, eat cocoanut in conjunction with foods that are rich in potassium phosphate.

FISH is not a desirable blood-building food. It is good food for the brain and nerves, because it contains that important nerve fat, lecithin. Some fish contain cancer germs. Fish is a good food first because it contains lecithin; secondly, because of the protein it contains; thirdly because of the ash.

ASPARAGUS is usually cooked. Anything cooked is dead food. Nearly all food we eat in its fresh state containing the seed, contains the vital principle. Be sure to crush the seeds when you eat foods containing seeds so you may masticate and utilize the vitamins in the seeds. If you cannot masticate and digest the seeds, you cannot utilize the vitamins.

CABBAGE is better in the form of sauerkraut. If you have a weak stomach and you eat cabbage in its raw state, you are liekly to suffer from gas generation. If you eat boiled cabbage, you will generate so much gas you will become uncomfortable. Red cabbage is better than white cabbage. Red cabbage contains more chlorine than white. Red cabbage should be eaten in the form of cole slaw.

CARROTS. You cannot find a better food than carrots whether you are sick or well; whether your digestion is weak or strong; you always find the salts you need in carrots whether it be chlorine, sodium, silicon or another salt. If you need sugar, you find it in carrots; if you need vegetable proteins to a small degree, you find it in carrots. The protein you find in carrots is easily digested and assimilated. You can eat carrots raw or boiled, but it is preferable you eat carrots raw. There is always some kind of salt you may need and this salt is more than likely in carrots.

CUCUMBERS. There is a great deal of sulphur in cucumbers. It is the most healing vegetable you can find. There is nothing so good for the blood, blood heat or congestion as cucumbers. If, however, you eat too much, the extra part of the cucumbers you cannot digest will be converted into gas. If there is a tendency to necrosis, eat cucumbers.

EGG YOLK is the nearest substance to the brain. Egg yolk, the brain, and the generative substance, are comparatively the same, from a chemical viewpoint. Excitable people, insane people, people who have lost their sexuality should eat plenty of raw egg yolk in an alkaline form. People who want to improve their complexion should use egg yolk. People who want to improve their hair should use egg yolk preparations or hair wash made of claret and egg yolk. This makes an excellent hair wash.

LENTILS are nutritious. Most people do not know much about lentils. We cannot eat lentils raw; they must be cooked.

SPINACH contains all the salts needed in your body, providing you do not overcook the spinach; providing you do not throw the juice into the sink.

Never eat too many radishes at one meal or you will suffer from gas. Carrots, raw spinach, goat's cheese and almond nuts are mong the very best foods for the purpose of obtaining vegetable salts for your tissues.

Dishes made from white flour, do not contain the vitamins. By right, you should not eat preparations made from white flour.

QUESTIONS AND ANSWERS

1. Are there any foods that will help eliminate pus from the system? Answer: Foods very rich in chlorine will help.

2. What affect do vitamins have on the chemical composition of foods? Answer: They are forever trying to establish processes of germination whether it be in the soil or in the soil of man, where germination processes take place. They have a great affect upon the chemical composition of foods. If there were no vitamins in food at any time, foods could not be worked up into living tissue. If there were no vitamins in the food, it would be impossible to build a vigorous sexual system. The vitamins are the life principles. They are taken up by the sexual system and utilized for purposes of reproduction. If food has been boiled that same food or seed can never germinate.

3. Do ox tails contain chlorine? Answer: Yes.

4. When a man suffers from chlorine excess should he eat freely of chlorine-containing foods in connection with a high protein diet? Answer: No. A sick man should not have a high protein diet. If you have chlorine to excess, omit chlorine-containing foods. If chlorine consumption is great, eat chlorine-containing foods in abundance, also the vitamins.

5. What are some of the foods that contain the heart salts? Answer: Goat's milk, evaporated or fresh; goat's cheese, goat's milk whey cheese, carrots and spinach.

6. What difference does it make if there is a high or low ash content? Answer: If the content is high it is more valuable to the human body because it is more easily digested. If the same food is rich in vitamins, it becomes doubly valuable to the human body because it can be metabolized.

7. What food elements are needed in arthritis deformans? Answer: If you suffer from arthritis deformans, you have simply waited too long., You are likely to die with it. Arthritis deformans means absolute sodium hunger, especially if it has continued for a long time. If the tissue salts are lacking in your tissues you are likely to suffer from arthritis deformans and as long as those salts are lacking, no doctor can cure you.

8. Are pigs poisonous and should people eat pork? Answer: Pigs are not poisonous. It may be perfectly true that pork contains substances that are not favorable, but this is also true in regard to cabbage, barley, wheat or almost any food. The pig is not a chlorine-excess animal. You could eat ham every day and never suffer from any kind of sickness if you eat it in proper combinations and not to excess.

9. Is there a possibility of ills of long standing being cured through diet? Answer: Yes. It is possible to eat foods and drink drinks of a curative nature according to the needs of your own constitution until your chronic ailment disappears. Diet cannot do everything but it is important as a curative agent. The doctor who pays no attention to diet is not a very desirable doctor. You had better not solicit his services.

10. Should the seeds of raisins be chewed and consumed? Answer: Yes, because you find vitamins in the seeds; but you should masticate them well. Seedless raisins do not contain vitamins.

11. Is it not necessary to give one acid to counteract another in the system? Answer: Yes. But that acid should be citric acid or formic acid, in food form. We must not give a man all sorts of acids and expect him to improve. Formic acid and citric acid, in food form, have a neutralizing effect upon other acids.

12. Can appendicitis be cured by diet? Answer: Yes, if it has not gone too far. If the appendix is decomposed, the best thing to do is scrape it out.

13. When there is itching in the palms of the hand and soles of the feet persistently, what chemical symptom may this be? Answer: Lack of potassium salt in the tissues; lack of sulphur in the tissues and lack of chlorine in the tissues or in the nerves.

14. Why may a certain portion of the body be cold while the rest is warm? Answer: Because of lack of chlorine or perhaps silicon.

15. What is the difference between the vitamins and ash content? Answer: If you burn a piece of wood what you have left is a few ashes. If you burn up a certain food you have certain ash left—this is the ash content of that food. The vitamins are the vital principles in a plant, seeds, milk or in a grain of wheat. Vitamins are the germ or embryo; it is the power of the young plant to take life to itself, grow and thrive. Every grain of wheat has a germ and this germ contains the vitamins. This germ represents about 1-1/2% of the whole grain in a grain of wheat; it is called the germ.

16. In what way will chlorine cure albuminuria? Answer: Chlorine works in the tissues; it works in albumin. It increases tissue metabolism or albumin metabolism.

17. Does a man who lives on vegetables and fruit get enough chlorine if he is vigorous? Answer: No. On a vegetable and fruit diet, it is simply impossible to get enough chlorine for any man whether he be sick or healthy. If a man is healthy and lives on this kind of diet for many years, he will eventually become sick. A healthy man, however, is able to utilize all the chlorine in the food that is obtainable.

18. Why do some people crave ordinary common salt? They want everything so salty no one else can eat it. Answer: One reason is because there is an excess of chlorine consumption. They need it and do not know where to obtain chlorine. Another reason is that the albumin is not doing its work because of lack of other salts or because there is a lack of chlorine salts. Still another reason may be perhaps a tendency to pus formation throughout the system as for instance in a tubercular man.

19. Can you by prescribing too much organic chlorine in Bright's disease, increase the ailment and thereby prevent a cure? Answer: In times of Bright's disease, organic chlorine is needed. A man who suffers from Bright's disease can never get enough organic chlorine. We must supply chlorine in abundance to such a patilent or he will not improve. It is important to cut out the albumin until the system reaches a point of albumin toleration again.

20. Is chlorine, found in common table salt, inorganic? And will this have the same effect as organic chlorine? Answer: Inorganic chlorine passes through the alimentary tract mainly. If you introduce inorganic chlorine into the arteries, you are interfering with the scheme of nature and you will eventually suffer. If you give your lacteals an opportunity, you will find that they refuse to take up inorganic chlorine. We need organic chlorine for the blood, secretions and tissues.

21. What elements are not obtainable in a vegetarian diet? Answer: Principally chlorine.

22. What chlorine foods would be of value to a person suffering from cataract? Answer: A chlorine diet would do nothing for cataracts.

23. What causes red, irritated eyelids? Is it due to acidity? How can it be eliminated? Answer: It may be due to many things as for instance, excessive sulphur consumption. It may be due to a Pargenic taint. It may be due to vegetable poison; it is seldom due to acidity.

24. How can we recognize nervousness or irritability caused by a lack of chlorine? Answer: Because of other symptoms that go with it and because it is a certain kind of nervousness and a certain kind of irritability. Chlorine hungry people or excess people are not only irritable, but ugly, revengeful, stormy, mean, cynical; and a very heavy cloud hangs over them and an anxiety they cannot explain.

25. Is chlorine, in the form of common table salt, harmful to the liver and other organs? Answer: It may be harmful if taken to excess, but not otherwise.

26. What is the cause of the collapse of a child who was never ill, yet suddenly had a collapse of her legs so she has not been able to walk since? Answer: The cause was in the cerebellum or else in the spinal centers. They gave out perhaps because they never were very strong and perhaps also because the parents did not know how to feed those spinal centers, cerebral centers or cerebellar centers.

27. What do ridges on the fingernails indicate? Answer: Lack of silicon.

28. What causes bow legs in babies? Answer: Lack of calcium, sodium and fluorine.

29. Will diet cure cataract? Answer: Yes, if it is supplied in time. Cataract requires lecithin and fresh warm milk from the goat.

30. How much common salt should be eaten with foods such as celery, radishes, nuts, cheese, etc.? Answer: When we suffer from autointoxication, we need more common salt than otherwise. If we are healthy and we eat plenty of celery, we do not need ordinary common salt for celery is rich in sodium which is the case with certain nuts and cheese such as goat's cheese, sheep's milk cheese or Roquefort cheese. Ordinary common salt is needed in times of autointoxication, fermentation and germ life in the intestines. Common salt passes through the alimentary tract and acts upon the walls of the stomach. It can do no harm. If a man suffers from obesity, he needs ordinary common salt in abundance. In the Desmogenic patient, the tissues are too active in sodium metabolilsm; he needs ordinary common salt in his diet to a great extent, otherwise, he may run short of chlorine and sodium and run into tuberculosis.

31. Can goiter be cured? Answer: There are four different kinds of goiters; one is caused by lack of iodine. This goiter requires iodine foods in abundance.

32. How can you regulate sodium between the tissues and the blood or can there not be too much sodium in the tissues and not enough sodium in the blood? Answer: The tissues are sometimes robbed and again the blood and the secretions may sometimes be robbed also. The Desmogenic patient sometimes suffers from indigestion, because the tissues rob the stomach or because there is not enough sodium in the secretions nor in the blood. The only way we can regulate this is to eat sodium foods in abundance.

FOODS AND CHEMICALS
PHOSPHORUS

INTRODUCTION

Children with insufficient phosphorus will suffer from scrofula. Phthisis is nothing than lack of phosphates in the body. It is just the same with the human body as with plants. Take the phosphates out of the soil, trees, fruits, vegetables and plants will suffer from disease. The agriculturist supplies the phosphates to the soil. We should supply phosphorus to the human body. When it is a question of crops, the agriculturist analyzes the soil and tells you that your soil lacks potassium phosphate or calcium phosphate; then you get the right kind of phosphate and sprinkle it into the soil and it becomes more congenial to the crops. We should handle human needs in a similar manner.

Phosphates are valuable for plant life and for soil vitality, also for growth of tissues. The most important are calcium phosphate, sodium phosphate and magnesium phosphate. Those are most important in the human organization. Those phosphates are tilling the soil in the tissues, bones and elsewhere. When there is a lack of phosphates, there is lack of vitality. You may think it important to study calories, protein, fat, sugar, water from a chemical standpoint; but, the study of the organic salts, as they act upon the human body, proteins, water, tissues, bones, nerves, vital organs and secretions is more important. Foods containing those salts are important for vitalization. If we test the blood or urine, what then? Do we know anything beyond those tests? If something is lacking, what are we going to do?

Suppose you find magnesium phosphate, albumin or sugar in the urine, what are you going to do then? Supply what? When sugar is refused by the tissues, eat foods rich in sodium chloride and potassium chloride and live in a high altitude.

When certain elements are not supplied, pus will form. Tubercular people are pus types. They become worse when the salts needed in the tissues are low. They may suffer from catarrh in the forehead, nose, stomach, chest, catarrh everywhere, because there is a lack of some of the organic salts. If those elements are not supplied, there will be not only catarrh but pus, swelling of the glands and pus formations. People who eat wrongly for 10 or 15 years, may develop pus diseases.

PHOSPHORUS IN THE MINERAL AND VEGETABLE KINGDOMS

With phosphorus in the protoplasm (even if there is life in the protoplasm), there can be no growth. Phosphorus is needed in protoplasm.

The larger the brain, the more phosphorus is required because more of it is burned up. If the brain is too large, intense or active, the brain is burning up phosphorus and the tissues are robbed. Then the patient may run into tuberculosis. This happens sometimes when a child is too highly developed. A child may be 60 years old in brain and 5, 6 or 7 years old in his body or he has an old head on young shoulders. The very best thing to do is to put that child to sleep and stop the brain from acting. Let the phosphorus go to the body. Give him a sandpile to play in and take him out of school, or you will bury him. That is why the consumptive should sleep much. When you put the brain to sleep, phosphorus goes to the body. Children who suffer from ricketts should be put to sleep so the phosphorus may go to the tissues.

PHOSPHORUS, ITS NATURE AND CHARACTERISTICS

When the heat in the brain becomes excessive, it affects the functions of the brain. When there is an excess of heat in the brain, there is a weakening of the functions in the brain. The physical functions of the body are transmuted or altered. When there is too much

heat in the brain, there is a wrong action in the tissues and functions of the body. You grow weak and irritable. You tremble and your nerves tremble. Be careful in regard to artificial heat so that it is not excessive. Never sit in an overheated room. The brain may become overheated. The temperature of the room should never be over 69 degrees, perhaps as low as 50 to 60. Room or atmospheric temperature is better for one at say 69 and for another at 65.

The heat point for the Exesthesic is low, because there is too high generation of heat in the nerves, brain and liver. The Exesthesic should be well dressed on the feet. They crave cool temperatures around the head however. The feet of the Exesthesic lady are often cold, but her head is overheated. There is greater generation of heat in the brain in all excitable, intense people. A person who is irritable should be sent to a higher altitude. Never permit too much heat to go to the brain; you can overheat the brain easily.

The head absorbs quicker than other parts of the body. If you take care of the physical functions there is no danger of paralysis. Be sure to cover your head in intense light and heat for the characteristics of phosphorus are such that it absorbs the hot sun rays easily. Always cover your head to protect it from the light and heat of the sun. It is better to go into the sun with a nude body than an uncovered head. If you suffer from the sun's rays, when as high as 105 degrees, be sure to cover your head or place green leaves in your hat.

You must protect your head. As long as you protect your head you are safe. If you have a patient suffering from excessive fever, protect his head and you save your patient. So soon as the fever heat in the body runs above 105 degrees, there is great danger. If the heat rises to 106 or more phosphorus melts. You cannot, as a doctor, test the brain temperature by putting the thermometer under the tongue. The heat is in the brain and the liver. If the heat rises to 105 with a thermometer under the tongue, the temperature has already reached 107 in the brain and spinal cord. Then you will lose your patient because you did not prevent an excessive brain temperature. When you apply heat to the body, you reduce heat in the brain. To prevent heat from going to the spinal cord and brain when the fever is high or in other words, save the phosphorus from melting, put your patient into a warm bath and you save him. Reduce the heat in the brain and liver by putting the patient into a warm bath, apply cold compresses on the neck or head and perhaps on the feet. Phosphorus melts at from 108 degrees to 111 degrees. In fact, it begins to melt at 104 deg.

Some people suffering from syphilis may have water on the brain because there is too much heat in the brain. If a man has too much heat in the brain, he drinks water like a fish. He perspires and his perspiration is mostly in the head.

When there is a lack of phosphorus, a person suffers from sterility. He loses sexual power. If a man lacks phosphorus, iron or oxygen, he will have weak children. If we lack phosphorus, we should not give rise to offspring because they will be feeble. Always supply iron, oxygen, phosphorus, sulphur and vitamins for transmission.

The phosphorus element has a great deal to do with vitalization, fertilization and the creation of offspring. If a man lacks phosphorus, he lacks transmissive power and has no right to become a father.

If a man has a great deal of phosphorus in his system and he has the faculty of veneration powerfully in the lead, he is prophetic. If a woman has spirituality in the lead and a great deal of phosphorus, she is mediumistic. She can sense your soul state as a bloodhound scents a criminal. She can even tell you your name. She takes it from your brain. This is mediumship. When the table begins to transmit messages, it is phosphorus àt work in the people around that table.

Fireflies are so named because they have much phosphorus. If we had sufficient phosphorus, we too could shine in the dark. The aura or light which is outside the body, is the result of phosphorus. When you have a great deal of phosphorus in your system, your soul becomes more illuminated. You have a light sphere around your body. When the spirit leaves the body, that light dies out; some believe it goes to heaven. That light is called the aura—is it the soul itself? If people have an abundance of phosphorus, it makes them more phosphorescent. If a man is dead and you hold up his fingers against the light, his fingers are black. What became of that former aura?

People with a great deal of phosphorus are highly evolved. People with very little phosphorus are of a low order. Take, for instance, the pig; it has only a spoonful of brain. The pig is not a very good philosopher. It does not have very much spinal matter, nor very fine nerve nets in the system. You find nothing but pork. All animals who do not have much phosphorus in the brain are of a low order. Evolution depends upon the gray brain substance. The more gray brain matter a man has, the more intelligent he is. The more gray matter he has, the more of a philosopher he is; the more interest he takes in other people. If a saint without very much phosphorus in her brain goes to church, she goes to sleep during the sermon. In her, the spirit may be willing but her flesh is weak. It is difficult to keep awake when we do not have very much phosphorus. Mental people are so wide awake that they can hardly ever fall to sleep. Highly-evolved men suffer from sleeplessness.

When phosphorus is introduced in food form, it causes growth in certain faculties. Put a man whose spirituality, veneration, ideality and all the spiritual faculties are weak on a heavy phosphorus diet and those faculties will develop when he calls them into action. When a man has a limited quantity of phosphorus in his brain, he has a low development of the occult, abstract faculties.

Phosphorus makes a man meditative. It produces what is called the subjective mind. A man with phosphorus in his system is more abstract. Phosphorus people are impractical. They seldom have any money.

Phosphorus is a bright element. Phosphorus people are wonderfully bright. A phosphorus man once wrote articles for the papers. When people went to see him, they were disappointed. His hat reached his shoulders; his whiskers were long; his shirt was sticking out behind when he walked; he was short, careless and indifferent and looked odd. Phosphorus always goes to extremes. People of the phosphorus type always have weak bodies, but are highly intelligent.

HOW TO INCREASE PHOSPHORUS IN THE BODY

Some of us may be of the Neurogenic constitutions. A Neurogenic boy with a very active brain who is going to school, and perhaps is the brightest child in school but low in vitality, should have something done for him so that all of his vitality does not go to his brain, because if it does, the child will eventually die or suffer from tubercular ailments, nervous prostration or some other ailment. His arms and limbs are so white that it appears as if they are made of plaster of Paris. He looks as though he had no blood in his body.

You may take a child like that to a medical specialist who tells you nothing can be done for him or he may prescribe medicine that will never increase his vitality nor give him an ounce of blood. We can never accomplish anything with medicine for such a child. We cannot get vitality from medicine, never build him up from medicine nor tonics. We must fall back on those foods that are placed at our disposal. In introducing foods, we must remember that no food can be taken up unless the body or the brain is exercised properly.

You know that phosphorus is used in the body, in the muscles and in almost all solid tissue. It is utilized in the blood and by the blood, and if a child sits in a classroom he cannot get enough fresh air and sunshine and cannot take up the phosphorus needed in the body.

If the brain is too active, the phosphorus goes to the brain; if the body is too active, the phosphorus goes to the body and the brain is robbed. If the sexual system is too active then the phosphorus goes to the sexual system or supports the sexual substance, increases passions and the man lives a wild life.

The phosphorus has three functions to perform; one is a mental function or brain function; the second is physical or tissue function and the third is a sexual or generative function, having to do with transmission, passion and with amatory love. The more passion a man has, the more phosphorus he draws toward the generative substance, the more phosphorus he burns up through that same passion. The more vigorous a man in muscle, the more he is out in active life in the sunshine and the more he moves about the more

phosphorus goes to the body or to the solid fibers, tissues and the more phosphorus being used up there. The man who has a large brain and a small body, the more active the brain and the more sluggish the muscles, the more that same phosphorus is burned up in the brain and the body suffers, then we have that kind of temperament or constitution we call Atrophic or tubercular.

For that reason we should remember always that phosphorus has various functions to perform, and it depends on our activity where that phosphorus goes. If the brain of the individual is most active as for instance in the Calciferic or Neurogenic or Atrophic people, the phosphorus goes to the brain and is burned up there. If the muscles themselves or the fibrous tissues are more active, the phosphorus goes to the muscles. If the generative system or sex function or passion is the most active, the phosphorus goes there to support that function.

When we are in vigorous action, in sudden action, as for instance, when we are taking physical exercises or when practicing athletics, we draw phosphorus to the muscles. That is why barley food is so valuable in building up muscle; because barley food yields its phosphorus to the muscles more readily than it does to other parts of the body. That is also why we can build muscle in a child more quickly on barley food— providing the child can handle it. When the child eats barley food, it must not have an acid stomach because if it is, barley preparations will make the stomach more acid.

There are some food elements that go with calcium; i.e., they carry calcium phosphates perhaps tricalcium phosphate. Milk for instance carries calcium phosphate in abundance. Thus some calcium phosphate foods support the bones more than any other part of the body. To get the benefit of those calcium foods or calcium phosphate foods, it becomes necessary to exercise accordingly.

A man who is quick and active will never build strong bones but a man who is slow, easy-going, very strong and makes great exertion when he does act, all of the tricalcium phosphate from foods that he eats. To develop bones, take all sorts of physical exercise and let them be slow and prolonged, never sudden. If you use vigorous effort all the time or if you carry a heavy load from morning until night and you are compelled to make strong and prolonged effort, you compel your bones to take up tricalcium phosphate. But when you are in quick action, when you use muscles quickly, rapidly or you engage in light physical exercise, very suddenly you compel your muscles to utilize phosphorus, fibrin and albumin. Muscles are principally protein or vegetable products, but bones are calcium products.

The bones are the strongest part of man and the stronger and larger the bones, the more slow and ox-like that man is in all his movements. That same man who is slow and easy-going, yet exercises a great deal of determination and effort in everything he does, and he compels his bones to take up the phosphates. The man who sits in a chair at a desk and studies all sorts of idealism, devotes himself to theosophy or religious philosophy—never uses any effort only writes, writes, writes—he uses the phosphorus in his brain. Meanwhile, his body becomes weaker and weaker; at last there is hardly anything left of him but his head. His head grows larger and larger and his body grows smaller and smaller. AT last there is but a big head and a little, frail body. He becomes a sort of a balloon. He likes the clouds. The more phosphorus that goes to the brain, the more impractical he becomes and the weaker his body becomes. Soon he goes above the clouds. where he belongs.

The calcium man is a solid man; a man of deep thought; a man of science; a man who does not believe anything until it is proven, a man who uses the phosphorus in the bones.

When we understand these principles, we understand why people can sit at the same table and eat similar foods, one becomes more and more muscular, the second becomes more and more bony and scientific and the third becomes more and more idealistic. The idealist cures by faith, while the Osseous cures by drugs. The idealist cures through the mind and the Osseous man cures in a material way.

When we send our children to school, first look them over and see what makeup they are. The education should begin in the backyard, in the sandpile, with a wheelbarrow and a spade with phosphorus children, while the education of some others should begin with very heavy physical exercises to develop bones. It may even be necessary to get a child to carry heavy planks,

so as to develop bones. The education of others can perhaps begin in the brain.

For instance, a child of a Carboferic constitution or perhaps Myogenic with a rather phlegmatic body, very active physical functions but rather dull, stupid brain cannot learn much in school. Mental exercises will never injure him. But, a child on the other hand, who looks as though he were made of alabaster, large intellect and strong development of the will section of the brain, weak development of the vital centers and backhead, a small, slender body, should not be sent to school. Every hour while he is in school, inside of four walls, he is using his brain and is simply preparing his coffin. The longer he is there, the sooner he will die.

Phosphorus has a vital and important intellectual function to perform in the brain, an important vital function to perform in the muscles, an equally important function to perform in the bones and in the sexual system. A man who lacks phosphorus is not capable of becoming a father or if he does, he will have a defective child. When phosphorus is not well supplied to the sexual system and to the generative substance, the offspring will be weak, no matter what that man may know about eugenics. If, at the time of conception, there is no phosphorus in the generative substance or if the phosphorus is used up in his brain principally or in the bones principally, his child will be defective.

Phosphorus has many important functions to perform: One is a generative function; another is an Osseous or bone-building function; another is a muscle-building or Myogenic or protein function and still another is a brain-building and brain-sustaining function. The question is, where do we want the phosphorus to go?

We must remember this question in regard to phosphorus because if it goes to the brain principally, it will weaken the entire body. The more phosphorus that goes to the brain, the weaker the man will be in a physical sense or the child, as the case may be. If phosphorus products are broken down rapidly, a weak liver will not throw them off equally at all times; hence, he will suffer from jaundice, low nutrition, acid stomach and other ailments. When the liver cannot carry them off and becomes over-flooded with phosphorus products, he is likely to suffer from yellow atrophy of the liver, from running of the bowels, persistent diarrhea that nothing will cure, bloating, sleeplessness, phthisis. At such a time, it becomes necessary to regulate the phosphorus function and send the phosphorus to the brain, to the muscles, to the sexual system, to the bones, then the trouble in the intestines and liver will soon disappear.

When suffering from broken down phosphorus, stop mental exercise, go to the hills, exercise slowly, go hunting or fishing. At any time when you suffer from phosphorus ailments, symptoms or diseases, go away from your stenography, from disagreeable surroundings, go to the hills and eat and drink foods that are rich in phosphorus and notice the results.

Water purifies itself by its own motion and the air purifies itself also by motion and sunshine. That is the way the air should be, purified before it acts on the human body.

PEOPLE WHO REQUIRE PHOSPHORUS FOODS

Why do people require phosphorus foods? We say that idiots require phosphorus food because their brain cells themselves are so sluggish that the brain cells may not make a vibration per month. How can a child like that understand anything? How can he utilize phosphorus? But we must supply it anyway and then call his attention to his environments and thus arouse his brain. We cannot use our eyes, ears, tongues, nor can we exercise emotion without utilizing phosphorus and developing brain. If you cannot get an idiot to understand anything, hit him so that it hurts and wake him up that way, and he will utilize phosphorus. When it hurts, you reach the feelings. You can reach him through the sensations. Arouse his brain and then supply phosphorus and it will do the work.

In any faculty that is weak, there is a low fire of phosphorus and therefore, that faculty cannot understand. What does a color blind man know about color? What does a man know about love who is weak in conjugality? He may think he is a good husband but his wife knows better. Among all faculties, if you or I have a weak faculty, the very best thing we can do is to wake that faculty up in some way and then

supply phosphorus. Do not try to develop your mind by mere suggestion, for that does not work. You cannot build the Masonic Temple out of moonshine, you must have stone and bricks, mortar and iron columns. So also with mental development. Do not try to make yourself courageous merely by thinking that does not work. Tackle a strong man and beat him. Make yourself feel it so that you feel it in your very bones and you call the faculty combativeness into action, which faculty phosphorus feeds, when the faculty is in action.

Phosphorus is used in every faculty seat of the brain. It is impossible even to develop a faculty without supplying phosphorus first. If you try to develop a faculty or any feeling or characteristic without supplying the material which is needed by the brain, it becomes erratic and instead of building it up, you weaken it.

People who imagine mind, memory, reason, emotion, prayer, concentration, etc., can be developed by mere suggestion and nothing else, do not know anything about the chemistry of man. For whenever we try to develop we should not only use that special feeling, characteristic, impulse or thought but should also supply the phosphorus or material needed.

There is phosphorus and phosphorus. The phosphorus that supports the sidehead; that which supports the intellect; phosphorus that supports the tophead; that which supports the concentration and will; phosphorus that supports the backhead are phosphorus in different combinations. The phosphorus that you find in honey, for instance, will build up your backhead. The more honey you eat and the more phosphorus you get of that kind, the more affectionate you become. Phosphorus, associated with sugar, for instance, develops parental love; phosphorus combined with calcium builds up firmness and the bones. The phosphorus you find in fruits builds up the moral faculties. Therefore, it is not a question only of phosphorus, it is a question of a special kind of phosphorus, when we wish to develop. What good is your prayer if you live on coffee, tea, spices and whiskey.

In one food as for instance beechnuts, you find phosphorus with calcium. In another food, spinach, you have phosphorus with potassium. In still another food, you find it combined with some other element or compound. Therefore when we understand all phosphorus functions and the various functions of the brain, dietetics become more understandable. Then as dietetians, we do not recommend a milk diet to everybody. We do not recommend a vegetable diet to all nor do we condemn a meat diet. We do not recommend a starvation diet either. Sometimes a man is sick and there is nothing left of him but skin and bones. If he goes to a sanitarium, they may starve him nevertheless. Think of starving a skeleton. We should build up such a man not starve him. There is a way of dieting without starving. We can give a man a diet by means of which the eliminative functions are active, yet not supplied with solid material. We can put a man on an eliminative diet and starve him by degrees, yet he may eat from morning until night as he is being starved.

Feebleminded people are in need of phosphorus. Their brain is not supplied with phosphorus nor is it taking up phosphorus. If you keep your child in school studying mathematics at last the brain will twist like a corkscrew and there comes a time when that child will not understand any mathematical problem at all. Lastly, it may die in an asylum. Atrophic people require phosphorus for the reason that phosphorus is being burned up too rapidly in the brain for which reason there is not enough going to the body. Sterility and impotence demand a phosphorus diet, also affection. In a warm climate and high altitude, under a phosphorus diet, you are able to overcome sterility and impotence.

Lawyers, doctors, students and ministers of the gospel who deliver sermons perhaps 2 or 3 times a day, may run into neurasthenia. Then what should we give them? Dope? Should we supply phosphorus for that which has been burned up in the brain? If you would take a drink rich in magnesium and eat food rich in magnesium, they would help eliminate all the phosphorus products so that tomorrow you would not suffer from ailments nor from gas. The stomach becomes sour because phosphorus products are so exceedingly sour that they make the stomach sour. If you talk much, you sour your stomach and tomorrow you cannot digest your food. If you have a small liver, you cannot afford to run into temper, because your liver is not equal to that temper. If you have a large liver, you may cultivate temper occasionally.

We cannot think, talk, cultivate emotion nor experience passion without burning up phosphorus. Phosphorus is the candle of intelligence that burns in the brain all the time.

The word phosphorus means light carrier. Phos means light; phorus means carrier. Carrier of light. That is what phosphorus is, viz., the intellectual lamp in the brain, burning, burning, burning. Phosphorus is the oil that supplies soul light. When phosphorus is no more supplied, that intellectual lamp goes out and then we are in the dark, like idiots.

Stopping Brain Breakdown

How should we take care of the brain? There are many things that we have to do. The cerebellum is a musculo-electrical dynamo, generating electrical messages to all the different cell structures of our body. Now we find that there are many things that are unfavorable to the cerebellum and that is why we have to consider how to stop breaking down. When we have constant colds in the head, this charges the cerebellum with too much blood. Whooping cough can cause a weakening of the cerebellum. So can malaria, exposure to cold, heavy lifting, excessive sex, great excitement, anxiety. Sunstroke affects the brain, as do fretting, stewing, studying, worrying, insomnia, pain, persistent work day and night. When the system is exhausted, long hours weaken the cerebellum beyond recuperation.

We cannot allow people to take too much of our time, gossiping, talking, overdoing the work that the brain is responsible for in our activities. Sicknesses use up the motor force, and when we lose this, we have to get back to the brain and the nerve foods.

When we have problems in the cerebrum, we may develop great fears of the opposite sex, fear of society, periodic headaches, listlessness, loss of ambition, inclination to nunnery or to the life of a hermit. The systic murmur of the heart is caused by cerebellum weakness and a feverish sex brain. In locomotor ataxia, the cerebellum is drained of its force, and the cells in the spinal cord undergo disintegration because of sexual taints.

Iron salts from the vegetable kingdom are favorable to the cerebellum. Certain kinds of sweets, natural sweets, phosphorus, vitalin, nerve salts, biosalts, sulphur foods, natural oils (as found in our foods and not in a concentrated form), nerve fats, parsley, parsley soups, the oat oils, silicon foods, sage tea, fresh air, sleep, rest, graceful muscle movements and raw egg shakes are good. We can take milk in a clabbered form and soups or broths, but not meat soups. Use sesame seed butter or almond butter in making soups and put more in at the table. Any nerve food in the form of a tonic, broth, soup, herb tea and so forth is indicated.

The medulla, or chest brain, takes care of the chest and its functions, the lungs, diaphragm, heart, vasomotor system, the arterial circulation, venous circulation and the oxydation of blood in the lungs. So long as the medulla is in a good state of health, the heart beats, throbs, pulsates; the lungs work and the blood current is active everywhere.

When the medulla is weak, the heart is weak and the lungs are feeble. When the medulla is severely damaged, the heart stops and no human invention can put it back into motion. From injuries of the medulla, millions of people have died simply because the heart stopped and the system was overcharged with carbonic acid gas. The medulla keeps the heart beating before birth and keeps it going until the thread of life is spun and the eyes close in death. A weakness in the medulla is indicated by a changeable pulse. The medulla is weak in the mental osseous people, phlegmatic people, mental ligamentous people. Those things favorable to the medulla are sulphur foods: onions, radishes, cauliflower and broccoli. Coconut and nutmeg calm the action of the medulla. Watermelon tea, sage tea and parsley tea are very good. We can take fish and fish broths.

We find that the sex brain is very closely related to the chest brain. Cold weakens the lining of the brain and spinal cord which weakens the sexuality. Excessive heat weakens the axis-cylinder cells of the brain and spinal cord and has a weakening effect on sexuality. Anything that uses up the cholesterol (the nerve and brain fat), will weaken the sexual system and the formation of red corpuscles in the blood. So will anything that uses up iron salts in the system and interferes with the aeration of the blood. Depletion of the sex brain causes cerebral neurosthenia, dropsy, hysteria—according to the nature of the sexual draining and the parts most affected.

Deep breathing favors salivation; hence, the necessity of proper breathing before and after meals. In cerebration or brain work, we consume a great deal of brain phosphorus, brain lecithin, sublimated sulphur food compounds, also certain organic salts: salts of sodium, chlorine, potassium, calcium, magnesium, iron, manganese and iodine—all of which are usually called "ash" or mineral elements by the chemists.

We find that four brain cells die each second. These dead cells must be replaced by new brain cells. "We live as we die," says the chemist. And nothing is more true. We must replace the old brain cells with new ones. We eat to live and we do this to keep the brain vigorously alive. If the brain is overworked, phosphorus appears in the urine. And if we do not supply phosphorus to the brain, soon our brains are dephosphorized, and the brain decays or brain trouble follows. We have to realize that there is a difference between phosphorus and phosphorus, fat and fat, chlorine and chlorine, fibrin and fibrin. The phosphorus that has passed through millions of refining processes in nature's mill of evolution, passing from the rock to the soil, from the soil to the trees and plants, from vegetables to animals, fish to birds, a thousand or perhaps a hundred thousand times before it enters the human brain, must logically be a more refined, purified, sublimated and evoluted phosphorus. The phosphorus in bone does not think, but the phosphorus in the brain can think. Why? Because it is super fine.

INFLUENCE OF AN EXCESSIVE AMOUNT OF PHOSPHORUS FOODS ON HEALTH

If phosphorus is broken down too rapidly a man becomes morbid. The more phosphorus a man burns up the more morbid he becomes and the more sour his stomach becomes and the more of a dyspeptic he will be. A dyspeptic has very little influence on anybody not even with the Almighty, because the prayer of a dyspeptic, in my opinion, does not go very high; it is a sour compound.

VOCATIONS FOR WHICH PHOSPHORUS PEOPLE ARE BEST ADAPTED

We have reference here to those kinds of phosphorus people who have it predominating in brain and body. There are some people who have a small body and a large head; they have the eyes low down in the face; they have a head shaped something like a balloon; they have a small body. Such people we call neurogenic or phosphorus people, which means nothing else than that the phosphorus is being attracted to the brain too rapidly and being burned up in the brain excessively. In other words, phosphorus consumption and metabolism are excessive in the brain. They are the people who are adapted for such vocations mentioned in this lesson. It is interesting to see where inclinations come from; it is interesting to see why a person takes up certain studies and why he succeeds in certain occupations.

HELPFUL HINTS

My points are taken in regard to the Neurogenic man or in regard to the tubercular man or any man who is forever using his brain. When calcium is acting upon the body, it takes a certain degree of phosphorus away from the brain and stops the brain action to a great extent. If a child is too active in brain, the body is not being built up. The girl, being too slender and boneless, must be put, not only on a phosphorus diet, but also on a diet rich in calcium. Calcium is lime, though not exactly, because lime is a calcium oxide and may also contain other elements. It is not right to call calcium by the name of lime, but sometimes it is. We hear doctors talk about lime hardening, not a strictly scientific expression.

Lecithin is a Greek word meaning egg yolk, raw egg yolk. Egg yolk is a compound of the greatest value to the brain and also to the generative system.

Whenever you wish to do your best, to use your brain tremendously; whenever you must have plenty of phosphorus for that brain of yours, make a drink containing from 3 to 7 raw egg yolks; drink that and you will be at your very best.

If you want to become a father and you want a really gifted child, see that your brain is well nourished and the generative substance is well supplied with vitalilty. Leave your books on eugenics in your library and steam up and you can accomplish more. We do not say anything against works on eugenics because they are good in their place, but what we mean is not to forget the food material needed in a certain case. Study eugenics, science, philosophy; we never know too much but whatever we do, let us not forget the food material which is needed in the human organization for certain purposes and by certain functions.

Ozone is brought down from the clouds every time it rains. During every electrical storm, ozone is brought low down. During and after an electrical storm, do not stay indoors, but go out and breathe and draw the ozone into yourself.

WHEN A PHOSPHORUS DIET IS NEEDED

There are always some symptoms, ailments and diseases by means of which we can determine positively and scientifically just when a phosphorus diet is needed. We have a few of those symptoms here but they are only a few, yet they indicate positively when a phosphorus diet is needed. We have in our possession perhaps a thousand symptoms, ailments and diseases not listed herein and which are not necessary to have unless we want to go into all the details of phosphorus.

Millions of men and women are taking treatments for sexual weakness today but never improve at all. Sexuality, to be improved, requires a rich phosphorus diet. Very few people know that the Almighty uses phosphorus for the purpose of developing a stronger sexualilty. Very few know that sulphur will give greater generative power and very few know that iron and oxygen are needed for that purpose. Supply phosphorus, sulphur, iron, oxygen, neurol and warmth, instead of going to specialists and thereby build up a stronger sexuality and give rise to greater offspring. Sometimes I look at people and think here is Mr. Weakling, anxious to marry; and here is this lady also anxious to marry; both may become father and mother in the course of time. She feels too weak and is afraid to marry and the man, perhaps, fears the results and hesitates. They may go to a doctor who may be interested only in the substance they have in their pocketbook. In a case like that eat abundantly of foods rich in iron, oxygen, phosphorus, sulphur and neurol and live in a congenial climate, when it is a question of developing a stronger sexuality.

When there is a dislike for exertion and work or when a person almost never makes an effort except under excitement, phosphorus is needed. You have heard people say, "Whenever I make an effort, I simply work on my nerves." They feel that way and speak that way simply because they are lacking in phosphorus. When we are burning up phosphorus too rapidly in the brain, nerves, muscles, bones and generative substance, you may be sure that sooner or later phosphorus will run low. If we do not know how to supply it, sooner or later, we become neurogenic and are not able to accomplish what we otherwise could.

Self efficiency. Businessmen, managers and railroad executives always speak about business efficiency, system. It has never occurred to these men that a suitable diet is necessary in order to increase business efficiency. Suppose you want to sell goods as a salesman. You would be able to use your brain more vigorously, to convince your prospects better, to make more sales, if you are under the influence of those food elements that give vim and snap to everything, including phosphorus. There is an important principle in business efficiency. You never can do your best as a salesman, manager, railroad executive without those elements in your blood, muscles, brain, that enable you to use all your energies to the very best advantage.

We do not care how strong self esteem and combativeness are if you lack phosphorus in brain and muscle you will feel a lack of self confidence; however powerful you may be; because when a man is weak, he is simply weak. When he has combativeness, when he is weak, then he is exceedingly nervous.

When phosphorus is lacking, a person looks old. On the other hand, when the vitamins are supplied, a man looks young. Therefore, an old man can make himself look young and a young man can make himself look old by diet alone.

When a man practices self abuse, he always weakens the phosphorus function and he weakens also the function of taking up neurol for the brain. The brain itself shrinks and the membranes become weakened and shrunken; he cannot take up phosphorus. Phosphorus metabolism is low in any man who abuses the sex function. I do not care whether a man goes to excess sexually or whether he practices self abuse, it leads to the same result or whether he eats foods that do not contain phosphorus, it brings the same result. If he falls back on a phosphorus diet, he cures his ailments and improves his appearance.

Phosphorus and fluorine and many other elements should be supplied in abundance in times of paralysis. When a child is slow in learning to walk or is clumsy, falls easily, phosphorus is needed. It requires a certain degree of strength to control your movements, to your feet and hands, to regulate the equilibrium of the body or the coordination of the muscles and tendons and if there is not enough phosphorus, there is weakness, awkwardness, clumsiness. Hence a person who lacks phosphorus is always clumsy. If he takes hold of something, he breaks it; if he pulls down a curtain, he jerks it down and breaks it; if he picks up a glass case, he falls in the stairway and breaks the case and his shoulder bone in the bargain.

The penmanship of a child that lacks phosphorus is clumsy and awkward because the child cannot control its fingers, the finger techinque is defective in the child or coordination of movements is not complete when phosphorus is lacking.

There are so many symptoms and peculiarities by which we know when phosphorus is needed. If a child does not like to study or if he studies too much and wants to study and read until he becomes a regular bookworm, phosphorus consumption is too great and nearly all the phosphorus goes to the brain. Then it is time to take the books away from him and lock them up. Send him into the backyard to a sandpile and give a shovel while the sun shines.

Remember when it is a question of phosphorus metabolism, we can always increase phosphorus metabolism at a time it is required. The sun cures. Let the sun fall upon the nude body. The sunlight increases phosphorus metabolism in the tissues when the body is nude. It is the same when we want to increase phosphorus metabolism or when a man is clumsy and awkward and lacking phosphorus in the brain. Take off his hat and let in the sunlight. The brain is stimulated to greater phosphorus metabolism. Keep the hat off and even shave the hair if necessary.

When a child wakes up and screams in the middle of the night, perhaps you call it colic, but it may be caused by a lack of phosphorus. When there is this lack, there are fleeting pains here there and everywhere. The more phosphorus is lacking, the more intense the pain.

Cow's milk contains phosphorus and calcium. Such milk is well suited for a man who is of a Calciferic constitution. A phosphorus and bony man is the man who should be given cow's milk in abundance. If a man is slender, has slender bones and he is in great need of development of muscles, cow's milk is needed because it contains potassium, chlorine, phosphorus and calcium. Some foods contain chlorine in an inorganic form as sauerkraut, which contains 13-14%, which is really nothing else than common table salt. Ham and many cheeses are very rich in chlorine but it is inorganic chlorine. In cow's milk, we have organic chlorine.

You think milk is sometimes very constipating. Cow's milk is exceedingly constipating but goat's milk or cheese is not constipating because goat's milk contains lactic acid in abundance. It also contains chlorine, sodium, potassium and only 5% of calcium of the salts. Every one of us should have a goat ranch and sell milk everywhere. It would be a great blessing. Goat's milk is exactly what children need. Do not boil goat's milk because you will kill the vitamins and alter the chemicals. Do not pasteurize it either. Feed children the natural product; never interfere with the Almighty's plan. Goat's milk is rich in potash and fluorine—the very salts and chemicals that make bacteria feel very uncomfortable.

PRINCIPAL PHOSPHORUS FOODS

WHEAT BRAN is rich in phosphorus but where is the person who can digest wheat bran? When wheat bran goes into the intestines, it takes up the water there and makes the intestinal walls dry. Instead of curing constipation, it increases it. Bran contains colloids. When it goes into the intestines, in heat and among germs, it becomes germ soil. We do not need to eat yeast either. We are told to eat yeast for the increase of vitamins, but we do not need the vitamins in yeast. We can get vitamins from nobler sources. It is true that yeast is full of vitamins but it is also true that these vitamins are born of fermentation and spores which are unfavorable to the human organization. Why not eat raw egg yolk for vitamins? There you do not find fermentative enzymes. In yeast you get germs and ferment; in egg yolk, you find life, organic salts and vitamins.

BARLEY is a food that deserves mention. In the various foods we find various food compounds. In barley, we find a great deal of phosphorus with silicon in abundance, also maltose or malt sugar, which is easily taken up by the muscles. Barley ferments easily. If the kidneys are weak, barley will affect them. A person with weak kidneys should never eat malt nor any barley food. Beer made of malt or barley should not be drunk by a person such as this.

If a child is growing and the muscular system is in a good condition but he is a little lean, you can build up muscle and flesh quicker on a barley diet than anything else because barley contains phosphorus, silicon, potassium, magnesium and maltose. It is a fine food for people who have strong kidneys and people who are lean.

BEANS contain nearly 39% of phosphorus and over 3% of ash. That is a fine food for growing children, providing they have good kidneys. If you give your children beans, peas and barley foods of various descriptions, they will build muscle, bone, nerves, brain and an efficient generative system and plenty of phosphorus will be supplied to all the functions.

Whenever there is gas, do not eat barley or beans. We cannot eat many foods at that time. Gas must absolutely be neutralilzed and sent out of the system, because I firmly believe that there is no indigestion at any other time except when there is gas in the system. I believe that gas is the only cause of indigestion. When there is gas in the system there is a lack of some organic salts.

When there is gas in the stomach, eat no food until that gas is neutralized. Gas is the meanest thing a patient has to fight. We have come to the conclusion, though I do not say I'm right, that about 70% of all diseases are caused by gas and acidity in the stomach. The intestines will stand still; they cannot act; there is no peristalsis in the stomach when there is gas pressing in every direction. The gas goes into the nerves, brain and the patient feels as though he is drunk and does not have control of the faculties and nerves. He cannot concentrate. You will live longer, become more efficient, merely by neutralizing intestinal gases.

The little baby suffers from gas and gray hair does not escape it. Even the growing youth is sometimes a gas factory. Doctors usually have a hard fight against gas even if they do not know that it is gas. The cause of indigestion, heart disease, gout, rheumatism, neuritis is gas and acidity. That weak brain, that lack of concentration, weak memory, weak sexual system, has its origin in gas and acidity. We actually believe that if we would only fall back on a basic diet at all times, and supply all those salts needed in the body, we could live perhaps 20 to 50 years longer. In fact, we do not know how much longer we could or could not live; but I believe if we master the question of diet, we may live as long as Carr, 152 years, perhaps even longer. Carr did not know anything about diet; he lived much on buttermilk and potatoes—a real gas diet.

FISH is a good food for the brain. Fish supplies neurol, phosphorus and sodium phosphate. The best fish you can buy is whiting. Remember that whiting is not whitefish. Do not eat whitefish any more than you can help or you may possibly suffer from cancer, as whitefish may carry cancer germs. Trout is also rather dangerous fish and likely to carry cancer germs.

In fish, we find phosphorus combined with a certain valuable fat, important to the spinal marrow, to the fatty substance in the nerves and to the brain. It is often needed in a nervous lady who is high-tempered, unstrung, intense, who burns up the fat and phosphorus in the nerves and brain, thereby suffering from neuralgia, burning nerves, burning nerve plexuses, hysterics and prostration. A fish diet often cures her. Whiting is a clean fish, even if it is found in dirty water.

LENTILS. Great physical workers should eat lentils. Phosphorus and potassium phosphate are found in lentils. Lentils support and build tissue. Dried olives—not ripe olives, but sundried olives, also olives treated by common salt—contain potassium, a certain

oleic fat, also phosphorus, which develops muscles and tissues. Give a man who suffers from paralytic symptoms olives in abundance.

We should always eat foods in such a form that we may obtain the organic salts. A food from which the organic salts have been taken, is a disease food. A food that has been overcooked, as for instance, cow's milk, subjected to 172 degrees of heat through pasteurization processes, that same milk has been altered in its organic salts and the vitamins have been killed. If you give your child such milk, you give your child dead food.

MILK. Cow's milk contains calcium, potassium, chlorine and phosphorus. Goat's milk contains fluorine, phosphorus, potash, a high percentage of chlorine, also lactic acid. This is a valuable food, because you find all the blood salts in goat's milk. Calcium phosphate, potassium chloride and sodium chloride are found in goat's milk and cheese. These are the very salts that are needed in the blood and by the blood and found in goat's milk in just about the exact proportion. This is why goat's milk is so very valuable. Human milk and goat's milk are very much the same except that human milk contains only 45/100 of 1% of organic salts while goat's milk contains almost 2% of organic salts or in other words, goat's milk contains many times as much organized salts as human milk. Cow's milk contains only 71/100 of 1% of organic salts and these are principally calcium. Goat's milk contains 1.74% organized salts, or several times as much organized salts as cow's milk. Some men say, "Milk is milk and that is all." But there is a chemical difference not generally know.

The phosphorus you find in cow's milk is perhaps that kind of phosphorus that builds bone, horns and hooves, needed by the calf. The baby needs brain. We do believe that you cannot build brain from cow's milk very successfully. We must fall back on vegetables, fish, egg yolk, rye and barley, in order to sustain and build an efficient human brain.

NUTS. Look at the percentage of salts found in nuts. In almonds, we find nearly 44% of the salts found in the ash. Almonds support your brain. Suppose you make an egg shake of raw egg yolk of some kind of alkaline liquid and then sprinkle grated almonds or walnuts into the drink. Eat a piece of baked whiting and a piece of whole rye bread and you have the best kind of brain food. Your brain from such a diet can solve knotty problems and elaborate the greatest inventions.

OATS. You should remember that all foods that you must cook are not so valuable as foods you can eat without cooking. **Do not cook egg yolk nor milk.** You do not need to cook nuts. There are many foods you can eat without cooking. Some foods must be cooked but in cooking them you destroy the vitamins. Then you get nothing but the dead elements. Of course, we need a certain degree of dead material but we should not forget we need life, life to sustain life. The weaker we grow, the more we need vitamins. In order to get vitamins, we must eat food that contain them. But this does not mean we should eat raw starch or raw potatoes.

RICE. Of course, we cannot digest raw rice. We find phosphorus and potassium, together with starch, in rice providing it is wild rice or unpolished rice. Never eat the ordinary polished rice because it is mainly starch.

RYE is an excellent brain food. Rye and barley are better brain food than wheat. Barley and rye require little digestive powers. Wheat is difficult to digest but rye yields its phosphorus easily, while wheat does not. It is almost impossible to take phosphorus out of wheat because it is so difficult to digest but a child, even with a weak stomach, could take phosphorus out of barley, rye, egg yolk and fish.

Clam broth, for instance, and whole rye bread would make a good phosphorus food. It is easy to take phosphorus out of clam broth and rye bread when the broth is hot and the bread well soaked in the broth. A rhinoceros could hardly extract the phosphorus from wheat bran, raw wheat and other wheat preparations.

Never give anyone cold food who has a weak stomach and never give such a patient heavy meals. Always bear this in mind: the weaker the stomach, the warmer the food should be.

FOODS AND CHEMICALS
<u>FLUORINE</u>

Fluorine is an important chemical element which helps the human organization. It is usually found in combination with calcium. Almost all foods that carry calcium also carry fluorine. Because it does not unite with oxygen, it becomes a protective element. Oxygen has two functions: 1. constructive and 2. destructive. Oxygen builds up and it tears down or destroys. That seems to be the work of oxygen in the universe. So soon as anything dies oxygen picks it to pieces, but if fluorine is present in tissue, fiber, bone or tooth, it is impossible for oxygen to do destructive work. Oxygen cannot decompose a bone or tooth if fluorine is present. That tooth or bone becomes lasting.

We should supply the fluorine foods to all children when they are growing; when the teeth are being formed; when the bones are growing; when all the solid fibrous tissues are being formed. Oxygen builds up and it also destroys us. If it were not for fluorine, our teeth, bones, solid tissue would not last very long.

There is a strong affinity between fluorine and calcium, but none between fluorine and oxygen. Those two elements are opposites. They are repulsive to each other, the same as people are repulsive who are of the Marasmic and Oxypheric constitutions.

Fluorine, sodium, sulphur and phosphorus are the elements that have a great deal to do with life. If any one of those elements is lacking, life is not complete.

Fluorine that has been organized into tissues is organic.

We are constantly eliminating some element. We are using sodium every day in the year. We break down chlorine every minute. We require fluorine every hour of the day. Certain diseases are burning up certain elements in our body. Calcium is used by many of the physical functions as, for instance, in the bones and teeth. Calcium, which is organized into bones, is organic; calcium used by the functions has not received any name. We call it functional calcium or free calcium.

Almost every element of all the 16 elements found in the human organization has two functions to perform, viz., 1. an organic function, 2. and a functional. This is also true in regard to fluorine. If there is a lack of fluorine in some bone, there may be excessive growth in some special part of the bone and not enough in another part; then bone metabolism becomes erratic.

If fluorine is lacking, there may be ulceration. If it were not for fluorine, calcium would fall apart like wall plaster. The skull of a man who died of syphilis will crumble into a hundred pieces. But take the skull of some other person, say of an Exesthesic, and that skull never breaks. The skull of a man who dies of syphilis is like wall plaster. When we get hold of a skull in which fluorine has been separated from calcium, we know the person died of syphilis.

Fluorine has an important function to perform in combination with calcium. Fluorine is an organization agent in bone. It acts upon calcium just about like cement and holds all the cells together. It holds together every little bone cell. The fluorine also builds a hard surface around the outside as a protection against oxygen and all sorts of bone enemies.

Bones and teeth have come to us from prehistoric times. I once had hold of a skull that was said to be 120,000 years old. It was the skull of an Egyptian woman. The anatomists fixed up a picture of her as they imagined her to look during life. They labeled it "This lady lived 120,000 years ago." We have proof that bones and teeth are almost indestructible with fluorine in combination with calcium.

The spleen cannot perform its function properly unless a certain amount of fluorine acts upon the spleen. There are certain spleen diseases which could be cured very quickly if you supplied the fluorine element in the form of food.

If children suffer from hip disease or decayed teeth, give them food rich in calcium and fluorine. Fluorine and calcium must act together in teeth, bone, feathers, hair and all sorts of elastic tissue. If we do not supply fluorine in connection with calcium, it is impossible to build good bone, teeth or solid tissue. For hip disease, supply foods rich in calcium, silicon, albumin and fluorine. Fluorine is a twin brother to calcium; it organizes lime and kills the germs that thrive in bone and joints.

You cannot build bone or teeth without material. You may call in a doctor when you are sick and his treatments may help, but do not forget the food your system needs. You cannot build good teeth and bones from coffee, doughnuts and cake. You cannot build a strong body with vegetarian dreams. You cannot become an efficiency expert by eating crullers, rolls, starch and candy. You cannot build muscles of cream nor motor nerves of butter.

If you suffer from varicose veins, eat fluorine and breathe fresh air and take exercises. When you give the veins exercise, you must massage upwardly toward the heart. Go in the same direction when you exercise, as the blood flows. The blood flows toward the heart. It flows from the arms toward the heart in the veins. It flows from the head to the heart in the veins. It flows from the feet to the heart in the veins. If you take massage always go in the same direction as the blood flows in the veins. Here is a valuable point for masseurs.

To build perfect bones and teeth, begin with fluorine before the teeth are gone. The right time to build teeth is when the child is between the ages of three and fourteen years.

There is no pus formation where fluorine is at work. Fluorine kills parasites. It prevents excess of heat in some special part of the system. On the other hand, if there is a lack of fluorine, there will be too much heat in one bone and not enough in another. One part will be feverish, another will be cold and some other part may suffer from something else. There is no equalization of heat, when there is a lack of fluorine.

Syphilis breaks down fluorine. When a man suffers from syphilis and a medical man cures him, he only kills the germs. Cure him with diet or he will never be cured. Medicine cannot drive a taint out. Supply the food elements that are necessary. In order to overcome syphilis, we must absolutely supply fluorine and keep supplying it until the miasm is gone. The only way to cure syphilis is by cell building. You must build a new man. You can never drive it out of the cell, because if a miasm is in the cell, that miasm will stay. You must build a new cell to take the place of the old one.

There is no food so valuable in times of pus formation or tuberculosis (which is nothing but a pus disease), as fresh goat's milk. It contains in greater quantities than any other milk. More fluorine is in the milk of Toggenburg goats than in the Nubian. Still less fluorine is in sheep's milk. Cow's milk contains only a trace of fluorine. People are giving cow's milk to their children and drinking it every day and yet we are told there are 40 million germs in one teaspoonful of cow's milk. The milk of the Saanen goat and of the Toggenburg is high in fluorine. You cannot find a better fluorine food for your babies.

We would never suffer from toothache if we had perfect enamel. No pus can form under the roots of the teeth if fluorine is supplied in abundance. There could be no decay of teeth.

There is one country of which it is said has not had one case of tuberculosis during the past 100 years and that country is using goat's milk in its national baby diet. They are feeding their children goat's milk. Don't you think it is time, here in America, to start using goat's milk? Everyone, everywhere, should have at least 2 Toggenburg or 2 Saanen goats. Consumptive hospitals should have at least 100, and they should have fresh air in abundance. Instead those consumptive patients are put inside four walls where there is dead air and given cream and egg white.

Fluorine works against tuberculosis pus formation; syphilitic pus formation and vaccination pus formation. Vaccination does not take so easily if you have plenty of fluorine in your body. You can vaccinate Exesthesic people yet the vaccine does not always take because they usually have plenty of fluorine in their bodies. There are certain constitutions in which vaccination does not take because fluorine is there to protect against pus. If we had any sense, we would not introduce tubercular, syphilitic nor vaccination pus into our bodies.

If a Pargenic falls, he may break his bones because they are brittle because of a lack of fluorine. If you are an osteopath and have a Pargenic patient you must be careful how you set the bones. Fluorine has everything to do with bone metabolism. Firmness is the faculty of bone building. A man who lacks firmness has soft bones or is almost bone-less. The Neurogenic man is weak in firmness and very strong in idealism; hence, he cannot build bone. Almost all Neurogenic people suffer from bone disease. They are always weak. There is something lacking in the tissues.

If your bones are small, if you suffer from weak bones or bone disease, supply fluorine. Fluorine protects calcium. You cannot build bones unless you do heavy work. Shoulder heavy planks and carry them a distance and you reach the bones. You cannot build heavy bones by sitting in an arm chair and dreaming about love and moonshine. If we increase fluorine, we increase bone formation. If we increase the capacity of the system to take up tricalcium phosphate, we can build bone.

A man 100 years old writes a book and says, the reason he lived so long is because he ate potatoes all his life. From this you conclude that potatoes are the best food for old age. Also a lady 105 years old says she lived that long because she never took a bath. We do not live long because we never take a bath nor because we eat potatoes. We live long because all needed elements are supplied in the body. Take fluorine and iron out of the diet of a beautiful young girl, and she will grow old at once. She will soon have many wrinkles in her face and will have no strength.

Fluorine preserves health, strength and vigor and makes us young. A lady goes to some beauty culturist and gets some of her "smear" and thinks she is beautiful but she fools no one but herself. I have nothing against beauty culturists. I believe every woman should do all in her power to stay young, beautiful and attractive. But she must fall back on the material supplied by the Almighty. The secret of youth is fluorine in abundance. If you fall back on a scientific diet, you find that you can retain vigor, strength and youthfulness and that you will look young when you are old. If you are 80, you will look 50, and while you live you can keep healthy.

If we know those 16 chemical elements that the Almighty has put into our system, we can defy sickness, death and old age for a long time and can maintain our health while we do live. If we live only 40 years and are healthy, we are better off than to live 70 years and be sickly all the time.

Vaccinosis (we do not mean vaccination), is a disease which is the result of vaccination. A man is vaccinated and it takes. Later some hidden disease develops in him and he does not know just what it is. He is simply sick. It is caused by and the after effect of vaccination.

You cannot feed sufficient fluorine to every constitution. For instance, it is impossible to give Pargenic people enough fluorine, because they suffer from fluorine hunger.

Fluorine acts upon the meninges and inflames them. When fluorine is excessive, they are fond of wines and fatty foods. They are always hungry, no matter how much they eat. They cannot remember; they have to reason out everything for themselves. They may suffer from religious mania. Their eyes are red. If you see a fluorine patient once, you will never forget him. Put a patient on a heavy fluorine diet, and he will develop a religious mania. Every man should pray; praying does not do any harm, but at the same time, we must not forget the element needed is fluorine.

When the meninges become inflamed, disease sets in at the surface of the brain, in the gray substance, resulting in insanity. We have many such patients in the asylums today. What is being done for those poor maniacs? We do not even know why these patients are there nor what has taken place in their systems. Excess or lack of the fluorine element is likely to result in insanity.

Fluorine patients tell me they feel as if they are divided in two. The vision is disturbed. Excess fluorine disturbs the eye structure.

A patient was taken to Macon, Missouri. The doctors there could do nothing. He was sent to other places and lastly brought to me. I placed that patient on a heavy fluorine diet and on foods rich in formic acid and he began to improve. But for this diet, he would be in the asylum today.

If we eat rightly, we will not suffer much. If we do not eat rightly, we will suffer. Diet will not do everything but anyone who has anything to do with human health, should study quantitative food chemistry and chemical diagnosis.

In a fluorine hungry patient, the mind is stupid. Motion makes him worse. The magnesium hungry patient is better when in motion but the fluorine hungry patient feels better when he sits down or lies down. Osteopathic treatments that reach the spinal respiratory center will help him. A doctor who was a fluorine hungry patient would forget his patients and what he had given them. He even forgot their address. Yet he was taking a memory course.

The fluorine hungry patient feels there is a dark mental cloud hanging over him; he feels that somebody is after him. He has a mean disposition; even if he tries to please, he feels ugly at heart. He feels as if he has not the normal use of his brain. I have experimented and found it possible to change disposition by diet.

One fluorine hungry patient thought that he heard voices for a long time. They may say there is a storm inside the brain. He knows it is not so, but at the same time, he knows it is there.

When fluorine is absolutely lacking, he may think he is a wonderful genius in regard to investments. He believes evil, ugly beings are living in him. He may say he has a good spirit and a very bad spirit inside that control him alternately. Then we wonder why such people commit crimes or suicide. There are various brain ailments when fluorine is not there to protect it. Those poisons begin to work on the brain and give rise to strange and unusual symptoms. These patients believe they have some wonderful power. They may think their tophead is in heaven and they can see what is going on there. We think those people are crazy, but it is simply toxins at work, because of lack of certain chemical elements. When you can diagnose the symptoms of several people who suffer from the same trouble you can see just exactly what element or elements are lacking.

Carbonic acid has its symptoms. Excessive coffee drinking has its symptoms. Look at a man who drinks whiskey or eats tobacco. Does he not become peculiar? Every poison has its disease symptom. Every toxin has its symptom. Germs generating their toxins in the body also produce their peculiar symptom. Lack of fluorine or excess of fluorine has symptoms.

That which we call characteristics is often the result of some chemical element, toxin, habit, food, drink, gas, etc. All those peculiarities of individuals we call imagination is not imagination but symptoms which the doctors seldom understand.

VOCATIONS FOR WHICH FLUORINE PEOPLE ARE BEST ADAPTED

The fluorine man is interested in revivals. Many people of the fluorine type become strongly interested in contemptible occupations.

Many specialists specialize in those functions that are disturbed in themselves. A doctor who suffers very much from indigestion becomes a specialist in digestion and diseases of the stomach. That holds good also in regard to those people who take up revivalism. They are afraid of the devil. A man may become a specialist in sexual diseases because he suffers from that ailment himself. That which we suffer from mostly, we study mostly.

The vibrating neurons in the brain cause diseases of the brain. A peculiar thing about fluorine patients is that they want to come in contact with the nude human body.

In the fluorine people, the faculty of spirituality is very active. If you want to develop psychic power, start in with a fluorine diet and that faculty will become very active.

A patient suffering from tuberculosis in any form, syphilis, scrofula or any pus disease, lacks air or has low oxidation. We cannot force one single speck more air into our lungs; however, all we can do is fall back on a diet that contains the salts that attract air from the atmosphere or go to a higher altitude. Then air is attracted into our system to a greater extent. A higher altitude is the one thing we need when we lack air.

When the air is more attenuated and we get into a higher altitude, there is greater effort of the respiratory centers. The medulla becomes more active and acts upon the lung cells and the whole respiratory system makes greater efforts at aeration.

A patient suffering from a tuberculosis ailment should be sent to a higher altitude not to a sanitarium room. Do not go into a sanitarium with such sickness. We cannot get air there, regardless of the altitude. You cannot change altitudes in a sanitarium. You cannot get fresh air within four walls and below a roof. You should not put a tubercular patient, a Pargenic patient, a scrofulous patient or any in whom oxidation is low, inside four walls. When you are in a sanitarium, you are below a roof and within four walls. The Almighty's sanitarium is best.

If the dura mater of the spinal cord becomes weakened, as it will in times of fluorine starvation, there is much danger of some kind of spinal disease. The dura mater lies close to the brain. Fluorine must be supplied so the function of the cerebral and spinal membranes will be protected at all times. If fluorine is not supplied, inflammation sets in or calcium is likely to harden, leading to brain trouble. This inflammation may go to the brain and cause insanity. Hence, fluorine is needed.

There is a bean called the caroba bean. It is very valuable if made into bread and all sorts of food preparations. This bean contains certain valuable principles that will drive out impurities from the system.

If syphilis gets the upper hand in the system of a Pargenic man because fluorine has been used up, this can be helped by sarsaparilla tea and by a high fluorine diet.

Pargenic impurity eventually results in tuberculosis. A young man of 18 or 20 years is reckless, consequently may contract a disease. He goes to a doctor who kills the germs but the taint remains. Suppose you have a glass of distilled water and you drop one dirty bug into the water then you kill the bug in the water with some drastic poison, is that water clean? Is there not a taint left in it? That is true also regarding sexual diseases—the germ is killed but the taint remains.

If a person suffers from venereal disease and the doctor simply kills the germ, the taint is left. The germ poison, impurity, taint or miasm is left and has gone perhaps into every cell of the brain, blood, nerves and all through the system. What was to prevent it? We must fall back on those materials which enable us to send that impurity out and build a new man. The taint remains until it is driven out. Just a few symptoms will enable us to know that a taint is there. The complexion may be coppery in a man who has a taint like that.

Another point is iodine, which we should remember in this connection. It has a great deal to do with oxidation. Iodine is fine for goiter. Also iodine is important when there is trouble with the generative function; there is also weakness in the cerebellum and trouble with the eyes when there is an iodine lack.

Pargenic impurity has its weak knees. There is likely to be ulcers in the long bones or trouble with the eyesight. There is a numbness in the thyroid gland and weakness in the cerebellum. The man has surly moods. He may not talk to his wife. He dislikes her. You see, there is reason for all those symptoms.

I was once almost forced to see a lady who had very peculiar symptoms and a strange disease. I did not want to go as I did not understand the sickness. I was talking to her for a couple of hours, when suddenly she wrinkled up her nose and wanted to know what that terrible smell was. "It smells," she said, "like a pigpen." I asked her if she had ever been near anyone who had syphilis. She said she delivered a baby two years ago that was decomposed and from that time she was not the same. She had that taint in her system. Then I knew what to do. If it had not been for that one symptom, I would not have been able to help her.

WHEN A FLUORINE DIET IS NEEDED

The spleen is hungry for fluorine. If you ever have a patient who suffers from this ailment, supply foods rich in fluorine. The spleen cannot perform its function without fluorine.

The hair falls out in bunches when fluorine is needed. All at once a whole bunch of hair falls out and maybe the eyebrows fall out also.

Fluorine and sodium are the two elements that enable us to utilize calcium. The calcium element cannot be organized without sodium and fluorine. Sodium keeps calcium in solution and fluorine organizes it. If there is a lack of fluorine, there will be too much calcium in this place and not enough in another place, nor can the calcium element be organized.

When a man's voice is goat-like in voice vibration, there is a lack of fluorine.

When there is a lack of fluorine, there is a tendency to pus formation. When there is a lack of fluorine, there is also a lack of oxygen; hence, the patient suffers from low oxidation in the tissues.

There are many different forms of rheumatism. Rheumatism caused by a lack of fluorine is characterized by numbness.

All children who lack fluorine are clumsy. The housewife who lacks fluorine will take a set of fine china dishes, carry them out and perhaps drop them on the floor.

Students deficient in fluorine cannot pass examinations, perhaps because there is a lack of fluorine, phosphorus and sulphur. It is better to throw the books aside and eat the right kind of food and get the thought factory in good condition first; then come back tomorrow. When there is a lack of oxygen in the system, the brain cannot act.

A young lady only 20 years of age is trying to live on doughnuts and coffee. After a few years, trouble develops somewhere in her system and she goes to a hospital. The surgeon cuts out something. After leaving the hospital, she is sick again. She needs another operation because her kidneys are loose. That surgeon never thought to ask what she ate. Coffee, tea, white bread, bacon, pie and other similar foods constitute the diet of that poor girl.

One lady in whom fluorine was lacking, told me she could hear roosters crow at great distances.

When lime in the body is not being organized, fluorine is lacking. Keeping calcium in solution is the function of fluorine and sodium.

When the fluorine element is absolutely lacking, it produces that kind of symptoms we describe here. When another element is lacking as for instance, sodium, there will be a combination of symptoms. These are "indirect" symptoms.

A fluorine-hungry patient can hardly wake up. You could almost carry him away, yet he does not waken.

A fluorine-hungry patient has trouble with walking, dancing or when he is in motion. Even though he does not speak, he is ugly just the same. Lack of fluorine interferes with literary ability and capacity and with the intellectual faculties. The Pargenic patient is a very poor speller. There is a swelling on the neck in Pargenic patients.

A patient I was examining told me that as he sat and looked at me, I looked as if I were 10 miles away. When a patient talks like that you know fluorine is lacking.

There are no healing properties in the bones in the fluorine-hungry patient. If you have a patient suffering from bone ailment, supply a fluorine diet. Fluorine organizes lime. Lime cannot be taken up by the bones when fluorine is lacking. Fluorine acts on the lime cells, helps to organize lime cells and makes the bones stronger.

When saliva runs from the mouth, it shows a streak of idiocy. When a man walks around with his mouth open and saliva runs from it, it is usually too late. You see such patients in the asylums.

There is a decomposed odor issuing from the body of a fluorine starvation patient.

The head of a fluorine-hungry patient is so sensitive that so soon as anything touches him, he gets sick and fussy. If you vaccinate a Pargenic man, you have something to answer for. A good doctor would not kill anyone.

A pain in the ball of the eye is one symptom that proves to you that you deal with a fluorine hungry patient.

The face, tophead and neck are greasy. If a Pargenic patient takes a bath, he becomes sick. When the discharges are yellow, the patient has the Pargenic impurity at work in his system. That miasm affects the bones, because when fluorine is not normally at work in the bones, there is also a lack of sodium in the system. Then when there is much moisture in the atmosphere, the bones swell and the patient is gouty. That same thing happens if you take a barrel of unslaked lime and place it where there is considerable moisture—the lime begins to swell. That happens also in the bones. All calcium patients are susceptible to moisture. That is the reason they should be placed in a dry atmosphere.

The tuberculosis patient, the Pargenic, the Isogenic, suffer from the same kind of calcium ailments. They should go to Southern California; I know of no better place. There is no moisture there. The sun is pouring down and boils the very bones. At the same time, there is a breezy current at night. During the day it is hot; yet no one sufferes sunstroke in Southern California. We have sunstroke in Chicago, but none in Southern California. That is the place we should have a sanitarium for that kind of patient.

If you put cold applications on a Pargenic man, his ailment is aggravated. I would not advise a Pargenic patient to go to that sanitarium where they turn the cold hose on nude patients. If there is anything a Pargenic, or

fluorine hungry patient cannot endure, it is cold applications and cold baths.

In the fluorine patient, the eyebrows are bushy, the hair is pointing in all directions. He is better in the morning but not in the evening. He says he feels a pain in his eyes going into his brain. Perspiration from the fluorine-hungry person is sour and the foot sweat is unendurable.

Some of those structures around the bones and many of those membranes, are more or less affected because of lack of fluorine.

I wish you would take a look at the tongue of the Pargenic patient. It is very dark and so thick that it fills the entire mouth. Oxidation in the bones and brain is always deficient in the Pargenic.

It seems there is no system nor order about a fluorine hungry patient. His wife has to take care of his belongings because he drops one article here and another there. He throws his hat in one corner and coat in another. He scatters things all over the house.

It takes him a long time to answer a question, but when his brain starts, it goes on by its own momentum.

He feels that no woman can be trusted and that no man can be relied upon. He has no faith in humanity. These symptoms are not exactly distinct fluorine hunger symptoms, but they are transcient symptoms; they come and go. They are not permanent. They are caused by something else in addition.

The teeth in the Pargenic man are never uniform; one tooth is too wide another is too narrow; one sticks this way, another that; one is too long another too short. The teeth and tongue tell the story. When he walks, he totters as if drunk. Then he may walk two or three blocks and totter again, perhaps even fall. The voice is deep down in his throat.

There are a few symptoms peculiar to the fluorine hungry patient. There may be others besides Pargenics who suffer from lack of fluorine. They have those same symptoms, perhaps in milder form.

PRINCIPAL FLUORINE FOODS

When we permit little children to run in the streets, what do they learn? Here is one body who has a bad habit which he teaches to your son. Every child perhaps has a bad habit which he teaches to your child while in the street. Thus your boy gains in criminal knowledge. When he comes home it is very likely you give him food that contains no fluorine nor sodium.

FOOD ANALYSIS EXPLAINED

BROTH, Cartileginous. All bone joints contain fluorine. When you buy a bone joint, be sure you get it from a young animal. Put all the greens you can into that water with the bone joint and let it simmer very slowly for about 6 hours. Do not cook over a fast fire and send the fluorine up to the ceiling where it is not needed. Save it for your bones. Get hold of greens growing in swamps; they are rich in fluorine. Seagrass is rich in fluorine. The seagrass that grows where the water is green is high in fluorine.

CABBAGE contains fluorine. As a general rule, we can say that all sorts of foods that contain lime also contain flurorine to a certain extent. You do not find much fluorine in cabbage. Red cabbage is rich in other salts as is white cabbage.

CAULIFLOWER. This is another kind of cabbage. There are many different species of cabbage, but all contain calcium and a small percentage of fluorine.

GOAT CHEESE contains fluorine. Anyone who eats cottage cheese should be sure his intestines are in good condition. The cottage cheese we get comes from cow's milk. Germs are very active upon cottage cheese; also upon the intestines. Cottage cheese always affects the intestines.

ROQUEFORT CHEESE is high in ash and low in fluorine.

COD LIVER OIL is medium in fluorine but high in ash.

FISH, BLACK BASS. All greenish fish contain a certain percent of fluorine, but if you cook the fish, the fluorine goes up into steam.

SPINACH. The hot-house spinach is not so good, because it is covered with manure and is full of germs. Do not eat spinach raised in hot houses.

QUESTIONS AND ANSWERS

1. What causes people to talk in their sleep? Answer: Intensity of nerve and brain.

2. What is the cause of excessive dreaming? Answer: Toxins in the brain or blood acting upon the brain cells.

3. What is indicated when a patient walks and strikes his foot against some obstruction and a cold sweat seems to break out from every pore? Answer: This is lack of combativeness or courage. His nerves are shocked.

FOODS AND CHEMICALS
MAGNESIUM

Magnesium enables the eliminative functions to carry on their work. There are three other elements also that enable the eliminative functions to carry on their work, viz., sodium, chlorine and potassium. If any one of these elements is lacking, there will be trouble with the bowels, liver, spleen, pancreas, portal system, blood or with some of the eliminative organs or functions.

If sodium is lacking there will be a special kind of constipation. If potassium is lacking, a certain kind of constipation will develop. If chlorine is lacking, there will be trouble with the stomach. The system will not be able to take care of the albumin. When chlorine is lacking, foods rich in albumin are likely to decay and form toxins. Any albumin not utilized will stay in the body, decay and produce poisons. If magnesium is lacking, constipation develops because magnesium is one of those elements that regulates and keeps the bowels alkaline and prevents gas from forming in the alimentary tract. If gas is generated, the stomach and entire alimentary tract will become acid. Perhaps that acid will reach the nerves and neuritis develops or terrible headache, because albumin toxins pass into the brain and produce pressure on the brain. Gas may very likely form in the alimentary tract and produce pressure on the heart, spinal centers, liver, spleen, stomach, arteries or veins, causing general disturbance of the function everywhere.

Sodium, potassium, chlorine and magnesium are very important and should not be removed from foods in process of manufacture. If these elements are supplied at all times, we will not be sick. We should know what chemicals there are in every kind of food. We should know what is lacking in bread, milk or in fact in anything we eat. We should know absolutely what all those foods contain.

MAGNESIUM, ITS NATURE AND CHARACTERISTICS

All foods that contain magnesium are alkaline. All foods that contain citric acid usually also contain magnesium. Those foods that contain magnesium and citric acid are highly antacid. They take up the acid in the system and convert it into a neutral salt. If you eat butter, cream, sugar, coffee and doughnuts when the stomach is acid, they will be converted into more acid.

When the stomach is acid, some foods will be converted into gas, causing disturbances. Some of those gases will pass up into the brain and may produce paralytic ailments. It may act upon the cerebellum so that it cannot perform its function. If that gas is pressing on the walls of the stomach, the stomach cannot digest food. It is impossible for the stomach to digest food so long as there is gas in the stomach.

The stomach has a certain movement, called peristalsis. Considerable gas in the stomach presses so that the stomach cannot move, cannot digest food, cannot perform its peristalsis movement, cannot pour its gastric juice over the foods. The food is left undigested. You feel a burning in the stomach at such a time or perhaps you feel as if you have a stone in your stomach. You feel uneasy, uncomfortable or bloated. You feel as if there is nothing to live for. Wrong eating has perhaps made more divorces than all other causes combined. The cooks are cooking people right into the hospital, saloon, asylum and into hell. If a man is mean, if he is irritable, beats his wife, drinks whiskey, stays out at night or carries on in an ungodly manner all the time, he has been eating wrong foods improperly prepared. If every wife would cook rightly, she could have all the love she wants.

When a man does not get the right kind of food, he is simply irritable.

A mother came to me in regard to her baby who suffered from crying spells. The stomach was as hard as a brick. I asked what the mother had been eating. She said eating good food as she was very particular about food. I asked again just what she had been eating. She said, "Oh, this morning I had my usual breakfast: a few pancakes, a cup of coffee with cream and sugar. Then I had a glass of orange juice and a piece of cake." "Well," I said, "Your baby suffers because you have been eating wrongly. Remember this—your milk must be alkaline, otherwise the baby will be sick and doctors will not be able to do any good for your baby."

The milk of the mother must be alkaline at all times. The mother should not eat the juices of oranges, lemons, limes nor anything acid. She must never get angry or tired for so sure as a mother gets tired, her milk will become acid. When she gets angry or nervous, the milk is affected. Another thing, the baby is using up the salts during gestation; he draws upon all of those salts from her, taking such salts out of her blood as iron, calcium, sodium, silicon and chlorine. Those are the salts that the mother must absolutely supply to the baby all the time. When the mother is through with gestation and lactation, she is about the same as an empty shell because those salts have been taken away from her blood and tissues. Therefore, she is likely to become acid. And do you think such a mother does not need something else than dope, serum, operations and chiropractic?

It is very difficult for the mother to have alkaline milk if those salts are lacking in her system; hence, she should eat foods rich in such alkaline salts so her milk will be alkaline. The baby cannot take care of the milk if it is not alkaline.

Oranges contain citric acid. Magnesium converts acid in the stomach to neutral salts, resulting in alkalinity. But the mother who eats oranges at a time like that will find that it affects her milk. Orange juice goes into the milk. Very quickly it passes into the milk and does not pass into the stomach. Oranges that contain seeds may be beneficial to a lady if she has no baby, if her stomach is acid. But at the time she has a baby, she must not eat oranges, because they affect the milk.

If there is too much sugar in mother's milk, it curdles and becomes subject to fermentation. The sugar will lay in the stomach and produce fermentation. If the mother eats too much sugar, her baby will surely suffer from stomach trouble.

When magnesium combines with oxygen, it becomes magnesia or magnesium oxide. Alba means white. Magnesium alba is nothing but white clay. White clay is used very considerably in medicine. If you use magnesia alba very excessively in a patient whose system is not very acid or whose stomach is not acid, you will create sickness in that patient. When magnesia alba is introduced into a stomach that is not highly acid, it forms a coating on the entire alimentary tract. Soon that will interfere with digestion. All this unorganized clay will form a coating on the alimentary tract which will interfere with digestion. Magnesia alba requires a very high acid medium to act upon. Citrate of magnesia is a citric white clay preparation. Be careful how you drink it.

There are many things given to children that should not be given them. It is very well to give a person magnesium when the stomach is very acid. If you suffer from a sour burning stomach and alimentary tract, you are in an acid condition and at such time, citrate of magnesia is beneficial. If there is not any acid in the stomach or in the alimentary tract anywhere, and you drink citrate of magnesia, just because you suffer from constipation, it will coat the alimentary tract. If you keep drinking it, it will do you that much more harm. Your intestines will lastly be like frozen hose. They cannot act. It does not make any difference what drastic drugs you take.

Potassium is excessively bitter but magnesium is tart. All sorts of foods that contain magnesium are tart. Almond nuts have a certain pungent taste. That is a magnesium taste. Endive has a pungent principle. That is magnesium. Citrate of magnesia, endive, almond nuts, have a tart or pungent taste and that is magnesium. All foods rich in magnesium have that tart or pungent taste. If you supply magnesium foods in abundance, the bowel contents will look almost like clay. Sometimes children will eat clay; this means they lack magnesium.

FUNCTIONS OF MAGNESIUM IN THE HUMAN ORGANIZATION

Mineral waters that contain magnesium and sulphur are laxative if you take them in great quantities. If those waters are taken at a time when the stomach is excessively acid, they will be beneficial. But if the stomach is not acid, they will do harm. It is better to eat foods containing magnesium and sulphur than to drink mineral water. Why drink mineral water to cure constipation when we can get foods that contain sulphur and magnesium, especially such mineral water that contain other minerals that are harmful?

We should always remember that man is organic. Everything we eat and drink should be organic.

If there is a lack of magnesium in the system, there is a certain stiffness in the various tissues and tendons. Here you can see that magnesium is lacking. Isogenic patients are often stiff. There is a lack of magnesium when the Isogenic patient suffers from constipation or when his tissues are stiff or when he suffers from gout. Then there is a lack of those important salts, sodium and magnesium. Some people take up more magnesium than others. All those who are elastic, quick, active in body and mind have more magnesium in their tissues. Sometimes the tissues are robbed of their salts. The tissues will rob the secretions and the blood of magnesium. In the Desmogenic man, the tissues are constantly taking magnesium out of the secretions and the blood, thus robbing the blood and the tissues. The Desmogenic is very likely to suffer from costive habits, notwithstanding the fact that there is a great deal of magnesium in the tissues, simply because the tissues, themselves, are robbing the blood and the secretions.

Phosphorus consumption is great in the neurogenic. The phosphorus products that are liberated during brain and nerve processes call for magnesium foods in abundance.

The phosphatic element is one of the most important elements there is. A chemist once told me that there was enough poison in his brain to kill 2 million people. You see it is phosphorus in the brain, nerves and in the system that is being burned up and thrown upon the liver, to take away from the body.

Magnesium helps eliminate and neutralize all poisons from the system.

When there is sleeplessness, there is a lack of magnesium; there is excess of phosphoric products. To overcome sleeplessness, take foods, drinks and tonics rich in magnesium.

All people who are excitable, high tempered or erratic, suffer from neurotic habits, high nerve tension or from psychotic habits. They should be given foods rich in magnesium. We have osteopathic doctors who talk about tension in the nerves, muscles and flexors and they remove that tension by means of certain treatments but they omit magnesium foods. Magnesium foods added to osteopathic treatments accomplish more. Magnesium relieves tension in the nerves, muscles, brain centers and flexors. Intense talking burns up phosphorus. When through talking, eat foods rich in phosphorus and magnesium. We do not know the value of eating. Magnesium foods affect the liver and eliminative organs and remove such phosphorus products that have been liberated during intense cerebration.

If you lack magnesium, you suffer from headache which is more severe because all such ailments are more intense when there is a lack of magnesium. When there is plenty of magnesium in the system, even though phosphorus is at work, you can be reposeful.

A function of magnesium is to keep the brain, nerves, flexors, motor nerves, spinal nerves and functions throughout the system cool; to cool a man down. When angry, take foods and drinks rich in magnesium and the temper will soon subside. Passion cools under the influence of magnesium. One function of magnesium is to regulate the nerves.

Magnesium aids in the construction of white fibers in the nerves, muscles and brain. If there is a lack of magnesium in the system, the fibers cannot function. Magnesium acts upon the albumin. All those various white fibers are manufactured out of chlorine and albumin, but magnesium must be there to act, otherwise, they will not be constructed.

Magnesium is an antidote to arsenic poisoning. A person should eat magnesium-containing foods in times of arsenic poisoning. If you give a person arsenic for any length of time, it will lodge in the liver and cannot be eliminated. If magnesium is not given in the form of food, it is impossible to get arsenic out of the liver. If the liver is exceedingly sluggish, adopt a magnesium diet to stir up the impurities and poisons in the liver and send the impurities, fermentation, acids and germs out of the system.

Many patients have been eating starch and sugar until they are sugar drunk. That is where we need magnesium to send that impuritiy out of the system. Magnesium is an antiacid; i.e., it works on acid. When acid is in the stomach, magnesium works on that acid and converts it into neutral salts. That is the function of magnesium. Those acids become neutralized. If magnesium has no acid to work on, it causes trouble.

Chlorine is hard on germs. Salty water makes the germs feel very uncomfortable. Chlorine will kill certain germs. Magnesium may not kill them, but it will wash them out. The germs hide themselves in the coating of the stomach and intestines. If they remain in the coating they are not washed out. They hide themselves in the coating of the stomach while magnesium is passing through. They seem to know how to protect themselves. Then when the good food comes along, they come out and feed. But if we take foods rich in chlorine, magnesium and sodium, those germs must go and we get better.

People who sit in seances and concentrate until they think they see spirits are drying up the oil in the corpus callosum. When that oil is exhausted, spooks are seen and raps from spirits are heard because the brain does not function normally. The hypnotist dries up that oil in his victim without knowing it; then he has him under his control. If you are under the influence of a hypnotist, say to yourself that he cannot have any influence on you; eat magnesium foods, and you will escape the evil mind of the hypnotist.

If we live on coffee, tea, white bread, cake, doughnuts and junk foods, and keep eating it, the magnesium will soon be entirely gone. Then we tremble from nervousness.

Magnesium acts favorably on all the eliminative organs, especially on the intestines. It helps the liver.

568

SYMPTOMS WHEN MAGNESIUM IS EXCESSIVE

If you live on magnesium food at a time when you do not need it, the brain and body become sluggish. When fatigued, disappointed in love, excessively passionate, eat magnesium foods in abundance for several days and you will feel very much better.

The more a person takes everything to heart, the less magnesium in the system because if magnesium were in the system, a person would not grieve. You can overlook disagreeable things if you eat foods rich in magnesium. Magnesium cleans and regulates the bowel. It enables the brain to accomplish what it should accomplish. It prevents tumors from growing. We have three elements to fall back on in times of tumor, viz.; magnesium, formic acid and fluorine.

A great deal of heat is generated in the human system. Iron, chlorine and sodium are sometimes broken down in the various organs, causing coagulation of the blood. If there is a lack of magnesium, the blood may centralize and form a tumor. In times of great brain energy, we could prevent brain tumors from forming and save the patient from insanity, merely by a formic acid diet. Even if the tumors have already formed, they may be scattered by the action of the formic acid. Give people who suffer from insanity caused by tumors in the brain a heavy formic acid diet and cold applications in abundance also an eliminative diet.

When there is a great deal of heat centralization in any part of the body, there is a tendency to thrombosis. People suffering from thrombosis or blood clotting, do not live long. If it forms in the brain, in some of the fibers, it leads to apoplexy and other ailments. Every doctor and nurse should fall back on diet in connection with their other methods of doctoring. The osteopath treats by osteopathy. The medical doctor prescribes drugs and operations. The hydropath gives cold baths. The physical culturist gives exercise. Certain mental scientists say, "Tell yourself there is no sickness." People should use them all and then add the proper diet. Diet will not do everything but it helps greatly.

Put a man on a meat diet and nothing but meat for a long time, and it will develop tuberculosis in less than 18 months, because there is no calcium in meat.

A heavy magnesium diet and nothing else for 4, 5 or 6 months, will weaken the brain and cause great stupidity, fear, dreadful dreams and weaken the perceptives.

The magnesium excess patient cannot discriminate. He is unable to see the difference in form, shape, outline or distances. Magnesium patients always forget where they place things.

SYMPTOMS WHEN MAGNESIUM IS DEFICIENT

A man gets so angry he has absolutely no control of himself when there is a lack of magnesium. As soon as he gets in a rush, he has a headache. A red color sends pain into the eyes.

They complain of clay-taste in their mouth. Press very strongly on a painful nerve and the pain disappears. Healers apply pressure in this case and they think they have great power.

We cannot increase magnesium in the body by taking magnesium drugs. Magnesium drugs are never taken up by the blood or tissues. Magnesium foods are taken up to a great extent if the patient lives in a cool climate.

PEOPLE WHO REQUIRE MAGNESIUM FOODS

People who have a red complexion. People who use the sexual instinct too strongly; people who are too active and generating too much heat in the brain; those who are too active in their passions and burning up certain salts and vital principles which are necessary for the body in a great many ways; hot-headed and excitable people; people who use the intellect too strongly; people who generate too much heat in the intellect; people who are intense; people who are sowing wild oats are all in need of magnesium. Magnesium will have a soothing and cooling effect.

A manager of a business, railroad, an executive, using their brains excessively, are in great need of magnesium. When the head burns; when there is heat in the nerves or liver, a magnesium diet is needed.

Nitropheric people do not require a high magnesium diet, because they hardly ever generate excess bodily heat. The skin is cold. You would think they were cold-blooded.

Magnesium has no constitution; at least, I have never found a magnesium constitution. I think the magnesium is simply there to act upon phosphorus products coming from the brain. Magnesium is eliminative rather than constructive.

INFLUENCE OF AN EXCESSIVE AMOUNT OF MAGNESIUM FOODS

Constructive nutrition is disturbed when there is an excess of magnesium. If there is a normal supply of magnesium in the body, a man is more even minded.

DISEASE TENDENCIES OF PEOPLE IN WHOM MAGNESIUM IS IN EXCESS

There are disturbances in the nerves, brain, sensory functions, motor functions, heart functions, impulsive functions and in the various functions of the body. The nerve fibers in the mucous membrane cannot transmit impulses, which result in disturbance of the function of the mucous membrane. Magnesium is important for digestion and nutrition. If magnesium is lacking in the body, the nerve and brain impulses cannot be transmitted properly, nor consecutively to the mucous membrane. The uterus and sexual functions are disturbed.

Paranois is the inability of the white brain substances to transmit impulses; because magnesium is acting in excess on the white brain substances which become pulpy. Then the patient is weakminded, so to speak.

People of an oxypheric constitution generate more heat than they need. If there is magnesium in excess in a constitution like that, boils appear. All at once you find adhesions.

The magnesium element has so much to do with phosphorus metabolism that if magnesium is not abundantly supplied to the body, all those phosphorus poisons and products are not eliminated. If magnesium is not supplied to eliminate those phosphoric poisons, gas generation results. Then many ailments peculiar to those elements develop.

A patient may become exceedingly fleshy in the central section of the body. This goes on for some time, then he may become emaciated, then weakening of the function occurs; then he dies. Be careful when there is excessive obesity in the bowels.

The system cannot take up nutrition and the patient becomes emaciated. There is no better cure for obesity than rushing the food through the alimentary tract. Such a lady patient will lose in flesh every day. If she will fall back strongly on chlorine or salty foods, she will also grow thin. You do not need anyone to reduce you, you can reduce yourself. Remember also your temperament, because some people are so constituted that even if they do not eat much food, they grow stout just the same.

If magnesium is lacking in the body, cell action in the brain becomes excessive. Suppose the brain cell fibers act only about once per month, how much energy could you get out of such a man? But suppose the brain fibers vibrate a thousand times per minute or more, there is where we get intensity. That is what takes place in one of those Exesthesic ladies of excessively high tension. If anything goes against her, she goes into hysterics. She is hard to live with. It is mostly the emotional faculties that are so active in Exesthesic people. It is great vibration in the various brain cells, nerves, liver and elsewhere.

When there is great activity in the brain, body, various functions of the brain and body; when the feelings are intense; when the brain is on fire, so to speak—magnesium food is required. When these brain cells and functions are too hot we must cool them off with magnesium food. When there is great vibration in the brain cells, we need magnesium food to cool them off so the vibration is not so intense. Give these high-strung ladies a drink of grapefruit juice. Soon they settle down easily and are cooled off. Give a person who is using too much phosphorus grapefruit juice two or three times every day and he cools down and is able to sleep. If he goes home after having delivered a lecture without such drinks, he may not be able to fall asleep.

To cure sleeplessness, put hot applications on the stomach and cool applications on the forehead and drink plenty of juice of grapefruit. Cool him off and he will sleep. Every high-tempered man can cool himself with grapefruit juice and other magnesium foods or fruits rich in magnesium. Temper springs from destructiveness, combativeness, amativeness, cerebellum, ideality and approbativeness. One or all of these faculties have temper in them.

Children who scream are using up magnesium in the system; when they scream so that you have to carry them all night, they lack magnesium. You should give the mother of that little crying child foods rich in magnesium. You should supply magnesium in the nourishment of that baby. Another thing, you should keep that little fellow awake between 5 o'clock and 10 o'clock at night. If you do not do that and do not supply magnesium, he will grow weak crying; you will be nervous and irritable taking care of him; you will burn up your magnesium; your complexion will fade and your eyes lose their brightness; all because of a lack of magnesium. If a mother does not eat rightly, there will be trouble with the baby. If she suffers from gas, her child will suffer from gas. If she suffers from temper, the child will suffer from temper. If she is excitable, her bably will be also. She must eat magnesium-containing foods herself and give herself plenty of sleep between 9 and 5. She must prevent that baby from getting gas into his stomach. The baby is affected by mental and physical states of the mother.

VOCATIONS FOR WHICH MAGNESIUM PEOPLE ARE BEST ADAPTED

Magnesium makes the fingers more skillful; there is greater elasticity, similar to silicon. Silicon makes the fingers more flexible and all the senses more alert. Magnesium has its influence on finger technique. When magnesium is normally supplied, there is greater finger skill; greater elasticity in the various members of the body; also greater communication in the brain between brain center and brain center, between the various faculties and between various functions of the body.

HELPFUL HINTS

Epsom salts have a powerful affect upon germs, impurities and poisons accumulated in the intestines but do not take them frequently.

Avoid too much citrate of magnesia or the intestines will become weak and the bowels will become coated with a clay coating. The alimentary tract will become coated. The peristaltic action will be weakened. If you take epsom slats, there will be greater peristaltic action in the intestines today but tomorrow, the bowels will stand still. It will be impossible to move the excreta or get the peristalsis into action. It is much better to increase the peristaltic action of the stomach by eating the right kind of food. Magnesium helps to carry off the impurities from the system; it takes care of the bowel.

Sodium is one of the eliminative salts. Chlorine acts upon the intestines. Magnesium is another one of those intestinal salts for giving perfect elimination. Eat foods rich in sodium, chlorine, magnesium and potassium, and put hot applications on the stomach; use the Swedish massage movements to cause greater action in the bowels; sleep in abundance; take the right kind of exercise; go to the hills occasionally for plenty of air and your constipation will be cured.

Some people use internal baths or colon irrigation; this is dangerous. Employ a doctor or first-class nurse who understands the construction of the intestines to give you an internal bath. If you take merely a hot water injection into the bowels, you will drive all the gas from the intestines up into the stomach and then up into the brain. After you take an inside bath, you feel drowsy because you have sent that gas up into the brain. Take a drink of peppermint tea and put the juice of limes into it and fill your stomach full so that no gas can be carried up into the stomach. Take three quarts water as hot as you can stand it, the hotter the better; two tablespoons of salt, put a little glycerine and soapsuds into the injection, inject it slowly lying on the right side. Let the water run in slowly, then shut it off; shut off the stream about three or four minutes, then let it run in slowly. When all the water shall have been injected, hold it ten or fifteen minutes, do a little exercising so that the water can do its work, then take plenty of time to evacuate all the water and impurities. Do not be in a rush. Do not do it in half an hour. The bowels cannot act fully in less than two hours. You should stay two hours and let Nature act; then you are doing the wise thing.

571

Magnesium hunger develops greater vibration in the brain cells; vibration in the nerve cells; rapid heart and pulse. The Exesthesic lady prefers to take a train or automobile where there are great vibration and noise; she needs more air. That is why the Exesthesic lady likes to ride in an automobile. If she gets sick or grows weak from walking, there is a lack of magnesium.

WHEN A MAGNESIUM DIET IS NEEDED

A direct symptom is one that is produced directly; an indirect symptom is brought about by magnesium in connection with some other element also lacking. A latent symptom appears only at stated intervals. It may appear for two or three weeks and then not again perhaps for two or three years. Transient symptoms may appear today then next week then in two or three weeks and appear constantly at those special times.

Gas generation is a symptom. Many elements as for instance, sulphur, produce gas generation. Lack of sodium or magnesium, produces gas, so will excess of magnesium; lack or excess of potassium produces gas; lack or excess of iron produces gas. Sulphur produces gas when it is in excess. These are indirect gas symptoms, because there are other elements that have the same symptoms. But there is a difference between gas and gas; viz., in one case of gas a person feels bloated for which he may take a salty drink. In another case, he may take a salty drink and it does not touch the gas. In other cases, bicarbonate of soda will break down that gas; or hot applications in other cases; or some other remedy helps to break down the gas. Gas and acid are different. Gas is one of the indirect symptoms of magnesium.

When magnesium is lacking there is always tenacity in the secretions. A man spits and the mucus is so tenacious that it reaches the floor. When magnesium is lacking, there is gas in the stomach. The stomach becomes hot. You can break down that gas by drinking juice of limes or the juice from sour oranges. If you drink that juice and the gas is broken down and you spit, the spit will hang from you mouth to the floor. It is a white froth. The white froth is not magnesium itself, but it is phosphorus. You see, it is not magnesium that is tenacious, but there is a tenacity when it is lacking. When there is magnesium, there is not that kind of mucus.

That is always an indication that magnesium is lacking and phosphorus has the upper hand. Frothiness means excess of phosphorus consumption. In the urine, it means that phosphorus products are broken down.

When phosphorus appears in the urine, you may be sure that it is not phosphorus lacking in the system, but it is magnesium that is lacking. Magnesium should be there to clean out all sorts of phosphorus products.

Phosphorus excess is known by sour bowels; there is a sour odor all over the body in the urine, excreta, secretions. If you wash and wash with soap, you still have a sour odor. You cannot scrub off that sourness.

When magnesium is exhausted, there will be disturbances of the digestive function. When the teeth are developing, certain salts are extracted from the blood and broken down, if magnesium is not supplied. Gas pockets will form in the intestines or perhaps the stomach. In one single corner of the stomach, there may be a gas pocket, and the gas is pressing downwardly, outwardly, sidewardly. It sets the heart trembling. Cancer may develop.

Some ladies are so nervous that they do not know what to do with themselves. It is phosphorus at work, which gets the upper hand when magnesium is lacking. The nervous system is on fire.

In July and August, when there is danger of heart disease, magnesium is needed. Eat a heavy magnesium diet during July and August.

PRINCIPAL MAGNESIUM FOODS

Magnesium tonics and drugs are beneficial only when the stomach is sour throughout, but at no other time. It is the magnesium tonics and drugs that are unorganized. The human system lives on and craves organic elements.

FIGS are rich in such sugar that is easily taken up by the body. Figs are high in all of those salts contained in the body. Spinach and almonds contain nearly all the salts that are needed by the body (with the exception of two). Use salt on almonds and one more element is supplied.

GRAPEFRUIT is high in magnesium. If you are excitable or high tempered, eat grapefruit. Grapefruit has a cooling and soothing effect upon the brain. If you are disappointed, eat grapefruit.

ALMONDS contain over 3% magnesium. Almond nuts and other foods high in magnesium are laxative. Do not eat the skin of almonds. Almonds are rich in starch.

BLACK WALNUTS contain potassium chloride.

RYE. Eat whole rye preparations and whole barley dishes.

BARLEY contains 12.5 magnesium and is rich in phosphorus. Here you find a better food for your tired brain, nerves, hot liver and restless disposition.

CHERRIES are a good nerve and brain food. The white cherry is high in phosphorus and rich in magnesium.

APPLES are rich in malic acid; hence, not very good for anyone with the exception of highly alkaline temperaments. There are three constitutions of people who can eat apples.

QUESTIONS AND ANSWERS

1. What causes an apparently well person to feel very short, like she was only about two feet tall? Answer: That is a magnesium-hunger symptom; sometimes they may also feel tall.

2. If epsom salt is not good for constipation, what could one take to increase action in a dropsical person? Answer: It is good for constipation. You should give a dropsical person foods rich in chlorine and potassium.

3. Does peppermint tea contain magnesium? Answer: It contains principally potassium.

4. In taking an enema, should one lie on the right or left side? Answer: Lie on the right side because the water flows more easily into the transverse colon.

FOODS AND CHEMICALS
SULPHUR

SULPHUR IN THE MINERAL AND VEGETABLE KINGDOMS

Sulphur is one of the most important of the chemical elements. If it were not for sulphur, we would not be here. There would be no life without sulphur. There would be nothing but death. Sulphur has a great function to perform in its relation to life.

SULPHUR—ITS NATURE AND CHARACTERISTICS

The sulphur patient is sensitive to atomospheric gases, to heat, cold, to external and internal conditions. Sulphur is remarkable for its changes, its peculiarities, also for its capacity to adapt itself to other elemental conditions. That holds good also in regard to the Exesthesic lady. She is exceedingly adaptable. At the same time, she is a great deal like sulphur

characteristics. There is a great similarity between the characteristics of the sulphur element and the characteristics of the sulphur lady. She has those peculiar sulphur characteristics; she changes with the weather. In other words, atmospheric gases and conditions have a great affect on her.

Whenever sulphur enters into the human body to excess or into any metal, there is but little strength. The steel is not so good if it contains considerable sulphur and carbon. The rails are brittle so that a sudden jerk in the locomotive may break them. If there is a great deal of carbon and sulphur in any metal there is not great strength. That holds good also in regard to the sulphur lady. She does not have a great deal of strength nor endurance. The sulphur lady is of such a nature that she needs intervals of rest. She can work for awhile, then she must rest. She should go out into the fresh, open air. If you have a sulphur lady for a stenographer, you must not keep her sitting still all the time, day after day, week after week. If you do, you will kill her. Sulphur is an element of variation. This is true of the sulphur lady.

FUNCTIONS OF SULPHUR IN THE HUMAN ORGANIZATION

There cannot be life without sulphur in the protoplasm. Take the sulphur out of the protoplasm and you have dead protoplasm. Take the sulphur out of the egg yolk and there is no life in the egg. Take the sulphur out of the human being and he will soon die. If there is a lack of sulphur, there will be a lack of bile; there will be ailments with the liver function. There will be a lack of lecithin for the brain. You will suffer from nervous prostration in the course of time, if sulphur is not supplied. If the sulphur is broken down too rapidly, you will run into nervousness or there will be a weakness in the sexual system. If there is a lack of sulphur, there will also be a lack of life in the generative substance and that man will be impotent. The lady is said to be sterile also. Neither can produce life.

Man is the life giver. He has greater power to secrete life than the lady. He is more able to utilize sulphur in the generative substance. It is because he is created as he is that he can utilize sulphur to a greater extent. He is the one to start life, and the woman is the one to continue it. In both instances, sulphur is needed. If sulphur consumption is too great in a mother, she is unable to become pregnant; she is sterile. If a man is not able to utilize sulphur in sufficient quantities and incorporate it into the generative substance, he is impotent.

Because sulphur has so much to do with the flow of bile when there is a deficiency of sulphur, the patient suffers from constipation. Here we have one kind of constipation caused by lack of sulphur in the liver. Also in the various functions. When there is a sufficient amount of sulphur acting upon the liver, there will be a greater flow of bile in the alimentary canal and intestines which will become more active.

A strong mental temperament or a brainy man has great intensity and is burning up sulphur too rapidly. When insufficient sulphur acts on the liver, its function becomes sluggish; resulting in constipatin. Constipation may be due to a lack of lubricant in the form of some needed fat. In still another, it may be due to a lack of sulphur. Some may have an excess of fatty acid. Constipation has many causes.

When a doctor gives a patient some strong drug for constipation, it is not always wise. He should supply that which is needed in the system. In order to do that, it becomes necessary to understand human types.

I supplied a sulphur diet to a man who had been drinking grape juice for 3 years until his liver became enlarged. He told me that he had been drinking one quart of juice a day for this time. He drank it because he wanted to improve his complexion and because he wanted to live longer. I put him on a very heavy sulphur diet. That reaches the liver. That is what sulphur does when it is abundantly supplied where there is enlargement of the liver, it decreases the size of it. Sulphur food is exceedingly good for the promotion of bile and liver action. In cases like that, it is important to supply sulphur foods.

The generative substance can never be supplied in normal quantities unless a certain amount of sulphur is supplied in foods. Remember that sulphur food must not be cooked. Sulphur is a peculiar element.

The mental man, the muscular man, the Exesthesic, the Nervi-Motive are all exceedingly susceptible to all kinds of moisture. A great many animals and people who are strongly developed in the cerebellum, are exceedingly sensitive to all sorts of atmospheric conditions. Such people feel it in their bones. They say that it is going to rain before it does. They cannot give any reason, but they feel it some way. When a man has that kind of development, he is a better weatherman than a meteorologist.

The sulphur lady is sensitive to all kinds of currents and gases in the atmosphere because the sulphur element is a little too active in her. If you eat too many sulphur foods you will feel as if you were drunk. You are not yourself. There is something peculiar at work within. You do not have full control of your feelings nor your brain. You cannot remember dates or names. We should not eat sulphur foods to excess because we will not have full control of our faculties. If we eat a normal amount of sulphur, we feel more vigorous. If we eat a little more, we feel stimulated. If we eat too much, memory fails. You can weaken the best memory in the world by four meals of sulphur food. Cooked sulphur will have a bad effect, even one meal, because it is more rapidly converted into gas.

If we eat an excess of sulphur, especially cooked sulphur, it will be rapidly converted into gas so that it interferes with oxidation. If it is converted into gas it enters the red corpuscles of the blood and fills the hemoglobin so that it can carry no oxygen.

Coal gas, sulphur gas and other gases will pass into the red corpuscles of the blood. It will stay there so that the iron in the hemoglobin of the red corpuscles becomes useless and we suffer from lack of free oxygen both in the blood and tissues.

Excessive sulphur results in low oxidation and anemia will result. We may think that diet has nothing to do with it, but it certainly has. Sulphur is always slow in its action. It is accumulative; it increases. In other words, if you eat a meal rich in sulphur, you will not suffer tonight but you will later on. Suppose you eat sulphur today and increase it at each following meal—it is cumulative. The more sulphur you eat the more you retain and the more you will suffer later on after it has reached its cumulated volcanic action.

If you suffer from sulphur symptoms, there is nothing better than ozone and cold wind. That holds good for Exesthesic ladies. They should go where they can get sufficient ozone and where it is windy. When a patient suffers from sulphur symptoms, he wants to be fanned. When you suffer from sulphur symptoms, you feel relieved when the cold strikes you. That is why they want the windows open and the air very cold. They like to take a cold swim in the morning—then they feel better. The medical man says the sulphur lady is imaginative. He cannot understand her symptoms and ailments, but it is not imagination. This is where we deal with the chemistry of man, with the symptoms peculiar to the various elements such as iron, sulphur, oxygen, carbon, etc. Each has its own characteristic.

The man who eats sulphur foods becomes filled with sulphur gas. The food is converted into gas.

Keratin contains sulphur. If there is not much sulphur in the hair, it is black. The red-haired person has more sulphur in the hair because sulphur consumption is greater. They usually always have more temper. There is greater responsiveness in any one having red hair. If one gets angry, he is intensely angry.

Sulphur patients usually fall into the hands of nerve specialists who may doctor them for a long time. They never think of sending them to a different climate where they can get fresh, cold air in abundance. The sulphur lady already has sulphur symptoms. You find sulphur products in the Exesthesic patient.

Unless the doctor knows about sulphur constitutions, he cannot measure the sulphur in the system because it disappears everywhere. When you perspire, there is sulphur. Sulphur is passing away all the time from the body. You find sulphur in the secretions.

If children suffer from excessive sulphur consumption, there will be eczema. It appears on the face, chest and other parts of the body. If you eat too much sulphur food at one time, there will appear little red pimples on the forehead or perhaps on the top of the head or under the arm. These pimples will itch. Soon eczema appears and the doctor gives you ointment to smear on your skin. But it seldom occurs to you or to your doctor that you have been eating too much sulphur foods.

If a patient suffers from syphilis and you put him on a heavy sulphur diet, there is a running sore in the middle of some long bone, an ulcer, which keeps running. The more sulphur food he eats, the more the ulcer runs. Sulphur is driving the syphilis out of the body.

All such foods that are rich in sulphur, very high in potash, can drive a miasm out of the body. When a patient comes to you with a running ulcer, if you heal it, you are retaining that impurity in the body. When you see any impurity or eruption anywhere at the surface of the body that is not the result of a special diet, leave it alone. That is another way of curing it.

You have volcanoes in the bowels of the earth. You have also volcanoes in your sulphur girls. When the sulphur lady is young, she is likely to fall into bad habits. The sulphur girl needs watching, not because she is bad, but because she is intense. Sulphur is at work in the liver, nerves, sex brain. You should never let a sulphur lady become a stenographer. She should go up into the hills. She should have variation. Let her sit still at a machine and she will soon be sick.

There is a great sensitiveness of nerves in the sulphur lady. She can live five years in six months. She is highly strung. Sulphur increases as it works. It gets worse and worse. That is the nature of sulphur. If there is too much sulphur—if there is not enough sulphur or if it is broken down too rapidly, the relative ailments are about the same.

A sulphur diet will have its affect on the hair. It is possible to change the hair color and skin color with a continuous sulphur diet, but not all at once. A lady I know had a birthmark which I removed by putting on a heavy sulphur diet. We can make the hair dark by introducing more nitrogen into the body and living in a warm climate. A high sulphur diet and a cold climate always make the hair and skin lighter.

Sulphur has to do with the regulation of temperature in the nerves. In all brain centers that have anything to do with sensation, sulphur is necessary. There are certain centers in the body called heat centers. They are in the wrist, ankles, small of the back and neck. When a person suffers from cold all those centers should be protected. A lady who suffers from sexual weakness cannot sleep well. She should not go without warm covering around her neck, wrists and ankles. If we supply a diet rich in sulphur and neurol in great quantities and place such a patient in a climate like Southern California, we can improve her.

You never yet found a pugilist among Exesthesic men. A Desmogenic pugilist could whip 20 Exesthesic men easily. Great sulphur consumption never produces great strength.

Sulphur and carbon make instruments brittle and almost useless. The same thing is true in the human organization. The sulphur lady can never use her brain as well as the Calciferic man. The Isogenic can study for hours without fatigue. Look at Edison. That is always the case when a man has a great amount of calcium in his constitution. But the Exesthesic man can never study like the Calciferic or Isogenic can. An Exesthesic cannot do a great deal of scientific or philosophical work, because his brain would give out.

The sulphur lady has a small-sized liver. I assisted in six autopsies on Exesthesic people and we found the liver was small in each one. The liver in some types is three times as large as other types. The Isogenic manufactures brain substances faster than the Exesthesic. The Exesthesic man is weaker sexually than the Isogenic.

Wherever life is at work, there is sulphur in action. If you cook an egg, you kill the life principle. Life cannot stand great heat or cold. Even a very high altitude will have its effect on life. There are certain animals that never breed in high altitudes. We can stay in a certain altitude a certain length of time and the altitude, which is not good for us, must be left. Great heat favors life. Any warm climate has a constructive effect upon the vital organs. If a person at the same time will supply himself with foods containing the vitamins, he will gain youthfulness. Send a girl to Southern California and her charms will come back. She will increase her matrimonial possibilities, especially if she will fall back upon those foods that give her the elements she is in need of. But if she lives on bacon, sausage, pie, cake, pastry, doughnuts, coffee and tea, she will lose her charms, even in California.

If you cook sulphur food, it is mainly converted into gas. Boiled sulphur is of no value. In some foods, for instance, German sauerkraut, you can boil the sulphur and it does not hurt it. When you have a great deal of chlorine and sodium in food to protect sulphur, you can eat sulphur in cooked form.

Without sulphur, there is no sensation. Sulphur itself has a great deal to do with nerve life and nutrition. When the sulphur element is lacking in the nerves and secretions, when it is not acting on the brain, there is a lack of sensation.

The sulphur lady may have her faults but she is very highly organized just the same. The sulphur type is one of the highest types. That is true of all people who have the sulphur element well organized into their tissue and acting upon the secretions and brain.

If you want to drive out a miasm from the body, remember that you must first fall back upon a heavy sulphur diet; also a potassium diet. Potassium has an influence upon certain miasms. The potassium and acid found in red currants or currant juice will drive miasms out of the body. Sulphur has its affect upon syphilis and will help drive it out. There are certain elements that we must fall back on in times of diseases. If a man suffers from syphilis, he needs a heavy sulphur, chlorine, fluorine and iron diet. In the course of time, that man would improve constitutionally.

Phosphorus is used in the soul or psychical process in mental life and soul expression. The intellectual man uses phosphorus very much. The Atrophic man who may be as weak as a baby may be materialistic, may not believe in anything, but he is scientific and philosophical, though there may be no soul life in him nor about him.

Your wife may have the mental side of her nature well developed. The intellectual process does not crave very much sulphur. But the mental processes require a great deal of sulphur. Sulphur has a great deal to do with phosphorus and with the psychical processes. Sulphur and phosphorus unite in mental life and expression. Where sulphur is active in an organization, you may be sure that you find soul life and emotion. Where only phosphorus is at work, where only the intellect and will faculties are at work, there you find the materialistic mind. Wherever sulpur consumption is great, the mental life is great, also there is a greater soul, or at least, the soul is more active.

If you experiment on a man of high soul life and take away from his diet all sulphur foods, that man falls in soul intelligence. His soul and social faculties sink. I did it once. I measured his head and tophead, which measured 15 inches when I started the experiment. When I was through, it measured 13-1/2 inches. It had shrunk 2 inches. The backhead had sunk also. you have the soul at work in the backhead and in the tophead. A man strong in those brain parts believes in religion. He does good in the world. When all those faculties are strongly developed, they crave sulphur. There also you have phosphoro-psychical processes at work. But in the materialist, you do not find so much sulphur at work nor so much soul life.

A man with nothing else than intellect is nothing but reason. He reasons away heaven, hell and everything else. Reason demands reason, but the soul does not need reason. It is no use to argue religion with a materialist. To be religious, a man needs a soul first.

The soul is more active in one man than in another. The soul is more active in a woman than a man. As a general rule, men do not go to church to any great extent. The church is usually full of women. Women, as a rule, are more religious than men. If a mother was not religious, what would the next generation be?

What would become of morality? The Almighty grafts religion into the race through the mother.

When there is a lack of sulphur, the soul is sick. A man is sick in the brain. There you have sickness that cannot be cured with any medicine nor any kind of treatments. There you need something else.

A great many men will fall in love with the Exesthesic lady. Exesthesic ladies are very attractive. We become fascinated by her, but if a man marries her, he finds it difficult to live with her, because she is too highly developed for him. Ladies like that do not belong here below. They belong in heaven. There are too many disagreeable things here below. She is blamed too much. In the Exesthesic lady, you have a lady like a harp with a thousand strings. She is certainly interesting. In her, sulphur consumption is great.

When sulphur consumption is great and a person eats too many sulphur foods, the excess is converted into gas. Gas and acid are retained in the body. The sulphur lady is always acid. It is gas of a sulphur nature that enters into the red corpuscles and interferes with oxidation of the blood and makes her exceedingly nervous and irritable. She suffers from nervous diseases. Those nervous ailments cannot be cured by anything else than a basic diet and ozone. The sulphur lady needs ozone and cold wind. There is nothing better for sulphur acid or gas than double oxygen or ozone. Oxygen is an element that works in conjunction with sulphur. Where sulphur is active, oxygen will also be active. Also, oxygen is required in abundance. The greater the sulphur consumption in the body, the more oxygen we need. The more sulphur food we eat, the more ozone we need, also cold wind to play upon us and the more exercise we need. Sulphur always comes to the surface of the body in times of great sulphur consumption.

When sulphur and phosphorus are at work, a great deal of phosphorus is broken down; also sulphur—then magnesium is needed.

The sulphur lady is not exactly a nervous lady. She is uneasy. There is too much heat in her nerves. If a man marries a sulphur lady, he should take her to the hills.

Nitropheric people are affinities to sulphur people, not physical, so much as mental affinities. The Nitropheric makes the Exesthesic an excellent mental affinity, but they do not give rise to vigorous offspring. If a sulphur lady marries an Isogenic man, she has better children, but she will quarrel with him.

When there is electricity in the atmosphere the Exesthesic feels uncomfortable. If she gets irritable, look for a thunderstorm. It is interesting to compare these things. You will be surprised at those laws at work unseen, in the very atmosphere and soul of man.

Sulphur types are always highly emotional.

CONSTITUTIONS IN WHICH SULPHUR IS INHERENT

Sulphur is excessive when too much is taken up and too much is broken down. If a Carboferic person eats a high sulphur diet, there would be no sulphur symptoms, because Carboferic people cannot take up and utilize sulphur. When sulphur is taken up and utilized in the body and the supply becomes excessive, certain sulphurous products are formed in the system, which results in sulphur symptoms.

At all times when there is excess of sulphur there is a love of change and variety. At one time there is complaint, at another optimism, at a third time, pessimism. At one time a lady is in high spirits, high health and perhaps in a few hours, she feels uncomfortable and there is always much temper. At one time love rules at another, she could tear out the heart of her husband. At one time she is full of fear, at another she is courageous and still another time she is timid as a rabbit. She can be peaceful, then quarrelsome. one time she jumps with joy then becomes very depressed. At one time she is as proud as a Spaniard, then she condemns herself and her every action and feels as little as an earthworm. She is an exclusive and another time familiar, then liberal, then selfish. At one time she is economical perhaps even stingy.

This is sulphur or changeableness and variety. The sulphur lady is something like the moon, she has all sorts of changing characteristics and yet she herself is not changeable. You know it is not in the soul of the lady it is not in the will nor in the reason of the lady that all of this takes place. It is in the disposition or in the temperament. They say people are temperamental when in fact the only temperamental lady we have is the Exesthesic and it happens only when sulphur is in excess.

Sulphur consumption is the very thing that produces such characteristics. At one time the sulphur lady would punish you, at another she would forgive you. At one time she is kind and then cruel. She is like the moon. At one time she loves her husband devotedly and at another perhaps 5 or 10 minutes, she takes him by the hair. She does not mean any harm by it because such actions are simply sulphur characteristics—nothing else than passing explosions, a little steam going up that's all. She is something like the fireworks on the 4th of July. Fireworks make considerable noise but there is no harm in them. So also in regard to the sulphur lady. There is considerable mental fireworks or considerable powder, but no battle. She means no harm for she is harmless.

She is also very proud and easily hurt. If anyone is an actress, she is. If you are married to a sulphur lady, you do not need to go to the theatre; you have one right in your home. She is just as true as she can be and just as well meaning as she can be. This holds good also in regard to the Exesthesic man. He has that kind of changingd and varying characteristics. At one time he thinks his girl is the finest woman in the world and maybe in 2 hours he does not want her or at least he wants her to stay away. Tomorrow he may be just as deeply interested in her again. A sulphur man loves by turns. This does not only hold good in regard to characteristics, but it holds good in regard to diseases also.

The diseases of the sulphur lady are just as varying as her characteristics. The diseases are constantly changing, newer and newer symptoms come up. She has all of those symptoms varying in a short time and the physician who attends to her cannot understand what is the matter or what kind of sickness she suffers from.

In the Calciferic man, the diseases are very pronounced and very chronic, which means very distinct, but diseases in the sulphur lady hide just the same as sulphur does. Sulphur is an element that hides itself, its symptoms and peculiarities so that the physician who attends the lady does not know from what she suffers.

You know sulphur is an element that is sleepy and sluggish in the morning and the sulphur ladies are also. They do not like to wake up. They sleep best in the morning and in the evening, they are active and wide awake. The real day commences about 11 o'clock. And if she eats breakfast at 8 o'clock, she may be sick or bothered with her stomach, liver, pancreas, bile or some function in the body.

In the morning, the sulphur lady is usually hard to please. By noon, she feels good natured. It is difficult for her to love her husband in the morning but she can love him in the evening. It is not she; it is the sulphur. She is sick but she cannot help herself because she is under the influence of sulphur. There is something unexplainable that is holding her and she does not know what it is.

Sulphur is fitful, volcanic; that is what the sulphur lady is also. She does things by fits and starts; she is a lady of variation. She certainly is interesting. She is deep, fastidious, sometimes volcanic. The husband who understands her nature, knows she is under the influence of sulphur and pays no attention. It is a theatre to him and she is the actress. You see, when we understand human nature, we make allowances; we say to ourselves, this is why that man acts this way—they are under the influence of sulphur.

A great many sulphur patients have a counting mania. When they suffer from nervous trouble, they may lie in bed and count every flower on the wallpaper. Sulphur inflames the faculty of calculation and they are compelled to count, count, count and keep counting. They are only fair in mathematics; it is just a sort of counting mania. Many of them when they become nervous through the excess of sulphur, have spells of ill humor but they do not mean any harm. Say nothing to the sulphur wife; simply let her go on and act until she is through and soon she acts differently. She will come throw her arms around you and kill you and say you are the finest husband in the world, then she cries and wants to make love. She is peculiar in the sense that in times of peace, she makes war; in time of war, she wants peace. When everything is peaceful and joyful, she wants trouble and when war commences, when the husband gets angry and feels like fighting, she becomes cured and implores for forgiveness. That is sulphur, it is not she, it is the sulphur.

She usually always has dry hair that crumbles and draws itself together like elastic. You can pull it out like a rubberband, and when you let go it curls. It does not break because it is very strong. She usually always has an excellent growth of hair between the ages of 14 to 32. After 32 her hair begins to fall.

A great many sulphur patients complain about an iron taste in the mouth due to the great deal of sulphur in the system. That sulphur which is not utilized is converted into gas, which will pass into the red corpuscles of the blood enter into the hemoglobin and prevent the normal iron function of the blood. This is the reason she has that iron taste in the mouth. When she has that taste, she also runs short of oxygen. Then she rushes to the windows and throws them open very suddenly and holds her mouth open as if she is dying from oxygen hunger. She cannot get enough air because sulphur gas as taken possession of the hemoglobin and prevents the red corpuscles from oxidizing the blood. Sometimes she has an inky taste; she feels as though she has been drinking ink. This is the same symptom.

In summer, during July and August, when it is very sultry, she is not able to get enough air. The liver becomes too sluggish and she craves something sour. Then she goes to the grocery store and buys canned pickles. In July and August, sulphur ladies eat piekles.

She has a strong development of ideality. It is ideality and also sulphur that prevents her from becoming happy in the full sense. If she has a fault or shortcoming, she does not want anyone to know it and she does everything possible to prevent other people from knowing anything unfavorable about her, about her husband or about her children. When the liver, stomach, kidneys, pancreas, spleen, blood and brain all become too hot, the Exesthesic person may drink beer. He feels relieved, goes to bed and perspires until the entire bed is wet. Then the heat is converted into steam. If the heat were not converted into steam, he might go crazy or get sick or commit some terrible act.

We cannot prescribe alike for all people because one man needs something that another man does not need. It is just the same in regard to work. For instance, hard, sedentary work will weaken a Myogenic man and make him more sick but it will help the Calciferic man. The Calciferic man is a calk all his life in the sense that he can handle milk, but the Myogenic man cannot drink and digest milk. A milk diet cures the Calciferic man and makes the Myogenic man sick. If you are a doctor and you get hold of two patients, one Myogenic and the other Calciferic, the one you may cure and the other you may kill on a milk diet. Milk is a bad food for the Myogenic man but it is curative to the Calciferic.

SYMPTOMS WHEN SULPHUR IS DEFICIENT

The sulphur patient gets so very hungry, she must eat. She feels as though something is going to happen; she trembles; and rushes to the table and eats quickly. Then she feels better only to feel worse in about an hour or two. That is a sulphur symptom. Sulphur is in a rush. If you are in love with a sulphur lady, she will rush you to the altar because she cannot wait.

Sulphur cannot wait. There is a vein of impatience in a person of a sulphur type. There is also more or less tension. Tension in the eyes and eyeballs, tension in the neck, drawing in the neck, spleen and stomach. The stomach may feel like lead. There may be drawing tension in the throat so they cannot talk. They may feel as though there is something in the throat, a ball, which the doctor calls Globus Hysterious. This ball is nothing but tension. They may suffer from tension in the sexual system, tension in the uterus. Fibroids may form in that organization, necessitating operations. Then the sulphur lady is hauled over to a hospital and operations performed for tumors. They send her home and say she is cured. If there is a piece left of the organ, tumors form again. The sulphur lady is under the influence of tension all the time. Tension in the brain, emotions, passions and everywhere.

This is why a naturapath is a better doctor for the sulphur patient, because the manipulations are soothing. Give her the kind of food and treatments that overcome tension and drives the sulphur products out of her system. Diet will do more than treatments and drugs combined.

She needs air in abundance. She likes to sleep at an open window where it is fresh, cool and breezy. Whenever there is too much sulphur in the system, there is a closing of the capillaries everywhere at the surface of the skin. Cold air to the nude body results in evaporation of sulphur gas and this gives relief. This is also why a sulphur patient likes a cold bath in the morning.

She feels refreshed. She likes to go to the hills or to stand at the seashore and see the stormy sea at work. It makes her feel romantic. When she sits still, there is always tension at work, flatus develops, gas in the stomach and in the intestines, in the blood and brain or in all combined. It is gas and sulphur products which are the foundation of all that tension.

Sulphur is peculiar in the sense that it works upon the nerves, capillaries, skin, liver, spleen and the portal system. The liver and skin hold sulphur. I do not know that the red corpuscles retain sulphur, but the spleen, pancreas, skin and many secretions do.

Anoxyemia means that there is not enough oxidation in the blood; hypoalonemia means that not enough of the salts are supplied to the blood.

The transmission of nerve impulse from the brain is fitful; nerve pressure is increased which affects the blood vessels. As soon as there is greater nerve pressure in the brain, all the blood vessels throughout the entire body are affected and as the nerve impulse transmitted by the nerves and by the brain are fitful, there is an unequal function throughout the entire body. It affects all the functions; i.e., digestion is poorer at one time than at another. One time the heart is more vigorous than another time. One time the spleen is on strike, another time the arteries and veins are affected or perhaps some other function of the body. Because of fitfulness in brain impulsion or nerve impulsion, there is a fitfulness in physical functions of the body and that gives rise to all such peculiar symptoms. It affects the blood vessels; it produces high nerve pressure. High intracranial pressure expands all the blood vessels. When there is high nerve pressure, there is also high blood pressure. Therefore if you go to a specialist, it may or may not mean anything. It may be caused by high nerve pressure, high brain pressure or by lack of certain blood salts. When blood salts are excessive, the blood function becomes erratic and the specific gravity of the blood is changed.

Blood tests made may or may not amount to anything. It depends on the constitution of the one who suffers from high blood pressure. Very severe work, excitement, anger, jumping, running or dancing increases the blood pressure, especially when greatly exhausted. If you drink ice-cold water, the blood pressure is raised. If there is expansion of the brain cells in the brain, the blood vessels in the body enlarge, resulting in high blood pressure in every artery and vein. If you go to a doctor and he tells you you have high blood pressure; what does it mean? He can tell you that there is high blood pressure and that is all. There are many causes for this.

Sulphur changes in color almost all the time. If you look at sulphur today, you find it has a certain color; if you look at it tomorrow, it may have changed color. So do Exesthesic or sulphur people. The complexion is changing all the time. Their complexion cannot be improved.

Some people say there is a heart in the solar plexus and some say there is also a second brain. The epigastric plexus is sensitive to all temperatural changes and to varying states of mind. It is only in certain people that the epigastric plexus is sensitive and the sulphur lady or the Exesthesic lady is the one who is sensitive. If she is shaken or frightened or if anything happens to her, she does not throw her hand to her heart but to the solar plexus because the epigastric plexus is more sensitive under the influence of high sulphur consumption.

The vocal organs are in a state of dryness in Exesthesic people. A lady who is a lecturer, of an Exesthesic type, needs a gass of water on the table to sip from because her throat becomes dry. This is a constant tendency in the Exesthesic lady. She cannot talk regularly nor persistently without feeling the effects of the speech, conversation or argument in the throat. The homeopathic doctor who deals in potencies, tells us that pulsatilla and chamomilla patients are exceedingly sensitive; they cry easily. He tells us that ailments like those which we have been going over, require that kind of drugs. He claims that such drugs cure that kind of patient. Such patients have that kind of characteristic; namely, what we call sulphur characteristics.

The nervous system, the sensory nerves, portal system, liver, colon, spleen and virilia are usually always the seat of trouble in Exesthesic people, and the real cause is excessive sulphur consumption.

Remember you should give a sulphur lady raw sulphur food and air in abundance, a high altitude, pleasing, soothing treatments and foods rich in sodium, iron, magnesium and manganese; do not forget ozone, because it has a wonderful affect on the red corpuscles of the blood. When there is too much sulphur in the system and when gases affect the red corpuscles ozone drives out such gases, thus increasing oxidation so the patient may recuperate.

HOW TO REDUCE SULPHUR IN THE BODY

We have four different methods of reducing sulphur in the body and while we give this advice, we know how very difficult it is to carry it out. For instance, when a man is high tempered and we tell him to control his temper, that may seen very good advice but to him, it is not. Perhaps he is trying every day to control his temper. This is also the case in regard to reducing sulphur in the system. We say here, omit foods rich in sulphur. It is very good advice but the man cannot do it. We may tell him to go to the moon and get well, but he cannot go, therefore he cannot get well. That kind of advice is not good. We must tell the man, woman or child how to get well. If a man is a criminal, we must not only tell him what to do in order to avoid being put into jail, but we must place him in favorable surroundings where it is easier for him to be good. This is also true in regard to reducing of sulphur in the body.

The main thing is to omit foods rich in sulphur and another thing to do is to eat all such foods rich in magnesium, sodium and iron. These are the important food salts we should introduce. The next best thing to do is send the patient to a high altitude where it is about 2,000 to 6,000 feet above sea level where there is plenty of ozone in the atmosphere. If you do this, there will be no temper to control, no passion to avoid, no fretting, no nervousness, no irritability, because everything will be adjusted as the man or woman is placed in the proper altitude and given the right kind of food.

HOW TO INCREASE SULPHUR IN THE BODY

Sulphur is increased by eating sulphur food. You cannot eat cooked sulphur foods (except carrots and sauerkraut) without a disturbance of some kind. If a certain percentage of acid is present in a food, malic acid, tartaric acid, salicylic or acetic acid or other kind of acid, and perhaps 8-12% of common salt (sodium and chlorine), you may cook sulphur food, eat it and perhaps feel good.

If you eat sulphur-containing food when there is gas generation in the stomach or intestines, you will be worse tomorrow. If you eat German sauerkraut, properly prepared and cooked, you can digest it and get sulphur normally, without generating gas. Boiled sulphur food cannot be utilized by your body, because that food does not contain enough chloriodium. If you eat cauliflower, salt it well, then you will not suffer from gas because those salts will prevent sulphur food from being converted into gas in the stomach. Try it sometimes when you are bloated. Take a teaspoonful of salt in cold, distilled water, and notice how the gas will pass down and flatus will disappear.

When there is a great deal of sulphur gas in the intestines, it is impossible to sleep. You wake up at midnight and your brain is so active it works like a factory and you cannot stop it. You think, think, think and in the morning at about 5 a.m., you become sleepy. Then you fall into a restless sleep and if you wake up at 7 a.m., you may feel angry. You are not yourself. Tomorrow perhaps you will suffer from headache. If you suffer from sleeplessness because of sulphur gas in the intestines, take a teaspoonful of salt in a glass of water.

There are so many facts in regard to diet and metabolism of the greatest importance that every physician and nurse should know. Cooked sulphur food generates gas when there is a deficiency of chlorine in the system. If we want to increase sulphur in the body, we should eat foods rich in raw sulphur.

In a climate which is warm and stuffy, we are always able to retain more sulphur. People who live in a warm, rather stuffy climate, always are more prolific because the sulphur element is more utilized in this climate. Hence, people multiply very rapidly in a warm climate. In a cold climate, the race may die out.

To increase sexual capacity, eat sulphur foods. Another element very important is phosphorus. The Almighty has arranged everything so that sulphur and phosphorus must work with oxygen, carbon, nitrogen and hydrogen, in order to produce results. Without sulphur in the egg yolk, no chick is born.

Without sulphur in the ovum or spermatosoa, no babe is born. To increase generative power, eat foods rich in sulphur and phosphorus and live in a warm climate.

To increase sulphur in the system, live in the emotional brain and strongly in the feeling. When you get lazy, indolent, sleepy, then you increase sulphur in the system.

PEOPLE WHO REQUIRE SULPHUR FOODS

When we want to stimulate a man, tone him up, bring out his efficiency, make him think more and use his brain capacities and emotions to a greater extent, we should give him raw sulphur food, phosphorus food and iron foods.

INFLUENCE OF AN EXCESSIVE AMOUNT OF SULPHUR FOODS

It is unfavorable to health, simply because of gas generation. The gas that passes into the red corpuscles of the blood prevents the iron or hematin from taking up oxygen. A man who has sulphur gas in his system is not able to take up a normal amount of oxygen. Give an Atrophic man an excessive sulphur diet and he will die of consumption, because he cannot utilize oxygen.

Disposition. An excessive amount of sulphur food makes every feeling, emotion, passion, love feeling or states of mind spasmodic. Such a person does everything by jerks. In the morning he wakes up happy, then in a few minutes he is unhappy. Next he is moody and ugly then kind and genial. Sulphur is an element of variation.

A spasmodic disposition is one that comes and goes by spells. A man who has too much sulphur in the system, takes a glass of water so suddenly that he spills the contents. He is jerky in brain also. Such a lady may be good, well-meaning, beautiful, have a great many virtues, yet she spoils most of her virtues by her erratic disposition.

What is disposition and where do we get it? Is it not because in the child certain chemical elements become more active than certain other elements? Is it not because some chemical elements become so active they affect the mind, producing moods, tendencies, habits and permanent states of mind or what we call disposition? When a man is spasmodic in everything, we say he has a spasmodic disposition; another man is pessimistic in everything he does and says, and we say he has a pessimistic. An Oxypheric man has an optimistic disposition. A Medeic man is always pessimistic. He has the pessimistic faculties in the lead and a hereditary taint in the blood. If a man has an optimistic disposition, his faculties become optimistic also. On the other hand, if a man's disposition is pessimistic, he always develops pessimistic faculties. If he becomes a preacher, he tells us that we are all going to hell. If the optimistic man becomes a preacher, he tells us we are all going to heaven, that all roads lead to heaven. The pessimist has an angry God and a hot hell.

This is nothing else than chemical elements acting upon brain and function. How very, very important it is for all who have anything to do with character, improvement, development, to study those laws and principles that lead to health and development.

INFLUENCE OF A DEFICIENT AMOUNT OF SULPHUR FOODS

Disposition. It leads to sterility, weakness in brain, nerve and function. If there is not enough of it in the body, it leads to sickness. We should have so much and no more. If you and I have a normal amount of sulphur in our system, we are healthy, but that which is normal for you may not be normal for me and it may not be normal for others. There is where it is a question of types of people. One type of patient needs more sulphur than another.

If there is a deficient amount of sulphur in the system, the disposition becomes temperamental or the man becomes emotional, erratic, spasmodic, moody and does not know just what he wants. Feed the Exesthesic lady right and she is an angel at times; feed the Nervi-Motive woman right and she is also good. Feed anyone right and we have an improved person. Feed each man right and he is more likely to go upwardly toward heaven; but feed him wrong and he is likely to go the other way.

CHEMICALS IN FOODS THAT PEOPLE WITH EXCESS SULPHUR SHOULD EAT

He should expose the body to air and wind as often as possible. The sulphur lady should live in the hills and have a little tent on top of the building where she can expose her body to the air, wind and sun everyday. Gas-producing foods are sugars, starches, fats and all sorts of cooked sulphur foods. I may say, in addition, that there are some drinks that are gas producers such as tea, coffee and chocolate.

VOCATIONS FOR WHICH SULPHUR PEOPLE ARE BEST SUITED

Sulphur people are more adapted for certain vocations than others. Their talents run toward decorations.

PRINCIPAL SULPHUR FOODS

HORSERADISH is one of the highest sulphur-containing foods.

CARROTS. Remember that carrots are a food that can be boiled without becoming gas producing. You can obtain sulphur for your brain and generative substance from carrots without adding salt to them. You can eat them raw or boiled because they are rich in salts.

SPINACH. You can cook spinach and get sulphur food without detrimental gas-producing results, and thus obtain sulphur for brain, nerves and function. But you cannot do that with other foods.

FIGS. Never eat sulphured figs; eat sundried figs. Sulphured figs have a bad affect upon the kidneys and will always generate gas. Never eat sulphured fruits of any kind. It pays to pay attention to how fruits are sundried. Always wash any food fiorst that has been sundried, because it may contain germs, creepers, dust, disease.

COCOANUT is difficult to digest for some people, but excellent food for the brain. For some reason, which I do not know, cocoanut builds up the chest. It increases the mammary glands enormously. You do not need to pay out any money for bust developers because you can develop your chest with cocoanut, breathing exercises and cold douches to the chest. Some foods have a greater affect upon some parts of the body than others. Cocoanut builds up the chest and will also sustain the fatty substance in the lungs.

For instance, horseradish has a stimulating affect upon the vital organs and skin function, but a bad affect upon the nerve ends in the stomach. If you eat horseradish for 2 or 3 years, you will lastly suffer from incurable indigestion, and no doctor can cure you. Horseradish will ruin the digestive function.

APPLES are rich in sulphur and phosphorus but they are rich also in malic acid. Malic acid has a detrimental affect upon the stomach and liver, especially the liver. We have been told that apples are excellent for health. We have heard that a man who eats 12 apples per day keeps the doctor away. Let us change that saying to the following: "A man who eats 12 apples a day will soon go to the hospital." Apples are so full of malic acid that this acid will ruin the liver and stomach. Of course, I know some apples are favorable, as for instance, the Delicious, Astrachan and others that are not saturated with malic acid.

CUCUMBERS are good when you suffer from congestion, blood fever, headache, caused by congestion in the brain. Then eat cucumbers. If you suffer from fever, eat cucumbers.

FOODS AND CHEMICALS
MANGANESE

Manganese is one of the elements in the human body, tissues, secretions and utilized by the functions.

MANGANESE, ITS NATURE AND CHARACTERISTICS

Manganese has the same relative influence on the human tissue as it has on metal ware, and as it has on metals, in general. If the human body is well supplied with it, the various tissues, cells themselves and the nerves become more ductile, tensile, elastic. If the manganese element is lacking in the tissues, nerves and cells there will be stiffness in the cells also. It will not only be stiffness but also inactivity in the cells. The man is dull in his reasoning; his memory is poor; he is not able to express his ideas nor handle his knowledge so successfully. His mind is somewhat dull; he is stupid; his mentality, receptivity or brain cells do not respond.

If the manganese element is lacking in the schoolboy or girl, they are not able to understand. The teacher thinks they are not up to the mark, that there is a loose screw or something lacking in the child. Manganese has a very important affect upon the brain, as we will see later.

If manganese is lacking in the brain, there is never that conscious vibratory action in the cells themselves; there is never the response, transmission of knowledge from cell to cell. There is a certain photographic process going on in the cells themselves. A man said that he had reached the limit in his investigation and said that the brain cells themselves never last longer than about 6 months. The fact of the matter is that the life of a cell is only 6 weeks. This is the length of life of almost any cell. So soon as a cell dies, a new one must take the place of the one that died. You can readily perceive that when cells die by the millions, almost every day, there must be some kind of photographic process going on in the brain, that those associations, experiences, facts that we have learned must be remembered for if they were produced by those dead cells we could never remember or learn anything. We learn, perhaps, a certain fact at the age of 7 and remember that fact at the age of 10, 15, 20, 30, 60 or even 100 years, showing that facts and knowledge are not forgotten although cells die each day.

How does it happen that a man can remember a certain fact all his life, considering that cells die by the millions every fleeting moment? How is it that we remember that which we learn, considering cells die all the time? There must be something behind the cells, knowledge in the cells, the memory in the cells, the feeling in the cells, the passion or impulses in the cells. Yet, these cells are dying every moment. Although the cells die, we retain our memories.

Here is where manganese comes in to help the living, pulsating soul to carry out that photographic process by mean of which transmission of knowledge takes place from cell to cell. All the cells are engaged in that same photographic process which is carried out by means of the manganese element. If you lack manganese, there will be a weakness in this process so you cannot learn, memorize answer questions even if you have the knowledge, because the cells are too slow in acting. The brain itself must act in unison and quickly. The cells themselves must act at one and the same time; they must act in harmony one with the other and perhaps a million or ten million must act at one and the same time. If we do not have manganese that process of transmission cannot be done. It is the manganese element that enables all of those cells to act synergically or in harmony.

FUNCTIONS OF MANGANESE IN THE HUMAN ORGANIZATION

I have not experimented much with manganese. When I experimented I did so on the most intellectual people I could find. I know that manganese is more in demand in people who are of the Nervi-Motive constitution, and it is in more demand in people who are Neurogenic or in all people who use their brain more than muscles. Manganese is not much in demand by a man who is a mere physical worker. In experimenting with these people I selected one young woman who was a student in a university and a young woman who was very bright in

certain lines of studies, but different from those lines which the young woman was taking up.

We are not generally informed regarding that which we call rheumatism and gout. We would be surprised to learn how different gout is in different types of patients. Gout has many different symptoms. For instance, in one gouty patient appears perspiration always at night. Such gouty patients are simply floating in perspiration. There are such patients so dry that you could not press one single drop out not even if you boiled your patient. Why should there be such differences in various gouty patients or in rheumatic patients? Why should there be such a difference between gout and gout? We find in one patient a lack of sodium as a cause of gout in another a lack of lime salts as a cause or lack of silicon or lack of manganese.

In each case, in studying the various ailments and symptoms, we must understand the differences in symptoms, then we know what special elements are lacking in each case. As we go on, we will notice the peculiarities of those patients who suffer from excess manganese and those who suffer from a lack of it.

If a man suffers from some kind of venereal miasm, we cannot do anything better than to give him foods lrich in sulphur, manganese and fluorine. It is not easy to cure a man who suffers from sexual disease without supplying all of those food elements in his general diet. You may be able to kill the syphilitic germs you may be able to drive the germs out of the system but you cannot drive out the taint because the taint is left in the body of that man in the cells, blood, brain. That miasm is the thing you cannot drive out with medicine. You may kill the germ but you cannot drive the bacterial toxin out of the system with anything else than with certain food salts. If we supply the various food salts from day to day, and keep it up from year to year, eventually we can reconstruct that man. That is the way to cure.

To cure, you must build a new man. That is the only way you can cure. Build yourself new; a new stomach, new heart, new bones, brain, organs throughout. That is the only way you can get cured by methods of cell processes, development, sublimation and purification.

Osseous and ligamentous tissue oxidation is increased by manganese. A Calciferic man, a bony man, who is constantly using the brain, thinking, reasoning, philosopher, inventor—he is breaking down tissue salts and nerve salts every fleeting moment. If it were not for the presence and influence of manganese in his tissues, the osseous and ligamentous tissue oxidation would become so low that he would become diseased eventually in his bones and ligaments. This is arthritis or gout. When the salts are lacking in the body, it results in heart disease, chronic rheumatism, gout, acidosis and many other diseases.

The principal cause is an insufficiency of oxygen because in an insufficiency of oxygen, there is also an insufficiency of vegetable salts in the various structures of the body. Oxygen cannot do its work and the oxygen process is the life process in the body, cells and blood.

Oxygen is a peculiar element; it builds us up, but it also destroys just as quickly. Oxygen has two functions to perform, viz., one upbuilding, constructive, anabolic function; the other is a destructive function (catabolism). When there is something wrong in the body, when the heart gives out, oxygen begins to carry us away. When there is any trouble in the bones, oxygen is again at work. The same thing takes place in the stomach, intestines and everywhere else. We either must live or else die. This is the work of oxygen. Oxygen is building us up and also constantly killing us. This is one reason the chemist said that we live as we die and when we quit living, we quit dying. When we quit dying, we quit living.

Manganese influences the oxidation process and the upbuilding processes in plants.

Manganese does not go through the blood. Iron goes through the blood; potassium goes through the tissues; but manganese acts on the nerves. This is one of the functions of manganese.

Another very remarkable fact regarding manganese and fluorine is that chemists—when they analyze and estimate the amount of phosphorus, potassium, chlorine, sodium, sulphur, calcium and other elements—do not analyze nor estimate manganese nor fluorine, but leave those two elements out.

We should remember that man is a living, thinking being. You may put unorganized metal into a radiator but when you have to do with a man, you must not give him unorganized metals. Give him those elements he needs in organized food form.

One peculiarity about manganese is that it is present in only a few foods and even in those foods it is present only in the smallest quantity. We find 0.02% is very high in California walnuts and almonds, the highest percentage of manganese in any food form.

Gout and rheumatism produced by excess of manganese never bothers a man in the daytime but always at night. As soon as he sits down, it aches here, there and everywhere.

The manganese excess patient should have a warm diet. Some patients should have a cold diet; some should have a stimulating and tonic diet; some should have negative foods, or foods that grow under the ground. Still other patients should have a fruit diet and so on.

SYMPTOMS WHEN MANGANESE IS DEFICIENT

When manganese is lacking, the brain shrinks in the cranium, resulting in peculiar symptoms. All old people run short of that important element. I am sure everyone who is growing old is in the greatest need of manganese and that if it is not supplied, he will eventually become feeble minded or insane. When he sits still, it seems his legs have no life. They are not numb, but they have no feeling. You may pinch them but he cannot feel it. That is the reason he wants to be in action and on his feet. This is the only patient who develops epileptic symptoms without having epilepsy. The patient does not fall but has the symptoms.

Whenever he moves he groans or when he makes any kind of effort, as if the effort is very hard. His head feels like a bushel basket. He goes to the mirror to see whether his head is large. He may feel as though he is going crazy. It seems that there is a lack of communication between one part of the brain and another part; lack of communication between one faculty in one hemisphere and another in the same hemisphere; lack of communication between brain and body. He does not know just what is going on in the body. There is a lack of consciousness between body and brain.

HOW TO REDUCE MANGANESE IN THE BODY

There is not very much danger of getting too much manganese in the body, but it may possibly happen.

When we first think of an element and about the peculiarities and characteristics, we cannot perhaps see the reason why there should be an element that qualifies us to adapt ourselves to night and darkness, the same as manganese does. If we did not have manganese in the body, we could not adapt ourselves to the dark nor to change of positions in the dark; we could not sleep, could not rest, the nerves would become uneasy, restless and we would be in constant trouble. We could not do what we should do in the dark, viz., rest, sleep and be comfortable.

If you have read the reports of people who work at night, steadily, year in and year out, you know such people usually suffer from brain trouble, because they draw too heavily upon the manganese supply. They violate nature. If you are a night worker, you should always eat foods rich in manganese, because the element is broken down at night when you are at work. If you lack manganese in the nerves, you get up about 2 o'clock and start thinking. This is what a manganese patient will do. He will be up at night, perhaps 2, 3 or 4 o'clock and start his brain working like a factory; he evolves wonderful ideas. When it begins to get daylight, he falls asleep from exhaustion. If he could then sleep until about 11 in the daytime, he would feel more recuperated and would repeat the same habit at night again. That breaks down the manganese element still more.

Osteopaths, chiropractors and others among manipulative and therapeutic lines, may think they can adjust everything in regard to the bones, nerves and nerve centers or the various physical organs in the body; they may speak learnedly about technique, diagnosis and adjustment. We give them credit for wonderful adjustments and cures, yet I want to tell you that unless you supply manganese element you can adjust night and day and continue to adjust, yet you will never get your patients adjusted nor cured. This holds good to all kinds of doctors. If the element is not supplied, treatments do not do very much good no matter what they are. We cannot cure a patient, if we do not supply the element needed. We should give him treatments but we must not forget diet; must not forget the chemical elements that the Almighty put into the body to do the work.

HOW TO INCREASE MANGANESE IN THE BODY

The reason we should use the intellectual faculties more is because these are the faculties that require manganese to a greater extent than the emotional. All people who are great intellectual geniuses and who use the intellect and reason to a great extent, are drawing heavily upon the manganese element and will eventually suffer from disturbances caused by the lack of manganese.

PEOPLE WHO REQUIRE MANGANESE FOODS

I have not found very many people who have manganese in excess. This is the reason I say all people require manganese foods. Usually young men and women, as a rule, are well supplied with manganese and are more active and graceful. When a man grows older, the manganese element cannot be assimilated; he is stiff in the various cells, fibers, joints and cords in the body.

INFLUENCE OF AN EXCESSIVE AMOUNT OF MANGANESE FOODS

I wonder if we know what disposition means? Is there any difference between temperament and disposition? A temperament is a system of functions, faculties and organs. Disposition is a prevailing state of mind. A permanent prevailing state of mind, acting both upon the body and the mind, produces a certain kind of attitude, both physically and mentally. Disposition is in the feelings, in the heart, soul, the very chemistry of the man, while temperament is in the organs and functions of the man. Temperament has very little to do with disposition, but disposition is partially chemical and partially hereditary.

Under certain conditions and certain states of mind existing in the parents at the birth of a child, the child is given a certain kind of chemistry and a certain kind of disposition. The child is perhaps optimistic all the time and we say the disposition is optimistic. We cannot very well say that he has an optimistic temperament. We may say he has an Osseous temperament, Lymphatic temperament or a Vital temperament, as the case may be, but we cannot say he has an optimistic temperament or a pessimistic temperament. Disposition refers to states of mind, soul, emotional states, more or less. If we cultivate a certain state of mind from day to day for 20, 30 or 50 years, eventually we may develop what may be called an acquired disposition. It is not easy to change a disposition.

INFLUENCE OF A DEFICIENT AMOUNT OF MANGANESE FOODS

The Almighty created us in such a way that there should be a certain sprinkling of manganese acting upon the nerves and brain. If that little sprinkling is lacking there will be trouble and sickness. The manganese element has a great deal to do with the continuance of certain states of the mind. This holds true in regard to the manganese element for it has to do with the feelings; it makes them more permanent. A man who lacks manganese cannot be depended on. He cannot depend on himself nor on his own love. He is a scatterbrain in love, work, studies. The manganese element has to do with the control and direction of soul impulses, or states of mind, and when it is lacking, the person is erratic in disposition, whatever his temperament may be.

This is not only true in regard to love, but in regard to eating, drinking, studying, reading and other habits. If a man who lacks manganese reads a book, he reads only the headings. He looks at the beginning and the end, then he is through with that book. He may be highly educated or learned, but there is nothing consecutive nor reliable about him. He is fitful in love, war, moneymaking, study, work, promises, position; you can never trust him.

DISEASE TENDENCIES OF PEOPLE IN WHOM MANGANESE IS IN EXCESS

Flatus. This comes on so quickly that the patient does not know when it comes. It could be in a few minutes of time. Now she is perfectly well—in 5 minutes she s spotted and bloated and feels as though she would burst from flatus; sudden, disagreeable flatus, caused by a sudden generation of gas.

Apoplexy never can be cured without increasing the manganese element. That holds good in regard to excess manganese, which develops apoplectic symptoms; it must be decreased. It is not apoplexy, however, it is only that kind of symptom developed by excess manganese.

Perhaps sometimes the patient will believe that something is pinching him and keeps pinching him in the arm, neck, head or nerves.

The patient may suffer from toothache and goes to the dentist, but the dentist can find nothing. Doctors are likely to say it is in the imagination. The patient goes home and has had no help. The fact of the matter is there is something wrong with the nerve centers. They lack manganese. This is the trouble. Eat plenty of nuts and you will get well. A nut diet cures you and all your nervousness will disappear—not all at once—but in the course of time.

Cracking in the ears and brain is a manganese-hunger symptom.

HELPFUL HINTS

Manganese element has a great deal to do with the function we call "synergy." If the faculties are working together, there is greater harmony among the faculties. One faculty can work more successfully with another. When we think, study or do any kind of work, we use all forty faculties. We do not use only the faculties of the brain, but also the nerves, muscles and senses throughout the body. We can walk and reason at the same time; we can dance and play at the same time; we can do many things at one time, but when there is a lack of the manganese element, a person can only do one thing at a time. And when there is considerable noise around him, he cannot do anything.

Manganese has a great deal to do with concentration. It is not concentration, because concentration is an act of the will, to a great extent, but it is unitization—synergy. There is greater power of synergy in a person in whom manganese is well supplied in the diet. You will say that this is a function of the brain. Intelligence is always in the gray substance. The gray substance always does the thinking. Take the gray substance out of one or more brain centers and see what you can do. The intelligence is in the gray brain. The soul function action in that gray matter we call a faculty. How are these soul faculties going to work? How is one faculty to know what another is doing?

We have never been told anything about brain telegraphy by any psychologist. There are fibers going from the body and up into the various parts of the brain; they are called communication fibers. They are called projecting fibers. If we destroy these fibers in the external capsule, we would not know what is going on in the body. We would become motionless and have no control of mind over body.

The communication fibers that run from one part in the same hemisphere to another part in the same hemisphere, are called intracommunication fibers, and these fibers that run from one faculty to another in an opposite hemisphere, are called intercommunication or interhemispherical communication fibers. All communication fibers are under the control of manganese. Hence also when we lack manganese, we are deficient in brain telegraphy or in soul telegraphy.

The manganese element is there for the purpose of unitizing and harmonizing all the various functions of brain, faculties, soul and body.

When a patient comes to you who suffers from gout and rheumatism, he may say that in the daytime he feels good, but at night as soon as he lies down, or when it gets dark, he aches. When he tells you this, you know it is lack of manganese. Manganese-hungry persons are worse when sitting down. They stiffen up and soon, when they try to rise, they must get up very slowly because they are so stiff they have lost all their strength. They must start in very, very slowly.

There are many different kinds of gout. Did you ever hear of a gout or rheumatism which aches only when you lie down? It aches in a certain bone. This is a manganese symptom because whenever a patient is still and whenever it is dark, his gout or rheumatism bothers him. The pain starts in as soon as it is dark.

WHEN A MANGANESE DIET IS NEEDED

Look at the handwriting of a patient who lacks manganese. The writing is shaky. The writer does not have control of his fingers. Most older people lack manganese.

Shrinkage of the brain happens in old people also. Old people cannot adjust themselves to motion. Lack of manganese has the same effect. The brain shrinks and the man cannot adjust himself to sudden motion. He feels like falling.

The manganese-hungry patient suffers from Angina pectoris, tremors and sudden, strong appetite for food.

As soon as there is a lack of manganese, there is traction, drawing, pressure in the nerves everywhere in the body. There are rigid eye muscles; one eye muscle draws back or contracts; the other does not; it draws the eye sideward. A patient like that has many peculiar sensations.

Iron, when lacking in the body, results in hysterics. This holds good in regard to manganese also.

I have seen patients look as though they were made of moonshine—white, pale and anemic. The skin had a glossy, shiny appearance; the patients perspired at night to such an extent that it seemed as if they were being dissolved in water.

Cold weather does not affect them but hot weather does. The manganese patient suffers from valvular insufficiency, which is really in the cardiac nerves. Any diseases a man, woman or child may suffer from when there is a lack of manganese is always in the nerves and produced by the nerves. When there is manganese hunger, all sorts of manganese ailments appear.

A patient who suffers from heart disease caused by manganese hunger goes to the doctor and the doctor probably gives him digitalis instead of nuts.

The manganese patient is never thirsty. He looks old—has many wrinkles in the skin—like wrinkled tissue paper. His nerves are uneasy; he is restless, cannot sit still; he must be on the move all the time.

He cannot look long at anything for things begin to dance. When the manganese patient sits down, he feels a draft somewhere and he begins to look around at windows.

PRINCIPAL MANGANESE FOODS

When the chemists make a quantitative food analysis they do not tell us how much manganese or fluorine is found in the various foods. They usually say "a trace." We do not like that. We do not like to have a man tell us "considerable"; we want to know how much or how little and we want it in figures.

All of the analyses we have made of all the elements have been put into figures. All such elements that have found their way into the human body and do not belong there, must find their way out also because anything that does not belong in the body, it makes a double effort to throw it out. This is where pain comes in. If you swallow something and you get it down into your throat, you will be surprised to notice the effort you are compelled to make in getting that foreign substance out of the throat.

When you are given drugs, they must be thrown out which requires vitality. For that reason, I never like drugs. Of course there are harmless drugs and those that contain elements we have in the body in vegetable form. Drugs that have a certain affect on the body, viz., teas which are beneficial and certain foods that contain certain chemical elements, should not be forgotten.

Egg yolk is about the same as eating brain substance or the same as eating life. If there is a lack of manganese in egg yolk, you will not get many chicks, and those you do get will not live long.

The most skillful chemist should be at the head of our cookery departments; chemists who understand organic chemistry, quantitative food chemistry and types of people. These chemists should superintend skilled cooks. Some day, the greatest doctors, specialists and chemists will be in our kitchens and the greatest scientists that we can produce will take charge of

our food supply. Then we will have health. They we can go into a restaurant and eat and feel safe. This will be in the future, however. Now you go into a restaurant and after eating, you go to a doctor who may know no more what is wrong with you than you do, because he does not study food, food manufacture or human types. He studies poisons but does not study that which goes into the body. If you go to a doctor who does not study food and you ask him what to eat, he perhaps tells you to eat what you please.

Peppermint leaves act upon the stomach and intestines, acidity and dull digestion. A cup of peppermint tea with the juice of one lime and a few senna leaves makes one of the very best laxatives you can find for a certain kind of acidity, gas generation and constipation.

The foods mentioned in this lesson are the foods and the only foods I know of that are rich in manganese and the best are:

CALIFORNIA WALNUTS. They are higher in manganese than any other food.

RAW EGG YOLK. You find vitamins in abundance in raw egg yolk and in nuts. If you are running low in life force, growing weak, old and feeble or suffer from manganese symptoms, I know of no better foods than these. Use plenty of egg yolk and also nuts especially California walnuts. Taken together with an ordinary diet with rye bread in abundance, and some kind of broths, you certainly have a highly constructive diet—a recuperative diet. Take them in connection with a basic diet, a manganese diet, then get the right kind of medical treatments, osteopathic treatments or other treatments and you will be sure to build up your body.

NASTURTIUM FLOWERS contain more manganese than the leaves.

Manganese is something like sulphur; it acts on the principle of life and acts in connection with the vitamins which are at work wherever manganese is at work. Vitamins are at work wherever sulphur and phosphorus are at work. They are a sort of trinity (Manganese, sulphur and phosphorus). They act on the generative substance, brain, life and on life processes. Wherever manganese is at work, there vitamins are at work also.

FOODS AND CHEMICALS
<u>NITROGEN</u>

FOOD ANALYSIS EXPLAINED

BEANS contain 24.3% protein and all brain and potash salts, principally potassium phosphate. They are very rich in protein and are muscle building. Muscles contain 17% nitrogen.

CHEESE contains 16% nitrogen.

EGG WHITES give 13% protein. Eggs contain a little more than 15% nitrogen.

MACKEREL (lean) contains 16 - 25% protein.

PEAS contain 23% protein and all the salts needed for the human system, principally potassium phosphate.

LENTILS hold 25% protein and contain all the salts with the exception of silicon and sulphur.

MEATS. In meats, we find from 16-25% protein and principally potassium phosphate.

DRIED STURGEON contain 32% protein also potassium phosphate and mostly all the salts.

FLANK (lean) contains 13% up to 27% protein usually 13-21% also potassium phosphate.

DRIED BEEF holds 47% protein and down to 24% also potassium phosphate.

CHUCK contains 13-22% protein and principally potassium phosphate of the salts.

SMOKED HERRING contains 36.9% protein also phosphorus, potassium, sodium and calcium.

WALNUTS contain 17% protein and 53% fat.

NUTS are principally fat from 67-83% fat.

PORTERHOUSE STEAK is principally water.

BUTTER NUTS contain 27.9% protein also potassium phosphate.

ALMONDS hold 25% protein, are rich in most of the needed salts; contain principally potassium phosphate; are muscle and brain building. Fish is also a brain food. Almonds contain the brain salts. When almonds are salted, they aid the digestion of starch. Do not eat almonds by themselves to any great extent as they may poison the stomach. They should be ground and sprinkled on other foods.

RAW PEANUTS contain a little more than 29% protein, are rich in vitamins and contain potassium phosphate in abundance. Do not eat roasted peanuts.

PIGNOLIA NUTS hold 33.9% protein. They are rich in potassium phosphate and are brain building.

STRING BEANS are rich in potassium phosphate and sodium. People should eat plenty of string beans, pineapple, strawberries and raspberries—all are rich in sodium.

POTATOES contain 2% ash; only about 13% of potatoes is protein; 60-70% is water and sugar is found to the extent of 21%. There is a very small percentage of potassium phosphate. Potatoes should be eaten only by children. People over 45 should not eat potatoes.

DUTCH CHEESE holds 29-47% protein. It is principally calcium among the salts. It is difficult to digest.

COW'S MILK contains from 3-4% protein. Scientists have been protein crazy for nearly 100 years. Excess of protein is killing many people. We find calcium and potassium in cow's milk, but hardly any iron.

PROTEIN FOODS are rich in nitrogen; contain from 13-17% nitrogen.

Infants' food may contain 89% of the cheapest kind of sugar; many times as much sugar as mother's milk. It may result in floating, gas, hip disease, bone and teeth troubles.

Much more calcium is found in cow's milk than in goat's milk. Goat's milk contains more iron.

COMPARISON OF GOAT & COW MILK

Contains	Cow's Milk (%)	Goat's Milk (%)
Water	85-87.20	87-89.39
Protein	3.55	2.78
Fat	3.70	3.84
Sugar	4.88	4.25
Ash	0.71	1.74
Potassium oxide	24.67	44.58
Sodium oxide	9.70	7.18
Calcium oxide	22.50	5.99
Magnesium oxide	3.05	2.48
Iron	0.55	2.00
Phosphorus	28.40	13.78
Sulphur	0.30	2.42
Silicon	0.04	None
Chlorine	14.28	31.00
Fluorine	None	0.66

Goat's milk contains lactic acid to the extent of 0.12-1.65%. It acts upon the alimentary tract. Goat's milk is closest to mother's milk.

Human milk contains 2.36% protein and much potassium.

Goat's milk contains 2.78% protein, a little more than mother's milk and all the blood salts; it also contains potassium chloride, calcium phosphate and sodium chloride.

REMARKS

All foods high in nitrogen build muscle. The Myogenic, Calciferic, Desmogenic and Nitropheric are protein types. These types are able to hold nitrogen in the system. Nitrogen principally takes up starch.

The person who lives on a high protein diet is likely to suffer from kidney disease.

Too much sugar, protein and fat cause fermentation and autointoxication in the stomach. The brain worker does not need much protein food. He should have brain food, alkaline salts especially magnesium, also vitamins.

Those parts of an animal which are exercised, contain more protein and more of the salts. Therefore, tough meat is more valuable than the tender meats; it is also the cheapest.

QUESTIONS AND ANSWERS

1. Do all foods high in nitrogen build muscle? Answer: No. If a certain nitrogen-containing food is too high in nitrogen a certain type, for instance, the Neurogenic, Pathetic or Carboferic may not be able to utilize the nitrogen in the food at all. A Nitropheric man or lady cannot digest a high proportion of nitrogen. Nitropheric people or people of a delicate constitution should eat foods that are low in nitrogen in order to gain strength. If they eat high nitrogen foods, they lose in strength, because they will suffer from protein poisoning and autointoxication. Foods that contain perhaps only 2% of nitrogen are more nourishing to them. We must know the difference between type and type and between nitrogen food and nitrogen food. The nitropheric constitution is a starch constitution with free nitrogen at work in the system. The Neurogenic constitution is a brain and nerve constitution, with very low power of nitrogen metabolism.

2. How can you determine whether a patient has a lack or excess of nitrogen in the system? Answer: If a patient lacks the nitrogen element, he has nitrogen-hunger symptoms; if a patient has an excess of nitrogen, he has nitrogen-excess symptoms. We know the patient by his symptoms and we know each element by its symptoms.

592

IV

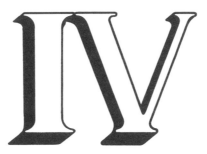

The proof is in the healing

The following pictures and case histories are from my patient files. While it may be true that a case history or personal testimony is not sufficient to establish objective evidence of improvement or healing, we find that "a picture is worth a thousand words."

The pictures that follow demonstrate the effectiveness of the natural regimen I use with patients, as drawn from the teachings of V. G. Rocine.

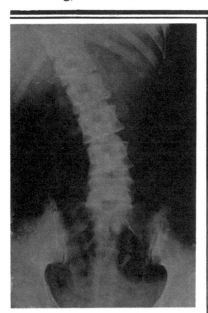

X-ray before.

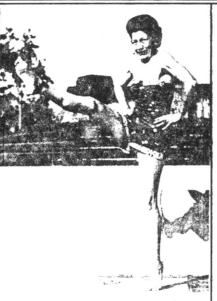

E.N. in her 70s; once a cripple.

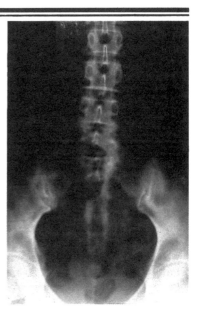

X-ray after.

E. N., FEMALE, IN HER 80s.
Complaints: Arthritis, bone spurs, pain.
History: Patient had been to chiropractors and different kinds of doctors including an orthopedic surgeon. X-rays showed 14 calcium spurs on the spine. No one helped her. One doctor said only bone surgery could help, while another said she would be bedridden the rest of her life. She came to me in extreme pain, bent over and somewhat to the right, head below the shoulders.

Testimony: When I first saw Dr. Jensen, I asked if he could do anything for me and he said he didn't know. He gave me an iris analysis and then started me on an elimination program with a diet and supplements of goat whey, carrot juice and veal joint broth every other day. I took colonics and sweat baths for four months.

He started adjusting my spine then, and after eight months under Dr. Jensen's care, my spine straightened and I was discharged from any further treatment. X-rays showed the spurs were gone and my spine was straight. I was 41 years of age at the time, and now, almost 40 years later, I have had no recurrence of my pains or my spinal troubles. My spine has remained straight over all these years.

V. G., MALE, AGE 39.

Complaints: Glomerulonephritis, Edema.

History: Patient noticed swelling in ankles and feet in 1975; went to Veterans Administration Hospital and was diagnosed as having glomerulonephritis. He was told that nothing could be done to help and was sent home with the understanding that he only had a few weeks to live.

Testimony: With the help of my wife and family, I arrived in San Diego, CA on January 7, 1977, and was taken to Dr. Jensen's Ranch. At that time, I needed help to walk. My weight was 175 pounds with a bloated abdomen, and my legs were swollen bigger than my head. After I saw Dr. Jensen, he put me on a program of work, exercise and eating all I could, except no citrus, bread, head lettuce, wheat or oatmeal. I took a few supplements, Kneipp baths, grass and sand walks for circulation. In the first month, I lost 32 pounds and was feeling very well. Then I had my first healing crisis. I lost 12 pounds in 3 days. I had diarrhea, fever and vomiting, averaging 30 trips to the bathroom each day—day and night. Two months later, I returned to my home. My weight was about 141 pounds and my body was slender again. In past years, I had bowel movements not more than twice a week, but now I have regular bowel movements one a day for sure and once in a while I have two. After I left the Ranch, I had another healing crisis at home. I had an extremely high fever and thought I was actually going to burn up. I had diarrhea and vomiting again for 3 days, and lost another 10 pounds. Maybe 3 or 4 pounds came back. Now, 5 years later, I feel wonderful!

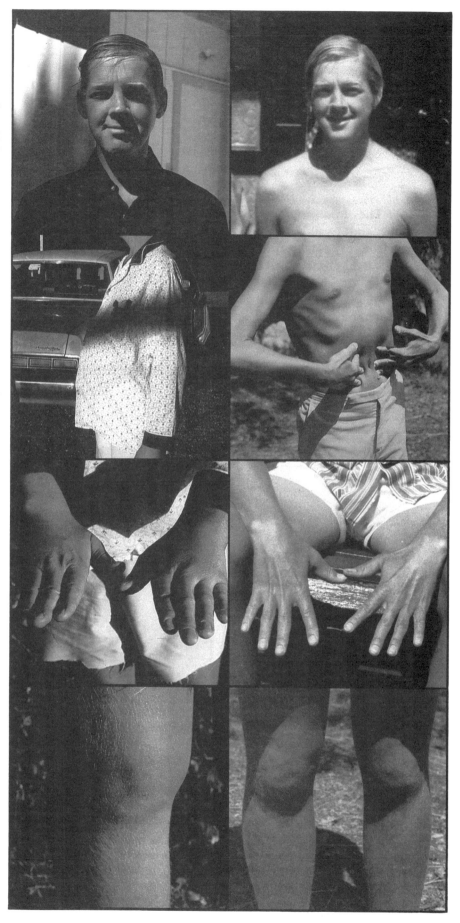

E. P., FEMALE, IN HER 70s.

Complaints: Arthritis, extreme pain.

History: Onset of arthritis pain began 2 years before first visit. Patient's doctor at that time diagnosed osteoarthritis on the basis of X-rays, and told her that 5 of her 7 neck vertebrae had degenerated. She was put in a neck brace and took Percodan and Bulazolidin for pain, a steroid named Phenylbutazone weekly and Ascriptin daily. She was told to eat anything she wished, that diet had nothing to do with arthritis.

Testimony: When I first came to Dr. Jensen, I couldn't move my neck; I couldn't drive a car; I couldn't cook. The only time I would be out of pain was when I took this drug. The pain was unbearable. And Dr. Jensen said, you've got to get off drugs or I cannot treat you. He gave me a seven-day cleansing treatment...with colemas, twice a day, broth and nutritional supplements. No medicines. Within a week, I found myself free of pain and feeling very well without drugs. And after that he gave me a food regimen to follow—no bread, no wheat, no citrus juices. He insists on a mixed green salad every day and chicken or fish for protein. Now, I travel; I drive; I work in the kitchen—I do everything. I had a healing crisis a month and a half after starting with Dr. Jensen. I developed a fever of 105 degrees, a terrible headache and brought up a lot of phlegm for 3 days. He told me I would have a crisis and I did. I can hardly believe it lasted only 3 days, and then I felt so good again, just as Dr. Jensen said I would. I'm even taking aerobics! I joined a gym, and Dr. Jensen said do it but be careful of the jumping and moving your neck to any extremes. I can hardly believe I had such a crippling malady, went on and then off of drugs, and became completely well again—all in my 70s. On TV, I said, "I was at the point of suicide because of the pain. Dr. Jensen saved my life!"

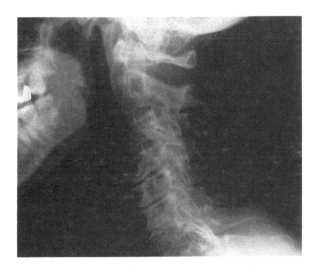

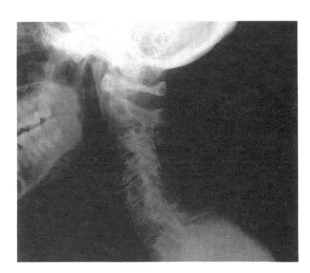

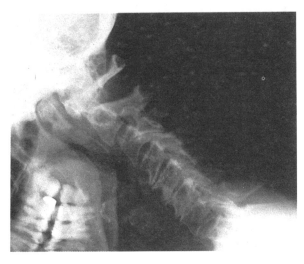

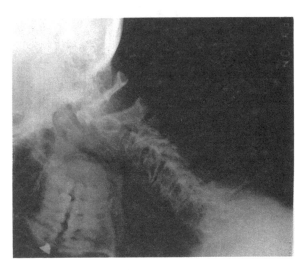

Before: March 1981. Calcium spurs due to arthritis.

After: September 1983. Complete relief reported.

R. M., MALE, AGE 64.

Complaint: Open, running ulcers on heel, instep and outside ankle of right foot; heel and instep of left foot; swollen ankles. (Blood pressure 80/58.)

History: Leg problems began two years prior to visit, treated without success by several doctors. Kidney stone attack in 1976, taken care of with nutritional supplements. Diarrhea for previous 7-1/2 years (7 or 8 bowel movements per day); no relief from either over-the-counter or prescription remedies. Patient's paternal grandfather died of gangrene, mother and one brother died of colitis.

Testimony: When ulcers first appeared on my legs two years before seeing Dr. Jensen, I remembered my grandfather who had gangrene. Doctors first amputated his feet, then his legs below the knees, then the rest below the hips, unable to stop the gangrene. He died of it two years later. I went to doctors but had no improvement. I was advised that my feet should be amputated, but felt that would not solve the problem. When I first came to see Dr. Jensen in December 1979, he put me on a special diet. My bowel improved but my feet and ankles grew worse. Then I went through the tissue cleansing program, and the results were almost miraculous. The ulcers cleared up in 7 days and continued to improve as I stayed on the doctor's health and harmony food regimen. Now, two years later, I am completely free of any leg or foot problems.

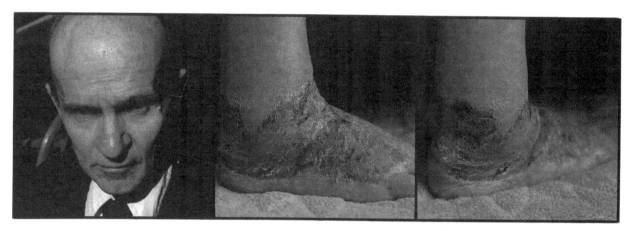

Foot ulcers at time of first visit.

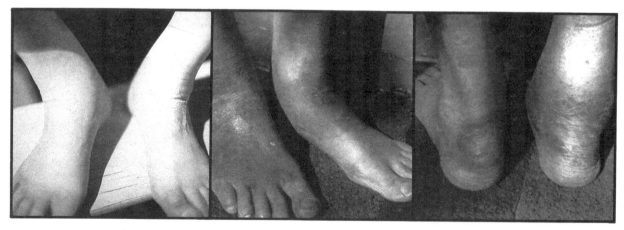

Continued improvement from correct diet 20 months after initial visit.

Feet after 7 days of tissue cleansing.

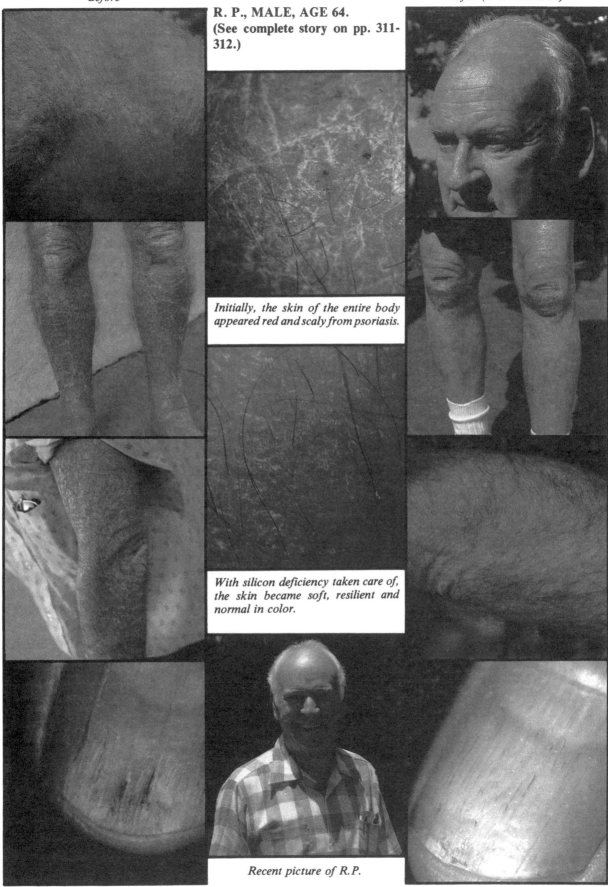

Before

After (4 months later)

R. P., MALE, AGE 64.
(See complete story on pp. 311-312.)

Initially, the skin of the entire body appeared red and scaly from psoriasis.

With silicon deficiency taken care of, the skin became soft, resilient and normal in color.

Recent picture of R.P.

597

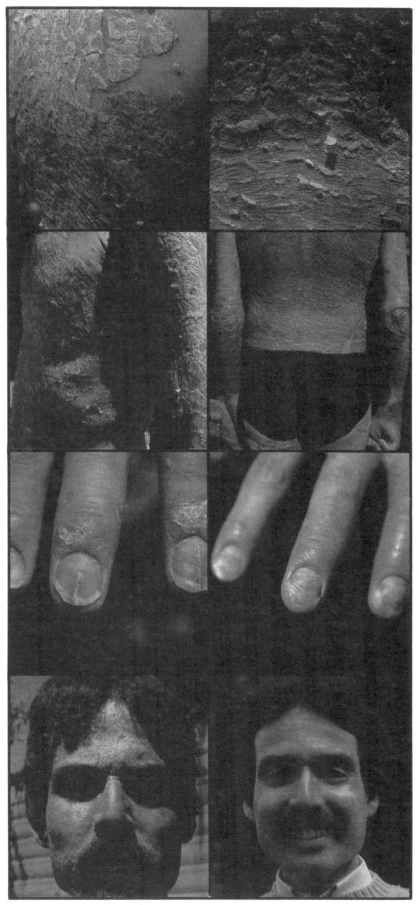

Stages in the course of taking care of psoriasis by nutrition and tissue cleansing. (1,2,3,4)

M. Z., MALE, AGE 27.

Complaints: Psoriasis, diabetes and arthritis.

History: Scaling of scalp and facial skin under beard began 7 years before patient's first visit. Doctor diagnosed problem as psoriasis but could do nothing for it. After 4 years, fingernails began showing pits and creases, then the following year, diabetes was diagnosed. About 6 months later, fluid in the knee and inflammation of the elbow were diagnosed as symptoms of psoriatric arthritis. Twenty aspirin per day were taken for arthritis pain; insulin shots were taken for diabetes; and the psoriasis became worse week by week.

Testimony: After taking the 7-day cleanse with colemas and taking special supplements, I could dress and undress without the difficulty I had before from arthritis. I was able to wear shoes for the first time in 9 months. After 2 months more, I was able to reduce my insulin intake because the diabetes was better. The psoriasis also improved. From the time I first saw Dr. Jensen in June 1980, I've made steady progress, but the doctor tells me I have another 5 years of work to do. Still, I'm very pleased with the improvement I've made so far, especially in my mental attitude—enough to go back to college!

Natural healing methods work slowly but surely to restore tissue. (5,6,7,8)

598

In conclusion

I have not attempted to keep photographic records of all my dramatic cases or many more would be presented here. And, there are many more. I might add that I also have thousands of less dramatic cases where patients have overcome diseases by nutrition and right living. The preceding photographs demonstrate the value and effectiveness of nutrition in overcoming disease, which is all I intended to do in this section.

We find, according to Dr. Rocine, that nutrition—together with an understanding of the chemical types of people and their temperaments—is a powerful tool in the healing art. I have proven this in over 50 years of sanitarium practice. The proof is in the healing.

It is not easy to change food habits ingrained for 20 years and take on a right way of eating and living, but it can be done. My patients have demonstrated that it can.

We find that it is necessary to find a doctor who has a wholistic perspective, who believes in prevention and who knows nutrition. There is no therapy, no healing art that can bring about complete healing without nutrition.

There is no magic "silver bullet" or single chemical element that can cure a disease or heal an organ by itself. Every disease eventually affects every organ in the body, depleting chemical elements that must be replaced. While one or two organs may be affected more than others in a particular person with a particular disease, we must realize that all other organs increase their level of activity in an attempt to compensate for the lowered activity of the weakest ones. In doing so, they all use more of the chemical elements and all tend to become depleted—some more so than others.

Each organ attracts the chemical elements it needs from the bloodstream, provided that we are eating the right foods to provide those elements and provided that we are digesting and assimilating well. What we must know, then, are what chemical elements are needed by each organ and what foods supply them to the body.

Therefore, we must seek out the laws of a good nutritional intake as a basis for preventing disease, developing good health and reaching toward high-level well-being.

Specifically, we need to use tonics, soups, broths, juices, specialty foods high in certain chemical elements, nutritional supplements and a proper food regimen to take care of any chemically-depleted organs. To keep physically well, it is necessary to maintain the right chemical balance in the body through a proper nutritional lifestyle. When we put all this together, it spells *good health*.

I have traveled to many countries all over the world, searching out the oldest living persons in places like the Hunza Valley of Pakistan; Vilcabamba, Ecuador; Turkey and the Caucasus Mountains of the USSR. I wanted to find out how these men and women—many of them over 120 years of age—had lived so long without succumbing to disease.

In every case, I found that the longevity of these people was due, in large part, to eating nutritious foods grown in soil rich in the chemical elements—pure, whole, natural foods. There were other factors contributing to their health and longevity, but proper nutrition was the basic foundation. When we stop and think that the great majority of the world population dies prematurely from diseases that develop due to chemical deficiencies in the diet, nutrition suddenly takes on a whole new perspective.

We must realize that good nutrition is the path of life, the simple most important factor in good health, a sound mind and a long life. There is no substitute for proper nutrition and no therapy or healing art that can keep a malnourished body free of disease.

We are what we eat—and what we do not eat. The body molds to the foods we put into it—for better or worse.

The later years of man should be years of peace, wisdom and joy. With the proper foods, we can live life to the fullest, all the years of our lives.

Index